CARDIAC MECHANO-ELECTRIC FEEDBACK and ARRYTHMIAS

From PIPETTE To PATIENT

CARDIAC MECHANO-ELECTRIC FEEDBACK and ARRYTHMIAS

From PIPETTE To PATIENT

PETER KOHL MD, PhD, RSRF
Reader in Cardiac Physiology
Director of the Cardiac Mechano-Electric Feedback Lab
Oxford University Laboratory of Physiology, Oxford
Adjunct Associate Professor
Medical Biotechnology Center
University of Maryland, Baltimore
Fellow and Tutor in Biomedical Sciences
Balliol College, Oxford

FREDERICK SACHS, PhD
Distinguished Professor of Biophysics
Center for Single Molecule Biophysics
Department of Physiology and Biophysics
State University of New York at Buffalo, NY

MICHAEL R. FRANZ, MD, PhD, FACC
Professor, Department of Pharmacology
Georgetown University Medical Center
Director, Arrhythmia Service
Nation Capital Veteran Affairs Medical Center, Washington, DC

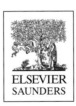

ELSEVIER
SAUNDERS

ELSEVIER
SAUNDERS
An imprint of Elsevier

The Curtis Center
170 S Independence Mall W 300E
Philadelphia, Pennsylvania 19106

Cardiac Mechano-Electric Feedback and Arrhythmias: From Pipette to Patient   1–4160–0034–8
Copyright © 2005, Elsevier Inc. All rights reserved.

NOTICE

Library of Congress Cataloging-in-Publication Data
Kohl, Peter.
    Cardiac mechano-electric feedback and arrhythmias : from pipette to patient / Peter Kohl,
Frederick Sachs, Michael R. Franz. – 1st ed.
      p. cm.
    ISBN 1–4160–0034–8
    1. Heart–Contraction. 2. Arrhythmia 3. Heart conduction system. 4. Biological control systems. I. Sachs,
Frederick. II. Franz, M. R. (Michael R.), 1949-III. Title.
QP1132.K64 2005
612.17–dc22   2004065902

Publishing Director: Anne Lenehan
Editorial Assistant: Vera Ginsburgs
Project Manager: David Saltzberg

Printed in the United States of America

9 8 7 6 5 4 3 2 1

CONTENTS

SECTION IV

Cardiac Mechano-Electric Feedback in Normal Physiology

SECTION V

Cardiac Mechano-Electric Feedback as a Pathogenic Mechanism

Stretching Our Views of Cardiac Control

The transduction of electrical impulses into changes in the rate and mechanical force of muscle contraction, known as excitation–contraction coupling (ECC), is a fundamental concept essential to both a basic and clinical understanding of the heart. Modulators of ECC, and hence of cardiac muscle performance, include neurohumoral transmitters such as catecholamines, as well as many other regulators, notably those that affect intracellular calcium handling. This affects actin–myosin interactions and adjusts hemodynamics in accord with changing requirements on a beat-by-beat, year-by-year basis.

The complementary concept that cardiac mechanical function changes that occur in response to neural and hormonal influences impact on the excitatory and conductive electrical properties of the heart, i.e., mechano-electric coupling or feedback (MEF) is a less established idea whose role in normal and pathological physiology has become an exciting new chapter in contemporary biology. Mechanisms and pathways whereby mechanical events, changes in tension and force, and spatial displacement alter the heart's electri-

cal properties are now recognized as an important dimension for development of new approaches in therapeutic cardiac control.

The figure provides a simplified but conceptually useful view of this emerging bi-directional dynamic. Although the left-to-right pathway, ECC, is a familiar element in current therapeutic strategies, the right-to-left pathway, MEF, has only recently begun to be explored as a topic of medical interest. However, although it has become well established that dysfunction in pathways of ECC is important in a number of cardiac pathologies (e.g., in various cardiomyopathies), there are only a few clues for a parallel influence of factors in pathways of MEF. This situation appears likely to change as greater attention is given to mechanisms involved in acute and chronic processes of cardiac remodeling. These include some of the most common forms of heart disease such as dilative failure, atrial fibrillation, and post-infarction scarring. Although we now suspect MEF to play a role in both electrical and mechanical pathological remodeling, direct evidence of this has remained elusive. Thus, although much basic

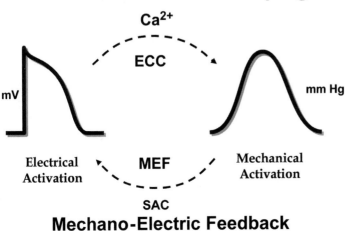

Electro-Mechanical Coupling

Ca^{2+}

ECC

mV

mm Hg

Electrical Activation

MEF

Mechanical Activation

SAC

Mechano-Electric Feedback

Simplified conceptual view of the complementarity in coupling between electrical activation of contraction and the influence of mechano-electric feedback (MEF) in cardiac muscle. Electrical activation and excitation–contraction coupling (ECC) are believed to be mediated by convergence of signaling pathways altering cellular calcium (Ca^{2+}) levels, resulting in activation and alterations in actin–myosin interactions. Pathways by which mechanical influences and changes in tension, length, and directional displacement alter cardiac electrical function are believed in many cases to be mediated by stretch-activated ion channels (SAC), which affect intracellular electrical potential and excitation. *(Modified from a figure provided by Michael Franz, with permission.)*

information is becoming available on topics such as how MEF may facilitate normal physiological processes, we still have few clues on how they may be applied in prevention or reversal of disease.

This book represents an important step in documenting the elusive yet important role of MEF. Here, assembled in one source, are the current thoughts and findings of many of the leading investigators in the field. As one reads the pages that follow, it becomes apparent that MEF is indeed a topic whose "time to shine" has arrived, and that this volume contributes much to lighting this path. The three editors are among the field's pioneers, and their selection of topics has resulted in an excellent summary of much of the world's current thinking. The book continues the momentum established by their leadership of a number of important international symposia on MEF that addressed many of the field's outstanding questions in forums encompassing most of its working investigators. The synthesis and distillation of these efforts have contributed much to the pages that follow by providing coverage of important concepts that proceed from basic physiology and move toward an integrated understanding of cardiac control and the exploration of new targets of largely unexplored therapeutic potential.

Classic studies on MEF and how it might contribute to well established events are discussed, such as the Bainbridge response, the function of stretch-activated channels, and the fatal phenomena of commotio cordis. In addition, new approaches by many of today's cutting edge MEF exponents employ a wide range of molecular, biophysical, and genetic tools. Thus, the various sections of the book detail not just the potential impact, influence, and implications of MEF, but they also provide clues to future directions.

The core concepts of cardiac MEF are covered in the initial sections of the book, and there are many interesting additional clinical presentations. Highlights are likely to be different for each reader. For this observer, the chapters that explore chronic influences, as well as the more well-known acute influences of MEF, and those that pertain to atrial fibrillation and other arrhythmias, were highlights. Here is the groundwork that illustrates how changes in MEF may determine disease reversibility and refractoriness to various thera-

pies. Other unique and fascinating topics include how MEF responses vary in different cardiac cell types, (e.g., cardiac myocytes versus cardiac fibroblasts), and several that touch on new questions about the submembranous cardiac cell architecture.

The network of filamentous cytoskeletal proteins has recently been recognized as important in diseases as varied as inherited monogenic arrhythmias and rare forms of cardiomyopathy. Yet, we have little idea of how these phenotypes arise at a cellular or physiological level. Are they parts of the MEF response mediated by alterations in process, such as the organization or anchoring of cell surface receptors and signaling complexes, or even interactions among various ion channel subunits that may be involved? Lastly, this reader noted several intriguing new approaches in studies that deal with still mysterious topics, such as how changes in transcellular electrical and physical communication influence expression of specific proteins that, in turn, determine "who says what to whom" in the close world of in situ cardiobiology.

In conclusion, I'd like to express the personal view that further discoveries concerning the integration of pathways of cardiac mechanical and electrical control, between ECC and MEF, are likely to provide new clues to the treatment and prevention of many forms of recalcitrant cardiac disease, especially those causative of life-threatening arrhythmias. Given that bias, it also seems worth suggesting that work on cardiac MEF, within all its extensions in man, should be supported nationally and internationally with elevated level of priority than has been the case recently. Despite decades of attempts at developing efficacious therapies for disturbances in the heart's electrical system, effective treatment and prevention options are few, and either problematic with respect to efficacy and side effects or increasingly more difficult to justify on a cost-effectiveness/resource utilization basis. The imperative for improvements in arrhythmia therapy is, nevertheless, but one of a number of reasons that speak to a need to expand fundamental and model studies on cardiac control to improve clinical translation and therapy. This book presents an excellent view of how such progress can be successfully achieved, and it illustrates its potential applications.

PETER M. SPOONER, PhD
BALTIMORE
MARCH 2005

PREFACE

Cardiac Mechano-Electric Feedback: From Pipette to Patient

• • • •

Peter Kohl, Frederick Sachs, and Michael R. Franz

The heart is a mechano-sensitive organ.

Stretching of cardiac tissue affects a wide range of structural and functional characteristics including gene expression, protein turnover, connective tissue properties, electrical and mechanical coupling, contractility, and electrophysiology. This book focuses on mechanically induced changes that, directly or indirectly, affect heart rate and rhythm.

Effects of stretch in man range from heart rate responses to changes in venous return, mechanical induction of premature ventricular beats (e.g., during cardiac catheterization) and tachyarrhythmia (e.g., *commotio cordis*), to chronic rhythm disturbance during cardiac volume or pressure overload and the use of mechanical intervention (e.g., pre-cordial thump) to reset dysrhythmic hearts.

Documented reports of cardiac mechanosensitivity date back well over a century. One of the earliest descriptions of mechanical effects on cardiac function is from 1763, when Akenside gave an account of heart rhythm disturbance after a chest impact.[1] His case report involved severe tissue trauma, however, and it was not until 1882 that Riedinger and colleagues highlighted that, under certain conditions, chest impacts may induce arrhythmia in the absence of structural damage—*commotio cordis*.[2] In 1915, Bainbridge reported his famous observation of a mechanically-induced increase in cardiac beating rate,[3] and five years later, Schott described "pre-cordial percussion" as an effective means of keeping Stokes-Adams sufferers conscious during periods of complete atrio-ventricular block.[4]

The notion of cardiac mechanosensitivity rings a bell with any life sciences student who had an opportunity to conduct practical classes involving Langendorff heart preparations that, quite literally, can be kick-started when quiescent by a finger tap. Similar taps are employed by cardiac surgeons to restart a heart upon weaning from induced arrest.

What are the underlying mechanisms of these phenomena? Are there tools to study them quantitatively? Is there a conceptual framework for cardiac mechanosensitivity?

The last question may, perhaps, best be approached on the basis of regulation theory, which would view mechanosensitivity not as a peculiar, but a necessary, property of any electrically controlled mechanical system. As illustrated in the figure, electro-mechanical control (excitation–contraction coupling, ECC) must be accompanied by a feedback pathway (mechano-electric feedback, MEF) to form a regulatory loop. This concept was first applied to stretch-induced augmentation of spontaneous and ectopic automaticity in atrial and ventricular multicellular preparations by Kaufmann and Theophile (a.k.a. Ravens) in 1967, who labeled their observations as a manifestation of "*mechano-elektrische Rückkoppelung*"—MEF.[5]

The mechanisms underlying cardiac MEF have begun to be explored by both intracellular and extracellular electrical recording techniques. The latter, monophasic action potential recordings, are most helpful in studying stretch effects in the intact heart.[6] Transmembrane recordings, most notably patch clamping, have identified stretch-activated ion channels[7] in

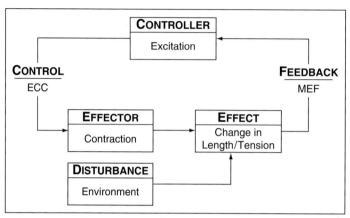

Simplified scheme of the cardiac electro-mechanical regulatory loop. The process of electrical excitation controls cardiac contraction via excitation–contraction coupling (ECC). The resulting changes in cell length and/or tension affect the process of excitation via mechano-electric feedback (MEF). MEF occurs independently of whether a mechanical effect is caused by cardiac contraction itself, or through changes in the mechanical environment of the heart; in the absence of MEF, the system would therefore not be stable. (*From Kohl P, Hunter P, Noble D: Stretch-induced changes in heart rate and rhythm: Clinical observations, experiments and mathematical models. Prog Biophys Mol Biol 71(1):91–138, 1999, with permission.*)

many cardiac cells, including pacemaker cells, atrial and ventricular myocytes, and fibroblasts. Their clinical relevance is starting to emerge,[6] aided significantly by the identification of a first selective blocker for these channels.[8] Advanced optical imaging and molecular techniques have helped to further establish cellular calcium handling and second messengers, such as nitric oxide, as key players in cardiac MEF.

While acute stretch effects are well documented, chronic cardiac pathology involving mechanically induced electrical and structural tissue remodeling is more complex and multifactorial, making it difficult to establish a causal chain of response.

There is strong evidence to suggest that chamber dilatation plays a key role in the development of atrial fibrillation. Similarly, arrhythmogenesis in heart failure and ventricular overload have been linked to the changed mechanical environment. In keeping with this concept, clinical interventions that reduce cardiac distension (such as diuretics and afterload-reducing agents or active and passive cardiac assist devices) and cardiac resynchronization therapy have beneficial effects, not only on pump function, but also on cardiac electrophysiology. Future studies hold the promise of revealing more specific pathways of these phenomena, as there is virtually *no* aspect of cardiac

function that is insensitive to the heart's mechanical environment.[9]

Cardiac mechanosensitivity and its effect on electrical function undoubtedly form a very complex system. Increasingly, fragments of this jigsaw are falling into place, as illustrated by the chapters in this book. There are, however, still large gaps to be filled, and we are far from a comprehensive understanding of the detailed mechanisms, physiological role, and clinical relevance of MEF.

The editors are indebted to the many contributors who investigate and clarify the role of MEF. Their work is truly interdisciplinary and translational, and it emphasizes the importance of a field that has gone relatively unnoticed for many decades. Research into MEF has developed from many different perspectives, from *E. coli* to cardiac myocytes, from computer modelling to clinical observations, from hitherto under-appreciated causes of cardiac arrhythmias to potentially providing new therapies.

In presenting the combined insight from basic science and clinical research, this book provides an up-to-date account of the current state of the MEF puzzle. There are potentially far-reaching cardiovascular health implications of a better understanding of the heart as an integrated electrical and mechanical closed-loop system. The editors hope that the readers will be as provoked as we are and that this text will stimulate further study into the many undiscovered facets of the mechanosensitive heart.

References

1. Akenside M: An account of a blow upon the heart, and of its effects. Philos Trans R Soc Lond 53:353-355, 1765.
2. Riedinger F: Über Brusterschütterung. In: Festschrift zur dritten Saecularfeier der Alma Julia Maximiliana Leipzig. Verlag von F.C.W. Vogel: Leipzig. pp 221–234, 1882.
3. Bainbridge FA: The influence of venous filling upon the rate of the heart. J Physiol 50:65–84, 1915.
4. Schott E: Über Ventrikelstillstand (Adams-Stokes'sche Anfälle) nebst Bemerkungen über andersartige Arhythmien passagerer Natur. Deutsches Archiv für Klinische Medizin 131:211–229, 1920.
5. Kaufmann R, Theophile U: Automatie fördernde Dehnung seffekte an Purkinjefäden, Papillarmuskeln und Vorhoftrabekeln von Rhesus-Affen. Pflügers Arch 297(3): 174–189, 1967.
6. Franz MR, Cima R, Wang D, et al: Electrophysiological effects of myocardial stretch and mechanical determinants of stretch-activated arrhythmias. Circulation 86:968–978, 1992.
7. Sachs F, Sigurdson W, Ruknudin A, et al: Single-channel mechanosensitive currents. Science 253:800–801,1991.
8. Bode F, Sachs F, Franz MR: Tarantula peptide inhibits atrial fibrillation. Nature 409:35–36, 2001.
9. Kohl P, Hunter P, Noble D: Stretch-induced changes in heart rate and rhythm: Clinical observations, experiments and mathematical models, Prog Biophys Mol Biol 71(1):91–138, 1999

CONTRIBUTORS

Maurits Allessie, MD, PhD
Professor, Department of Physiology, University of
Maastricht, Maastricht, The Netherlands.
*The Substrate of Atrial Fibrillation in Chronically
Dilated Atria*

Angelo Auricchio, MD, PhD
Professor, Division of Cardiology, University
Hospital, Magdeburg, Germany.
*Cardiac Resynchronization Therapy for Patients with
Heart Failure with Ventricular Conduction Delay*

Clive M. Baumgarten, PhD
Professor of Physiology, Internal Medicine
(Cardiology) and Biomedical Engineering,
Department of Physiology, Medical College of
Virginia, Virginia Commonwealth University,
Richmond, Virginia.
*Cell Volume–Sensitive Ion Channels and Transporters in
Cardiac Myocytes*

Donald M. Bers, PhD
Professor and Chair, Department of Physiology,
Loyola University Chicago, Maywood, Illinois.
*The Response of Cardiac Muscle to Stretch: The Role of
Calcium*

Meenakshi A. Bhalla, MD
Internal Medicine Resident, Department of
Medicine, SUNY at Buffalo GME Consortium,
Buffalo, New York.
*Natriuretic Peptide and Sudden Cardiac Death in
Patients with Congestive Heart Failure*

Vikas Bhalla, MBBS
Postdoctoral, Heart Failure Research Fellow,
Department of Medicine, Division of Cardiology,
Veterans Affairs Medical Center, University of
California San Diego, San Diego, California.
*Natriuretic Peptide and Sudden Cardiac Death in
Patients with Congestive Heart Failure*

Frank Bode, MD
Senior Physician, Medizinische Klinik II,
Universitaets Klinikum Schleswig-Holstein Campus
Luebeck, Luebeck, Germany.
*Stretch Channel Blockers: A New Class of
Antiarrhythmic Drugs?*

Thomas K. Borg, PhD
Carolina Distinguished Professor and Chair,
Department of Cell and Developmental Biology and
Anatomy, University of South Carolina, Columbia,
South Carolina.
*Cardiac Fibroblasts: Origin, Organization, and
Function*

Christian Boulin, PhD
Unit Coordinator, Senior Scientist, Scientific Core
Facilities, Services and Technology, European
Molecular Biology Laboratory, Heidelberg, Germany.
Antiarrhythmic Effects of Acute Mechanical Stimulation

Günter Breithardt, MD
Professor of Medicine (Cardiology), Department of
Cardiology and Angiology, University of Münster,
Münster, Germany.
*Drugs Interacting with Mechano-Electric Feedback:
Proarrhythmia, Remodeling, and Apoptosis*

Daniel Burkhoff, MD, PhD
Associate Professor of Medicine, Department of Medicine, Columbia University, New York, New York.
Cardiac Assist Devices: Effects on Reverse Remodeling

A. John Camm, QHP, BSc, MD, FRCP, FESC, FACC, FAHA, FCGC, CStJ
British Heart Foundation Prudential Chair in Cardiology, Department of Cardiac and Vascular Sciences, St. George's Hospital Medical School, London, United Kingdom.
Atrial Fibrillation and Dilated Cardiomyopathy

Peter Carson, MD
Associate Professor of Medicine, Department of Cardiology, Georgetown University Hospital; Chief, Coronary Care Unit, Department of Cardiology, Washington Veteran's Administration Medical Center, Washington, District of Columbia.
Neurohormonal Antagonists in Relation to Sudden Death in Heart Failure

Barbara Casadei, MD, DPhil, FRCP
Reader in Cardiovascular Medicine; Senior Fellow of the British Heart Foundation, Department of Cardiovascular Medicine, University of Oxford; Honorary Consultant in Cardiovascular Medicine, John Radcliffe Hospital, Oxford, United Kingdom.
Non-neural Component of Respiratory Sinus Arrhythmia

Patricia J. Cooper, MSc, Cand PhD
Senior Research Assistant, The Cardiac Mechano-Electric Feedback Lab, Laboratory of Physiology, University of Oxford, Oxford, United Kingdom.
Mechanical Modulation of Sinoatrial Node Pacemaking

Harry J.G.M. Crijns, MD, PhD
Professor of Cardiology; Head, Department of Cardiology, Cardiovascular Research Institute Maastrict, Academic Hospital Maastrict, Maastricht, The Netherlands.
Electro-Mechanical Remodeling in Hypertrophy

Dirk W. Donker, MD
Resident in Cardiology, Department of Cardiology, Cardiovascular Research Institute Maastrict, Academic Hospital Maastrict, Maastricht, The Netherlands.
Electro-Mechanical Remodeling in Hypertrophy

Harish Doppalapudi, MD
Fellow, Department of Cardiology, University of Alabama at Birmingham, Birmingham, Alabama.
Mechanical Modulation of Defibrillation Efficacy by Preload Changes

N.A. Mark Estes III, MD
Director, Cardiac Arrhythmia Center; Director, Cardiac Electrophysiology and Pacemaker Laboratory; Department of Medicine, Tufts-New England Medical Center, Boston, Massachusetts.
Ventricular Fibrillation Secondary to Nonpenetrating Chest Wall Impact (Commotio Cordis); Sudden Death Caused by Chest Wall Trauma (Commotio Cordis)

Michael R. Franz, MD, PhD, FACC
Professor, Department of Pharmacology, Georgetown University Medical Center; Director, Arrhythmia Service, Nation Capital Veteran Affairs Medical Center, Washington, District of Columbia.
Preface: Cardiac Mechano-Electric Feedback: From Pipette to Patient; Mechanical Triggers and Facilitators of Cardiac Excitation and Arrhythmias; Stretch Channel Blockers: A New Class of Antiarrhythmic Drugs?; Mechano-Electric Feedback: New Directions, New Tools

Eric Honoré, PhD
Director of Research, Institut de Pharmacologie Moléculaire et Cellulaire, Centre National de la Recherche Scientifique, Valbonne, France.
Potassium-Selective Cardiac Mechanosensitive Ion Channels

Peter J. Hunter, PhD
Professor, Bioengineering Institute, University of Auckland, Auckland, New Zealand.
Distributions of Myocyte Stretch, Stress, and Work in Models of the Normal and Infarcted Ventricles.

Raymond E. Ideker, MD, PhD
Jeanne V. Marks Professor of Medicine, Department of Medicine; Professor, Department of Physiology, Department of Biomedical Engineering, University of Alabama at Birmingham, Birmingham, Alabama.
Mechanical Modulation of Defibrillation Efficacy by Preload Changes

Michiel J. Janse, MD
Professor, Experimental and Molecular Cardiology Group, Academic Medical Center, Amsterdam, The Netherlands.
Mechano-Electric Feedback in Atrial Fibrillation

Jonathan M. Kalman, MBBS, FRACP, PhD, FACC
Professor of Medicine, Department of Medicine, University of Melbourne; Director of Cardiac Electrophysiology, Department of Cardiology, Royal Melbourne Hospital, Melbourne, Australia.
Mechanically Induced Electrical Remodeling in Human Atrium

Pamela Karasik, MD
Assistant Professor of Medicine, Department of Cardiology, Georgetown University Hospital; Assistant Chief of Cardiology, Veterans Affairs Medical Center, Washington, District of Columbia.
Mortality from Heart Failure: Hemodynamics Versus Electrical Causes

David A. Kass, MD
Abraham and Virginia Weiss Professor of Cardiology; Professor of Medicine; Professor of Biomedical Engineering, Department of Medicine, Division of Cardiology, Johns Hopkins University Medical Institutions, Baltimore, Maryland.
Passive Ventricular Containment: A New Treatment Concept for Dilated Cardiomyopathy

Angie M. King, BA
Research Assistant/Lab Manager, The Cardiac Mechano-Electric Feedback Lab, University Laboratory of Physiology, University of Oxford, Oxford, United Kingdom.
Antiarrhythmic Effects of Acute Mechanical Stimulation

Paulus Kirchhof, MD
Fellow, Department of Cardiology and Angiology, Hospital of the University of Münster; Fellow, Institute for Ateriosclerosis Research; Project Leader, Interdisciplinary Center for Clinical Research, University of Münster, Münster, Germany.
Drugs Interacting with Mechano-Electric Feedback: Proarrhythmia, Remodeling, and Apoptosis

André G. Kléber, MD
Professor, Department of Physiology, University of Bern, Bern, Switzerland.
Effects of Mechanical Signals on Ventricular Gap Junction Remodeling

Stefan Klotz, MD
Postdoctoral Research Fellow, Department of Medicine, Division of Circulatory Physiology, Columbia University, New York, New York.
Cardiac Assist Devices: Effects on Reverse Remodeling

Peter Kohl, MD, PhD, RSRF
Reader in Cardiac Physiology, Director of the Cardiac Mechano-Electric Feedback Lab, Oxford University Laboratory of Physiology, Oxford; Adjunct Associate Professor, Medical Biotechnology Center, University of Maryland, Baltimore; Fellow and Tutor in Biomedical Sciences, Balliol College, Oxford.
Preface: Cardiac Mechano-Electric Feedback: From Pipette to Patient; Mechanical Modulation of Sinoatrial Node Pacemaking; Antiarrhythmic Effects of Acute Mechanical Stimulation; Mechano-Electric Feedback: New Directions, New Tools

Andrew Kramer, PhD
Scientific Fellow, Basis Research, Cardiac Rhythm Management, Guidant Corporation, St. Paul, Minnesota.
Cardiac Resynchronization Therapy for Patients with Heart Failure with Ventricular Conduction Delay

Max J. Lab, MD, PhD
Professor, National Heart and Lung Institute, Imperial College; Senior Research Investigator, Clinical Research Centre, Medical Research Council, London, United Kingdom.
Regional Stretch Effects in Pathological Myocardium

Ulrike Laitko, PhD
Postdoc, Department of Neurosciences, Ottawa Civic
Hospital; Ottawa Health Research Institute, Ottawa,
Ontario, Canada.
*The Mechanosensitivity of Voltage-Gated Channels May
Contribute to Cardiac Mechano-Electric Feedback*

Mark S. Link, MD
Associate Professor of Medicine; Co-Director of the
Cardiac Arrhythmia Laboratory, Department of
Medicine, Tufts-New England Medical Center,
Boston, Massachusetts.
*Ventricular Fibrillation Secondary to Nonpenetrating
Chest Wall Impact (Commotio Cordis); Sudden Death
Caused by Chest Wall Trauma (Commotio Cordis)*

Alan Maisel, MD
Professor of Medicine, University of California;
Director, CCU and Heart Failure Program, VA
Healthcare, System San Diego, California.
*Natriuretic Peptide and Sudden Cardiac Death in
Patients with Congestive Heart Failure*

Vladimir S. Markhasin, MD, PhD, DSc
Professor, Chief Researcher, Laboratory of
Mathematical Physiology, Institute of Immunology
and Physiology, Ekaterinburg, Russia.
*Mechano-Electric Heterogeneity in Physiologic Function
of the Heart*

Barry J. Maron, MD
Director, Hypertrophic Cardiomyopathy Center,
Minneapolis Heart Institute Foundation,
Minneapolis, Minnesota.
*Ventricular Fibrillation Secondary to Nonpenetrating
Chest Wall Impact (Commotio Cordis); Sudden Death
Caused by Chest Wall Trauma (Commotio Cordis)*

Andrew D. McCulloch, PhD
Professor and Vice Chair of Bioengineering,
University of California, San Diego, La Jolla,
California.
*The Effects of Wall Stretch on Ventricular Conduction
and Refractoriness in the Whole Heart*

Elliot McVeigh, PhD
Principal Investigator, Laboratory of Cardiac
Energetics, NHLBI, National Institutes of Health,
DHHS, Bethesda, Maryland.
*Evolving Concepts in Measuring Ventricular Strain in
the Human Heart*

Robert W. Mills, Cand PhD
Graduate Student Researcher, Department of
Bioengineering, University of California, San Diego,
La Jolla, California.
*The Effects of Wall Stretch on Ventricular Conduction
and Refractoriness in the Whole Heart*

Catherine E. Morris, PhD
Professor, Department of Medicine, University of
Ottawa; Senior Scientist, Department of
Neuroscience, Ottawa Health Research Institute,
Ottawa Hospital, Ottawa, Ontario, Canada.
*The Mechanosensitivity of Voltage-Gated Channels May
Contribute to Cardiac Mechano-Electric Feedback*

Joseph B. Morton, MB, BS, PhD
Senior Fellow, Department of Medicine, University of
Melbourne; Cardiologist, Department of Cardiology,
Royal Melbourne Hospital, Melbourne, Australia.
*Mechanically Induced Electrical Remodeling in Human
Atrium*

Sanjiv M. Narayan, MB, MD, MRCP
Assistant Professor, Department of Medicine,
University of California; Director of
Electrophysiology, Department of
Medicine/Cardiology, VA Healthcare System,
San Diego, California.
*The Effects of Wall Stretch on Ventricular Conduction
and Refractoriness in the Whole Heart; Natriuretic
Peptide and Sudden Cardiac Death in Patients with
Congestive Heart Failure*

Martyn P. Nash, PhD
Senior Lecturer, Bioengineering Institute, University
of Auckland, Auckland, New Zealand.
*Distributions of Myocyte Stretch, Stress, and Work in
Models of the Normal and Infarcted Ventricles*

Michel Ovize, MD, PhD
Professor of Physiology, INSERM E 0226,
Laboratoire de Physiologie Lyon-Nord, Université
Claude Bernard-Lyon I and Service d'Explorations
Fonctionnelles Cardiovasculaires, Hôpital Louis
Fradel, Hospices Civils de Lyon, Lyon, France.
Mechanical Versus Ischemic Preconditioning

Amanda Jane Patel, PhD
Senior Research Scientist, Institut de Pharmacologie
Moléculaire et Cellulaire, Centre National de la
Recherche Scientifique, Valbonne, France.
*Potassium-Selective Cardiac Mechanosensitive Ion
Channels*

Karin Przyklenk, PhD
Professor, Departments of Emergency Medicine and
Anesthesiology, University of Massachusetts Medical
School, Worcester, Massachusetts.
Mechanical Versus Ischemic Preconditioning

Michael J. Reiter, MD, PhD
Professor of Medicine-Cardiology, University of
Colorado Health Sciences Center, Denver, Colorado.
*Volume and Pressure Overload and Ventricular
Arrhythmogenesis*

Espen W. Remme, PhD
Research Scientist, Institute for Surgical Research,
Rikshospitalet University Hospital, Oslo, Norway.
*Distributions of Myocyte Stretch, Stress, and Work in
Models of the Normal and Infarcted Ventricles*

John Jeremy Rice, PhD
Research Staff Member, Functional Genomics and
Systems Biology Group, IBM T.J. Watson Research
Center, Yorktown Heights, New York; Adjunct
Faculty Member, Department of Biomedical
Engineering, The Johns Hopkins University,
Baltimore, Maryland.
*The Response of Cardiac Muscle to Stretch: The Role of
Calcium*

Frederick Sachs, PhD
Distinguished Professor of Biophysics, Centre for
Single Molecule Biophysics, Department of
Physiology and Biophysics, State University of New
York at Buffalo, New York.
*Preface: Cardiac Mechano-Electric Feedback: From
Pipette to Patient; Stretch-Activated Channels in the
Heart; Membrane–Cytoskeleton Interface and
Mechanosensitive Channels; Mechano-Electric Feedback:
New Directions, New Tools*

Jeffrey E. Saffitz, MD, PhD
Paul E. Lacy and Ellen Lacy Professor of Pathology
and Immunology, Department of Pathology,
Washington University School of Medicine, St. Louis,
Missouri.
*Effects of Mechanical Signals on Ventricular Gap
Junction Remodeling*

**Prashanthan Sanders, MBBS (Hons),
PhD, FRACP**
Clinical and Research Associate, Service de
Rythmologie, Hôpital Cardiologique du Haut-
Levêque, Bordeaux, France.
*Mechanically Induced Electrical Remodeling in Human
Atrium*

Ulrich Schotten, MD, PhD
Assistant Professor, Department of Physiology,
University of Maastricht, Maastricht, The
Netherlands.
*The Substrate of Atrial Fibrillation in Chronically
Dilated Atria*

**Abdulhalim Salim Serafi, MBChB, MSc,
FESC**
Assistant Professor, Medical Department, Umalqura
University; Consultant Cardiologist, Cardiology
Department, Alnoor General Hospital, Kingdom of
Saudi Arabia; Research Registrar, Cardiology
Department, Bristol Royal Infirmary; Doctoral
Student, Cardiology Department, University of
Bristol, United Kingdom.
*Wall Stress and Arrhythmogenesis in Patients with Left
Ventricular Hypertrophy, Dilation, or Both*

Steven N. Singh, MD
Chief of Cardiology, Veterans Affairs Medical Center;
Professor of Medicine and Pharmacology, Georgetown
University, Washington, District of Columbia.
*Mortality from Heart Failure: Hemodynamics Versus
Electrical Causes*

Olga Solovyova, PhD
Head, Laboratory of Mathematical Physiology,
Institute of Immunology and Physiology,
Ekaterinburg, Russia.
*Mechano-Electric Heterogeneity in Physiologic Function
of the Heart*

Peter M. Spooner, PhD
Executive Director, D.W. Reynolds Cardiovascular
Clinical Research Center, Johns Hopkins University;
Associate Professor, Division of Cardiology, Johns
Hopkins University Medical Institutions, Baltimore,
Maryland; Director (Emeritus), Arrhythmia, Ischemia
and Sudden Cardiac Death Research Program,
National Heart, Lung and Blood Institute, NIH,
Bethesda, Maryland.
Foreword: Stretching Our Views of Cardiac Control

Thomas M. Suchyna, PhD
Doctor, Department of Physiology and Biophysics,
Hughes Center for Single Molecule Studies, SUNY at
Buffalo, Buffalo, New York.
*Membrane–Cytoskeleton Interface and Mechanosensitive
Channels*

Borys Surawicz, MD
Professor Emeritus, Department of Medicine, Indiana
University School of Medicine, Indianapolis, Indiana.
*Is the U Wave in the Electrocardiogram a Mechano-
Electric Phenomenon?*

Peter Sutton, PhD
Associate Director, Hatter Institute, Department of
Cardiology, University College Hospital; Senior
Lecturer, Department of Physiology, University
College London, London, England.
*Load Dependence of Ventricular Repolarization;
Termination of Arrhythmias by Hemodynamic
Unloading*

Toru Suzuki, MD, PhD
Specially Appointed Faculty Member, Departments of
Clinical Bioinformatics and Cardiovascular Medicine,
The University of Tokyo, Tokyo, Japan.
*Stretch Effects on Second Messengers and Early Gene
Expression*

Peter Taggart, MD, DSc, FRCP
Reader in Cardiology, Hatter Institute, Department
of Cardiology, University College Hospital, London,
United Kingdom.
*Load Dependence of Ventricular Repolarization;
Termination of Arrhythmias by Hemodynamic
Unloading*

John V. Tyberg, MD, PhD
Professor, Department of Medicine and Physiology
and Biophysics, University of Calgary, Calgary,
Alberta, Canada.
*Mechanical Modulation of Cardiac Function: Role of
the Pericardium*

John Vann Jones, PhD, FRCP
Professor, Department of Cardiology, Bristol Royal
Infirmary, Bristol, United Kingdom.
*Wall Stress and Arrhythmogenesis in Patients with Left
Ventricular Hypertrophy, Dilation, or Both*

Paul G.A. Volders, MD, PhD
Co-Principal Investigator, Department of Cardiology,
Cardiovascular Research Institute Maastricht,
Maastricht University; Medical Doctor, Department
of Cardiology, Academic Hospital Maastricht,
Maastricht, The Netherlands.
Electro-Mechanical Remodeling in Hypertrophy

Ed White, PhD
Reader in Cellular Cardiology, School of Biomedical
Sciences, University of Leeds, Leeds, United
Kingdom.
*Temporal Modulation of Mechano-Electric Feedback in
Cardiac Muscle*

Tsutomu Yamazaki, MD
Professor, Department of Clinical Bioinformatics, Graduate School of Medicine, University of Tokyo, Japan.
Stretch Effects on Second Messengers and Early Gene Expression

Shamil Yusuf, BSc (Hons), MbChb (Hons), MCOptom, MRCP
British Heart Foundation Research Fellow in Cardiology, Department of Cardiac and Vascular Sciences, St. George's Hospital Medical School, London, United Kingdom.
Atrial Fibrillation and Dilated Cardiomyopathy

Markus Zabel, MD
Registrar, Head of Cardiac Electrophysiology and Rhythmology, Medical Cardiology and Pulmologie, Free University, Berlin, Germany.
Mechanical Triggers and Facilitators of Cardiac Excitation and Arrhythmias

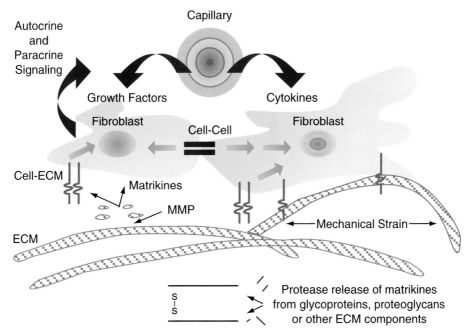

Figure 10–2 Schematic representation of the dynamic interaction among components of the acellular extracellular matrix (ECM) and the cardiac fibroblasts. MMP, matrix metalloproteinases; s-s, fibronectin disulfide bond.

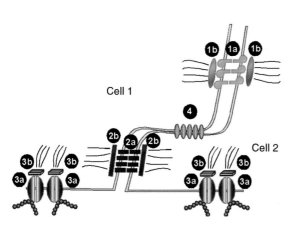

Figure 11–1 The cell membranes of two adjacent cardiomyocytes are connected by fascia adherens junctions *(1)*, desmosomes *(2)*, and gap junctions *(4)*. The surface membranes are connected to extracellular matrix proteins through cell adherens molecules *(3)*. Fascia adherens junctions consist of the transmembrane-spanning Ca^{2+}-dependent adherens proteins (N-cadherins, *1a*) that are anchored in a submembranous scaffold *(1b)* consisting of several proteins (plakoglobin, catenins). The submembranous complex binds to the microfilaments of the cytoskeleton (actin). Desmosomes are formed by the transmembrane-spanning proteins desmocollin and desmoglein *(2a)* and are anchored in a submembranous scaffold of plakoglobin and desmoplakin *(2b)*. The latter proteins are bound to intermediate filaments (desmin). Gap junctions *(4)* consist of clustered gap junction channels each formed by two juxtaposed hemi-channels (each formed by six connexin proteins). The extracellular matrix is connected to integrin *(3a)* through fibronectin. Intracellularly, integrins bind to cytoskeletal proteins through a number of intermediate proteins *(3b)* that cluster integrin molecules and can induce intracellular signals when activated by extracellular mechanical stimuli.

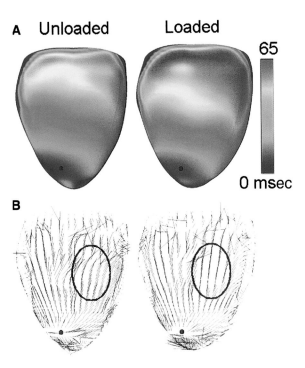

■ **Figure 14–2** Activation time fields *(A)* and conduction velocity vector fields *(B)* before and during application of 30 mm Hg ventricular volume load in isolated rabbit heart, using methods from Sung and colleagues.[29] The *small solid circle* indicates the approximate position of pacing. The ellipses outline a region in which the apparent direction of conduction has been changed by application of load.

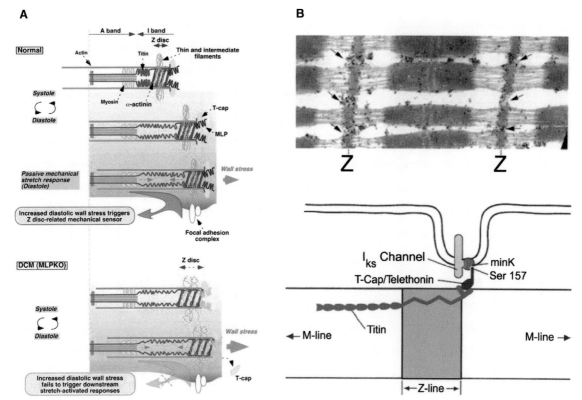

■ **Figure 28–4** *A,* Proposed working model of the cardiac stretch sensor machinery. *Top,* Normal conditions. Titin, anchored between Z-disc and M-line, exhibits elastic "molecular springs" (I band). Titin is able to store force generated by systolic compression (systole), and it largely determines passive myocardial stiffness (diastole). With increasing diastolic wall stress, the titin/MLP/telethonin (T-cap) complex is stretched and mechanical load is sensed. *Bottom,* Loss of the MLP/T-cap complex in knockout mice (MLPKO) causes a defective stretch-sensor function, ultimately leading to dilative cardiomyopathy (DCM), which, in turn, enhances wall stress and mechanical stretch stimuli. *B,* Model for the titin/T-cap/minK complex in cardiac myocytes. *Top,* Detection of T-cap by immunoelectron microscopy in skeletal muscle. T-cap is clustered where membrane structures corresponding to T-tubules and terminal cisternae contact the Z-line periphery *(arrows). Bottom,* Summary of known interactions of titin, T-cap, and minK (=KCNE1). T-cap connects the myofibrillar apparatus to the sarcolemma at the Z-line periphery. Phosphorylation of the C-terminal tail of the T-cap by yet unidentified kinases may regulate the stability of the complex. *(A, Reproduced from Knöll R, Hoshijima M, Hoffman HM, et al: The cardiac mechanical stretch sensor machinery involves a Z disc complex that is defective in a subset of human dilated cardiomyopathy. Cell 111:943–955, 2002, with permission; B, reproduced from Furukawa T, Ono Y, Tsuchiya H, et al: Specific interaction of the potassium channel β-subunit minK with the sarcomeric protein T-cap suggests a T-tubule-myofibril linking system. J Mol Biol 313:775–784, 2001, with permission.)*

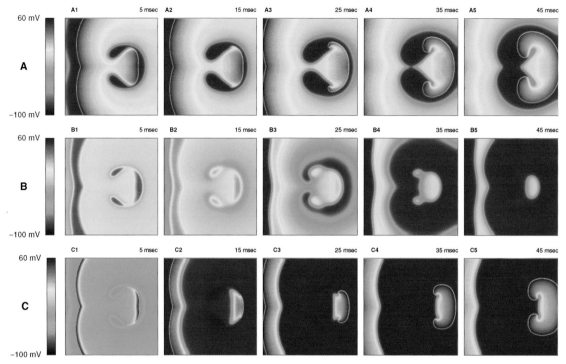

■ **Figure 33–6** Two-dimensional model (2.5 × 2.5 cm) of ventricular myocardium, consisting of 251 × 251 single-cell models[40] (transmembrane voltage is color coded; see Reference 41 for mesh implementation). *A,* Control figure-of-eight re-entry activity. *B,* Mechanical stimulation, modeled by activation for 5 msec of SAC_{CAT} (reversal potential, −10 mV; see Chapter 8 for equation), causes depolarization of tissue in the excitable gap and terminates re-entry. *C,* Mechanical stimulation of tissue after simulated ischemic sensitization of SAC_K to stretch shifts net mechanically induced reversal potential to more negative levels (here −35 mV), which prevents depolarization of resting tissue and shortens action potential duration, rendering mechanical stimulation incapable of instantaneously terminating re-entry. *(Illustration courtesy of Dr. Alan Garny, the Cardiac MEF Lab, University of Oxford.)*

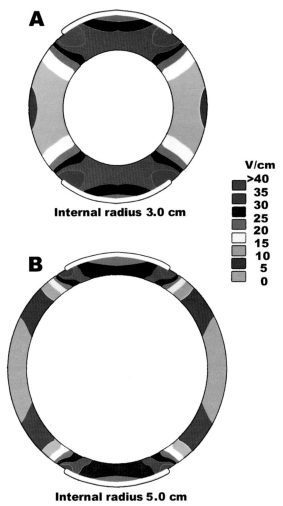

■ **Figure 35–3** Computer simulation of effect of cardiac dilation on potential gradient field produced by a 200 V shock. Each circle represents a cross section of the left ventricle. The defibrillation electrodes are curved discs, applied to the top and bottom portions of the heart, and have the same surface area in *A* and *B*. The volume of myocardium is the same in *A* and *B*. *A*, The internal radius of the heart is 3.0 cm; *B*, the internal radius is 5.0 cm. The central portions represent the blood-filled chamber. The conductivity of the myocardium is assumed to be 0.003 S/cm, and the conductivity of the blood is 0.0065 S/cm. The color key depicts the resulting potential gradients with yellow and red corresponding to regions of least potential gradient and purple representing areas of greatest potential gradient. The low-gradient area is considerably larger for the dilated heart *(B)*. *(Reproduced from Hillsley RE, Wharton JM, Cates AW, et al: Why do some patients have high defibrillation thresholds at defibrillator implantation? Pacing Clin Electrophysiol 17:222–239, 1994, with permission.)*

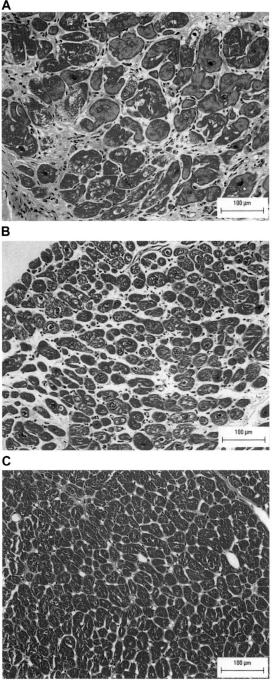

■ **Figure 37–4** Normalization of the myocyte diameter in LVAD-supported hearts. Histologic samples representative for end-stage heart failure *(A)*, LVAD-supported hearts *(B)*, and normal hearts *(C)*.

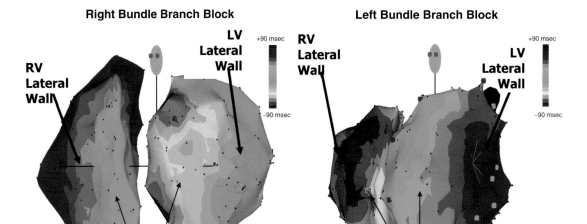

Figure 38-1 Isochronal plot (red: −90 msec; blue: +90 msec) obtained from patients with right (RBBB; *left*) and left (LBBB; *right*) bundle branch block. In RBBB, the left ventricular (LV) breakthrough site is in the septum, from which activation slowly spreads toward the anterior region, with the right ventricular (RV) lateral wall and the outflow tract being activated last. Total RV activation time in RBBB is always significantly longer than in LBBB. The endocardial spread of activation was similar in both patient populations. Patients with LBBB have a single RV anterolateral breakthrough site. The LV is activated late with respect to the start of QRS, starting from the septum, followed by inferior and finally lateral and posterolateral walls.

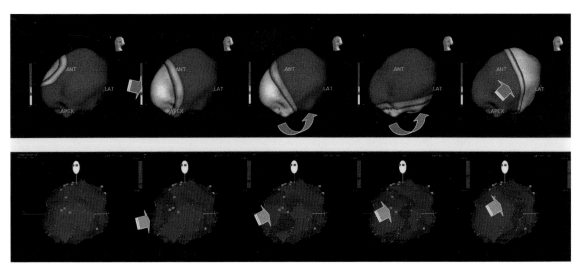

Figure 38-2 Transmural (*top;* color coding: white, −5 mV; purple, +5 mV) and endocardial (*bottom;* color coding: red line indicates progression from −87 to +22 msec) left ventricular (LV) activation in a patient with left bundle branch block QRS morphology. The endocardial activation proceeds uniformly and directly to the lateral and posterolateral wall, ending at the basal region near the mitral valve annulus. In contrast, the transmural activation does not cross from the anterior wall to the lateral wall, but it reaches the lateral or posterolateral regions by propagating inferiorly around the apex and across the inferior wall. This apparent conduction block occurs in the absence of any observable structural defects in the region, such as ischemic scarring, and thus appears to be a functional line of block.

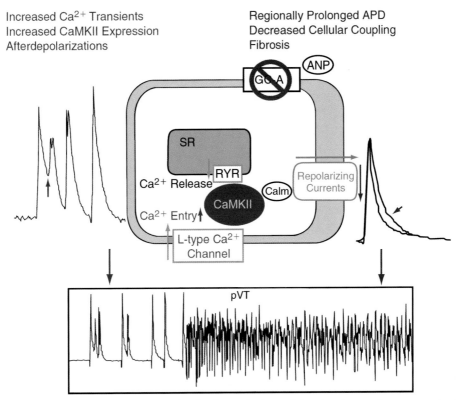

Increased Ca^{2+} Transients
Increased CaMKII Expression
Afterdepolarizations

Regionally Prolonged APD
Decreased Cellular Coupling
Fibrosis

ANP

GC-A

SR

RYR

Ca^{2+} Release

CaMKII

Calm

Ca^{2+} Entry

L-type Ca^{2+}
Channel

Repolarizing
Currents

pVT

■ **Figure 39–2** Electrophysiologic consequences and molecular mechanisms of chronic volume and pressure overload in a mouse model of deletion of the atrial natriuretic peptide (ANP) receptor guanylyl cyclase A (GC-A).[3] The net repolarizing current of the cardiac action potential is reduced, as reflected by prolonged ventricular action potential duration (APD). Cardiac hypertrophy, increased cell size, increased interstitial fibrosis, and the preponderance of the stretch signal in the left ventricle increase regional inhomogeneity of APD. Focal cardiac fibrosis also forms potential re-entrant circuits. These processes create a substrate for functional re-entry (right side of scheme). In addition, Ca^{2+} transient amplitude is increased, and expression levels of Ca^{2+}–calmodulin-dependent protein kinase II (CaMKII) are increased. These changes are triggers for afterdepolarizations and the occurrence of polymorphic ventricular tachycardias (pVT; left side of scheme and bottom). The combination of this CaMKII-dependent trigger for arrhythmias and a functional substrate for re-entry allows for spontaneous occurrence of pVT with bradycardia. In this model, pharmacologic blockade of CaMKII suppresses ventricular arrhythmias. Similar mechanisms of arrhythmias were identified in models with increased expression of CaMKII or CaMKIV.[23] RYR, ryanodine receptor; SR, sarcoplasmic reticulum; Calm, calmodulin.

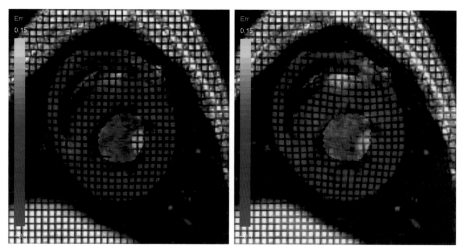

■ **Figure 40–1B** Two time frames of systolic contraction in a paced canine heart. The color bar represents the amount of radial thickening at each location computed from the tag deformation; yellow represents 15% thickening (top of the color bar), and blue represents 15% thinning (bottom of the color bar). The *left panel* is at the first onset of contraction; the *right panel* is 40 msec later. Note the transmural gradient thickening observed in the anterior septum (12 o'clock position in the left ventricle). This early contraction is likely from an activation that escaped from the paced atrium into the septum. *(Data provided by Dan Ennis, National Heart Lung and Blood Institute.)*

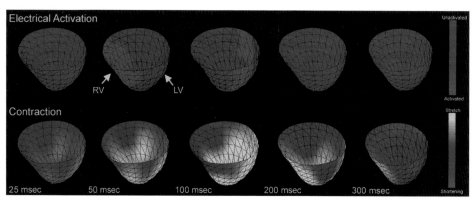

■ **Figure 40–3** An example of coregistered mechanical contraction data and electrical activation data obtained from myocardial tagging and a 128-electrode sock array in a canine heart with left bundle branch block. The surface on which the color is rendered represents the epicardial surface of the left (LV) and right (RV) ventricles. The blue color in the electrical activation data (top) shows the locus of points on the surface that have been activated after RV pacing. The yellow color in the mechanical map of circumferential strain (bottom) shows a prestretch of the LV free wall at 100 msec, followed by contraction (blue).

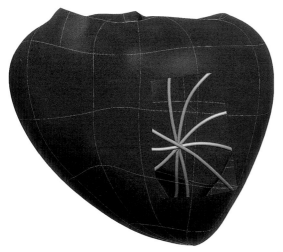

Figure 41–2 Porcine ventricular geometry and rotation of the transmural myocyte orientation from roughly −60 degrees at the epicardial surface to +90 degrees at the endocardial surface (with respect to the circumferential direction; positive angles counterclockwise).

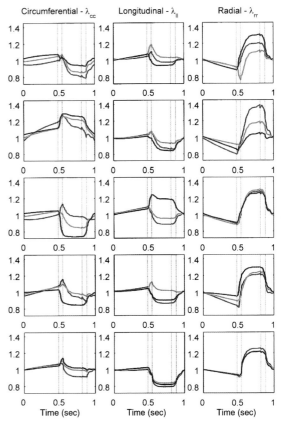

Figure 41–5 Circumferential *(left)*, longitudinal *(center)*, and radial *(right)* stretch ratios, during the cardiac cycle at five circumferential locations around the equator of the ventricles, as indicated by the diagram in the corresponding row of Figure 41-6. *Red, green,* and *blue lines* represent subendocardial, midwall, and subepicardial locations, respectively. *Gray bands* indicate the isovolumic contraction and relaxation phases of the cardiac cycle.

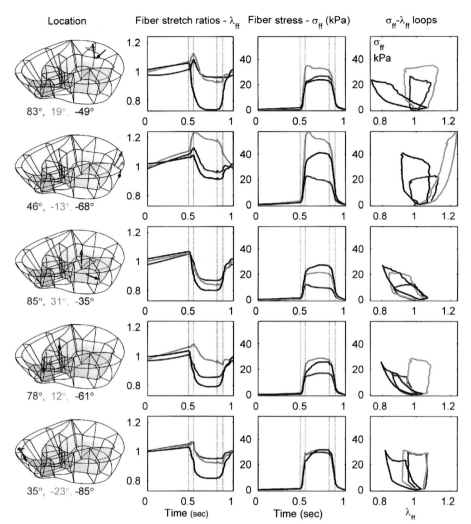

■ **Figure 41–6** Transmural sarcomere stretch ratio and stress during the cardiac cycle at five locations around the equator of the ventricles, illustrated on the *left* with fiber directions indicated by *arrows* and angles relative to the circumferential axis. *Red, green,* and *blue lines* represent subendocardial, midwall, and subepicardial locations, respectively. The *second column* shows the fiber stretch ratio through the heart cycle. The *third column* shows the developed fiber stress. The *right column* illustrates the resulting fiber stress–stretch loops. *Gray bands* indicate the isovolumic contraction and relaxation phases of the cardiac cycle.

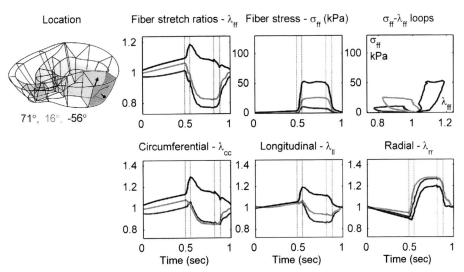

■ **Figure 41–7** Stretch and stress results in a left ventricular free wall anterior region *before* it is subject to infarction. The region is highlighted in purple on the *left,* with fiber directions indicated by *arrows* and angles relative to the circumferential axis. The *top row* shows fiber stretch ratio and stress through the heart cycle and the resulting fiber stress-stretch loops. The *second row* shows corresponding stretch ratios in cardiac wall coordinates. *Red, green,* and *blue lines* represent subendocardial, midwall, and subepicardial locations, respectively. *Gray bands* indicate the isovolumic contraction and relaxation phases of the cardiac cycle.

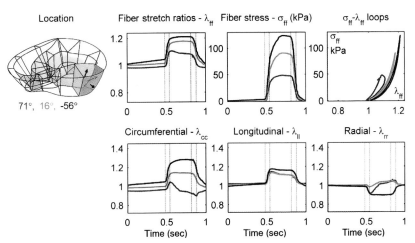

■ **Figure 41–8** Stretch and stress results from a left ventricular free wall anterior region subject to infarction. The region is highlighted in purple on the *left,* with fiber directions indicated by *arrows* and angles relative to the circumferential axis. The *top row* shows fiber stretch ratio and stress through the heart cycle and the resulting fiber stress-stretch loops. The *second row* shows corresponding stretch ratios in cardiac wall coordinates. *Red, green,* and *blue lines* represent subendocardial, midwall, and subepicardial locations, respectively. *Gray bands* indicate the isovolumic contraction and relaxation phases of the cardiac cycle.

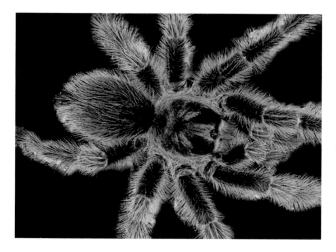

■ **Figure 42–1** The Chilean tarantula *Grammostola spatulata*. (From Bode F, Sachs F, Franz MR: Tarantula peptide inhibits atrial fibrillation. Nature 409:35–36, 2001, with permission.)

(SUB-CELLULAR) MECHANISMS OF CARDIAC MECHANO-ELECTRIC FEEDBACK

• • • •

CHAPTER 1

Stretch-Activated Channels in the Heart

• • • •

Frederick Sachs

BACKGROUND

Mechanosensitive ion channels fall into two categories: stretch-activated (SAC) and stretch-inactivated channels (SIC). SAC open with increases in stress (membrane tension), whereas SIC are tonically active and close with increased stress. SAC are much more common than SIC, whereas both types are lumped into the general category of mechanosensitive channels (MSC). (MSC does *not* refer specifically to the bacterial MSC, denoted MscL or MscS [mechanosensitive channel large or small].[1]) MSC is a phenomenological term, not a structural term.

In addition to channels that are directly sensitive to mechanical stress, there are channels activated by increased cell volume (volume-activated channels). These channels may be mechanically sensitive themselves, or they may be activated by secondary processes. These include increased Ca^{2+} and the decrease in ionic strength brought on by swelling (see Chapter 3).

Many channels with previously characterized gating properties have been shown to be mechanosensitive. These channels include *Shaker,* voltage-dependent calcium and sodium channels (see Chapter 4), cyclic adenosine monophosphate,[2] *N*-methyl-D-aspartate channels,[3] and the antibiotic alamethicin.[4]

However, not all channels are mechanosensitive, and many channels, such as *N*-methyl-D-aspartate, are only weakly modulated by tension. This chapter arbitrarily reserves the term MSC to refer to channels whose probability of being open can be significantly and reversibly changed with physiologically relevant stimuli. An example of SAC activity is shown in Figure 1–1.

There are no direct data on the stretch sensitivity of channels in organelles, but indirect data[5,6] suggest that these may exist, and that Ca^{2+} release channels are par-

ticularly significant candidates. Transporters may also be stretch sensitive.

Recent articles suggest that stretch activates Na^+-H^+ exchange, increasing cell Na^+ and thus Ca^{2+} through Na-Ca^{2+} exchange.[7–9]

STRUCTURE

There is no generic molecular structure associated with MSC. The only eukaryotic mechanosensitive channels that have been cloned and reconstituted are those of the K^+-selective TREK-1 family (see Chapter 2) and a Ca^{2+}-activated K^+ channel from chick heart.[10] The common cationic SAC has not been cloned. The lack of homology among MSC was accurately demonstrated in *Escherichia coli* where the two most common MSC have no significant sequence homology: one is a pentamer, and the other is a heptamer.[1,11] Site-directed spin labeling and cross-linking have shown that MscL opens like an iris; the alpha helices of the transmembrane segments tilt and flatten, making the channel larger in diameter and thinner.[12,13]

EVOLUTION

MSC developed early in living cells.[14] They are found in bacteria, archaea, fungi, higher plants, and animals.[15,16] This primitive evolutionary origin probably reflects the need to solve a universal problem: volume regulation.

Osmotic pressure is such a powerful stimulus that a small difference in transmembrane osmolarity can produce membrane lysis (~10 mN/m), which means death. For example, *E. coli,* once dried out on the seashore and then rained upon, had to adapt to drastic changes in osmotic pressure. As organisms became more com-

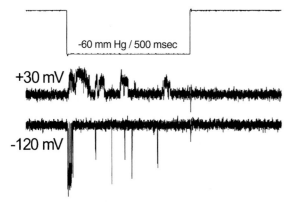

■ **Figure 1–1** Cationic stretch-activated ion channel activity from a cell-attached patch in chick heart cells. The channels were stimulated by suction in the pipette as shown in the top trace. The activity is shown at two membrane potentials. The channels inactivate with time and have voltage-sensitive kinetics.

plicated, the ability to carry on metabolism in a closed membrane made volume regulation an essential requirement and might have given rise to more specialized ion channels.

In animals, the epithelia are subjected to large volume flows. In the kidney, for example, the water flux across the cell may be a cell volume every 20 sec. Influx and efflux rates must be continually matched. However, no ion selective channel can regulate cell volume. The movement of a single charged species across the membrane quickly changes the membrane potential ($V = Q/C$) and blocks the flow of additional ions.

Mechanosensitive channels can sense the swelling that results from changes in osmotic pressure, but the regulation itself must be passed on to transporters capable of moving neutral species. These species may be uncharged molecules such as taurine or sugars, ion pairs such as KCl, or mixed fluxes of K^+ and Cl^- through nonselective or separate channels (see Chapter 3). The large conductance channels of bacteria such as MscL and MSC do not distinguish well between anions and cations, and hence can serve both as sensors and regulators. The low homology between the known MSC and volume-activated channel candidates suggests that the sensors have evolved independently multiple times. That voltage-dependent channels are stretch sensitive is another clue (see Chapter 4).

GENERAL PHYSIOLOGIC FUNCTIONS

Once mechanosensitive channels evolved to handle volume regulation, they probably were recruited to serve other purposes. For example, they may indicate to plants that roots should grow down whereas the stems should grow up. Protozoa, such as *Paramecium,* have dual mechanical senses; the anterior is Ca^{2+} selective and the posterior is K^+ selective.[17] Stimulation of the posterior by a predator causes the ciliary beat rate to increase, causing the animal to run away, and stimulation of the anterior causes the animal to back up to avoid beating its "head" against a wall.

Inheriting this kind of mechanosensitivity from our ancestral free-living microorganisms, we developed the senses of touch, hearing, local gravity (the vestibular system), feedback for the voluntary musculature, and a system for monitoring filling of the hollow organs (blood pressure, gastric and bladder filling, etc.).

Some of these senses, such as hearing and the specialized touch receptors, use fibrous proteins to efficiently transfer forces from the macroscopic cell structure to the channels,[18] whereas the less differentiated receptors, such as those from bacteria,[19,20] astrocytes, and presumably other cell types such as striated muscle (including heart), seem to activate through stress in the lipid bilayer (see Chapter 5). Evidence is accumulating that the channels used in some of the specialized receptors are of the transient receptor potential or the *Caenorhabditis elegans* touch receptor *mec* family that is homologous to endothelial Na^+ channel.[18,21]

WHAT MAKES CHANNELS MECHANICALLY SENSITIVE?

The key to what makes channels mechanically sensitive seems to be a significant change in channel dimensions (in the plane of the membrane) between the open and closed states. Open SAC are wider than shut SAC. This size does not refer to the size of the pore but to the outer physical dimensions where the protein meets the lipid. (For the specialized receptors, such as cochlear hair cells and nematode touch receptors, the channels appear to open, not using bilayer tension, but by having a gate pulled for a significant distance, perhaps 4 nm, by fibrous proteins.)

For tension-sensitive channels, at a given tension, T, the energy difference between the open and closed states is $\Delta G = T*\Delta A$, where ΔA is the difference in membrane area between the closed and open states. Also, there may be secondary energy terms arising from thinning of the channel as it enlarges.[13,20] (This is equivalent to the common Poisson constant in mechanics, where stretching causes thinning to maintain a constant volume.) In addition to bilayer tension, there may be local effects of curvature that can be modified by amphipaths.[20] Curiously, some channels only open when the membrane is concave, and others only open when it is convex, although the tension should be the same in both cases.[22]

WHAT IS MEMBRANE TENSION, AND HOW IS TENSION GENERATED?

Although tension sounds like a simple concept, the cell cortex is not mechanically homogeneous, and the definition of tension becomes obscure. Because it is a fluid, the lipid bilayer is the simplest component. It would have a homogenous tension, free of shear stress. However, the cytoskeleton supports the bilayer by adding a binding energy to the lipids, and the cytoskeleton supports static and time-dependent shear stresses in three dimensions (see Chapter 5). The extracellular matrix is another component of the cell cortex that is likely to have an effect on membrane mechanics, but the magnitude of its contribution is unknown. Finally, the connective tissue outside cells has a strong influence on the stresses that reach the cortex. The cytoskeleton is not required for mechanical sensitivity, because bac-

terial MSC can be functionally reconstituted into artificial lipid bilayers.[20] In what follows, the term *membrane tension* is used in its sloppiest, most general, form: some kind of average tension in the cell cortex.

In most quantitative experiments, tension is generated in a patch pipette by applying hydrostatic pressure (suction). This causes the membrane to bulge and the tension to increase, but MSC are not sensitive to the applied pressure; they are sensitive to the tension. According to Laplace's law, the tension in a patch of uniform curvature (a spherical cap) is $T = Pr/2$, where P is the *trans*membrane pressure and r is the radius of curvature. With patch pipettes, SAC open significantly at pressures 25 to 50 mm Hg or 3000 to 6000 Pa. (Note that for elastic membranes, the tension is nonlinearly related to the pressure.[16]) The formulation of membrane tension using Laplace's law ignores the effects of the membrane bending stiffness and the presence of the cytoskeleton.

To permit the pressure and tension units to make more intuitive sense, Table 1–1 provides conversions. A useful scale factor is that the lytic tension of a lipid bilayer or a red cell is about 10 dyne/cm, which is equal to 10 mN/m.

Limitations of Patch Measurements of Stretch-Activated Channels

Patches cannot be formed without a massive reorganization of the cell cortex,[23,24] and there is a substantial resting tension caused by adhesion of the membrane to the glass.[25] This tension may be half the lytic tension.[26] With these factors in mind, it is important to know whether we can judge the contribution of SAC to the resting conductance of a cell in situ. It is a question

TABLE 1–1	Common Units for Pressure and the Tension in a Patch with a 1-μm Radius of Curvature			
P (atm)	P (mm Hg)	P (Pa)	P (cm H$_2$O)	T (mN/m)
1.00	760	101,325	103	200
atm, atmosphere; P, pressure; T, tension.				

that cannot be answered with a patch recording but requires whole-cell or larger scale recordings.

The absolute calibration of tension in a patch is difficult and rarely performed. Calculating the tension requires knowledge of patch geometry and the stress–strain properties of the membrane. Furthermore, the applied pressure is usually not accurately calibrated. The meniscus of the solution–capillary interface at the upper end of a patch pipette applies a resting pressure that must be offset. The best calibration is to find the pressure that eliminates fluid flow from the open pipette tip. Despite these difficulties, absolute tension calibrations exist for MscL in artificial bilayers. The midpoint of the gating curve is at about 10 mN/m and a sensitivity corresponding to a change in area of approximately 20 nm^2.[27] (Planar bilayers cannot be used for stressing MSC. There is excess lipid at the partition, and capillary forces holding the bilayer to the partition maintains a constant tension regardless of membrane curvature.)

Channel Density

Patch recordings show the activity of only a few MSC, suggesting a density of approximately one per square micrometer. There are no known tissues with a much greater density, including the cochlear hair cells. In any case, the patch clamp is not a reliable tool to measure channel density. The area that is sampled is small and may not be representative. For example, in adult striated muscle (including cardiac muscle), SAC may be located in the T-tubules, where they are not accessible to a pipette.[28] Furthermore, channels can stick to the glass walls of the pipette and not appear in the cap that spans the pipette.[29]

Stimuli

Attention to stimulus detail is important when attempting to compare experiments. As opposed to voltage- or ligand-gated channels, mechanical channels have no trustworthy whole-cell current counterparts. Osmotic stress is commonly labeled a "mechanical" stimulus, and perhaps in some sense it is, but the effects are different from the effects of direct stress. Hu and Sachs[30] showed that in chick heart cells, direct mechanical stress activated a cation conductance, whereas osmotic stress activated an anion conductance. Similarly, Kohl's group[31,32] reports that stretching sinus node cells of the rabbit increases the spontaneous pacemaking rate, but swelling decreases it (see Chapter 8).

Voltage clamp is the most accurate method to study channel currents, but it is difficult to voltage clamp and stretch cells. Pulling on isolated heart cells is particularly tedious, because the force probes either do not stick or damage the cells[28,33] (see Chapter 9). In addition, the process of isolating cells with proteolytic enzymes removes the extracellular connections that normally transmit forces among cells. Thus, even when probes are glued to the "surface" of an isolated cell, it is important to know what may happen in situ. Answering that question requires the use of specific pharmacologic agents on intact tissues and organs.

PROPERTIES OF NONSELECTIVE CATIONIC CHANNELS IN THE HEART

Despite the experimental demands of work on MSC, we have managed to glean some knowledge about them. The following sections intersperse data on heart with data on other systems, because there is a shortage of cardiac data.

As mentioned previously, there is no simple homology among MSC. There can be multiple types of mechanical channels in single cells, much as there are many types of voltage-gated channels in a single cell. In early embryonic chick heart cells, for example, there are five different MSC, and the relative numbers change during development.[34] In young embryos (7 days), there are multiple nonselective cationic SAC (SAC$_{CAT}$) and K$^+$-selective SAC (SAC$_K$). One SAC$_K$ appears to be a maxiK channel.[35] As the embryo gets older (17 days), the cells express only two channel types: the high conductance (90 pS) SAC$_K$ and a lower conductance (20 pS) SAC$_{CAT}$.[30] Developmental changes in MSC function are undoubtedly present in the mammalian heart as well. There is at least one successful experiment demonstrating SAC in fetal ventricular cells.[36] However, there are no published experiments showing single-channel recordings of MSC in adult ventricular cells. This dearth of data on adult cells may fit the hypothesis that adult SAC are located in T-tubules.[28] In neonatal cells or cells in culture, the T-tubules are not fully developed; hence, the channels are accessible to a patch clamp.

A deliberate search for SAC in rat atria produced only SAC_K channels (probably of the 2P domain family; see Chapter 2). This finding is also compatible with the T-tubule hypothesis, because atrial cells do not have T-tubules. These results are in conflict with earlier data from the same preparation showing nonselective and K⁺-selective currents. However, there were little single-channel data in these experiments.[37] More experiments are clearly needed.

Permeation Properties

The K⁺-selective MSC, as expected from other K⁺ channels, are highly selective for K⁺ over other cations, and the conductances are relatively large. For example, the conductance of mouse TREK-1 is approximately 50 pS in K⁺ saline. The channel displays a strong outward rectification that results from external Mg^{2+} block and from an intrinsic voltage-dependent gating. In chick heart, the cationic channels are approximately 25 and 50 pS and the K⁺ channels are approximately 100 and 200 pS.[34] These numbers obviously depend on the permeant ion species and are provided only as rough guidelines.

Time-Dependent Behavior of Mechanosensitive Channels

In general, MSC responses inactivate with time, although they have mostly been studied with constant stimuli. In the extreme case of steady-state stimulation, there may be no response because the channels are fully inactivated.

In the heart, the only knowledge of the dynamic properties of single channels came from atrial SAC_K channels.[38] However, there are dynamic whole-cell recordings of MSC from rat and chick heart. In the study by Zeng and colleagues[28] on rat ventricular cells, the stretch-sensitive currents did not show much inactivation. However, in the Bett and Sachs[39] study and the Hu and Sachs[30] study on chick cells, inactivation was common. In the adult rat heart cell study of Bett and Sachs,[40] mechanical stimuli displayed hysteresis.

Initially, the cells were insensitive to mechanical stimulation. Deformation produced no current. However, if the cells were repeatedly stimulated, mechanosensitivity suddenly appeared. The transition was associated with a sudden inward current as though something (possibly parallel cytoskeletal links) had broken (Fig. 1–2). The endogenous protection of MSC from stress in the resting cell is important when comparing studies on different cells or tissues or even when comparing results on a single preparation at different times. The observed mechanical sensitivity can depend on the history of stimulation and probably on the metabolic history as well. Cellular data suggest that repeated stretching would be more effective in exposing large mechanical effects than short-term stimulation. Stretch may cause the fusion of vesicles with the plasmalemma, changing the local stress and perhaps delivering new channels to the surface.[41] Vesicle fusion may also play a role in the excretion of atrial natriuretic peptide.[42]

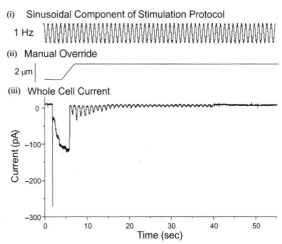

(i) Sinusoidal Component of Stimulation Protocol

1 Hz

(ii) Manual Override

2 μm

(iii) Whole Cell Current

■ **Figure 1–2** Prolonged stimulation exposes mechanosensitivity in rat ventricular cells.[40] An isolated cell was squeezed sinusoidally against a coverslip using the side of a patch pipette (2 μm, 1 Hz) while recording the whole-cell current. After 1 to 2 minutes of continuous stimulation, ending about 2 sec into the recording, a spike of inward current appeared, followed by a sustained inward current (apparently the saturated value of the mechanosensitive current). The mean position of the stimulation pipette was then lifted 2 μm, and the cell began to respond in phase with the stimulus and then inactivated. *(From Bett GCL and Sachs F: Whole-cell mechanosensitive currents in rat ventricular myocytes activated by direct stimulation. J Memb Biol 173:255–263, 2000, with permission.)*

Currently, it is unclear how SAC in the heart respond to sustained stimuli such as osmotic stress (see Chapter 3). However, inferential data using SAC blockers such as Gd[3+] or GsMTx-4 suggest that osmotic stress does lead to sustained low-level activation.

Resting Activity

The resting activity of SAC in cells cannot be measured with single-channel recording. However, with specific pharmacologic blockers, measurements can be obtained at the whole-cell level. The most precise measurements to date used whole-cell currents with a permeablized patch clamp of isolated rabbit atrial cells (Fig. 1–3). The SAC_{CAT} blocker GsMTx-4 had no effect on the action potential, suggesting that under auxotonic conditions, there is little resting SAC activity.[43] Consistent with this result, monophasic action potential recordings in the intact heart showed that GsMTx-4 had little effect on the action potential when the heart was mechanically unloaded.[44]

PHARMACOLOGY OF STRETCH-ACTIVATED CHANNELS

Given the wide variety of MSC, it is not surprising that there is no universal "blocker." However, one of the most general pharmacologic effects is that the lan-

thanides, notably Gd[3+] and La[3+], can block many MSC, ranging from bacteria to humans.[45] Gd[3+] sensitivity, although often used as a signature of MSC channels, is not reliable, because it has significant reactivity with other channels such as voltage-dependent Ca^{2+} channels. Furthermore, Gd[3+] readily precipitates many physiologic anions including PO_4^{3-}, HCO_3^-, and proteins[46]; therefore, it cannot be used in physiologic conditions. The active form of Gd[3+] is unknown. Gd[3+] can have valences of +2 or +3 and can form various hydrates. Although there have been reports of Gd[3+] effects when it was administered in blood, the origin of these effects is not clear. (In Gd[3+]-based magnetic resonance imaging contrast agents, the Gd[3+] is chelated, not free.)

Amiloride[45] and the cationic antibiotics such as streptomycin have been used to block cationic SAC_{CAT}.[47] But again, these agents are not specific for SAC. In general, the pharmacology of SAC cannot be generalized yet, because there have been few tests. Some SAC are sensitive to "specific" ion channel reagents such as tetrodotoxin and diltiazem.[34]

Amphiphilic compounds such as arachidonic acid, chlorpromazine, general anesthetics, and lysolipids can affect MSC[20] (see Chapter 2) but can hardly be considered specific. The amphiphiles appear to act by affecting local membrane curvature. This allows MSC to be activated (or inactivated) in the absence of global tension. However, the sensitivity of MSC to amphipaths makes them vulnerable to modulation by amphiphilic members of the signal transduction pathways, such as inositol phosphates and lysolipids. The pharmacology of MSC is improving with the discovery of a specific inhibitory peptide isolated from tarantula venom,[48,49] which is now available commercially. (For more details see the Peptide Institute Web site: www.pepnet.com.)

This peptide, GsMTx-4, blocks SAC in a number of cells including chick heart; rat heart and astrocytes; and rabbit, sheep, and dog ventricular cells. It is capable of blocking stretch-induced atrial fibrillation in rabbit heart at less than 200 nM.[44] GsMTx-4 seems remarkably specific, with no significant effects found on other channels. For example, Figure 1–3 shows action potentials from an isolated rabbit atrial cell exposed to GsMTx-4 at doses up to eight times that required to block SAC in rat astrocytes. The action

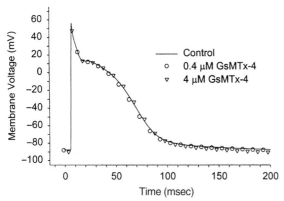

■ Figure 1–3 Action potentials recorded from isolated rabbit atrial cells are unaffected by GsMTx-4 *(Baumgarten and Clemo, unpublished data)*.

potential is unaffected. Apparently, GsMTx-4 affects none of the channels or transporters that generate the action potential.

GsMTx-4 does reduce swelling-induced currents in the heart and astrocytes,[49] suggesting that GsMTx-4 may be useful to treat hypertrophy where these currents are tonically active (see Chapter 3).

In a surprising observation, Clemo and colleagues[50] found that *spontaneous depolarizations* (SD),[43] first reported by Nuss and colleagues,[51] were blocked by GsMTx-4. SD commonly occur in failing hearts and are distinguished from *delayed afterdepolarizations* by the effect of increased extracellular Ca^{2+}: delayed afterdepolarizations are potentiated and SD

are inhibited. SD are not affected by the common drugs that affect voltage-dependent channels. The origin of SD is not established, but their *de facto* sensitivity to GsMTx-4 suggests that they are produced by SAC. We clearly have much to learn about the role of SAC in the heart.

Intracellular Ca^{2+} Effects of Stretch-Activated Channel Activation

Heart cells, like other cells,[6] increase their permeability to Ca^{2+} with mechanical stimulation. This influx is large enough to produce Ca^{2+} waves (Fig. 1–4[43,52]).

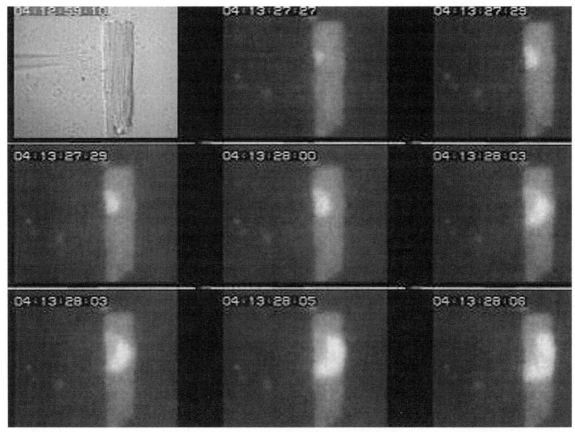

■ **Figure 1–4** Ca^{2+} waves induced in adult rat ventricular cells by gentle pressing with a fire polished pipette. The cells were loaded with Fluo-3AM, but the first frame is in Differential Interference Contrast. The initiation of these waves was blocked by removal of extracellular Ca^{2+} or the addition of Gd^{3+} to block the channels. The time code is hour:minute:second:frame. *(Sachs F. Mechanoelectric Transduction. In Zipes D, Jalife J [eds]: Cardiac electrophysiology: From cell to bedside. Philadelphia, Saunders, 2004, 96–102, with permission.)[43]*

The effect of mechanical stimulation is blocked by Gd^{3+}, suggesting that it results from SAC_{CAT} activation close to Ca^{2+} release sites. Mechanical forces can produce a direct Ca^{2+} influx through SAC_{CAT} and can increase intracellular Ca^{2+} using Na^+ influx and Na^+-Ca^+ exchange. This coupling provides many possible pathways for membrane stress to modify excitation and contraction—that is, mechano-electric feedback (MEF).

As a final caveat to those new to MEF, there is another coupling pathway that probably does not involve MSC, and that is auto- and paracrine activation of purinergic receptors. All cells release adenosine triphosphate on mechanical stimulation so that P2X and P2Y receptors may indirectly serve as mechanical transducers.[53]

Summary

MEF translates variations in mechanical compliance, such as scarring or heterogeneity of relaxation, into changes of electrical activity. Electrical and mechanical heterogeneity are maximal during repolarization, when the chambers are still under systolic pressure. This pressure produces a bulge, or aneurism, in a weakened part of the wall resulting in excitation during the vulnerable period, a prelude to tachyarrhythmias.[54]

The most likely, rapidly responding transducers for MEF are the mechanosensitive ion channels (although the mechanical effects on Ca^{2+} binding also are rapid; compare with Chapter 22). Unlike many other ion channels, the sensitivity of MSC seems not to be regulated by expression density—all cells have a low density ($\sim 1/\mu m^2$). The mechanical sensitivity is most likely modulated by the cytoskeleton and by amphipaths such as arachidonic acid (see Chapter 2). MSC are modulators of electrical activity, not the prime movers. Blocking MSC does not have a large effect on the action potential unless cells are stretched.

The complexity of cytoskeletal modulation of MSC is emphasized by work on touch reception in *C. elegans*. Saturation mutagenesis exposed about 12 genes involved in transduction. These critical proteins included tubulin, collagen, and membrane proteins of the mec/endothelial Na^+ channel family.[21] The fibrous proteins appear to be responsible for transferring external forces to the channels. We should expect that in the heart, the genotype of mechanical transduction is

similarly complex. Chronic remodeling of the heart undoubtedly involves changes in mechanical sensitivity through cytoskeletal modifications.

The development of specific pharmacologic agents for MSC, such as GsMTx-4, should allow us to examine the contribution of MSC to cardiac function. They may also represent a new class of antiarrhythmic drugs. Interesting times are ahead.

References

1. Chang G, Spencer RH, Lee AT, et al: Structure of the MscL homolog from Mycobacterium tuberculosis: A gated mechanosensitive ion channel. Science 282:2220–2226, 1998.
2. Vandorpe DH, Morris CE: Stretch activation of the Aplysia S-channel. J Membr Biol 127:205–214, 1992.
3. Paoletti P, Ascher P: Mechanosensitivity of NMDA receptors in cultured mouse central neurons. Neuron 13:645–655, 1994.
4. Opsahl LR, Webb WW: Transduction of membrane tension by the ion channel alamethicin. Biophysical J 66:71–74, 1994.
5. Kondratev D, Gallitelli MF: Increments in the concentrations of sodium and calcium in cell compartments of stretched mouse ventricular myocytes. Cell Calcium 34:193–203, 2003.
6. Niggel J, Suchyna TM, Sigurdson W, Sachs F: Mechanically induced calcium movements in astrocytes and C-6 glioma cells. J Membr Biol 174:121–134, 2000.
7. Baartscheer A, Schumacher CA, van Borren MMGJ, et al: Increased Na^+/H^+-exchange activity is the cause of increased $[Na^+]_i$ and underlies disturbed calcium handling in the rabbit pressure and volume overload heart failure model. Cardiovasc Res 57:1015–1024, 2003.
8. Cingolani HE, Perez MG, Pieske B, et al: Stretch-elicited Na^+/H^+ exchanger activation: The autocrine/paracrine loop and its mechanical counterpart. Cardiovasc Res 57:953–960, 2003.
9. von Lewinski D, Stumme B, Maier LS, et al: Stretch-dependent slow force response in isolated rabbit myocardium is Na^+ dependent. Cardiovasc Res 57:1052–1061, 2003.
10. Tang QY, Qi Z, Naruse K, Sokabe M: Characterization of a functionally expressed stretch-activated BKca channel cloned from chick ventricular myocytes. J Membr Biol 196:185–200, 2003.
11. Bass RB, Strop P, Barclay M, Rees DC: Crystal structure of *Escherichia coli* MscS, a voltage-modulated and mechanosensitive channel. Science 298:1582–1587, 2002.
12. Betanzos M, Chiang CS, Guy HR, Sukharev S: A large iris-like expansion of a mechanosensitive channel protein induced by membrane tension. Nat Struct Biol 9:704–710, 2002.
13. Perozo E, Cortes DM, Sompornpisut P, et al: Open channel structure of MscL and the gating mechanism of mechanosensitive channels. Nature 418:942–948, 2002.
14. Martinac B, Kloda A: Evolutionary origins of mechanosensitive ion channels. Prog Biophys Mol Biol 82:11–24, 2003.
15. Hamill OP, Martinac B: Molecular basis of mechanotransduction in living cells. Physiol Rev 81:685–740, 2001.
16. Sachs F, Morris CE: Mechanosensitive ion channels in non-specialized cells. Rev Physiol Biochem Pharmacol 132:1–77, 1998.

17. Naitoh Y: Mechanosensory transduction in protozoa. In Colombetti G, Lenci F (eds): Membranes and Sensory Transduction. New York, Plenum Press, 1984, pp 113–134.

18. Corey DP: New TRP channels in hearing and mechanosensation. Neuron 39:585–588, 2003.

19. Hase CC, Le Dain AC, Martinac B: Purification and functional reconstitution of the recombinant large mechanosensitive ion channel (MscL) of *Escherichia coli*. J Biol Chem 270:18329–18334, 1995.

20. Perozo E, Kloda A, Cortes DM, Martinac B: Physical principles underlying the transduction of bilayer deformation forces during mechanosensitive channel gating. Nat Struct Biol 9:696–703, 2002.

21. Ernstrom GG, Chalfie M: Genetics of sensory mechanotransduction. Annu Rev Genet 36:411–453, 2002.

22. Bowman CL, Lohr JW: Mechanotransducing ion channels in C6 glioma cells. GLIA 18:161–176, 1996.

23. Ruknudin A, Song MJ, Sachs F: The ultrastructure of patch-clamped membranes: A study using high voltage electron microscopy. J Cell Biol 112:125–134, 1991.

24. Wan X, Juranka P, Morris CE: Activation of mechanosensitive currents in traumatized membrane. Am J Physiol 276:C318–C327, 1999.

25. Opsahl LR, Webb WW: Lipid-glass adhesion in giga-sealed patch-clamped membranes. Biophysical J 66:75–79, 1994.

26. Akinlaja J, Sachs F: The breakdown of cell membranes by electrical and mechanical stress. Biophysical J 75:247–254, 1998.

27. Sukharev S, Sigurdson W, Kung C, Sachs F: Energetic and spatial parameters for gating of the bacterial large conductance mechanosensitive channel, MscL. J Gen Physiol 113:525–539, 1999.

28. Zeng T, Bett GCL, Sachs F: Stretch-activated whole-cell currents in adult rat cardiac myocytes. Am J Physiol Heart Circ Physiol 278:H548–H557, 2000.

29. Ruknudin A, Song M, Auerbach A, Sachs F: The structure of patch clamped membranes in high voltage electron microscopy. Proceedings of the Electron Microscopic Society of America 47:936–937, 1989.

30. Hu H, Sachs F: Mechanically activated currents in chick heart cells. J Membr Biol 154:205–216, 1996.

31. Cooper PJ, Lei M, Cheng LX, Kohl P: Selected contribution: Axial stretch increases spontaneous pacemaker activity in rabbit isolated sinoatrial node cells. J Appl Physiol 89:2099–2104, 2000.

32. Lei M, Kohl P: Swelling-induced decrease in spontaneous pacemaker activity of rabbit isolated sinoatrial node cells. Acta Physiol Scand 164:1–12, 1998.

33. White E: Length-dependent mechanisms in single cardiac cells. Exp Physiol 81:885–897, 1996.

34. Ruknudin A, Sachs F, Bustamante JO: Stretch-activated ion channels in tissue-cultured chick heart. Am J Physiol 264:H960–H972, 1993.

35. Kawakubo T, Naruse K, Matsubara T, et al: Characterization of a newly found stretch-activated $K_{Ca,ATP}$ channel in cultured chick ventricular myocytes. Am J Physiol 276:H1827–H1838, 1999.

36. Craelius W, Chen V, El-Sherif N: Stretch activated ion channels in ventricular myocytes. Biosci Rep 8:407–414, 1988.

37. Zhang YH, Youm JB, Sung HK, et al: Stretch-activated and background non-selective cation channels in rat atrial myocytes. J Physiol (Lond) 523:607–619, 2000.

38. Niu W, Sachs F: Dynamic properties of stretch-activated K^+ channels in adult rat atrial myocytes. Prog Biophys Mol Biol 82:121–135, 2003.

39. Bett GCL, Sachs F: Activation and inactivation of mechanosensitive currents in the chick heart. J Membr Biol 173:237–254, 2000.

40. Bett GCL, Sachs F: Whole-cell mechanosensitive currents in rat ventricular myocytes activated by direct stimulation. J Membr Biol 173:255–263, 2000.

41. Kohl P, Cooper PJ, Holloway H: Effects of acute ventricular volume manipulation on in situ cardiomyocyte cell membrane configuration. Prog Biophys Mol Biol 82:221–227, 2003.

42. Bilder GE, Schofield TL, Blaines EH: Release of atrial natriuretic factor. Effects of repetitive stretch and temperature. Am J Physiol 251:F817–F821, 1986.

43. Sachs F. Mechanoelectric Transduction. In Zipes D, Jalife J (eds): Cardiac Electrophysiology: From Cell to Bedside. Philadelphia, Saunders, 2004, 96–102.

44. Bode F, Sachs F, Franz MR: Tarantula peptide inhibits atrial fibrillation during stretch. Nature 409:35–36, 2001.

45. Hamill OP, McBride DW: The pharmacology of mechanogated membrane ion channels. Pharmacol Rev 48: 231–252, 1996.

46. Caldwell RA, Clemo HF, Baumgarten CM: Using gadolinium to identify stretch activated channels: Technical considerations. Am J Physiol 275:C619–C621, 1998.

47. Belus A, White E: Streptomycin and intracellular calcium modulate the response of single guinea-pig ventricular myocytes to axial stretch. J Physiol (Lond) 546:501–509, 2003.

48. Oswald RE, Suchyna TM, McFeeters R, et al: Solution structure of peptide toxins that block mechanosensitive ion channels. J Biol Chem 277:34443–34450, 2002.

49. Suchyna TM, Johnson JH, Clemo HF, et al: Identification of a peptide toxin from Grammostola spatulata spider venom that blocks stretch activated channels. J Gen Physiol 115:583–598, 2000.

50. Clemo HF, Hackenbracht JM, Patel DG, Baumgarten CM: Swelling-activated cation current causes spontaneous depolarizations in failing ventricular myocytes. Biophysical J 82:270A–271A, 2002.

51. Nuss HB, Kaab S, Kass DA, et al: Cellular basis of ventricular arrhythmias and abnormal automaticity in heart failure. Am J Physiol Heart Circ Physiol 277:H80–H91, 1999.

52. Sigurdson WJ, Ruknudin A, Sachs F: Calcium imaging of mechanically induced fluxes in tissue-cultured chick heart: Role of stretch-activated ion channels. Am J Physiol 262:H1110–H1115, 1992.

53. Neary JT, Kang Y, Willoughby KA, Ellis EF: Activation of extracellular signal-regulated kinase by stretch-induced injury in astrocytes involves extracellular ATP and P2 purinergic receptors. J Neurosci 23:2348–2356, 2003.

54. Franz MR, Bode F: Mechano-electrical feedback underlying arrhythmias: The atrial fibrillation case. Prog Biophys Mol Biol 82:163–174, 2003.

CHAPTER 2

Potassium-Selective Cardiac Mechanosensitive Ion Channels

• • • •

Amanda Jane Patel and Eric Honoré

S tretch-sensitive K^+ channels play a key role in mechano-electric feedback (MEF) and cardiac arrhythmias. Opening of K^+ channels increases the resting membrane potential and reduces the action potential duration, thus dramatically affecting cell electrogenesis. The TREK channels are members of the novel structural class of K^+ channels comprising four transmembrane segments (TMS) and two P domains in tandem (2P). TREK-1 is expressed in cardiac myocytes and is opened by membrane stretch and cell swelling. This chapter reviews the molecular and functional properties of the TREK channels and discusses their possible pathophysiologic role in the heart.

INTRODUCTION

Several mechanosensitive K^+-selective channels (SAK) are found in both atrial and ventricular myocytes. In neonatal rat atrial myocytes, K_{ATP} channels are opened by negative pressure applied to a patch of the plasma membrane.[1] The mechanosensitivity of the cardiac K_{ATP} channel is enhanced by the channel opener pinacidil, whereas it is inhibited by internal adenosine triphosphate (ATP) and tolbutamide. The mechanosensitive K_{ATP} channels in neonatal rat atrial myocytes are also reversibly opened by cellular swelling with a hypotonic solution.[1] Interestingly, K_{ATP} channels recently have been associated with *commotio cordis*.[2] K_{ATP} channels would act as arrhythmia-sustaining rather than arrhythmia-triggering entities.[3] In adult rat atrial and ventricular myocytes, however, stretch fails to modulate the activity of K_{ATP} channels.[4] A mechano-gated $K_{Ca2+,ATP}$ channel has also been reported in cultured chick ventricular myocytes.[5] This channel is opened by intracellular Ca^{2+} and ATP, but blocked by external tetraethylammonium (TEA) and charybdo-

toxin. This mechanosensitive K^+ channel may thus correspond to a BK channel. Membrane stretch similarly augments the muscarinic K^+ channel activity in rat atrial myocytes.[6] In the absence of acetylcholine (ACh), K_{ACh} channels are not active and negative pressure fails to activate these channels. With ACh in the pipette, applying negative pressure (0 to −80 mm Hg) to the membrane causes a reversible, pressure-dependent increase in channel activity in cell-attached and inside-out patches (in the presence of internal guanosine triphosphate). The atrial muscarinic K^+ channels are modulated by stretch, independently of receptor/G proteins, probably through a direct effect on the channel protein/lipid bilayer.[6] By contrast, rabbit atrial K_{ACh} channels are rapidly and reversibly inhibited by membrane stretch.[7] The heteromeric Kir3.1/Kir3.4 and the homomeric Kir3.4 channels expressed in *Xenopus* oocytes possess similar mechanosensitivity in response to hyposmolar stress. Kir3.4 is thus a stretch-inactivated K^+ channel and may be physiologically relevant in atrial volume–sensing and other responses to stretch.[7] The mechanosensitivity of GIRK (Kir3) channels is mediated primarily by channel–phosphatidylinositol 4,5-bisphosphate (PIP_2) interaction, with protein kinase C (PKC) playing an important role in modulating the interaction probably through PIP_2 hydrolysis.[8] Voltage-gated K^+ channels are also modulated by membrane stretch. For instance, the archetypical voltage-gated channel *Shaker* exhibits either stretch activation when the open channel probability (Po) is low (i.e., at negative potentials) or stretch inactivation when Po is high (i.e., at depolarized potentials).[9] Finally, as initially identified in 1987 by Morris and colleagues, stretch opens large conductance, Ca^{2+}-independent, arachidonic acid (AA)–sensitive, K^+ channels (K_{AA}) in both atrial and ventricular myocytes.[4,10-15] The SAK/K_{AA} channels belong to the novel class of mammalian 2P domain K^+ channels (see Reference 16 for review). The next section reviews the molecular and functional properties of the cardiac SAK/K_{AA}/2P channels.

THE ENDOGENOUS CARDIAC SAK/K_{AA} CHANNELS

The patch clamp technique was used to identify and characterize the SAK/K_{AA} in molluscan, chick, and rat cardiac myocytes.[4,10-15,17-19] SAK are opened at the whole-cell level by applying a positive pressure to the interior of the cell through the patch pipette.[4] The cardiac SAK/K_{AA} channels are K^+-selective outward rectifiers with a large single-channel conductance (in the range of 100 pS in a symmetrical K^+ gradient). The density of these channels is about 0.2/μm^2.[18] The pressure to induce half-maximal activation is −12 mm Hg at +40 mV in cell-attached patch.[4] The latency for activation is 50 to 100 msec, with a time to peak of about 400 msec.[18] Stretch activation is not maintained, and a time-dependent decrease in current amplitude occurs within 1 sec.[18] A time-dependent adaptation is also observed at the whole-cell level when isometric displacement is applied to chick heart cells.[20] This adaptation is caused by channel inactivation.[21] SAK/K_{AA} channel activity is independent of intracellular Ca^{2+}. The probability of opening is mildly voltage dependent, with greater channel activity at depolarized potentials.[4] Mechano-activation persists on patch excision demonstrating that cell integrity is not required for stretch activation.[4] TEA (10 mM), 4-aminopyridine (4-AP) (5 mM), apamine (10 nM), nifedipine (10 μM), quinidine (100 μM), tetrodotoxin (10 μM), ouabain (100 μM), vanadate (1 mM), glibenclamide (10 μM), tolbutamide (10 μM), and 4,4′-diisothiocyanato-stilbene-2,2′-disulfonic acid (DIDS) (100 μM) fail to affect the rat atrium SAK/K_{AA} channels.[4,10-15,17-19] These channels are inhibited by gadolinium (Gd^{3+}) in chick heart cells, whereas they are resistant in rat atrium.[4,19] However, Gd^{3+} is highly nonspecific and technically difficult to use because of precipitation with divalent or polyvalent anions. The SAK and K_{AA} channels share the outward rectification, the single channel conductance (about 100 pS), the mean open time (about 1.4 msec), the burst openings, the K^+ selectivity,

and the insensitivity to known organic channel inhibitors. Pressure activation of SAK/K_{AA} channels occurs in the presence of albumin, a fatty acid binding protein, demonstrating that pressure and AA activate the K^+ channel through separate pathways.[4]

Interestingly, both the SAK and the K_{AA} channels are opened by intracellular acidosis, further suggesting that they correspond to the same channel.[4,10] The SAK/K_{AA} channel is more sensitive to pressure at acidic pH, analogous to the effect of pH on AA-activated K^+ channel activity. The SAK/K_{AA} channels in rat atrium are additionally opened by clinical doses of volatile general anesthetics including chloroform, halothane, and isoflurane.[14] The cardiac SAK/K_{AA} channel also is apparently directly activated by intracellular ATP in the millimolar range.[13] The response to intracellular ATP is rapid and occurs in isolated patches, which appears to preclude the action of a kinase. In rat ventricular cardiomyocytes, the SAK/K_{AA} channel is additionally activated by extracellular ATP through the phospholipase A_2 (PLA_2) pathway.[22] The purinergic-dependent activation of cyclic PLA_2 requires the simultaneous activation of both p38 mitogen-activated protein kinase (MAPK) and p42/44 MAPK by a cyclic adenosine monophosphate (cAMP)–dependent protein kinase and a tyrosine kinase–dependent pathway, respectively.[22] The SAK/K_{AA} channel in rat atrial myocytes is inhibited by protein kinase A (PKA) activation with cAMP or by addition of the β_1-adrenergic receptor agonist isoproterenol.[14]

THE MAMMALIAN 2P DOMAIN K^+ CHANNELS

Mammalian K^+ channel subunits can be divided into three main structural classes comprising two TMS, four TMS, or six/seven TMS.[16] The common feature of all K^+ channels is the presence of a conserved motif called the P domain (or K^+ channel signature), which is part of the K^+ conduction pathway. The two TMS (including the inward rectifiers) and six/seven TMS (including the voltage-gated outward rectifiers, SK and BK channels) classes comprise a single P domain, whereas the most recently discovered class of four TMS subunits is characterized by the presence of a tandem of P domains.[16] Functional K^+ channels are tetramers of pore-forming subunits for the two and six/seven TMS classes and dimers in the case of the four TMS class.[23]

The class of mammalian four TMS K$^+$ channel subunits includes 15 members so far (Fig. 2–1). Although these subunits display the same structural motif with four TMS/2P, an extended M1P1 extracellular loop with both amino and carboxy termini intracellularly, they share rather low sequence identity outside the P regions. This structural motif is associated with unusual functional properties. The 2P domain K$^+$ channels can be subdivided into six main structural and functional classes (see Fig. 2–1): (1) the weak inward rectifiers TWIK-1, TWIK-2, and KCNK7 (functional expression of KCNK7 has not been reported); (2) the acid-sensitive 2P domain K$^+$ channels TASK-1, TASK-3, and TASK-5 (functional expression of TASK-5 has not been reported); (3) the lipid-sensitive mechano-gated 2P domain K$^+$ channels TREK-1, TREK-2, and TRAAK; (4) the halothane-inhibited 2P domain K$^+$ channels THIK-1 and THIK-2 (functional expression of THIK-2 has not been reported); (5) the alkaline-activated 2P domain K$^+$ channels TALK-1, TALK-2, and TASK-2; and (6) the spinal cord 2P domain K$^+$ channel TRESK (see Reference 16 for review). Evidence for heteromultimers has been provided for TASK-1 and TASK-3.[24,25] The next section concentrates on the functional and physiopathologic properties of the four TMS/2P domain lipid-sensitive mechano-gated TREK/TRAAK K$^+$ channels.

TREK/TRAAK CHANNELS

Pattern of Expression of TREK/TRAAK Channels

The genomic organization of TREK-1 (1q41), TREK-2 (14q31), and TRAAK (11q13) is similar, suggesting that they may have arisen by gene duplication from a common ancestor.[26] TREK-1, TREK-2, and TRAAK are consistently found in the human brain.[26] Besides the central and peripheral nervous systems, important expression is also found for human TREK-1 in the ovary and the gastrointestinal tract, for TREK-2 in the pancreas and the kidney, and for TRAAK in the placenta.[26–28] TREK-1 and TREK-2 splice variants with amino acid extensions in the amino terminal domain have been identified.[29,30] Interestingly, the TREK-2 splice variant TREK-2b is highly expressed in the kidney and pancreas, whereas TREK-2c is found in the brain.

Both mouse and rat TREK-1 are found in the heart.[14,31] Reverse transcriptase-polymerase chain reaction (PCR) analysis indicates that TREK-1 is present in atria, ventricle, and septa of adult rat hearts.[14] The presence of TREK-1 at the plasma membrane of rat cardiomyocytes was confirmed by immunostaining with a polyclonal antibody.[14] However, TREK-1 was not found in human heart using semiquantitative PCR.[32,33] Human TREK-2 and TRAAK, rat TREK-2, and mouse TRAAK are similarly absent from the heart.[26,32,34] A TRAAK splice variant (HKT4.1b) that

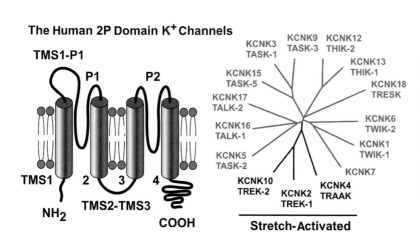

■ **Figure 2–1** *Left,* Membrane topology of a four-transmembrane segment (TMS) 2P domain K$^+$ channel. A functional channel is a dimer of subunits. *Right,* Phylogenetic tree of human 2P domain K$^+$ channels. So far 15 subunits have been cloned forming six structural and functional subfamilies. TREK-1, TREK-2, and TRAAK are stretch-activated K$^+$ channels.

contains an extra 26 amino acids in the amino terminal domain, however, was apparently detected in the human heart using Northern blot analysis.[35] Clearly, the fine expression of TREK/TRAAK channels in specialized cardiac cells, such as the pacemaker cells or the conductive tissue, needs to be carefully evaluated in the human heart.

Biophysical Properties of TREK/TRAAK Channels

TREK-1, TREK-2, and TRAAK channel activity is elicited by increasing the mechanical tension in the cell membrane and is independent of intracellular Ca^{2+} and ATP[26,28,34,36,37] (Fig. 2–2). The single-channel conductances are about 50 and 100 pS in a physiologic and symmetrical K^+ gradient, respectively.[26,28,36,38] Channel activities are characterized by a typical flickering behavior. Rectification strongly affects the functional role of an ion channel in cell electrogenesis. For instance, the inward rectifiers are more conductive at negative membrane potentials because of internal block at depolarized potentials by intracellular Mg^{2+} and polyamines. In contrast, outward rectifiers allosterically open at depolarized potentials. Outward rectification is caused by specific gating mechanisms (including voltage-dependent gating), and also by the difference in K^+ concentration between the intracellular and extracellular media. In the absence of gating, the I-V curve of a K^+-selective channel in a physiologic K^+ gradient is predicted to rectify outward current because current flows more easily from the side of high-permeant ion concentration (i.e., the intracellular side). This outward rectification, called the Goldman–Hodgkin–Katz, or open channel rectification, is the signature of leak K^+ channels. In a symmetrical K^+ gradient, the I-V curve of such a channel is expected to become symmetric. For TREK-1 channels, several mechanisms contribute to the strong outward rectification: (1) the open rectification caused by the physiologic K^+ gradient; (2) an extracellular Mg^{2+} block at negative membrane potentials; and (3) an intrinsic voltage-dependent gating mechanism.[30,39] The outward rectification also is observed at the single-channel level in the presence of extracellular Mg^{2+}. On depolarization, TREK-1 presents both an instanta-

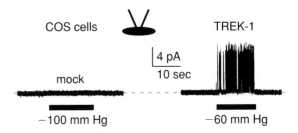

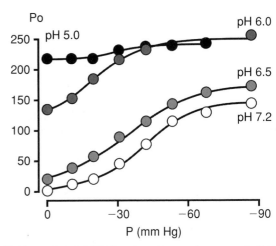

■ **Figure 2–2** TREK-1 is activated by membrane stretch. CV-1 origin SV4o (COS) cells were transiently transfected with the complementary DNA encoding TREK-1, and channel activity was monitored at +50 mV in the cell-attached patch configuration. Mechano-gated K^+ channels are absent in mock transfected COS cells. Mechanosensitivity of TREK-1 persists on patch excision in the inside-out patch configuration. The dose–effect curve between channel activity and negative pressure is described by a sigmoidal relation. At intracellular pH 7.2, 50% of TREK-1 channels are opened at a patch pressure gradient of –36 mm Hg. Intracellular acidification gradually shifts the dose–effect curve toward more positive values, and ultimately at pH 5.0 all channels are opened in the absence of stretch. Intracellular acidosis converts mechano-gated TREK-1 channels into constitutively active K^+ channels.

neous and a time-dependent component.[39] The activation time course follows a single exponential, and the time constant decreases linearly with depolarization. In a symmetrical K^+ gradient, a large inward tail current is recorded on repolarization. An obvious function for background or leak K^+ channels is to bring the resting membrane potential to a value close to E_K about −90 mV. Resting K^+ channels thus will tend to limit repetitive activity because membrane hyperpolarization increases distance to the threshold of cell firing. If K^+ channel Po is high, cells will be voltage clamped at E_K, and thus might become completely inexcitable. Rectification mechanisms modulate the influence of K^+ channels at rest and, consequently, tune excitability. Outward rectification will favor the opening of the channel at depolarized potentials and will increase their role in the repolarization of the action potential. Opening of TREK-1 channels at depolarized potentials thus will tend to decrease the action potential duration and stimulate repetitive activity. It has been proposed that phosphorylation/dephosphorylation of S333, a PKA site in the carboxy terminal domain of TREK-1, is responsible for the interconversion between voltage-dependent and leak phenotypes of rat TREK-1 expressed in *Xenopus* oocytes.[30] Our own results, however, do not confirm the role of this residue for mouse TREK-1 expressed in mammalian cells.[39]

In the inside-out patch configuration, positive pressure is significantly less effective than negative pressure in opening channels, suggesting that a specific membrane deformation (convex curving) preferentially opens these channels.[36,37] The relation between channel activity and pressure is described by a sigmoidal relation with half-maximal activation at −36 mm Hg (Fig. 2–2).[34,36,37] At the whole-cell level, TREK-1 and TRAAK are modulated by cellular volume.[36,40] When the osmolarity of the external solution is increased, the basal TREK-1 and TRAAK current amplitudes are reversibly decreased.[36,40] Both the number of active channels and the sensitivity to mechanical stretch are strongly enhanced after a treatment of cell-attached patches with the cytoskeleton disrupting agents colchicine and cytochalasin D.[37] Similarly, excising patches in the inside-out patch configuration produces an almost 10-fold increase in channel activation by stretch.[37] These data suggest that mechanical force may be transmitted directly to the channel through the lipid bilayer and does not require the integrity of the cytoskeleton.[36,37] The cytoskeleton could act as a tonic repressor of channel activity and allow a dynamic tuning of the stretch sensitivity of the channels. Decreasing internal pH shifts the pressure–activation relation of TREK-1 and TREK-2, but not TRAAK, toward positive values and ultimately leads to channel opening at atmospheric pressure[37] (see Fig. 2–2). Acidosis essentially converts a TREK mechano-gated channel into a constitutively active channel.[26,37] In contrast, TRAAK is opened by intracellular alkaline pH.[41] TREK-1 also is gradually and reversibly opened by heat. A 10°C increase enhances TREK-1 current amplitude by about sevenfold.[40] Finally, TREK-1 has been shown to be directly and reversibly inhibited by hypoxia,[42] although this finding has not been confirmed by our own group (Buckler and Honoré, in press).

Pharmacology of TREK/TRAAK Channels

TREK and TRAAK channels are insensitive to the classical K^+ channel blockers including TEA (10 mM), 4-AP (3 mM), Ba^{2+} (1 mM), charybdotoxin (1 µM), and apamine (10 µM), although they are reversibly blocked by Gd^{3+} (30 µM in the presence of AA) and amiloride (2 mM).[36-38,43] TREK-1, TREK-2, and TRAAK are opened by the neuroprotective agent riluzole (100 µM), whereas sipatrigine (10 µM), another neuroprotective compound, potently inhibits TREK-1 and TRAAK.[44,45] TREK-1 is blocked by local anesthetics including bupivacaine (1 mM) and tetracaine (0.1 mM), whereas together with TREK-2, unlike TRAAK, it is opened by clinical doses of volatile general anesthetics including ether, chloroform, halothane, and isoflurane.[27,46,47] Ca^{2+} antagonists penfluridol (2.5 µM), mibefradil (2.5 µM), and La^{3+} (100 µM) block TREK-1.[48] Finally, high concentrations of glibenclamide (200 µM) reversibly inhibit TREK-1.[48]

TREK-1, TREK-2, and TRAAK are reversibly opened by polyunsaturated fatty acids (PUFAs) including AA[26,34,36,38] (Fig. 2–3). The activation is observed in excised patch configurations and in the presence of cyclo-oxygenase and lipoxygenase inhibitors indicating that the effect is independent of AA metabolism.[36,38] The threshold concentration is 100 nM, and the effect does not saturate at concentrations as high as 100 µM.[34,38] The activation induced by PUFA is critically dependent on the length of the carbonyl chain[34,36,38] (see Fig. 2–3). The long chain PUFA, including AA and docosahexaenoic acid

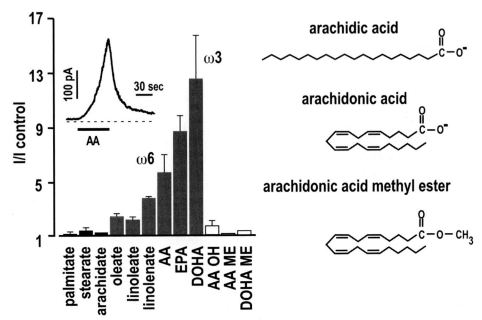

■ **Figure 2–3** Polyunsaturated fatty acids open TREK-1. Channel activity was monitored in the whole-cell configuration at 0 mV. Fatty acids were applied at the concentration of 10 μM. Polyunsaturated, long chain, negatively charged lipids open TREK-1, TREK-2, and TRAAK.

(DOHA), are the most effective. The extent of saturation is critical because long chain saturated fatty acids are ineffective[36,38] (see Fig. 2–3). Besides the length of the carbonyl chain and the unsaturation, the negative charge of the carboxyl function is critical for channel activity.[36,38] Substitution of the carboxyl function of AA or DOHA with an alcohol or a methyl ester function prevents channel activation[36,38] (see Fig. 2–3). Activation of TREK and TRAAK channels by PUFA in the excised patch configuration indicates that the effect is direct by interacting either with the channel protein or by partitioning into the lipid bilayer, or both.[36–38,43] Micromolar concentrations of AA open TREK and TRAAK channels with onset and offset kinetics that are in the order of minutes.[36,38,43]

Considering that TREK and TRAAK channels are mechano-gated and that activation of these channels by AA does not saturate at high doses, it is possible that the effects of PUFA might be related to a membrane alteration resulting in a change in curvature.[36,43] If such an effect occurs, chemically unrelated compounds

known to modify membrane curvature should mimic the effect of AA. Anionic amphipaths including trinitrophenol (TNP) have been shown to cause erythrocyte crenation (obtain more spherical shape), whereas cationic amphipaths such as chlorpromazine (CPZ) and tetracaine increase the typical discoid form (cup formers) and reverse the membrane effects of crenators[49] (Fig. 2–4). The bilayer-couple hypothesis assumes that these effects derive entirely from interactions within the bilayer and are independent of the cytoskeleton.[49] Anionic amphipaths preferentially insert in the outer leaflet (presumably because of the natural asymmetric distribution of negatively charged phosphatidylserines in the inner leaflet) and generate a convex positive curvature of the membrane[49] (see Fig. 2–4). In contrast, positively charged amphipaths are expected to preferentially insert in the inner leaflet of the bilayer, thus generating a concave negative curvature.[49] Assuming that TREK and TRAAK channels are preferentially opened by negative compared with positive mechanical pressure (i.e., convex negative

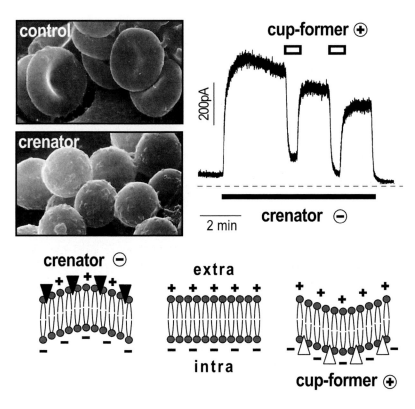

Figure 2–4 Anionic amphipaths (including arachidonic acid) drastically alter the shape of erythrocytes (membrane crenation)[49] *(left)*. Anionic amphipaths (crenators) are openers of TREK-1 (recorded in the whole-cell configuration at 0 mV), whereas cationic amphipaths reverse channel activation (cup formers) *(right)*. Anionic amphipaths preferentially insert in the external leaflet of the bilayer, whereas cationic amphipaths insert in the inner leaflet, thus differentially altering the membrane curvature *(bottom)*. The bilayer is naturally asymmetric with an excess of negatively charged phosphatidylserines in the inner leaflet.

curvature), it is expected that anionic amphipaths would open, whereas cationic amphipaths would close, the channels. Indeed, TNP, an anionic amphipath, opens TREK channels, whereas CPZ and tetracaine reverse TREK-1 opening by TNP or AA[36,37] (see Fig. 2–4). Although the bilayer-couple hypothesis qualitatively accounts for the opening TREK and TRAAK channels by PUFA, the possible existence of a specific binding site on the channel protein itself cannot be entirely ruled out.[36,37]

Extracellular lysophospholipids (LP) including lysophosphatidylcholine (LPC), unlike phospholipids, open TREK and TRAAK channels.[26,43] The threshold concentration for opening is 100 nM and, again, no saturation is obtained at high concentration.[43] At low doses, AA and LPC produce additive activation. The effect of LP is critically dependent on the length of the carbonyl chain (longer than 10 carbons) and the presence of a large polar head (choline or inositol).[43] Activation is independent of the saturation status of the lipid, the charge of the polar head, or the presence of an

acetyl group at position 2.[43] Considering that TREK and TRAAK channels are opened by neutral LP, the bilayer-couple hypothesis, which is based on the charge of the molecule (as described for PUFA), cannot explain LP activation.[50] It has been postulated rather that the conic shape of the molecule is the important parameter conditioning the stimulation by extracellular LP.[43] Interestingly, intracellular LP inhibit TREK channel activity.[43] This effect may be related to the concave curvature of the membrane expected if LP insert in the inner leaflet without flipping to the external leaflet of the bilayer.

The Carboxy Terminal Domain of TREK Is Critical for Channel Gating

Deletional analysis demonstrates that the carboxy terminal, but not the amino terminal domain and the extracellular M1P1 loop, is critical for all stimuli active on TREK-1: stretch, intracellular acidosis, and temperature, as well as AA and LPC.[36,37,40,43] Chemical and mechanical activation might share a common molecular pathway.[37] Substitution of the carboxy terminal domain of TREK-2 with that of TASK-3 suppresses activation by both PUFA and intracellular acidic pH.[51] Interestingly, replacing the carboxy terminal domain of TRAAK with that of TASK-1 and TASK-3 did not affect the response to pressure, AA, or alkali, demonstrating that gating mechanisms are fundamentally different between the TREK and TRAAK.[41] A charged cluster (301KKTKEE306) in the proximal carboxy terminal domain of TREK-1 and TREK-2 (327-332) is essential for channel function.[51,52] Deletion of this region in TREK-2 impairs activation by AA and intracellular acidosis.[51] Protonation of a specific glutamate residue (E306) in the cytosolic carboxy terminal domain of TREK-1 (position 332 in TREK-2) is actually responsible for channel opening at acidic intracellular pH.[52] Another important region for pH_i regulation has been mapped in the carboxy terminal domain of TREK-2 (334GEIKAHAAEW343).[51] Deletion and chimeric analysis demonstrates that the carboxy terminal domain of TREK-1, but not the PKA phosphorylation site S333, is also responsible for voltage- and time-dependent gating.[39]

TREK-1 and TREK-2 activation, unlike TRAAK, is reversed by PKA and PKC stimulation.[26,31,36,38,40,43] PKA-mediated phosphorylation of Ser333 in the carboxy terminus mediates TREK-1 closing.[36] Interestingly, corticotropin induces, through a cAMP-dependent mechanism that is dependent on PKA, the expression of TREK-1 messenger RNA (although it blocks its function) in adrenocortical cells.[48] TREK-1 is additionally opened by sodium nitroprusside and 8-Br cGMP.[53] Mutation of the protein kinase G consensus sequence at S351 (previously called PKAII[36]) suppresses the stimulatory effect of cGMP.[53] Stimulation of the G_s-coupled receptor 5-HT4sR and the G_q-coupled receptors mGluR1 or mGluR5 inhibits TREK-1 and TREK-2 activity, but not TRAAK, whereas stimulation of the G_i-coupled receptor mGluR2 increases TREK-2 currents.[26,36,54] Recently, it was shown that diacylglycerols and phophatidic acids directly inhibit TREK channels and may be responsible for the down-modulation by group I metabotropic receptors.[54]

SAK/KAA/TREK/TRAAK AND CARDIAC FUNCTION

Heart rate significantly increases when atria are stretched (see Chapter 8). K^+ channels that open at suprathreshold depolarized potentials will not affect threshold, but will tend to facilitate recovery and repetitive refiring.[30,39] TREK-1, similarly to cardiac SAK channels, preferentially opens at depolarized potentials with complex outward rectification.[39] Opening of TREK-1 thus will tend to increase repetitive activity and will contribute to the facilitation of heart rate observed during atrial distension.

Stretch is the main stimulus of atrial natriuretic peptide (ANP) secretion.[55] ANP secretion is initiated by an increase in intracellular Ca^{2+}. Opening of TREK-1 by stretch may act as a negative feedback of ANP secretion by shortening action potential, thus decreasing intracellular Ca^{2+}.[14] β-Adrenergic stimulation, by inhibiting TREK channels, would stimulate ANP release from atrial myocytes, an effect that is indeed observed.[55]

In pathologic conditions such as ischemia, TREK-1 channel opening may become critical. Ischemic insult induces PLA_2 activation, PUFA and LP release, cell swelling, and intracellular acidosis.[16,50] All these alterations will contribute to open TREK-1 and will tend to repolarize the membrane potential, reduce intracellular Ca^{2+}, and thus protect ischemic cardiomyocytes. Interestingly, chemical ischemia induced by carbonyl cyanide p-trifluoromethoxyphenyl hydrazone (FCCP) strongly opens TREK-1.[52] On the contrary, the enhanced K^+ efflux through the open TREK-1 channels could be deleterious because it may trigger apoptotic cell death as previously reported for the background acid-sensitive TASK-1/-3 2P domain K^+ channels.[24] Interestingly, TREK-1 mice are more vulnerable to cerebral ischemia and epileptic insult.[56] Moreover, the neuroprotective effect of polyunsaturated fatty acids and lysophospholipids is lost in TREK-1$^{-/-}$ mice.[56] Finally, these knockout mice are also more resistant to general anesthesia by volatile anesthetics, including halothane.[56] The cardiovascular phenotype of these mice remains to be determined.

CONCLUSION

TREK-1, TREK-2, and TRAAK encode the mechano-gated, lipid-sensitive SAK/K_{AA} K^+ channels. TREK-1 is expressed at high levels in rodent heart, although its expression in human heart still needs to be established. Opening of TREK channels by membrane stretch is relevant to cardiac MEF. So far, no human mutation and associated pathology has been reported in the novel family of 2P domain K^+ channels. However, because of the unusual polymodal behavior of the TREK/TRAAK channels, it is anticipated that this group of ionic channels will have important implications for various disease states.

References

1. Van Wagoner DR: Mechanosensitive gating of atrial ATP-sensitive potassium channels. Circ Res 72:973–983, 1993.
2. Link MS: Mechanically induced sudden death in chest wall impact (commotio cordis). Prog Biophys Mol Biol 82:175–186, 2003.
3. Kohl P, Nesbitt A, Cooper PJ, et al: Sudden cardiac death by Commotio cordis: Role of mechano-electric feedback. Cardiovasc Res 50:280–289, 2001.
4. Kim D: A mechanosensitive K^+ channel in heart cells. Activation by arachidonic acid. J Gen Physiol 100:1021–1040, 1992.
5. Kawakubo T, Naruse K, Matsubara T, et al: Characterization of a newly found stretch-activated $K_{Ca,ATP}$ channel in cultured chick ventricular myocytes. Am J Physiol 276:H1827–H1838, 1999.
6. Pleumsamran A, Kim D: Membrane stretch augments the cardiac muscarinic K^+ channel activity. J Membr Biol 148:287–297, 1995.
7. Ji S, John SA, Lu Y, et al: Mechanosensitivity of the cardiac muscarinic potassium channel. A novel property conferred by Kir3.4 subunit. J Biol Chem 273:1324–1328, 1998.
8. Zhang L, Lee J, John SA, et al: Mechanosensitivity of GIRK channels is mediated by protein kinase C-dependent channel-phosphatidylinositol 4,5-bisphosphate interaction. J Biol Chem 279:7037–7047, 2004.
9. Gu CX, Juranka PF, Morris CE: Stretch-activation and stretch-inactivation of Shaker-IR, a voltage-gated K^+ channel. Biophys J 80:2678–2693, 2001.
10. Wallert MA, Ackerman MJ, Kim D, et al: Two novel cardiac atrial K^+ channels, IK.AA and IK.PC. J Gen Physiol 98:921–939, 1991.
11. Kim D, Duff RA: Regulation of K^+ channels in cardiac myocytes by free fatty acids. Circ Res 67:1040–1046, 1990.
12. Kim D, Clapham DE: Potassium channels in cardiac cells activated by arachidonic acid and phospholipids. Science 244:1174–1176, 1989.
13. Tan JH, Liu W, Saint DA: TREK-like potassium channels in rat cardiac ventricular myocytes are activated by intracellular ATP. J Membr Biol 185:201–207, 2001.
14. Terrenoire C, Lauritzen I, Lesage F, et al: A TREK-1-like potassium channel in atrial cells inhibited by b-adrenergic stimulation and activated by volatile anesthetics. Circ Res 89:336–342, 2001.
15. Sigurdson W, Morris CE, Brezden BL, et al: Stretch activation of a K^+ channel in molluscan heart cells. J Exp Biol 127:191–209, 1987.
16. Patel AJ, Honoré E: Properties and modulation of mammalian 2P domain K^+ channels. Trends Neurosci 24:339–346, 2001.
17. Hu H, Sachs F: Mechanically activated currents in chick heart cells. J Membr Biol 154:205–216, 1996.
18. Niu W, Sachs F: Dynamic properties of stretch-activated K^+ channels in adult rat atrial myocytes. Prog Biophys Mol Biol 82:121–135, 2003.
19. Ruknudin A, Sachs F, Bustamante JO: Stretch-activated ion channels in tissue-cultured chick heart. Am J Physiol 264:H960–H972, 1993.
20. Bett GC, Sachs F: Whole-cell mechanosensitive currents in rat ventricular myocytes activated by direct stimulation. J Membr Biol 173:255–263, 2000.
21. Suchyna TM, Besch SR, Sachs F: Dynamic regulation of mechanosensitive channels: Capacitance used to monitor patch tension in real time. Phys Biol 1:1–18, 2004.
22. Aimond F, Rauzier JM, Bony C, et al: Simultaneous activation of p38 MAPK and p42/44 MAPK by ATP stimulates the K^+ current ITREK in cardiomyocytes. J Biol Chem 15:39110–39116, 2000.
23. Lesage F, Reyes R, Fink M, et al: Dimerization of TWIK-1 K^+ channel subunits via a disulfide bridge. EMBO J 15:6400–6407, 1996.
24. Lauritzen I, Zanzouri M, Honore E, et al: K^+-dependent cerebellar granule neuron apoptosis: Role of TASK leak K^+ channels. J Biol Chem 278:32068–32076, 2003.
25. Czirjak G, Enyedi P: Formation of functional heterodimers between the TASK-1 and TASK-3 two pore domain potassium channel subunits. J Biol Chem 277:5426–5432, 2001.
26. Lesage F, Terrenoire C, Romey G, et al: Human TREK2, a 2P domain mechano-sensitive K^+ channel with multiple regulations by polyunsaturated fatty acids, lysophospholipids, and Gs, Gi, and Gq protein-coupled receptors. J Biol Chem 275:28398–28405, 2000.
27. Patel AJ, Honoré E, Lesage F, et al: Inhalational anaesthetics activate two-pore-domain background K^+ channels. Nat Neurosci 2:422–426, 1999.
28. Lesage F, Maingret F, Lazdunski M: Cloning and expression of human TRAAK, a polyunsaturated fatty acids-activated and mechano-sensitive K^+ channel. FEBS Lett 471:137–140, 2000.
29. Gu W, Schlichthorl G, Hirsch JR, et al: Expression pattern and functional characteristics of two novel splice variants of the two-pore-domain potassium channel TREK-2. J Physiol 539:657–668, 2002.
30. Bockenhauer D, Zilberberg N, Goldstein SA: KCNK2: Reversible conversion of a hippocampal potassium leak into a voltage-dependent channel. Nat Neurosci 4:486–491, 2001.
31. Fink M, Duprat F, Lesage F, et al: Cloning, functional expression and brain localization of a novel unconventional outward rectifier K^+ channel. EMBO J 15:6854–6862, 1996.
32. Medhurst AD, Rennie G, Chapman CG, et al: Distribution analysis of human two pore domain potassium channels in tissues of the central nervous system and periphery. Brain Res Mol Brain Res 86:101–114, 2001.

33. Meadows HJ, Benham CD, Cairns W, et al: Cloning, localisation and functional expression of the human orthologue of the TREK-1 potassium channel. Pflugers Arch 439:714–722, 2000.

34. Bang H, Kim Y, Kim D: TREK-2, a new member of the mechanosensitive tandem pore K+ channel family. J Biol Chem 275:17412–17419, 2000.

35. Ozaita A, Vega-Saenz de Miera E: Cloning of two transcripts, HKT4.1a and HKT4.1b, from the human two-pore K+ channel gene KCNK4. Chromosomal localization, tissue distribution and functional expression. Mol Brain Res 102:18–27, 2002.

36. Patel AJ, Honoré E, Maingret F, et al: A mammalian two pore domain mechano-gated S-like K+ channel. EMBO J 17:4283–4290, 1998.

37. Maingret F, Fosset M, Lesage F, et al: TRAAK is a mammalian neuronal mechano-gated K+ channel. J Biol Chem 274:1381–1387, 1999.

38. Fink M, Lesage F, Duprat F, et al: A neuronal two P domain K+ channel activated by arachidonic acid and polyunsaturated fatty acid. EMBO J 17:3297–3308, 1998.

39. Maingret F, Honoré E, Lazdunski M, et al: Molecular basis of the voltage-dependent gating of TREK-1, a mechano-sensitive K+ channel. Biochem Biophys Res Commun 292:339–346, 2002.

40. Maingret F, Lauritzen I, Patel A, et al: TREK-1 is a heat-activated background K+ channel. EMBO J 19:2483–2491, 2000.

41. Kim Y, Bang H, Gnatenco C, et al: Synergistic interaction and the role of C-terminus in the activation of TRAAK K+ channels by pressure, free fatty acids and alkali. Pflugers Arch 442:64–72, 2001.

42. Miller P, Kemp PJ, Lewis A, et al: Acute hypoxia occludes hTREK-1 modulation: Re-evaluation of the potential role of tandem P domain K+ channels in central neuroprotection. J Physiol 548:31–37, 2003.

43. Maingret F, Patel AJ, Lesage F, et al: Lysophospholipids open the two P domain mechano-gated K+ channels TREK-1 and TRAAK. J Biol Chem 275:10128–10133, 2000.

44. Duprat F, Lesage F, Patel AJ, et al: The neuroprotective agent riluzole activates the two P domain K+ channels TREK-1 and TRAAK. Mol Pharmacol 57:906–912, 2000.

45. Meadows H, Chapman CG, Duckworth M, et al: The neuroprotective agent sipatrigine (BW619C89) potently inhibits the human tandem pore-domain K+ channels TREK-1 and TRAAK. Brain Res 892:94–101, 2001.

46. Punke MA, Licher T, Pongs O, et al: Inhibition of human TREK-1 channels by bupivacaine. Anesth Analg 96:1665–1673, 2003.

47. Patel AJ, Honoré E: Anesthetic-sensitive 2P domain K+ channels. Anesthesiology 95:1013–1025, 2001.

48. Enyeart JJ, Xu L, Danthi S, et al: An ACTH- and ATP-regulated background K+ channel in adrenocortical cells is TREK-1. J Biol Chem 277:49186–49199, 2002.

49. Sheetz MP, Singer SJ: Biological membranes as bilayer couples. A molecular mechanism of drug-erythrocyte interactions. Proc Natl Acad Sci USA 71:4457–4461, 1974.

50. Patel AJ, Honoré E: Lipid and mechano-gated 2P domain K+ channels. Curr Opin Cell Biol 13:422–428, 2001.

51. Kim Y, Gnatenco C, Bang H, et al: Localization of TREK-2 K+ channel domains that regulate channel kinetics and sensitivity to pressure, fatty acids and pHi. Pflugers Arch 2001:952–960, 2001.

52. Honoré E, Maingret F, Lazdunski M, et al: An intracellular proton sensor commands lipid- and mechano-gating of the K+ channel TREK-1. EMBO J 21:2968–2976, 2002.

53. Koh SD, Monaghan KM, Sergeant GP, et al: TREK-1 regulation by nitric oxide and cGMP-dependent protein kinase. J Biol Chem 47:44338–44346, 2001.

54. Chemin J, Girard C, Duprat F, et al: Mechanisms underlying excitatory effects of group I metabotropic glutamate receptors via inhibition of 2P domain K+ channels. EMBO J 22:5403–5411, 2003.

55. Ruskoaho H: Atrial natriuretic peptide: Synthesis, release, and metabolism. Pharmacol Rev 44:479–602, 1992.

56. Heurteaux C, Guy N, Laigle C, et al: TREK-1, a K+ channel involved in neuroprotection and general anesthesia. EMBO J 23:2684–95, 2004.

CHAPTER 3

Cell Volume–Sensitive Ion Channels and Transporters in Cardiac Myocytes

• • • •

Clive M. Baumgarten

In addition to stretch-activated channels (SAC) that respond to purely mechanical stimuli (see Chapters 1 and 2), the heart possesses channels that are regulated primarily by a number of voltage- and ligand-gated channels and ion transporters that are modulated by cell volume. These pathways respond to osmotic cell swelling and shrinkage and to isosmotic cell inflation. Moreover, some of the volume-activated channels (VAC) become persistently activated in cardiac disease.

From an operational perspective, VAC and SAC are distinguished by the nature of the stimulus. The stretch caused by cell swelling is a more complicated perturbation than purely mechanical stretch. Nevertheless, both cell volume and stretch can alter membrane tension and the cytoskeleton and can trigger some of the same signaling cascades. As a result, the distinction between VAC and SAC is not absolute.

Insight into the role of volume-sensitive channels in cardiac physiology and pathophysiology is still emerging. Cardiac cell volume is not constant. Myocyte volume increases acutely with ischemia/reperfusion and chronically as part of cellular hypertrophy during disease-induced cardiac remodeling. Cell volume also is modulated physiologically by atrial natriuretic factor, autonomic stimulation, and pharmacologic agents, including nitrates and diuretics. Therefore, volume-sensitive channels and transporters play a role in both physiology and pathophysiology. This chapter explores volume-sensitive ion channels and transporters in mammalian heart and their regulation.

TRANSDUCING CELL VOLUME

A basic but largely unanswered question is: How is cardiac cell volume transduced into a biologic response?

The answer almost certainly depends on the volume-sensitive process considered. In several cases, participants in transduction and signaling are known, but a clear demarcation of the initial step(s) remains elusive. Although schemes for detecting volume changes have been considered, especially in the context of cell volume regulation, the enormous diversity of signaling elicited by a volume change and its tissue-specific nature have proven to be experimental and conceptual challenges. The following is a brief overview of several potential transduction mechanisms (see Reference 1 for review).

An obvious effect of osmotic swelling and shrinkage is dilution or concentration of cytoplasmic ions and regulatory molecules and a consequent change in ionic strength. Such perturbations can affect ion transport by altering ion gradients, the concentration of intracellular regulatory ions, surface potential, and binding affinities. Isosmotic cell inflation, which avoids changes in ion concentration and ionic strength, is an equally effective stimulus for several VAC, however.

The consequences of osmotic stress depend, at least in part, on whether a cell is intact or dialyzed by a patch pipette. Initially, water flux during an osmotic challenge exceeds the ability of diffusion from the pipette to maintain cytoplasmic ion content. As volume reaches a new steady state, however, the flux of water decreases, and ion concentrations again approach those in the pipette. Transport numbers for anion and cation fluxes between the pipette and cell may affect the steady-state volume obtained.[2]

Volume changes also modify membrane tension by stretching the cell or by altering membrane curvature. The resulting forces may directly regulate channels or membrane-bound signaling molecules (see Chapters 4 and 7). Specializations, such as caveolae, are proposed to serve as tension sensors that activate signaling. Because the sarcolemma has a much greater area than that required to encompass cell volume and is supported by the cytoskeleton, the effect of volume changes on membrane tension is difficult to quantify.

The cytoskeleton is deformed and undergoes reorganization in response to volume perturbations. Channels and transporters are structurally anchored in the membrane by specific cytoskeletal components, and their activity may reflect the state of the cytoskeleton. The cytoskeleton also anchors signaling molecules. It is clear that signaling cascades participate in the volume response, and they also may serve as volume sensors. Volume modulates signaling by altering the association of signaling molecules with their docking and adapter proteins and targets by mass action. Binding affinities can be altered by physical distortion of proteins, ionic strength, or the concentration of competing ions, and through macromolecular crowding. Macromolecular crowding reflects the idea that proteins do not behave ideally in solutions and that enzymatic reactions are influenced by the concentration of macromolecules that are neither substrate nor product. Inert macromolecules exclude kinases, phosphatases, and other signaling enzymes from a fraction of the cytoplasm. Thus, altering the concentration of inert macromolecules by even a few percent can significantly affect reaction rates and, thereby, the functions of target proteins.

VOLUME-ACTIVATED CHANNELS

$I_{Cl,Swell}$

The most extensively studied VAC is $I_{Cl,Swell}$ (or $I_{Cl,VOL}$), which is found throughout the heart in many species including humans.[3-5] Its basic properties are shown in Figure 3–1. $I_{Cl,Swell}$ is elicited by anisosmotic swelling in hyposmotic bath or hyperosmotic pipette solutions, isosmotic swelling caused by urea uptake, or cell inflation caused by positive pressure applied to the patch pipette.[6-9] The current is outwardly rectifying in physiologic or symmetric Cl^- gradients, time-independent over most of the physiologic voltage range, but it partially inactivates at strongly positive potentials.[10,11] Although Cl^- is the primary charge car-

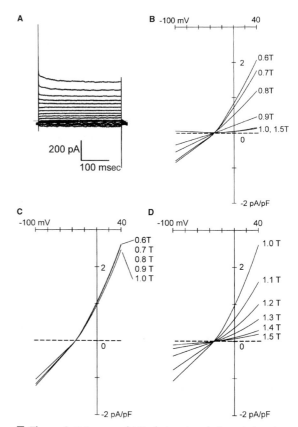

■ **Figure 3–1** $I_{Cl,Swell}$ and I-V relations in solutions designed to isolate Cl^- current with perforated patch. *A,* $I_{Cl,Swell}$ measured as difference current (0.6 − 1 T) in rabbit ventricle with steps to voltages between -100 and +60 mV from -80 mV. *B,* Activation of $I_{Cl,Swell}$ is graded. 9-anthracene carboxylic acid–sensitive currents during ramp clamps in 0.6 to 1 T and in 1.5 T in dog ventricle. *C,* Persistent activation of $I_{Cl,Swell}$ in 1 T in pacing-induced heart failure in dog. Swelling in 0.9 to 0.6 T does not elicit additional current. *D,* Osmotic shrinkage (1.1 to 1.5 T) inhibits $I_{Cl,Swell}$ in heart failure. Records obtained with perforated patch. *(Modified from Baumgarten CM, Clemo HF: Swelling-activated chloride channels in cardiac physiology and pathophysiology. Prog Biophys Mol Biol 82:25, 2003; and Clemo HF, Stambler BS, Baumgarten CM: Swelling-activated chloride current is persistently activated in ventricular myocytes from dogs with tachycardia-induced congestive heart failure. Circ Res 84:157, 1999, with permission.)*

rier, organic anions also permeate, and the permeability sequence is: $I^- > NO_3^- > Br^- > Cl^- > Asp^-$.[8,9] Tamoxifen and 4,4′-diisothiocyanatostilbene-2,2′-disulphonic acid (DIDS) distinguish between $I_{Cl,Swell}$ and both the cystic fibrosis transmembrane regulator

Cl⁻ channel (CFTR) ($I_{Cl,cAMP}$) and the Ca^{2+}-activated Cl⁻ channel and are selective blockers under conditions that isolate anion currents. Other less selective anion channel blockers in combination with volume perturbations often are used to identify $I_{Cl,Swell}$.[3,4,12] Activation of $I_{Cl,Swell}$ shortens action potential duration, depolarizes resting membrane potential and contributes to cell volume regulation and arrhythmogenesis.[3,4,12]

Background Cl⁻ current has the same biophysical properties and pharmacology as $I_{Cl,Swell}$ and has been attributed to the same set of ion channels.[4] Spontaneous activation of $I_{Cl,Swell}$ can occur with ruptured patches without an overt osmotic gradient and can contribute to background current.[7] This may result from washout of cytoplasmic regulatory molecules or spontaneous cell swelling. A Donnan system exists between the cytoplasm, which contains charged proteins, and mobile ions in the pipette; the resulting distribution of ions and water tends to cause cell swelling. In addition, swelling can result from differences in the permeability of various ions—that is, the distinction between tonicity and osmolarity.

$I_{Cl,Swell}$ appears to be both a VAC and SAC because it is sensitive to membrane shape or tension and mechanical stretch, as well as volume. One way to modify membrane tension and shape is with charged amphipaths. Anionic amphipaths preferentially insert into the outer membrane leaflet and induce convex curvature (crenation) that mimics swelling, whereas cationic amphipaths insert into the inner leaflet and induce concave curvature (cupping) that mimics shrinkage. In ventricle, $I_{Cl,Swell}$ is activated by crenators and is inhibited by cupping agents without changing cell volume.[6] Identical modulation of mechano-gated 2P K⁺ channels, TREK and TRAAK, by amphipaths is attributed to altered membrane tension. Although the actions of amphipaths are complex, these data suggest $I_{Cl,Swell}$ or an upstream signaling cascade senses membrane tension or shape.

The classic method for identifying SAC is by applying positive or negative pressure to a membrane patch. Whereas most investigators find only cation SAC by this method, Sato and Koumi[13] described an 8.6 pS Cl⁻ SAC in excised patches from human atrial myocytes. Activation occurs with positive pipette

pressure in the outside-out and negative pressure in the inside-out configurations, and open probability increases from 0.03 to 0.94 at 4.5 to 20 mm Hg. Cl⁻ SAC unitary currents are blocked by 9-anthracene carboxylic acid (9AC) and the stilbene derivative DIDS with the same potency as the VAC $I_{Cl,Swell}$ in these cells.

Mechanical activation of $I_{Cl,Swell}$ also is accomplished by stretching β_1 integrins with monoclonal antibody–coated magnetic beads.[14] Binding of beads without stretch, stretch of another membrane protein, and the magnetic field alone did not provoke current. Cl⁻ SAC was blocked by tamoxifen, a selective blocker of $I_{Cl,Swell}$,[14] and also by hyperosmotic shrinkage (Browe and Baumgarten, unpublished data). Thus, stretch and swelling both appear to regulate the same channel.

Clemo and colleagues[15,16] found that $I_{Cl,Swell}$ is persistently activated in ventricular myocytes from a canine rapid pacing dilated cardiomyopathy model, and similar results are obtained in ventricular myocytes from rabbit aortic regurgitation, canine infarct and peri-infarct zone cells, and human atrial myocytes from patients with right atrial enlargement.[3] An outwardly rectifying, tamoxifen- and 9AC-sensitive Cl⁻ current with I⁻ > Cl⁻ permeability is present under isosmotic conditions in heart failure and infarction myocytes, but not sham or control cells. $I_{Cl,Swell}$ in diseased myocytes is turned off by osmotic shrinkage (1.1 to 1.5 T), whereas osmotic swelling (0.9 to 0.6 T) does not activate more current. However, the maximal activated $I_{Cl,Swell}$ is approximately 40% greater in heart failure than control cells.[16]

The molecular identity of $I_{Cl,Swell}$ remains in dispute. Hume and coworkers[4] provided substantial evidence that ClC-3 underlies $I_{Cl,Swell}$ in heart. This view has been challenged by others who believe ClC-3 is an intracellular channel and noted that knockout of ClC-3 did not abolish $I_{Cl,Swell}$ in noncardiac tissue.[17] $I_{Cl,Swell}$ also can be elicited in cardiac myocytes from *Clcn3*⁻/⁻ mice, but its regulation and antibody sensitivity are distinct from that in *Clcn3*⁺/⁺, although several biophysical characteristics of the current appear unchanged.[18] ClC-3 knockout leads to up-regulation of message for other ClC channels and 35 unidentified proteins, which may contribute to the novel $I_{Cl,Swell}$. These data argue that distinct channel proteins may cause currents with an $I_{Cl,Swell}$ phenotype. Tissue-specific regulation, antibody sensitivity, and unitary conductance of $I_{Cl,Swell}$ have been documented previously.[3]

Activation of $I_{Cl,Swell}$ lags behind a volume change by approximately 1 minute, suggesting that signaling is required for stimulus transduction. The regulation of cardiac $I_{Cl,Swell}$ is complex, involving multiple signaling cascades, but some unresolved conflicts remain.

One of the first responses to swelling and stretch is activation of protein tyrosine kinase (PTK), which occurs in less than 5 sec.[19] Sorota[20] found that block of PTK with genistein or herbimycin suppressed stimulation of $I_{Cl,Swell}$ in dog atrial myocytes. Dialysis with ATPγS prevented block by genistein but did not spontaneously activate $I_{Cl,Swell}$ or preclude its inhibition by shrinkage. This result indicates that PTK is not sufficient to regulate $I_{Cl,Swell}$.

In contrast, differential effects of two PTK families, Src and epidermal growth factor receptor (EGFR) kinase, are found in human atrial and rabbit ventricular myocytes (Ren and Baumgarten, unpublished data).[21] Genistein and selective Src inhibitors substantially augment $I_{Cl,Swell}$, whereas selective inhibitors of EGFR kinase suppress it. Src blockers stimulate current only in osmotically swollen myocytes, and the current is blocked by tamoxifen, DIDS, and osmotic shrinkage. Moreover, the protein tyrosine phosphatase (PTP) inhibitor orthovanadate opposes the action of PTK inhibitors. Thus, phosphorylation and dephosphorylation of multiple tyrosines by PTK and PTP modulate $I_{Cl,Swell}$ but are not sufficient to activate $I_{Cl,Swell}$ in normotonic solution.[20,21]

The role of protein kinase A (PKA) also is controversial. Initial studies showed that neither organic nor highly specific peptide blockers of PKA inhibit $I_{Cl,Swell}$.[6,8] In contrast, Sorota[5] and coworkers manipulated cyclic adenosine monophosphate (cAMP) and described a rapid stimulation of $I_{Cl,Swell}$ that was PKA independent and a slower inhibition that was PKA dependent.[3] Their interpretation was questioned by Hume and coworkers,[4] who suggested that PKA might act instead by modulating a protein kinase C (PKC) site on ClC-3.

Duan, Hume, and coworkers[3,4] suggested that $I_{Cl,Swell}$ is activated by dephosphorylation of ClC-3 by ser/thr protein phosphatases (PP) and is inhibited when phosphorylated by PKC. Duan and colleagues[10] found that $α_{1a}$-adrenergic stimulation blocks $I_{Cl,Swell}$ by pertussis toxin-sensitive signaling. Inhibition of PKC precluded the effects of phenylephrine, and activation of PKC suppressed $I_{Cl,Swell}$. This group implicated ClC-3 ser-51, a consensus PKC site, as a critical residue.[22] Regulation of $I_{Cl,Swell}$ by α-adrenergic stimulation, PKC, and PP was confirmed in canine and rabbit myocytes from normal and failing hearts.[3] In control myocytes, PP2a is responsible for current activation, and $I_{Cl,Swell}$ is independent of $[Ca^{2+}]_i$. In heart failure myocytes, however, calcineurin (PP2b), a Ca^{2+}-dependent PP, also regulates $I_{Cl,Swell}$, and activation of $I_{Cl,Swell}$ is inhibited by PP2b blockers, cyclosporin A and FK506, and by 1,2-bis(2-aminophenoxy)ethane-N,N,N′,N′-tetraacetic acid acetoxymethyl ester (BAPTA-AM). In addition, block of extracellular signal regulated kinase 1/2 (ERK1/2) rapidly inhibits $I_{Cl,Swell}$ in failure myocytes. In contrast to these studies, activation of PKC was reported to stimulate rather than inhibit $I_{Cl,Swell}$ in canine atria.[23] However, the consensus is that PKC acts to inhibit $I_{Cl,Swell}$, whereas PP2a, PP2b, and ERK1/2 act to stimulate it.

Recent studies on $I_{Cl,Swell}$ activation by pulling on integrins revealed additional control mechanisms.[14,24] Stretch provokes autocrine/paracrine signaling, involving angiotensin I (Ang I) receptors and downstream activation of sarcolemmal nicotinamide adenine dinucleotide phosphate (NADPH) oxidase, and elicits a tamoxifen-sensitive Cl^- SAC with properties similar to $I_{Cl,Swell}$. Blocking Src, FAK, Ang I receptors, EGFR kinase, or NADPH oxidase prevents stimulation of Cl^- SAC. NADPH oxidase produces superoxide ($\cdot O_2^-$), which is converted to H_2O_2 by superoxide dismutase. Catalase destroys H_2O_2 and inhibits the Cl^- SAC, and a tamoxifen-sensitive Cl^- current is turned on by exogenous H_2O_2. In addition, the Cl^- SAC seen with integrin stretch is suppressed by osmotic shrinkage, and $I_{Cl,Swell}$ in hyposmotic media is inhibited by NADPH oxidase blockers and catalase, suggesting that signaling cascades are involved in the activation of these channels by stretch and osmotic swelling (Browe, Ren, and Baumgarten, unpublished data).

In addition to $I_{Cl,Swell}$, an inwardly rectifying Cl^- VAC, termed $I_{Cl,IR}$, is present in atrial and ventricular myocytes.[25] This channel slowly activates with a biexponential time course at negative potentials, exhibits

Cl$^-$ > I$^-$ > Asp$^-$ permeability, and is blocked by 9AC but neither tamoxifen nor DIDS. Osmotic swelling increases its amplitude and speeds activation; shrinkage causes inhibition. The current density of $I_{Cl,IR}$ is less than that of $I_{Cl,Swell}$, however. Based on its biophysical characteristics and the presence of transcripts, $I_{Cl,IR}$ has been attributed to ClC-2.

Nonselective Cation Volume-Activated Channels

Although most studies of VAC have focused on $I_{Cl,Swell}$, several weakly selective cation channels (CAT) also are activated by osmotic swelling, as shown in Figure 3–2. In rat atrial cells, the VAC$_{CAT}$ exhibits nearly equal permeabilities for Na$^+$, K$^+$, and Cs$^+$, and a P_{Ca}/P_K ratio of 0.13.[26] Its time course of activation closely follows that of the volume change. Swollen myocytes in symmetrical K$^+$ produced single-channel currents with a unitary conductance of 36 pS, and open probability increased on depolarization. Curiously, application of negative pressure to the patch pipette increased the open prob-

ability of the VAC$_{CAT}$ in some patches but decreased it in others. This channel has different single-channel biophysical characteristics than cationic SAC activated through stretch of a patch by negative pipette pressure (see Chapter 1), and it is insensitive to Gd^{3+}. However, osmotic swelling of guinea pig ventricular myocytes rapidly activates a VAC$_{CAT}$ with a nearly linear I-V relation that is blocked by Gd^{3+}.[27]

In contrast to these linear VAC$_{CAT}$, an inwardly rectifying VAC$_{CAT}$, termed $I_{CIR,Swell}$, is seen on osmotic swelling of rabbit and canine ventricular myocytes (Fig. 3–3).[2,15] This channel has a P_K/P_{Na} ratio of 6 to 8 and is blocked by Gd^{3+} and GsMTx-4,[2,15,28] both SAC blockers, but it is insensitive to Ba^{2+}, an inward-rectifier K$^+$ channel blocker. Importantly, $I_{CIR,Swell}$, together with $I_{Cl,Swell}$, are persistently activated in ventricular myocytes from rapid pacing and aortic regurgitation models of dilated cardiomyopathy and can be turned off in these failure myocytes by osmotic shrinkage.[15,16] $I_{CIR,Swell}$ appears to be responsible, at least in part, for spontaneous depolarizations that arise late in phase 4 and cause runs of tachycardia in myocytes from disease models; the spontaneous depolarizations and spontaneous

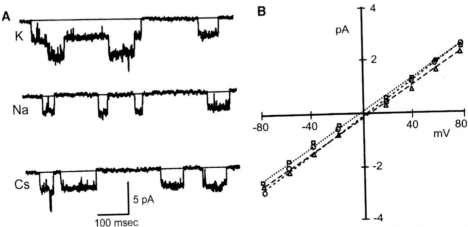

■ **Figure 3–2** Cation volume-activated channels in rat atrial myocytes do not distinguish among Na$^+$, K$^+$, and Cs$^+$. *A,* Unitary currents recorded at –60 mV from cell-attached patches on osmotically swollen cell (0.73 T) with 140 mM KCl, NaCl, or CsCl in the pipette. *B,* I-V relations from inside-out patch with either 140 mM KCl, NaCl, or CsCl in the bath and 140 mM KCl in the pipette were linear and reversed at 0 mV. Unitary current amplitude, reversal potential, and conductance were not significantly affected by choice of cation. *(Modified from Kim D, Fu C: Activation of a nonselective cation channel by swelling in atrial cells. J Membr Biol 135:27, 1993, with permission.)*

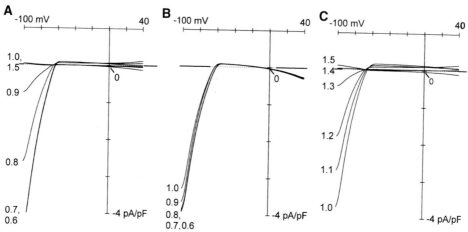

■ **Figure 3–3** Inwardly rectifying cation volume-activated channel, $I_{Cir,Swell}$, in dog ventricle measured as Gd^{3+}-sensitive current during voltage ramp with perforated patch. *A,* Activation is graded on osmotic swelling (0.9 to 0.6 T). *B,* Persistent activation of $I_{Cir,Swell}$ in pacing-induced heart. Swelling in 0.9 to 0.6 T elicits only a slight increase in current. *C,* Osmotic shrinkage (1.1 to 1.5 T) inhibits $I_{Cir,Swell}$ in heart failure. $I_{Cir,Swell}$ is blocked by the SAC antagonist GsMTx-4 but not by Ba^{2+}.[2] *(Modified from Clemo HF, Stambler BS, Baumgarten CM: Persistent activation of a swelling-activated cation current in ventricular myocytes from dogs with tachycardia-induced congestive heart failure. Circ Res 83:147, 1998, with permission.)*

activity are blocked by the SAC blockers GsMTx-4 and Gd^{3+} or by osmotic shrinkage.[3] Moreover, this current contributes to volume regulation in normal and heart failure myocytes,[2,15] and thereby may influence other volume-sensitive channels and transporters.

SWELLING EFFECTS ON VOLTAGE-GATED ION CHANNELS

I_{Ks}

Sasaki and colleagues[29] were the first to study the effects of cell volume on cardiac delayed rectifier K^+ current, I_K. On hyposmotic swelling (0.7 T) of guinea pig ventricular myocytes, they observed a 170% increase in I_K that was not separated into its rapid and slow components, I_{Kr} and I_{Ks}. They found that osmotic shrinkage (1.3 T) inhibits I_K by 44%,[30] a result confirmed by other reports.[31–33] These effects are as rapid as the volume changes; activation of I_K on swelling and recovery in isosmotic solution has a $t_{1/2}$ of 20 to 50 sec, and the response to osmotic

shrinkage is complete within 20 sec.[30,34] Analysis of tail currents and studies with selective I_{Kr} and I_{Ks} blockers indicate that augmentation of I_K on swelling is caused by the stimulation of I_{Ks} in the guinea pig[27,35,36] and canine[37] ventricle. Isosmotic cell inflation by positive pipette positive pressure (5 to 20 mm Hg) gives a similar enhancement of I_{Ks}.[34] In contrast to swelling, osmotic shrinkage inhibits both I_{Kr} and I_{Ks}.[33]

Swelling-induced activation of PTK[19] leads to enhancement of I_{Ks}. The broad-spectrum PTK inhibitor genistein, but not its inactive analog daidzein, blocks stimulation of I_{Ks} on cell swelling.[37,38] Genistein also reduced I_{Ks} under isosmotic conditions, suggesting that basal activity of PTK is needed to support I_{Ks}.[37,38] Caution is warranted, however, because of nonspecific effects of genistein. A smaller PTK-independent inhibition of isosmotic I_{Ks} also was seen with daidzein.[37] Neither lavendustin A nor tyrphostin A51, other PTK blockers, affected I_{Ks}, and both genistein and daidzein blocked stimulation of I_{Ks} by cAMP.[38] Taken together, these data raise questions about how genistein blocks activation of I_{Ks} by swelling.

Cardiac I_{Ks} arises from the 6TM1P Kv channel KCNQ1 (also termed KvLQT1 or Kv7.1) and an accessory subunit KCNE1 (MinK). KCNQ1 expressed either alone or with KCNE1 in COS-7 cells gives a twofold augmentation of current in 0.7 T, recapitulating the activation of I_{Ks} by myocyte swelling.[39] Homomeric and heteromeric channels are equally responsive to cell swelling, suggesting that KCNQ1 is the osmotically responsive component. In contrast to studies in native cells,[37,38] however, results in this expression system argue against involvement of PTK.[39] Swelling-induced current is not affected by genistein, orthovanadate, or AMP-PNP, a nonhydrolyzable adenosine triphosphate (ATP) analog. The native signaling cascade may not have been recapitulated in the expression system.

In contrast to PTK, blockers of PKC, PKA, and other ser/thr kinases did not prevent enhancement of I_{Ks} by osmotic swelling or isosmotic inflation of myocytes.[34,36,37] Disruption of the actin cytoskeleton with cytochalasin B and D and microtubules with vinblastine and colchicines also were ineffective.[34] Furthermore, increase of $[Ca^{2+}]_i$ is not a required component of the signaling cascade.[30,34,35,37]

I_{Kr}

The effect of swelling on I_{Kr} is distinct from that on I_{Ks}. Osmotic swelling of ventricular myocytes in 0.65 T was reported to decrease I_{Kr} by 25%,[35] but no change was seen in 0.76 T.[36] I_{Kr} also is suppressed by osmotic swelling in rabbit sinoatrial node (SAN) cells, which contributes to slowing of their spontaneous rate.[40]

Osmotic swelling reduces the sensitivity of I_{Kr} to several pharmacologic agents. Under isosmotic conditions, I_{Kr} is fully blocked by 0.2 μM dofetilide, but with swelling, 10 μM is required for full block, and 0.2 μM gives less than 50% inhibition.[35] A similar volume-induced reduction in sensitivity was shown for La^{3+}. Swelling also limits the ability of E-4031 to prolong action potential duration, but this is attributed to the effect of swelling on multiple plateau currents rather than a specific effect on I_{Kr}.[36] Cell volume–induced alterations in drug potency and efficacy may be important factors in antiarrhyth-

mic drug action during ischemia/reperfusion and other settings in which myocyte cell volume changes.[41] This may result from swelling-induced alterations in drug binding or, secondarily, because volume alters action potential trajectory, and thus other conductances.

$I_{Ca,L}$

The literature offers conflicting results on how osmotic swelling alters $I_{Ca,L}$. Stimulation of $I_{Ca,L}$ was reported in rabbit atrial,[42] SAN,[42] and ventricular[43] myocytes; inhibition was found in rat[44] and rabbit[43] ventricular myocytes; and no significant change was detected in guinea pig[29,36,45] and dog[37] ventricular myocytes. Augmentation of $I_{Ca,L}$ by swelling is supported by fura-2 measurements of diltiazem-sensitive Ca^{2+} influx in neonatal rat myocytes.[46] At least in rabbit ventricle, however, the effect of swelling on $I_{Ca,L}$ is biphasic. There is an initial increase followed by a decrease under perforated patch conditions.[43] Thus, the time after swelling at which measurements are made, as well as other experimental details, may contribute to the apparent discrepancies.[43]

In a detailed study, Matsuda and colleagues[42] compared osmotic swelling induced by 0.6 T bath or 1.4 T pipette solution and cell inflation produced by positive pipette pressure. In each case, $I_{Ca,L}$ increases by approximately 35%, and the swelling-induced currents are blocked by dihydropyridines. $I_{Ca,L}$ is augmented without changing the shape of the I-V relation, inactivation kinetics, or steady-state activation; the same percentage stimulation of peak $I_{Ca,L}$ is seen with Ba^{2+} as the charge carrier. Analysis of whole-cell current noise indicated that swelling causes an increase in open probability from 0.27 to 0.36 without altering unitary current amplitude or the number of active channels.

Several potential mechanisms for the stimulation of $I_{Ca,L}$ were ruled out.[42] Specifically inhibiting PKA with PKI and treatment with nonspecific ser/thr kinase inhibitors did not block the increase. Maximizing Ca^{2+} channel phosphorylation with cAMP and forskolin strongly stimulates $I_{Ca,L}$, but $I_{Ca,L}$ is further augmented on swelling. Inflating cells with pipette solutions strongly buffered with ethyleneglycoltetraacetic acid

(EGTA) or BAPTA also fails to interrupt the enhancement of $I_{Ca,L}$ with swelling.

One possible reason for the decrease in $I_{Ca,L}$ seen in some studies of ventricular cells is that T-tubules, where a large fraction of Ca^{2+} channels are located, are pinched off. This does not appear to be the case in rat ventricular myocytes, however, on the basis of experiments in which the membrane was stained with di-8-ANNEPS.[44] These authors observed severe membrane blebbing on swelling under ruptured patch conditions, which accompanied the marked suppression of $I_{Ca,L}$. In contrast, blebs are not significant during swelling under perforated patch conditions where the decrease in $I_{Ca,L}$ is smaller.[43]

Hyperosmotic cell shrinkage also modulates $I_{Ca,L}$. Shrinkage under ruptured or perforated patch conditions causes a reduction in $I_{Ca,L}$ amplitude and a slowing of inactivation.[31] Current amplitude decreases approximately 30% in 1.5 T, and the time constants for inactivation increase to 120 to 150% of control.

$I_{Ca,T}$

The effect of osmotic stress on $I_{Ca,T}$ has not been extensively studied. Pascarel and colleagues[45] showed that 0.7 T perfusion stimulates $I_{Ca,T}$ sixfold in guinea pig ventricle at a time when $I_{Ca,L}$ was unaffected. To measure $I_{Ca,T}$ in this preparation, it is necessary to increase $[Ca^{2+}]_i$ to 5.4 mM, and $I_{Ca,T}$ and its augmentation on swelling are abolished by 40 µM Ni^{2+}, which is sufficient to block $I_{Ca,T}$. These authors also provided evidence for involvement of the cytoskeleton. Disruption of the actin cytoskeleton with cytochalasin D or microtubules with colchicines prevents the stimulation of $I_{Ca,T}$. Taxol, a microtubule stabilizer, has no effect, however. No information is available about the effect of swelling on $I_{Ca,T}$ in atrial and SAN myocytes, where this current has a greater physiologic role.

Other Cation Channels

Although osmotic swelling is expected to dilute cytoplasmic K^+ as water flows into the cell and appropriate shifts of E_K are detected under some situations, I_{K1} appears to be unaltered by osmotic swelling[29,35–37,42] or cell inflation.[34,47] I_{to} also is relatively insensitive to volume changes. Only a 10% inhibition of I_{to} at +60 mV is seen on swelling in 0.6 T.[37] Finally, inflation of rabbit SAN myocytes does not significantly alter I_f.[42]

LIGAND-GATED ION CHANNELS

I_{K-ATP}

Van Wagoner[48] found that ATP-sensitive K^+ channels (I_{K-ATP}) in cultured neonatal and adult rat atrial cells are activated with a delay by hyposmotic (0.83 T) swelling under perforated-patch conditions. Mechanical stretch of cell-attached and inside-out patches by negative pipette pressure also provokes single-channel openings. The I-V relation for the VAC I_{K-ATP} is similar in amplitude and shape to the pinacidil-activated current (10 µM), and both are blocked by glibenclamide. Similar results were reported by others in both neonatal rat atrial[49] and guinea pig ventricular myocytes.[50] Activation is enhanced under ischemic conditions, and the extent of shortening of action potential duration in hyposmotic solution is much greater at 2 than 5 mM $[ATP]_i$. This suggests that osmotic activation of I_{K-ATP} may be particularly important during ischemia and reperfusion.

The mechanism of regulation of I_{K-ATP} by osmotic swelling is unknown. One possibility is disruption of the actin cytoskeleton. I_{K-ATP} is regulated by F-actin.[51] DNase I, which forms complexes with G-actin, thereby disrupting F-actin, and cytochalasin B both stimulate I_{K-ATP} by reducing its sensitivity to ATP.

I_{K-ACh}

Cardiac muscarinic K^+ channel activity is mechanosensitive. In the presence of cholinergic agonists, stretching patches with negative pressure increases open probability without altering agonist affinity[52]; this is not caused by mechanosensitivity of G_i because stretch augments channel activity even after maximal activation with GTPγS. The response to cell swelling is different, however. Inflation of rabbit atrial myocytes rapidly (<500 msec) inhibits carbachol-induced current by 15%.[53] To identify this mechanism, Ji and colleagues[53] expressed the components of the cardiac muscarinic K^+ channel, Kir3.1 (GIRK1) and Kir3.4 (GIRK4), in oocytes together with an excess of $G_{\beta\gamma}$ and osmotically swelled the oocytes in 0.5 T. Osmotic swelling reduces the Kir3.1/3.4 current by 18%, whereas currents from expressed Kir2.1, which is responsible for I_{K1}, are unaffected. Homomeric mutant Kir3.4 channels that are carbachol-sensitive and G protein–regulated also are inhibited by osmotic swelling,[53] as are homomeric Kir3.1 channels.[54] Recently, the role of PKC and phosphatidylinositol 4,5-bisphosphate (PIP_2) in the volume-sensitive regulation of Kir3.4 was studied in detail in the same expression system and native cells.[54] The volume sensitivity of Kir3.4 is abolished by inhibiting PKC. PKC is thought to regulate I_{K-ACh} through PIP_2 production. To test the role of PIP_2, PIP_2 binding to Kir3.4 was enhanced by replacing the binding domain of Kir3.4 with the homologous segment of Kir2.1 or by point mutations mimicking Kir2.1. Strengthening the interaction between PIP_2 and chimeric or mutant Kir3.4 eliminates both volume sensitivity and regulation by PKC.[54] In contrast, double reverse mutants of Kir2.1, which are thought to weaken its association with PIP_2, induce volume sensitivity in Kir2.1, an effect not present in wild-type channels. Zhang and colleagues[54] further demonstrated that block of PKC suppressed inhibition of I_{K-ACh} in native rabbit atrial myocytes.

PUMPS AND EXCHANGERS

Na⁺-K⁺ Pump

Osmotic swelling of ventricular myocytes rapidly stimulates the Na^+-K^+ pump, whereas osmotic shrinkage causes inhibition.[30,55] Whalley and colleagues[55] showed that this is caused by a volume-induced change in the affinity for internal Na^+. The $K_{0.5}$ for Na^+ decreases from 21.4 mM in isosmotic to 12.8 mM in hyposmotic (0.8 T) and increases to 39.0 mM in hyperosmotic (1.5 T) bath solutions, whereas the maximum pump current, I_p, and the Hill coefficient for

activation by Na^+ are unchanged. Altered affinity is attributed to dephosphorylation by PP1 on swelling and phosphorylation by PKC on shrinkage, and it was independent of Na^+ and Ca^{2+} entry.[56] PP1 is downstream of PTK, which is rapidly activated on swelling,[57] and phosphatidylinositol 3 kinase (PI3K), and inhibitors of PTK and PI3K blocked the response to swelling. Although there is agreement on the effect of osmotic swelling on the magnitude of I_p, details regarding the voltage-dependence of stimulation and its $[Na^+]_i$-dependence apparently differ in rabbit[55] and guinea pig[30] myocytes. Moreover, in guinea pig pump stimulation on swelling and activation of $I_{Cl,Swell}$ were mutually exclusive.[30]

The phosphorylation site that regulates the Na^+-K^+ pump during osmotic perturbations has not been identified, but a candidate is phospholemman (PLM). PLM is the founding member of the FXYD protein family, is homologous with the Na^+-K^+ pump γ-subunit, and is a muscle-specific Na^+-K^+ pump regulator that tightly associates with both the $\alpha_1\beta$ and $\alpha_2\beta$ pump isoforms ($\alpha_1\beta > \alpha_2\beta$).[58] Coexpression of PLM with either $\alpha_1\beta$ or $\alpha_2\beta$ reduces the Na^+ affinity twofold and slightly reduces the K^+ affinity, resulting in a reduction of I_p. Thus, a swelling-induced dissociation of PLM from $\alpha\beta$, perhaps caused by altered phosphorylation, could explain the effect of osmotic swelling on I_p. PLM is the major sarcolemmal target of PKA and PKC in heart. Interestingly, PLM also forms anion channels and is postulated to regulate VAC and cell volume.[59]

Notably, measurements of I_p with $[Na^+]_i$ fixed under whole-cell voltage clamp conditions do not fully reflect I_p in the intact myocyte. Swelling causes a persistent decrease of $[Na^+]_i$, whereas shrinkage causes an increase. $[Na^+]_i$ is regulated as a pump-leak system wherein Na^+ influx and efflux balance exactly in the steady state. If Na^+ influx is constant, alterations in pump Na^+ affinity during an osmotic challenge necessarily will cause $[Na^+]_i$ to change just enough to restore the pump rate back to its original value. Thus, the effect of swelling and shrinkage on Na^+ influx must ultimately control the pump rate and I_p. Nevertheless, the magnitude of the change in $[Na^+]_i$ required to adjust pump rate to match the leak will have consequences for other transport processes.

Na$^+$-Ca^{2+} Exchange

The Na$^+$-Ca^{2+} exchanger (NCX) also is modulated by cardiac cell volume. Hyposmotic swelling (0.5 T) decreases I$_{NCX}$, measured as the Ni^{2+}-sensitive current, by about 30%, whereas hyperosmotic shrinkage (1.3 T) stimulates the current by about 15%.[60] Volume-sensitive I$_{NCX}$ is blocked by Ca^{2+}-free bathing solution containing EGTA and by intracellular dialysis with the NCX inhibitory peptide, XIP. More intense osmotic shrinkage initially causes greater NCX stimulation, but the stimulation is transient, and I$_{NCX}$ decays over 5 to 10 minutes. A stimulation of NCX at the plateau potential also is found with more severe shrinkage (2.2 T).[31] The mechanism by which cardiac NCX is modulated by anisosmotic solutions is unclear, but may, in part, reflect altered [Na$^+$]$_i$.[31]

Na$^+$-H$^+$ Exchange

Whalley and coworkers[61,62] found that hyperosmotic shrinkage causes an alkalinization by 0.10 pH unit. They attributed alkalinization to Na$^+$-H$^+$ exchanger stimulation because the rate of pH$_i$ recovery from intracellular acidosis induced by brief exposure to NH$_4$Cl is enhanced by 60%, despite a nearly 50% increase in cytoplasmic buffer capacity in hyperosmotic media. In addition, changes in [Na$^+$]$_i$ are consistent with exchanger stimulation.[61] Reducing the gradient driving H$^+$ extrusion by decreasing [Na$^+$]$_o$ to 15 mM, or specifically blocking Na$^+$-H$^+$ exchange with dimethylamiloride (DMA), converts the alkalinization in hyperosmotic solutions to an acidification, and there is a DMA-sensitive increase in [Na$^+$]$_i$ on exposure to hyperosmotic solutions after blocking the Na$^+$-K$^+$ pump. The response to hyperosmotic shrinkage depends on the extent of the challenge, however. On doubling osmolarity, intracellular acidosis is observed rather than alkalosis.[62] Nevertheless, as judged by the rate of recovery of pH$_i$ from an NH$_4$Cl pulse, the Na$^+$-H$^+$ exchanger is progressively stimulated over the entire range of hyperosmotic solutions examined. Acidification with strong cell shrinkage is attributed to Ca^{2+} release from the sarcoplasmic reticulum and the competition between Ca^{2+} and H$^+$ for anionic binding sites. After blocking Ca^{2+} release with ryanodine, doubling osmolarity produces an increase in pH$_i$, as expected from stimulation of the Na$^+$-H$^+$ exchanger.

Whalley and colleagues[62] also studied the effects of hyposmotic swelling on Na$^+$-H$^+$ exchanger function. Although pH$_i$ is unchanged on myocyte swelling, the rate of recovery of pH$_i$ from an NH$_4$Cl pulse is significantly slowed, despite the decrease in cytoplasmic buffer capacity. Thus, osmotic swelling causes inhibition, and osmotic shrinkage causes stimulation of the Na$^+$-H$^+$ exchanger. Modulation of the Na$^+$-H$^+$ exchanger necessarily influences [Na$^+$]$_i$, but regulation of pH$_i$ is more complex and cannot be predicted from Na$^+$-H$^+$ exchanger function alone.

Alkalinization in hyperosmotic media and stimulation of H$^+$ efflux was confirmed in cultured neonatal rat cardiac myocytes by 2′,7′bis(2-Carboxylethyl)-5(6)-carboxyfluorescein acetoxymethyl ester (BCECF-AM) fluorescence.[63] In this system, stimulation of Na$^+$-H$^+$ exchange was Ca^{2+} dependent. Removal of extracellular Ca^{2+} and exposure to calmodulin and CaMKII antagonists blocked stimulation, as did an inhibitor of myosin light chain kinase. The effect of swelling and shrinkage on pH$_i$ in intact heart was determined by ^{31}P nuclear magnetic resonance.[64] Consistent with other studies, shrinkage and swelling increased pH$_i$ by 0.14 unit and decreased it by 0.02 unit, respectively. These authors concluded, however, that Na$^+$-H$^+$ exchange did not control pH$_i$ during a volume change because an Na$^+$-H$^+$ exchange blocker did not prevent osmolarity-induced alkalinization. Instead they attribute pH$_i$ changes to altered [HCO$_3^-$]$_i$. HCO$_3^-$ free perfusion prevented volume-induced pH$_i$ shifts.

Interestingly, mechanical stretch and hypertrophy also activate the cardiac Na$^+$-H$^+$ exchanger by an autocrine–paracrine mechanism involving angiotensin II receptors, endothelin A receptors, and PKC.[65] It is unclear whether this pathway also contributes to the responses to osmotic stress.

CONCLUSION

Substantial evidence indicates that cell volume modulates a variety of anion and cation channels and transporters in the heart and that the transduction processes are both diverse and complex. The resulting membrane currents and altered ion gradients affect cardiac function. Volume sensitivity adds an additional dimension to mechano-electric feedback.

Acknowledgments

This chapter was supported by grants HL-46764 and HL-65435 from the National Institutes of Health.

References

1. Baumgarten CM, Feher JJ: Osmosis and the regulation of cell volume. In Sperelakis N (ed): Cell Physiology Source Book: A Molecular Approach. New York, Academic Press, 2001, pp 319–355.
2. Clemo HF, Baumgarten CM: Swelling-activated Gd^{3+}-sensitive cation current and cell volume regulation in rabbit ventricular myocytes. J Gen Physiol 110:297–312, 1997.
3. Baumgarten CM, Clemo HF: Swelling-activated chloride channels in cardiac physiology and pathophysiology. Prog Biophys Mol Biol 82:25–42, 2003.
4. Hume JR, Duan D, Collier ML, et al: Anion transport in heart. Physiol Rev 80:31–81, 2000.
5. Sorota S: Insights into the structure, distribution and function of the cardiac chloride channels. Cardiovasc Res 42:361–376, 1999.
6. Tseng GN: Cell swelling increases membrane conductance of canine cardiac cells: Evidence for a volume-sensitive Cl channel. Am J Physiol Cell Physiol 262:C1056–C1068, 1992.
7. Sorota S: Swelling-induced chloride-sensitive current in canine atrial cells revealed by whole-cell patch-clamp method. Circ Res 70:679–687, 1992.
8. Hagiwara N, Masuda H, Shoda M, et al: Stretch-activated anion currents of rabbit cardiac myocytes. J Physiol (Lond) 456:285–302, 1992.
9. Vandenberg JI, Yoshida A, Kirk K, et al: Swelling-activated and isoprenaline-activated chloride currents in guinea pig cardiac myocytes have distinct electrophysiology and pharmacology. J Gen Physiol 104:997–1017, 1994.
10. Duan D, Fermini B, Nattel S: α-adrenergic control of volume-regulated Cl^- currents in rabbit atrial myocytes: Characterization of a novel ionic regulatory mechanism. Circ Res 77:379–393, 1995.
11. Shuba LM, Ogura T, McDonald TF: Kinetic evidence distinguishing volume-sensitive chloride current from other types in guinea-pig ventricular myocytes. J Physiol (Lond) 491:69–80, 1996.
12. Sorota S: Pharmacologic properties of the swelling-induced chloride current of dog atrial myocytes. J Cardiovasc Electrophysiol 5:1006–1016, 1994.
13. Sato R, Koumi S: Characterization of the stretch-activated chloride channel in isolated human atrial myocytes. J Membr Biol 163:67–76, 1998.
14. Browe DM, Baumgarten CM: Stretch of beta1 integrin activates an outwardly rectifying chloride current via FAK and Src in rabbit ventricular myocytes. J Gen Physiol 122:689–702, 2003.
15. Clemo HF, Stambler BS, Baumgarten CM: Persistent activation of a swelling-activated cation current in ventricular myocytes from dogs with tachycardia-induced congestive heart failure. Circ Res 83:147–157, 1998.
16. Clemo HF, Stambler BS, Baumgarten CM: Swelling-activated chloride current is persistently activated in ventricular myocytes from dogs with tachycardia-induced congestive heart failure. Circ Res 84:157–165, 1999.
17. Jentsch TJ, Stein V, Weinreich F, et al: Molecular structure and physiological function of chloride channels. Physiol Rev 82:503–568, 2002.
18. Yamamoto-Mizuma S, Wang GX, Liu LL, et al: Altered properties of volume-sensitive osmolyte and anion channels (VSOACs) and membrane protein expression in cardiac and smooth muscle myocytes from $Clcn3^{-/-}$ mice. J Physiol (Lond) 557:439–456, 2004.
19. Sadoshima J, Qiu ZH, Morgan JP, et al: Tyrosine kinase activation is an immediate and essential step in hypotonic cell swelling-induced ERK activation and c-*fos* gene expression in cardiac myocytes. EMBO J 15:5535–5546, 1996.
20. Sorota S: Tyrosine protein kinase inhibitors prevent activation of cardiac swelling-induced chloride current. Pflugers Arch 431:178–185, 1995.
21. Du XL, Gao Z, Lau CP, et al: Differential effects of tyrosine kinase inhibitors on volume-sensitive chloride current in human atrial myocytes: Evidence for dual regulation by Src and EGFR kinases. J Gen Physiol 123:427–439, 2004.
22. Duan D, Cowley S, Horowitz B, et al: A serine residue in ClC-3 links phosphorylation-dephosphorylation to chloride channel regulation by cell volume. J Gen Physiol 113:57–70, 1999.
23. Du XY, Sorota S: Protein kinase C stimulates swelling-induced chloride current in canine atrial cells. Pflugers Arch 437:227–234, 1999.
24. Browe DM, Baumgarten CM: Angiotensin II (AT1) receptors and NADPH oxidase regulate a Cl^- current elicited by β1 integrin stretch in ventricular myocytes. J Gen Physiol 124:273–287, 2004.
25. Duan D, Ye L, Britton F, et al: A novel anionic inward rectifier in native cardiac myocytes. Circ Res 86:E63–E71, 2000.
26. Kim D, Fu C: Activation of a nonselective cation channel by swelling in atrial cells. J Membr Biol 135:27–37, 1993.
27. Kocic I, Hirano Y, Hiraoka M: Ionic basis for membrane potential changes induced by hypoosmotic stress in guinea-pig ventricular myocytes. Cardiovasc Res 51:59–70, 2001.
28. Suchyna TM, Johnson JH, Hamer K, et al: Identification of a peptide toxin from *Grammostola spatulata* spider venom that blocks cation-selective stretch-activated channels. J Gen Physiol 115:583–598, 2000.
29. Sasaki N, Mitsuiye T, Noma A: Effects of mechanical stretch on membrane currents of single ventricular myocytes of guinea-pig heart. Jpn J Physiol 42:957–970, 1992.
30. Sasaki N, Mitsuiye T, Wang Z, et al: Increase of the delayed rectifier K^+ and Na^+K^+ pump currents by hypotonic solutions in guinea pig cardiac myocytes. Circ Res 75:887–895, 1994.
31. Ogura T, You Y, McDonald TF: Membrane currents underlying the modified electrical activity of guinea-pig ventricular myocytes exposed to hyperosmotic solution. J Physiol (Lond) 504:135–151, 1997.
32. Kasamaki Y, Guo AC, Shuba LM, et al: Potassium current and sodium pump involvement in the positive inotropy of cardiac muscle during hyperosmotic stress. Can J Cardiol 14:285–294, 1998.
33. Ogura T, Matsuda H, Shibamoto T, et al: Osmosensitive properties of rapid and slow delayed rectifier K^+ currents in guinea-pig heart cells. Clin Exp Pharmacol Physiol 30:616–622, 2003.
34. Wang ZR, Mitsuiye T, Noma A: Cell distension-induced increase of the delayed rectifier K^+ current in guinea pig ventricular myocytes. Circ Res 78:466–474, 1996.
35. Rees SA, Vandenberg JI, Wright AR, et al: Cell swelling has differential effects on the rapid and slow components of delayed rectifier potassium current in guinea pig cardiac myocytes. J Gen Physiol 106:1151–1170, 1995.

36. Groh WJ, Gibson KJ, Maylie JG: Hypotonic-induced stretch counteracts the efficacy of the class III antiarrhythmic agent E-4031 in guinea pig myocytes. Cardiovasc Res 31:237–245, 1996.

37. Zhou YY, Yao JA, Tseng GN: Role of tyrosine kinase activity in cardiac slow delayed rectifier channel modulation by cell swelling. Pflugers Arch 433:750–757, 1997.

38. Washizuka T, Horie M, Obayashi K, et al: Does tyrosine kinase modulate delayed-rectifier K channels in guinea pig ventricular cells? Heart Vessels (Suppl 12):173–174, 1997.

39. Kubota T, Horie M, Takano M, et al: Role of KCNQ1 in the cell swelling-induced enhancement of the slowly activating delayed rectifier K$^+$ current. Jpn J Physiol 52:31–39, 2002.

40. Lei M, Kohl P: Swelling-induced decrease in spontaneous pacemaker activity of rabbit isolated sino-atrial node cells. Acta Physiol Scand 164:1–12, 1998.

41. Wright AR, Rees SA: Targeting ischaemia—cell swelling and drug efficacy. Trends Pharmacol Sci 18:224–228, 1997.

42. Matsuda N, Hagiwara N, Shoda M, et al: Enhancement of the L-type Ca^{2+} current by mechanical stimulation in single rabbit cardiac myocytes. Circ Res 78:650–659, 1996.

43. Li GR, Zhang M, Satin LS, et al: Biphasic effects of cell volume on excitation-contraction coupling in rabbit ventricular myocytes. Am J Physiol Heart Circ Physiol 282:H1270–H1277, 2002.

44. Brette F, Calaghan SC, Lappin S, et al: Biphasic effects of hyposmotic challenge on excitation-contraction coupling in rat ventricular myocytes. Am J Physiol Heart Circ Physiol 279:H1963–H1971, 2000.

45. Pascarel C, Brette F, Le Guennec JY: Enhancement of the T-type calcium current by hyposmotic shock in isolated guinea-pig ventricular myocytes. J Mol Cell Cardiol 33:1363–1369, 2001.

46. Taouil K, Giancola R, Morel JE, et al: Hypotonically induced calcium increase and regulatory volume decrease in newborn rat cardiomyocytes. Pflugers Arch 436:565–574, 1998.

47. Du XY, Sorota S: Cardiac swelling-induced chloride current depolarizes canine atrial myocytes. Am J Physiol Heart Circ Physiol 272:H1904–H1916, 1997.

48. Van Wagoner DR: Mechanosensitive gating of atrial ATP-sensitive potassium channels. Circ Res 72:973–983, 1993.

49. Baron A, van Bever L, Monnier D, et al: A novel K$_{ATP}$ current in cultured neonatal rat atrial appendage cardiomyocytes. Circ Res 85:707–715, 1999.

50. Priebe L, Beuckelmann DJ: Cell swelling causes the action potential duration to shorten in guinea-pig ventricular myocytes by activating I$_{KATP}$. Pflugers Arch 436:894–898, 1998.

51. Terzic A, Kurachi Y: Actin microfilament disrupters enhance K$_{ATP}$ channel opening in patches from guinea-pig cardiomyocytes. J Physiol (Lond) 492:395–404, 1996.

52. Pleumsamran A, Kim D: Membrane stretch augments the cardiac muscarinic K$^+$ channel activity. J Membr Biol 148:287–297, 1995.

53. Ji S, John SA, Lu Y, et al: Mechanosensitivity of the cardiac muscarinic potassium channel. A novel property conferred by Kir3.4 subunit. J Biol Chem 273:1324–1328, 1998.

54. Zhang L, Lee JK, John SA, et al: Mechanosensitivity of GIRK channels is mediated by protein kinase C-dependent channel-phosphatidylinositol 4,5-bisphosphate interaction. J Biol Chem 279:7037–7047, 2004.

55. Whalley DW, Hool LC, Ten Eick RE, et al: Effect of osmotic swelling and shrinkage on Na$^+$-K$^+$ pump activity in mammalian cardiac myocytes. Am J Physiol Cell Physiol 265:C1201–C1210, 1993.

56. Bewick NL, Fernandes C, Pitt AD, et al: Mechanisms of Na$^+$-K$^+$ pump regulation in cardiac myocytes during hyposmolar swelling. Am J Physiol Cell Physiol 276:C1091–C1099, 1999.

57. Sadoshima J, Izumo S: Tyrosine kinases mediation of *c-fos* expression by cell swelling in cardiac myocytes. Heart Vessels (Suppl 12):194–197, 1997.

58. Crambert G, Fuzesi M, Garty H, et al: Phospholemman (FXYD1) associates with Na,K-ATPase and regulates its transport properties. Proc Natl Acad Sci USA 99:11476–11481, 2002.

59. Moorman JR, Jones LR: Phospholemman: A cardiac taurine channel involved in regulation of cell volume. Adv Exp Med Biol 442:219–228, 1998.

60. Wright AR, Rees SA, Vandenberg JI, et al: Extracellular osmotic pressure modulates sodium-calcium exchange in isolated guinea-pig ventricular myocytes. J Physiol (Lond) 488:293–301, 1995.

61. Whalley DW, Hemsworth PD, Rasmussen HH: Sodium-hydrogen exchange in guinea-pig ventricular muscle during exposure to hyperosmolar solutions. J Physiol (Lond) 444:193–212, 1991.

62. Whalley DW, Hemsworth PD, Rasmussen HH: Regulation of intracellular pH in cardiac muscle during cell shrinkage and swelling in anisosmolar solutions. Am J Physiol Heart Circ Physiol 266:H658–H669, 1994.

63. Moor AN, Murtazina R, Fliegel L: Calcium and osmotic regulation of the Na$^+$-H$^+$ exchanger in neonatal ventricular myocytes. J Mol Cell Cardiol 32:925–936, 2000.

64. Befroy DE, Powell T, Radda GK, et al: Osmotic shock: Modulation of contractile function, pH$_i$, and ischemic damage in perfused guinea pig heart. Am J Physiol Heart Circ Physiol 276:H1236–H1244, 1999.

65. Cingolani HE, Alvarez BV, Ennis IL, et al: Stretch-induced alkalinization of feline papillary muscle: An autocrine-paracrine system. Circ Res 83:775–780, 1998.

CHAPTER 4

The Mechanosensitivity of Voltage-Gated Channels May Contribute to Cardiac Mechano-Electric Feedback

• • • •

Catherine E. Morris and Ulrike Laitko

The stretch-activated cation nonselective channels (SAC_{CAT}), often described as "ubiquitous," have not been detected in the sarcolemma of adult mammalian cardiomyocytes (see Chapter 1). Their molecular identity also remains elusive.[1,2] In contrast, the cardiomyocyte sarcolemma has many identified voltage-gated channels (VGC), some of which are as susceptible to membrane stretch as SAC_{CAT}. The mechanosensitivity of VGC has been studied in native[3] and in recombinant preparations.[4] Thus, VGC are contenders as possible contributors to mechano-electric feedback (MEF). But as with SAC_{CAT}, the published record on the mechanosensitivity of VGC in native cells, including in cardiomyocytes, is sparse and presents some unresolved contradictions.

MECHANOSENSITIVITY OF VOLTAGE-GATED CHANNELS IN CONTEXT

The responsiveness of VGC to membrane stretch may be surprising if one assumes mechanosensitive gating signifies an evolved "design" for transducing membrane stretch. But that is probably the wrong way to think about the issue. For evolution to engineer a channel with conformational equilibria that exhibit no susceptibility to membrane deformations would be difficult. Membrane proteins interact with the surrounding lipid molecules, and it is known that the lipid composition of the bilayer strongly affects channel function.[5] Besides particular lipid–protein interactions that might translate far-field lipid tension into intramolecular strain, membrane proteins also inevitably feel local pressure applied to their surface. This effective pressure shows multiple abrupt variations as a function of depth across the several nanometer-thick bilayer; any perturbation that alters this pressure profile inevitably alters the conformational equilibria (Fig. 4–1, *top*), provided the different protein conformations have different shapes in the part of the protein that is bilayer embedded. From this standpoint it is not surprising that mechanosensitive gating is widespread among unrelated channels, with different manifestations from one channel type to the next.[10–12] As with any phenotypic trait, each instance of mechanosensitivity can be an opportunity or a liability ("physiology vs. pathology"), or, where the bilayer is protected against significant changes in tension,[13] mechanosensitivity can be a neutral trait.

VGC respond to membrane stretch over the same tension range[9,14] that activates stretch-activated potassium-selective channels (SAC_K) such as TREK[15] or the molecularly unidentified SAC_{CAT} mentioned earlier. Figure 4–1 *(bottom left)* illustrates recordings from oocyte membrane of the oocyte's endogenous SAC_{CAT} and a recombinant VGC. Both are activated by comparable stretch stimuli. "MscL," the bacterial osmotic valve channel, requires far *more* mechanical gating energy (~20 to 50 kT)[16]—an order of magnitude at least beyond the approximately 2 to 3 kT mechanical energy that dramatically increases Po in the prototypical VGC, *Shaker*[17] (T here is not tension but temperature; kT refers to thermal energy per molecule, i.e., to RT/[Avogadro's number]). Does this mean *Shaker* was designed as a highly specialized mechanotransducer and MscL was not? No. It means that the biological significance of mechanical gating energy is

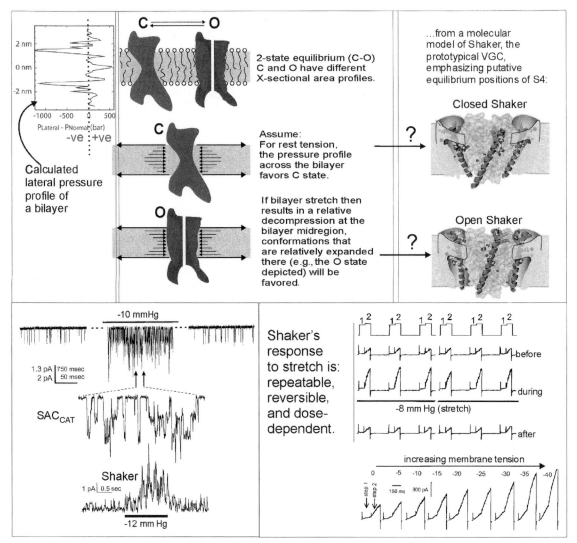

■ **Figure 4–1** Mechanosensitivity in *Shaker,* the prototypical voltage-gated channel (VGC). A lateral pressure profile from a molecular dynamics simulation[6] is aligned next to a sketch modified with permission from a Web page of R. Cantor, who has emphasized how general anesthetics and lipid composition affect the bilayer pressure profile, and hence the conformational equilibria of embedded membrane proteins.[7] An equilibrium reaction between two different conformations of a membrane-embedded protein is depicted. The conformations differ in the membrane-spanning region of the protein (e.g., *C* is smaller than *O* near mid-bilayer). Insofar as the different shapes of *C* and *O* make for different cross-sectional area profiles, *C* and *O* will be differentially favored whenever the lateral pressure profile of the bilayer changes. Bilayer stretch should change the lateral pressure profile, and hence the C-O equilibrium. *Far right,* Molecular models for closed and open *Shaker* channels (modified with permission from Ahern and Horn[8] with emphasis on the putative locations of the voltage sensor regions of the channel); note the shape differences in the part of the channel embedded in the bilayer. The two *bottom boxes* are extracted from Gu and colleagues.[9]

entirely specific to its context: Whereas the bacterial lifestyle routinely generates 20 to 50 kT mechanical gating energy for MscL channels (near-lytic membrane distension during osmotic swelling), 2 to 3 kT mechanical gating energy may seldom be experienced by *Shaker*-type channels in their native environments. If MscL responded to the moderate levels of bilayer tension that gate *Shaker*, it could not act as a safety valve, but it would cause the cell to continually leak. *Shaker's* gate (and probably that of other VGC) is kept closed by several kT (units of thermal energy per molecule) of conformational energy,[18] and although electrical energy (depolarization) is the normal source of energy for opening the channel, mechanical energy (bilayer stretch) also can appreciably increase the open probability of *Shaker* (see Fig. 4–1, *bottom right*). Note that stretch acts reversibly and in a dose-dependent fashion, as expected if stretch simply perturbs the normal equilibrium among closed and open states.

MECHANOSENSITIVITY OF VOLTAGE-GATED CHANNELS IN CARDIAC MYOCYTES

Cardiac cells deploy voltage-gated calcium (VGC_{Ca}), sodium, potassium, and cation-permeant (pacemaker) channels. The mechanosensitivity of L-type Ca^{2+} channels has been compellingly demonstrated in whole-cell recordings of rabbit atrial and sinoatrial node cells[3] (Fig. 4–2, *bottom*). Comparable mechanically enhanced L-type responses have been reported for many smooth muscle preparations,[19,20] including intact myocytes monitored by perforated patch, with bath perfusion (shear) as the mechanical stimulus.[21] As Matsuda and colleagues[3] point out, neither SAC_{CAT} nor mechanosensitive delayed rectifier or pacemaker currents were evident in their data (Fig. 4–3). The test conditions were, however, not optimal for observing the contributions from these channels (see Fig. 4–3), so this may not be the last word on those conductances. However, in another report,[22] delayed rectifier currents of guinea pig ventricular myocytes (reported as mechanosensitive in vascular endothelial cells) increased activity with osmotic swelling, but they were not consistently affected by whole-cell inflation. The L-type Ca^{2+} current in this preparation showed no

consistent response to either stimulus,[22] and Belus and White[23] found L-type current in ventricular myocytes to be insensitive to stretch. In smooth muscle,[21] both hydrostatic swelling and osmotic swelling augment L-type current, but it should be recalled that these do not represent identical stimuli (see Chapter 1).

Voltage-Gated Calcium Channels

Figure 4–2 shows mechanosensitive current through two types of recombinant VGC_{Ca} channels: N-type and L-type. Below that are data on native L-type current (rabbit sinoatrial myocytes). The results are encouragingly consistent among these preparations. Recombinant N- and L-type channels respond similarly to mechanical stimuli (increased peak current at all voltages, no detectable shift of I-V relations). For both N- and L-types, the stretch effect can be attributed to the α-subunit alone because it persists in the absence of coexpressed auxiliary subunits. We predict that the mechanosensitivity of cardiac L-type channel also will reside in the α-subunit.

N-type data are featured in Figure 4–2 because more aspects of VGC_{Ca} channel mechanosensitivity have been examined there than for L-type channels. Notably, with the membrane voltage clamped to a typical action potential waveform (as opposed to using step depolarizations), stretch reversibly increases the current with each spike (bottom of N-type section). Similar experiments are needed for L-type current in myocytes. Meanwhile, on the basis of N-type channel data, it could be expected that when a freely firing cardiomyocyte is stretched in situ, this could appreciably augment beat-to-beat variations in $[Ca^{2+}]_i$. Urgent questions include: Does sufficient stretch occur? If yes, over what parts of the sarcolemma does it occur? Unfortunately, membrane dyes that report on bilayer tension do not exist to noninvasively do for membrane mechanics what voltage dyes have done for the membrane potentials of cardiomyocyte arrays.[24]

To assess the role of L-type calcium channel mechanosensitivity during the cardiac action potential, further studies on Ca^{2+} signals and contractility, such as those of Yasuda and colleagues,[26] may help. When stretch reversibly increases the N-type peak current, it also accelerates the rate of inactivation[14]; if this applied

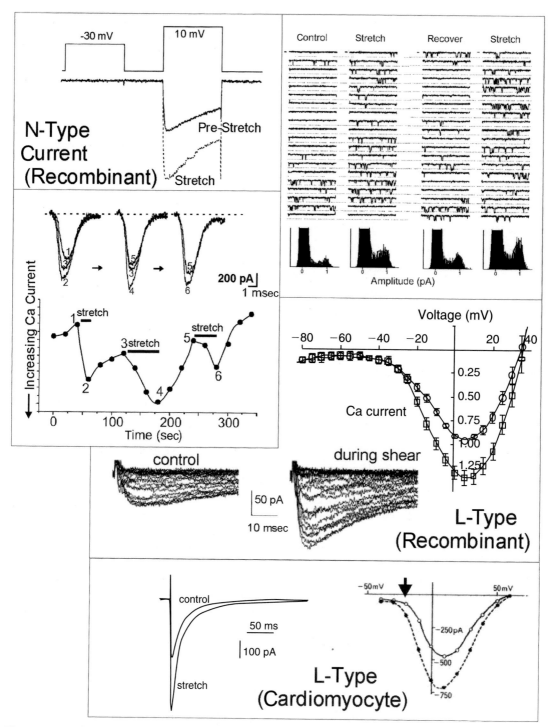

■ **Figure 4–2**   Mechanosensitivity of recombinant and native voltage-gated calcium channels. The N-type data are reprinted with some additional labels from Calabrese and colleagues.[14] Recombinant L-type current data are from Lyford and colleagues,[25] and the native current data are redrawn from Matsuda and colleagues.[3] See Figure 4–4 for discussion of *arrow*.

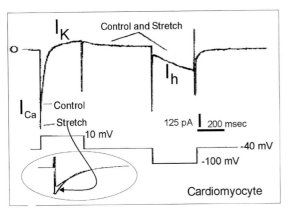

■ **Figure 4–3** Differential mechanosensitivities for voltage-gated channels in rabbit cardiomyocytes. Overlaid control and stretch traces are redrawn from Matsuda and colleagues[3]; an amplitude-compressed, time-expanded inset displays L-type I_{Ca} with and without stretch. The delayed rectifier (I_K) and pacemaker current (I_h) were unchanged in response to the same stretch that augmented L-type I_{Ca}. However, before ruling out stretch effects on I_h and I_K, it would be necessary to do tests at voltages nearer the foot of the activation curve for each.[9,14,42] Matsuda and colleagues[3] note that no SAC_{CAT} current was evident, based on having also used 50 mM Ca solutions. SAC_{CAT} has a low conductance in high Ca^{2+}, this would yield only small SAC_{CAT} currents (see Reference 27).

to L-type Ca^{2+} currents (inspection of traces in Matsuda and colleagues[3] leaves this unresolved; compare Figs. 4–2 and 4–3), it could help explain how so-called unloaded shortening protocols in rat cardiomyocytes increase peak $[Ca^{2+}]_i$ transients and accelerate their decay.[26] As Yasuda and colleagues[26] point out, the possibility that acute changes in cell stretch during this type of contractility experiment elicit mechanosensitive responses from L-type channels needs to be tested.

Other Voltage-Gated Channels Worthy of Attention

The cardiac sodium channel isoform, $Na_v1.5$, also is found in some smooth muscles. $Na_v1.5$ current in interstitial cells of Cajal (a smooth muscle cell type) increases with shear stress, possibly indicating mechanosensitivity.[28,29] Unlike VGC_{Ca} channels, however, these $Na_v1.5$ responses to shear have not been

checked against conditions where it is quite certain that membrane stretch is the operative stimulus (e.g., whole-cell inflation or patches subjected to stretch). Flow-induced effects on currents can be the secondary consequences of phenomena such as shear-induced adenosine triphosphate release or the washout of autocrine inhibitors.

If the α-subunit of the skeletal muscle sodium channel isoform ($Na_v1.4$) is subjected to membrane stretch, it irreversibly switches to fast-mode gating, accompanied by a left-shift in the voltage curves.[30,31] Intriguingly, this action of stretch is identical to that of coexpressing the α-subunit with auxiliary β-subunits. Even more intriguingly, β-subunits of Na_v channels are, in part, cell adhesion molecules.[32] Whether $Na_v1.5$ α-subunits show comparable mechanosensitivity is unknown. However, the correspondences between $Na_v1.5$ and $Na_v1.4$ behavior with or without β-subunits[33] suggest this needs checking. This is especially important because $Na_v1.5$ α-subunits may insert into the sarcolemma with a partial complement of β-subunits. Human cardiac α-subunits acquire $β_1$ but not $β_2$ in the endoplasmic reticulum[34]; therefore, newly inserted channels may be briefly β deficient. If this leaves them vulnerable to irreversible stretch-induced changes in gating, either in the endoplasmic reticulum (where ryanodine receptors, a variant of VGC_{Ca}, are reported to be mechanosensitive[35]) or the sarcolemma, the consequences could be significant.

We have begun to study recombinant pacemaker channels (hyperpolarization-activated cyclic nucleotide-gated, or HCN, channels) through macroscopic currents in cell-attached *Xenopus* oocyte patches (before, during, and after stretch). The HCN current is cation-selective and inwardly rectifying. It has a tiny unitary conductance and is generally evident only at substantially hyperpolarized voltages. Our preliminary finding (C. Morris, U. Laitke, W. Lin, unpublished results) is that the HCN current increases with stretch. What relation this bears to the hyperpolarization-activated, stretch-activated cation channel (an unidentified large unitary conductance channel) reported by Hisada and colleagues[36] for smooth muscle is unknown. Ventricular myocytes express two HCN isoforms,[37] and they also exhibit an inwardly rectifying, swelling-activated cation current that has tentatively been ascribed to SAC_{CAT} on the basis of toxin sensitivity.[38] Because SAC_{CAT} never turn up in single-channel recordings from these cells, it would be good to rule out pacemaker channel contributions to the swelling-activated ventricular myocyte current.

PROSPECTS

To rigorously test hypotheses about the mechanophysiology of VGC in heart, the underlying molecular biophysics must be clarified. If auxiliary subunits or particular subregions of the channels affect heart VGC mechanosensitivity, it may be possible to minimize, exaggerate, or otherwise manipulate stretch modulation of the VGC, whereas preserving their voltage-gating. Appropriately altered channel constructs could then be generated for physiopathologic testing in transgenic native cells, cardiomyocyte cell lines, or both. For L-type calcium channels, transgenic mouse approaches are possible,[39] but the literature suggests there would be daunting challenges. The prospects seem better for pacemaker channels, because the roles of HCN isoforms in targeted knockout mice and in sinoatrial cells isolated from these animals are published.[40]

If VGC mechanosensitivity turns out to be at least partially localized to a channel subregion, it would be fruitful to monitor, in mammalian cell lines, the mechanical behavior of minimal or chimeric recombinants (see Altier and colleagues[41] for discussion of L-type VGC$_{Ca}$ channels). However, no such mechanical gate may exist. For *Shaker* channels, voltage-dependent gating appears to be inherently mechanosensitive, as if the channel must expand in the bilayer whenever its voltage sensors move in response to membrane depolarization.[42]

Selectively ablating mechanosensitivity from VGC may or may not be possible, but focusing on voltage ranges where stretch and depolarization make energetically comparable contributions in myocytes is likely to provide insight about the possible physiologic significance of VGC mechanosensitivity. Figure 4–4 illustrates, for a *Shaker* mutant studied in oocyte membrane, what is meant by the range where stretch and depolarization are energetically similar. The membrane is stepped to a subthreshold potential (see *asterisks* in Fig. 4–4) that rarely opens a channel. Then membrane is stretched, and the same step elicits a macroscopic current. Comparable experiments have not been feasi-

ble for recombinant L-type current because blockers of oocyte SAC$_{CAT}$ also block L-type current. Cardiac myocytes, however, can be clamped by a perforated patch and mechanostimulated through carbon fiber pairs in the presence and absence of a dihydropyridine blocker of L-type current. Obtaining stretch-induced dihydropyridine-sensitive current from such a preparation during steps to voltages that without stretch are subthreshold would demonstrate the possible impacts of stretch on L-type current during the myocyte action potential.

CONCLUSIONS

In the context of cardiomyocytes, the term *mechanosensitive channel* should be used as a broad descriptor that includes some or all of the VGC. Currently, a reasonable hypothesis is that macroscopic mechanosensitive currents in cardiomyocytes arise from the combined susceptibilities to stretch of many channels, including unidentified non-VGC plus voltage-gated calcium, potassium, sodium, and pacemaker channels. Although VGC are mechanosensitive in native or recombinant systems, or both, it is unknown if there are physiologic or pathophysiologic consequences. What is incontrovertible is that the membrane tensions needed to augment VGC$_{Ca}$ channel activity or to accelerate voltage-gated potassium channel activation are no different from those needed to gate unitary SAC$_{CAT}$ and SAC$_K$ events. Moreover, many VGC are demonstrably present in adult cardiac sarcolemma, unlike SAC$_{CAT}$, which have been assiduously sought but not found.

Beyond that, there is confusion. Sinoatrial, but not ventricular, myocytes show mechanosensitive L-type current, although both express L-type channels in abundance. The laboratory reporting mechanosensitive L-type current detected no mechanosensitive cation current and observed no effects on other VGC. Because Ca^{2+} channel pore subunits (recombinant L- and N-type) are robustly mechanosensitive, the sinoatrial node L-type channel mechanosensitivity cannot be dismissed as an artifact. One might conclude that ventricular myocyte membrane channels are protected from stretch were it not that another laboratory reported macroscopic currents tentatively attributed to SAC$_{CAT}$.

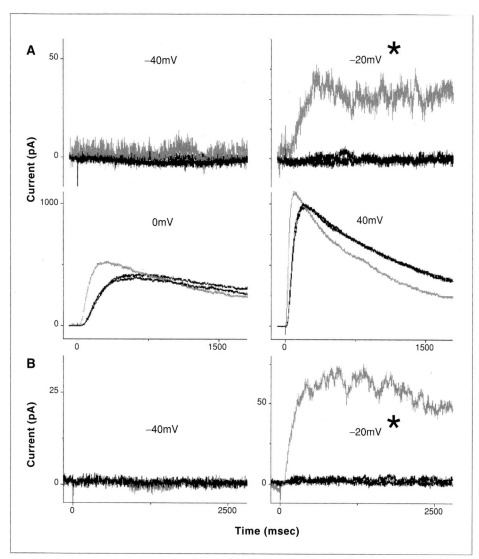

■ **Figure 4–4** Mechanosensitive responses near the foot of the activation curve. Before, during, and after stretch data sets *A* and *B* are for a mutant *Shaker* activation and inactivation both accelerate with stretch (reprinted from Laitko and Morris[42]). Data illustrate that there is a voltage range near the foot of the activation curve (close to −20 mV for this mutant) where stretch with depolarization elicits current when depolarization alone cannot. Based on the foot of the I-V relation of Figure 4-2 (see *arrow* added to that figure), similar responses for L-type current may occur in myocytes. This is worth closer scrutiny because during action potentials, proportionally the largest stretch-augmented I_{Ca} may occur before the upswing of voltage, generating a mechanically amplified positive feedback current.

The postulate that VGC contribute to MEF is undercut by reports that a pentavalent spider toxin blocks stretch-induced atrial defibrillation and a macroscopic ventricular swelling-activated cation cur-

rent, but has no discernible effect on cardiac action potentials. Deepening the conundrum further, however, the electrophysiologically characterized action of this toxin is to inhibit SAC_{CAT} channels, and these have not yet been found in adult mammalian cardiomyocytes.

More data are needed from experiments on cardiomyocytes. Especially valuable would be action potential clamp of, for example, sinoatrial node cells before, during, and after cell stretch, especially if stretch-dose data could be obtained. Then, as VGC mechanosensitivity is characterized biophysically (e.g., for recombinant pacemaker channels), the cardiomyocyte action potential clamp data would provide a particularly meaningful reference framework. It would provide a way to test the scope of the biophysically characterized mechanical effects in well-developed mathematical models of cell-specific cardiac action potentials.

The current understanding of how diverse VGC fashion cardiac action potentials represents an enormous effort over many decades. The possibility that mechanical load alters the output of VGC was first raised about 10 years ago, and it began to be seriously addressed in recombinant VGC about 5 years ago. Although it may be problematic to establish with full precision how VGC mechanosensitivity modulates cardiac action potentials, it would be foolhardy to dismiss lightly the possibility that such modulation exists and has a role in MEF.

References

1. Kanzaki M, Nagasawa M, Kojima I, et al: Report clarification (re: 1999 Science 285:882–886) Science 288:1347, 2000.
2. Juranka PF, Haghighi AP, Gaertner T, et al: Molecular cloning and functional expression of Xenopus laevis oocyte ATP-activated P2X4 channels. Biochim Biophys Acta 1512: 111–124, 2001.
3. Matsuda N, Hagiwara N, Shoda M, et al: Enhancement of the L-type Ca^{2+} current by mechanical stimulation in single rabbit cardiac myocytes. Circ Res 78:650–659, 1996.
4. Morris CE, Juranka PF, Lin W, Laitko U: Studying the mechanosensitivity of voltage-gated channels using oocyte patches. In Liu XJ (ed): Xenopus Protocols: Cell Biology and Signal Transduction (Meth Mol Biol series). The Humana Press Inc. Tototwa, NJ, 2004 (In press).
5. Tillman T, Cascio M: Effects of membrane lipids on ion channel structure and function. Cell Biochem Biophys 38:161–190, 2003.
6. Gullingsrud J, Schulten K: Gating of MscL studied by steered molecular dynamics. Biophys J 85:2087–2099, 2003.
7. Cantor RS: The influence of membrane lateral pressures on simple geometric models of protein conformational equilibria. Chem Phys Lipids 101:45–56, 1999.
8. Ahern CA, Horn R: Specificity of charge-carrying residues in the voltage sensor of potassium channels. J Gen Physiol 123:205–216, 2004.
9. Gu CX, Juranka PF, Morris CE: Stretch-activation and stretch-inactivation of Shaker-IR, a voltage-gated K+ channel. Biophys J 80:2678–2693, 2001.
10. Sachs F, Morris CE: Mechanosensitive ion channels in nonspecialized cells. Rev Physiol Biochem Pharmacol 132:1–77, 1998.
11. Morris CE: Mechanosensitive ion channels in eukaryotic cells. In Sperelakis N (ed): Cell Physiology Source Book, 3rd ed. San Diego, Academic Press, 2001, pp 745–760.
12. Hamill OP, Martinac B: Molecular basis of mechanotransduction in living cells. Physiol Rev 81:685–740, 2001.
13. Morris CE: Mechanoprotection of the plasma membrane in neurons and other non-erythroid cells by the spectrin-based membrane skeleton. Cell Mol Biol Lett 6:703–720, 2001.
14. Calabrese B, Tabarean I, Juranka P, Morris CE: Mechanosensitivity of N-type calcium channel currents. Biophys J 83:2560–2574, 2002.
15. Patel AJ, Lazdunski M, Honore E: Lipid and mechano-gated 2P domain K(+) channels. Curr Opin Cell Biol 13:422–428, 2001.
16. Chiang CS, Anishkin A, Sukharev S: Gating of the large mechanosensitive channel in situ: Estimation of the spatial scale of the transition from channel population responses. Biophys J 86:2846–2861, 2004.
17. Tabarean IV, Morris CE: Membrane stretch accelerates activation and slow inactivation in Shaker channels with S3-S4 linker deletions. Biophys J 82:2982–2994, 2002.
18. Yifrach O, MacKinnon R: Energetics of pore opening in a voltage-gated K(+) channel. Cell 111:231–239, 2002.
19. Langton PD: Calcium channel currents recorded from isolated myocytes of rat basilar artery are stretch sensitive. J Physiol 471:1–11, 1993.
20. Holm AN, Rich A, Sarr MG, Farrugia G: Whole cell current and membrane potential regulation by a human smooth muscle mechanosensitive calcium channel. Am J Physiol 279: G1155–G1161, 2000.
21. Chang XF, Zeng YJ, Hu JL: Mechanosensitive channel currents recorded in rat brain microvascular endothelial cells with whole-cell mode. Sheng Wu Hua Xue Yu Sheng Wu Wu Li Xue Bao (Shanghai). 32:529–532, 2000.
22. Sasaki N, Mitsuiye T, Noma A: Effects of mechanical stretch on membrane currents of single ventricular myocytes of guinea-pig heart. Jpn J Physiol 42:957–970, 1992.
23. Belus A, White E: Streptomycin and intracellular calcium modulate the response of single guinea-pig ventricular myocytes to axial stretch. J Physiol 546:501–509, 2003.
24. Rohr S, Salzberg BM: Characterization of impulse propagation at the microscopic level across geometrically defined expansions of excitable tissue: Multiple site optical recording of transmembrane voltage (MSORTV) in patterned growth heart cell cultures. J Gen Physiol 104:287–309, 1994.
25. Lyford GL, Strege PR, Shepard A, et al: •(1C) (Ca(V)1.2) L-type calcium channel mediates mechanosensitive calcium regulation. Am J Physiol 283:C1001–1008, 2002.
26. Yasuda S, Sugiura S, Yamashita H, et al: Unloaded shortening increases peak of Ca2+ transients but accelerates their decay in rat single cardiac myocytes. Am J Physiol 285:H470–H475, 2003.
27. Yang XC, Sachs F: Block of stretch-activated ion channels in Xenopus oocytes by gadolinium and calcium ions. Science 243:1068–1071, 1989.
28. Strege PR, Holm AN, Rich A, et al: Cytoskeletal modulation of sodium current in human jejunal circular smooth muscle cells. Am J Physiol 284:C60–C66, 2003.

29. Strege PR, Ou Y, Sha L, et al: Sodium current in human intestinal interstitial cells of Cajal. Am J Physiol 285:G1111–G1121, 2003.

30. Tabarean IV, Juranka P, Morris CE: Membrane stretch affects gating modes of a skeletal muscle sodium channel. Biophys J 77:758–774, 1999.

31. Shcherbatko A, Ono F, Mandel G, Brehm P: Voltage-dependent sodium channel function is regulated through membrane mechanics. Biophys J 77:1945–1959, 1999.

32. Isom LL: The role of sodium channels in cell adhesion. Front Biosci 7:12–23, 2002.

33. Baroudi G, Carbonneau E, Pouliot V, Chahine M: SCN5A mutation (T1620M) causing Brugada syndrome exhibits different phenotypes when expressed in Xenopus oocytes and mammalian cells. FEBS Lett 467:12–16, 2000.

34. Zimmer T, Biskup C, Bollensdorff C, Benndorf K: The beta1 subunit but not the beta2 subunit colocalizes with the human heart Na+ channel (hH1) already within the endoplasmic reticulum. J Membr Biol 186:13–21, 2002.

35. Ji G, Barsotti RJ, Feldman ME, Kotlikoff MI: Stretch-induced calcium release in smooth muscle. J Gen Physiol 119:533–544, 2002.

36. Hisada T, Ordway RW, Kirber MT, et al: Hyperpolarization-activated cationic channels in smooth muscle cells are stretch sensitive. Pflugers Arch 417:493–499, 1991.

37. Fernandez-Velasco M, Goren N, Benito G, et al: Regional distribution of hyperpolarization-activated current (If) and hyperpolarization-activated cyclic nucleotide-gated channel mRNA expression in ventricular cells from control and hypertrophied rat hearts. J Physiol 553:395–405, 2003.

38. Suchyna TM, Johnson JH, Hamer K, et al: Identification of a peptide toxin from Grammostola spatulata spider venom that blocks cation-selective stretch-activated channels. J Gen Physiol 115:583–598, 2000.

39. Song LS, Guia A, Muth JN, et al: Ca(2+) signaling in cardiac myocytes overexpressing the alpha(1) subunit of L-type Ca(2+) channel. Circ Res 90:174–181, 2002.

40. Stieber J, Herrmann S, Feil S, et al: The hyperpolarization-activated channel HCN4 is required for the generation of pacemaker action potentials in the embryonic heart. Proc Natl Acad Sci USA 100:15235–15240, 2003.

41. Altier C, Spaetgens RL, Nargeot J, et al: Multiple structural elements contribute to voltage-dependent facilitation of neuronal alpha 1C (CaV1.2) L-type calcium channels. Neuropharmacology 40:1050–1057, 2001.

42. Laitko U, Morris CE: Membrane tension accelerates rate-limiting voltage-dependent activation and slow inactivation steps in a shaker channel. J Gen Physiol 123:135–154, 2004.

CHAPTER 5

Membrane–Cytoskeleton Interface and Mechanosensitive Channels

• • • •

Thomas M. Suchyna and Frederick Sachs

Mechanosensitive channel (MSC) activity has been implicated in cardiac arrhythmias and other pathologies. MSC gating is controlled primarily by the mechanical properties of the membrane in which it is embedded. Unlike voltage- and ligand-gated channels, MSC function is highly dependent on the local "mechano-physical" environment. The mechanical properties of the membrane are modulated by its lipid composition and its interaction with the cytoskeleton and extracellular matrix (ECM). The attachments among cells in a tissue and stress in the tissue affect the membrane–cytoskeleton interaction and the cytoskeletal and ECM architecture.

Unfortunately, much of our understanding of the functional role of vertebrate MSC comes not from tissue studies, but from experiments on isolated cells where cytoskeletal architecture is affected by adherence to a rigid substrate such as a coverslip. Furthermore, single-channel gating properties have been investigated in membrane patches that are always exposed to unphysiologic stresses by adherence to the glass walls of the pipette. Detailed knowledge of the mechanics of the channels, the lipids, the cytoskeleton, and the ECM are necessary to obtain a better understanding of MSC function.

Before delving into the structure of the plasma membrane–cytoskeleton interface, it is helpful to review the basic physical properties of lipid membranes (see the next section). The following sections focus on the membrane–cytoskeleton interaction as a composite structure, exogenous agents that perturb this structure, and their effects on MSC gating.

MECHANICAL PROPERTIES OF A HOMOGENEOUS MEMBRANE

There are two categories of MSC: those activated by tension transmitted through an associated protein tether,[1] and those activated by the tension developed in the surrounding bilayer.[2] This chapter focuses mainly on the mechanical and gating properties of the latter category.

The lipid bilayer can be described as a two-dimensional fluid in which all channels are embedded and around which all supporting components of the cortical cytoskeleton (CSK) and ECM are arranged. A channel sensitive to bilayer tension will be intimately linked to the dynamic mechanical responses of the membrane. There are four major modes of deformation in a naked bilayer, as shown in Figure 5–1.

A fifth mode of deformation is membrane compression. Like most liquids, the membrane is relatively incompressible (10^9 to 10^{10} N/m^2; see Reference 3); therefore, this mode of deformation is not likely to be important under most physiologic conditions. The common assumption is that the lipid membrane is a constant-volume structure. Membranes will resist stretching because of the high surface tension of the polar lipid interface (~70 mN/m) that keeps head groups tightly packed (see Fig. 5–1, mode 1). The maximum area strain ($\Delta A/A$) that a lipid membrane can withstand in steady state without lysis is less than 4%.[4] To maintain constant volume, the membrane area change must be compensated by an appropriate decrease in thickness (~3.6% at the lytic tension). For small deformations (as in a Hookean spring), a linear relation exists between the membrane tension (T) and the area strain: $T = K_A \cdot \Delta A/A$, where K_A is the area expansion modulus (10^2 to 10^3 mN/m for biologic membranes), ΔA is the change in area, and A is the initial area. Membrane expansion occurs during hypotonic swelling and during pressure changes applied to membranes in a patch pipette. Later in this chapter we describe a method for measuring changes in membrane capacitance to estimate the change in area

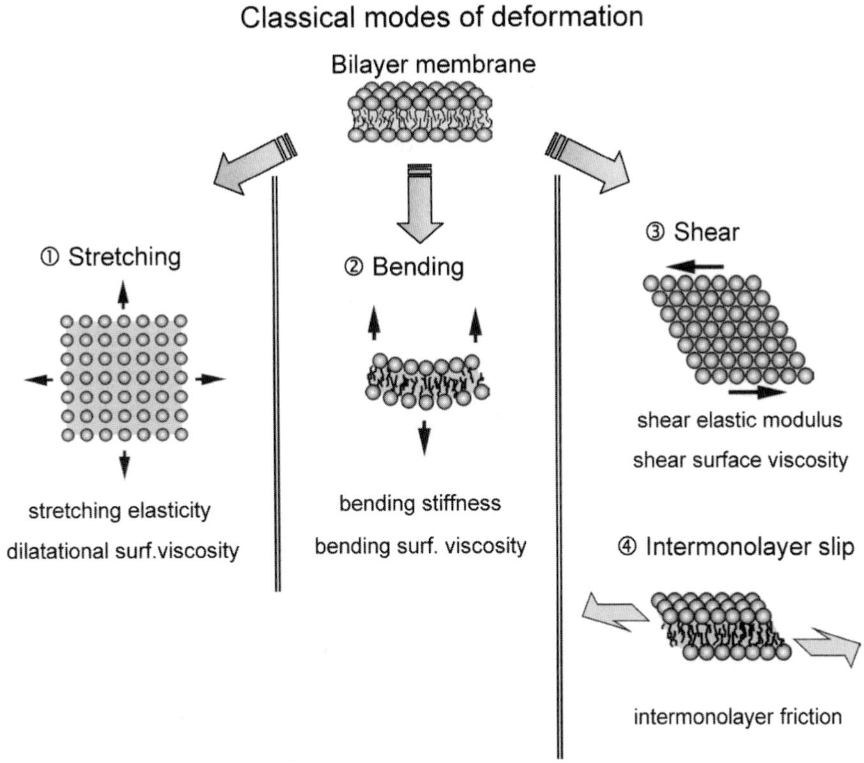

Classical modes of deformation

Bilayer membrane

① Stretching

stretching elasticity
dilatational surf.viscosity

② Bending

bending stiffness
bending surf. viscosity

③ Shear

shear elastic modulus
shear surface viscosity

④ Intermonolayer slip

intermonolayer friction

■ **Figure 5–1** Four physiologically relevant modes of deformation that may affect mechanosensitive channel gating. *(Courtesy Rumiana Dimova, Lipids and Membrane Mechanics, Max Planck Institute of Colloids and Interfaces, Golm; http://www.mpikg-golm.mpg.de/th/people/dimova/courses/handouts/l3handouts.pdf)*

that occurs when a patch is stretched. For a constant volume membrane, the change in capacitance with stretch is twice the change in area because the thickness must decrease.

The membrane can resist bending (see Fig. 5–1, mode 2), because membrane curvature causes stretching of one monolayer and compression of the other. However, the energy to bend a bilayer is so small that unsupported bilayers (and red cells) undergo large fluctuations in curvature. Membranes also have a natural curvature because of differences in the area occupied by the head groups and the acyl chains[5] (see "Membrane Modifiers: Amphipaths, Polyvalent Cations, and Peptides"). The bending stiffness depends on the degree of coupling, or shear between the bilayers (see Fig. 5–1, mode 4, intermonolayer slip). The viscous drag may be negligible for slow deformations, but it can have large dynamic effects.[6]

All of the deformations in Figure 5–1 are sensitive to the concentration of cholesterol, the degree of saturation, the length of acyl chains,[7–9] and the physical characteristics of the head groups. The shear and bending rigidity increase as cholesterol concentration, lipid saturation, and chain length increase. Components such as saturated sphingolipids may aggregate (into a new phase), forming ordered domains called rafts.[10] Rafts and membrane strain are important in the formation of caveolae.[11,12] Proteins adjacent to or within rafts will experience different mechanical stresses from those in the fluid portions of the membrane. In addition, interaction of the bilayer with the cytoskeleton can significantly increase the shear and bending rigidity (see "Mechanics of Heterogeneous Membranes: Cortical Cytoskeleton Support").

For a channel to respond robustly to membrane stress, it must undergo a significant change in dimensions between the closed and open states (see Chapter 1 and Reference 13). Figure 5–2A shows the major types of conformational changes that a channel may undergo during a transition between the closed and open states. The general forces that are generated in a two-dimensional bilayer and lead to the channel conformational changes in Figure 5–2A are summarized in Figure 5–2B. Far-field membrane tension—that is, stretch-ing—favors states that are larger in area, where the energy change is proportional to the area of the channel (the square of a linear dimension; see Fig. 5–2A, label a). There also is interfacial line tension between the channel and the surrounding boundary lipids that is proportional to the perimeter of the channel. As with the change in area under tension, large perimeters are favored over small perimeters, but this effect is lin-

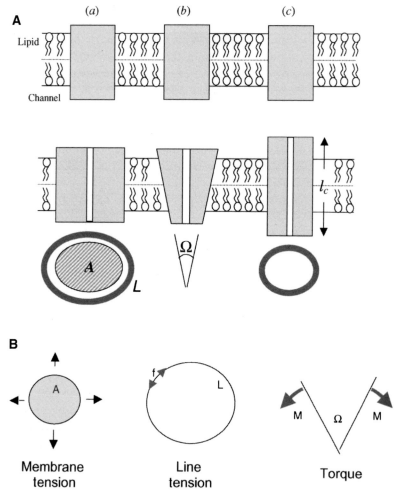

■ **Figure 5–2**   A, Three basic types of mechanosensitive channel (MSC) deformation during transition between closed and open states. a, A change of area A occupied by the channel in plane of the membrane also changes the length L of the border between the channel complex and surrounding lipid where the line tension f resides; the "shape" of the complex does not change. b, A change of shape of the MSC expressed as a body angle Ω; average in-plane area of the complex does not change. c, Change of the length l_c of the MS complex normal to the membrane; it can lead to changes in line tension f at the border with lipid. B, Generalized forces (membrane tension, line tension, and torque) that lead to the conformational changes shown in A. (From Markin VS, Sachs F: Thermodynamics of mechanosensitivity: Lipid shape, membrane deformation and anesthesia. Biophysical J 86:370A, 2004, with permission.)

ear to the channel dimensions. Line tension is produced by the difference in area expansion modules between the protein channel and the surrounding lipids. Line tension reflects all of the physical chemical properties of the bilayer such as thickness, bending rigidity, hydrophobic mismatch with the channel, and other properties. The corresponding decrease in membrane thickness that occurs during stretching also can create a hydrophobic mismatch between the transmembrane domains and the boundary lipids that could induce a conformational change (see Fig. 5–2A, label c).

In addition to the area and linear strains, membrane curvature (spontaneous or pressure induced) can produce transmembrane torque on the channel (see Fig. 5–2A, label b).

The channel conformational changes and the membrane forces that produce them that are most relevant to the open probability (Po) of eukaryotic MSC is a major focus of current research.

MECHANICS OF HETEROGENEOUS MEMBRANES: CORTICAL CYTOSKELETON SUPPORT

The bilayer and CSK should be considered a composite structure. The physical modes of deformation described earlier are either intensified or buffered depending on the strength and arrangement of the membrane's interaction with the CSK. Thus, stretch-activated channel gating properties (activation and inactivation) are dependent on the strength of interaction between the CSK and membrane.[14-16] The cortical CSK is a thin (200 nm; see Reference 17) protein lattice that provides support and governs the interaction of the membrane with the deeper cytoskeleton. Adhesion of the CSK to the membrane creates a mechanical composite with increased bending modulus and shear rigidity.[4]

For example, red blood cells have no deep cytoskeleton, only the cortical CSK that increases the elastic shear modulus to 10^{-2} mN/m. Thus, unlike homogeneous lipid bilayers, red blood cells recover rapidly from large extensions.[18] In addition, the higher bending modulus affects the spontaneous curvature so that red blood cells are resistant to nar-

row neck budding of spicules.[19] The CSK also strengthens their membrane, which otherwise would be broken into vesicles in the normal circulatory shear flow.

In isolated adherent cells, there are only a few strong focal adhesion attachment sites confined to discrete cell–cell and cell–ECM binding sites. On the nonadherent surfaces, strong focal adhesion attachments have a density of only 0.2 to 1 μm^2.[20] The bulk of membrane–CSK adhesions are rapid, dynamic processes where the bonds re-form continuously.[21]

Bilayer adhesion to the CSK has been investigated by measuring the amount of force necessary to pull a bilayer tether away from a cell. The calculated adhesion energy density of fibroblasts is relatively small ($\sim 9.1 \times 10^{-19}$ J/μm^2), corresponding to a few hundred binding interactions per μm^2.[22] Thus, bilayer deformations are controlled primarily by many weak protein–lipid surface interactions, with different domains experiencing different amounts of stress depending on the degree of cytoskeletal adhesion and the rate of change of stress.[15] However, it is important to recall that, in general, biologic membranes are fluid, so there can be no tension gradients at equilibrium.

CSK interactions with the membrane are facilitated by a web of membrane-associated proteins (e.g., integrins, small GTPases, dystroglycan) and fibrous elements (e.g., spectroplakins, Ezrin-Radixin-Moesin [ERM] proteins, vinculin) that cross-link the membrane-bound components to the major filamentous proteins. A number of molecular signaling agents affect the strength of this interaction: phosphatidylinositol 4,5-bisphosphate (PIP2), lysophosphatidic acid, Ca^{2+}, and intermembrane receptor kinases that are activated by external signals.[22-24] PIP2 is central to controlling dynamic membrane–cytoskeletal interactions such as membrane ruffling and filopodia extensions, and the formation of more permanent structures such as microvilli and focal adhesions.[25] Increased levels of PIP2 increase membrane–cytoskeleton adhesion energy and strengthen the CSK by recruiting proteins for actin cross-linking, bundling, nucleating, and capping. Most of the cytoskeletal proteins that associate with the membrane have cationic binding sites that favorably interact with the negatively charged PIP2 lipids.

The CSK cross-linking proteins are especially important elements in the regulation of MSC gating properties. They localize ion channels and transporters, and their rodlike structure contains flexible domains that allow them to absorb mechanical stress.[26,27] They also are critical components for formation and stabilization of structures such as caveolae, microvilli, T-tubules, and costameres. These macroscopic structures may have physical properties that focus or buffer mechanical forces transmitted to channels. In particular, two families of cross-linking proteins, spectraplakins and ERM, have been reported to interact with various channels and transporters, either directly or through auxiliary subunits.

COSTAMERIC MEMBRANES AND T-TUBULES

The costameric/T-tubule system, present in both skeletal and cardiac muscle cells, is a region of cytoskeletal—membrane interaction that illustrates many of the concepts described earlier. Costameres are regions rich in CSK cross-linking proteins (spectrin, dystrophin, titin) located at the Z-lines (Fig. 5–3). They have strong adhesion to the sarcolemma and the ECM.[28] The sarcolemma in the intercostameric regions is weakly attached to the CSK and balloons outward during muscle contraction.

Costamere interaction among adjacent muscle fibers acts to distribute forces laterally among the fibers. In skeletal muscle cells, dystrophin colocalizes with costameres[29] and is responsible for the tight adhesion between the costameric proteins and the sarcolemma.[30] In dystrophin-deficient muscle cells, the membrane–costamere adherence is much weaker and the shear elasticity of the membrane is significantly less,[31] leading to membrane microlesions and hyperactive MSC.[14] In the heart, dystrophin is not localized to the costameres,[32] but rather mutations that specifically disrupt dystrophin in the heart and lead to weakening of the ventricular wall and dilated cardiomyopathy.[33]

Titin is another member of the spectraplakin family that, because of its functional interactions and its location in the sarcomere, plays an important regulatory role in mechanical deformation of the sarcolemma. Titin has multiple isoforms of variable length depending on the muscle in which it is expressed.[34] It is a huge rod-shaped protein that connects the costameres (Z-disks) to the I-bands and functions as a molecular ruler for sarcomere length (see Fig. 28–4A). It has numerous spectrin repeats that can reversibly unfold to absorb excess stress between the contractile apparatus and membrane during overload.

Titin interacts with KvLQT1 channels and localizes them to the T-tubules.[35] KvLQT1 may be mechanically sensitive[36] (see Chapter 3), and titin may be the mechanical link that affects KvLQT1 gating through its interactions with the auxiliary channel subunits MinK and T-cap (see Fig. 28–4B).

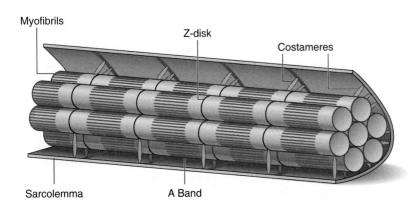

Myofibrils

Z-disk

Costameres

Sarcolemma

A Band

■ **Figure 5–3** Structure and distribution of costameric elements (multiprotein cortical cytoskeleton complexes) around the Z-disks, at the location of T-tubules along muscle fibers.[28]

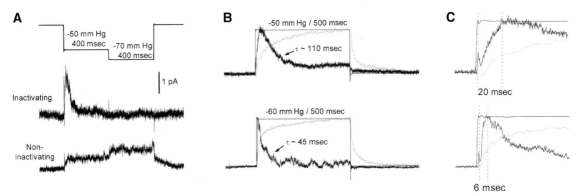

■ **Figure 5–4** MSC activation and inactivation analyzed with high-speed pressure stimuli and patch capacitance. *A,* The current from inactivated cation-selective MSC (MSC$_{CAT}$) does not respond to increased stimulus, but channels with a disrupted inactivation mechanism do respond. *B,* Average inactivating MSC$_{CAT}$ currents (black indicates normalized) shown for rat astrocytes *(top)* and chick heart cells *(bottom)* with the corresponding ΔC_p records (gray) and the pressure stimulus (square pulse). The patch potential is held at −90 mV in both cases. The kinetics of chick heart MSC inactivation and activation (*C,* expanded view) are approximately three times faster than those observed for astrocyte MSC. In both cases, the activation rate appears to roughly follow the rate of capacitance change, which again is more rapid in chick heart cell patches.

Costameres are located at the sites where T-tubules enter the fibers. T-tubule membranes have a high cholesterol content and high local curvature with a diameter of only 200 to 300 nm. The sarcolemma at the Z-line, and within the T-tubule system, contain most of the Ca^{2+} handling components (L-type Ca^{2+} channels, Na^+-Ca^{2+} and Na^+-H^+ exchangers) and many voltage-gated channels.[37] The strong cytoskeletal interactions, high cholesterol concentration, and titin's ability to absorb tension would suggest that channels in the T-tubule regions are "mechano-protected." In contrast, the intercostameric sarcolemma might be particularly mechanosensitive when subjected to high local curvature during contraction and to stretch when the resting sarcomere length is exceeded.

However, these assumptions about mechano-protected and mechanosensitive regions of the sarcolemma need to be treated with caution. The high curvature of T-tubules may place the channels under resting stress, and the tubules are in such intimate relation with the contractile apparatus that they may be highly stressed during contraction. Channel gating in the T-tubules may also be modulated by direct interaction with CSK elements. Finally, the sarcolemma is highly invaginated with caveolae that can increase in number or reversibly unfold when stretched.[12]

The question of how the ultrastructure of the membrane affects MSC gating has been a focus of investigation since Morris and Horn[38] raised the issue of seeing MSC currents in patches, but no equivalent whole-cell currents. In oocytes, MSC are easily observed in patches, but a variety of mechanical deformations did not produce significant whole-cell currents.[39] Zhang and colleagues[40] suggested that the excess membrane of microvilli in the intact oocyte were absent in the patch. The excess membrane area in the whole oocyte buffered the expected tension. However, they found that channels could be activated in blebs that lack CSK. The mechano-protection in situ could have been a result of excess membrane caused by folding or cytoskeletal buffering. In cardiac ventricular cells, the discrepancy is reversed where cation currents were recorded from adult rat cells,[41] but no single-channel currents were observed. It was proposed that MSC in adult cells are located in the T-tubules, and hence are inaccessible to pipettes. It also could be because of cytoskeletal disruption or strong mechano-protective properties.

GATING OF CATION-SELECTIVE MECHANOSENSITIVE CHANNELS: RELATION TO MEMBRANE TENSION AND CYTOSKELETAL INTEGRITY

Cation-selective MSC (MSC_{CAT}) are found in all tissues of the body. In the heart, excessive mechanical stress can activate these channels, leading to increased background and transient cytoplasmic Ca^{2+} levels.[42,43] MSC_{CAT} activation is followed by a rapid, voltage-sensitive, inactivation phase during a maintained pressure stimulus[16,44,45] (Fig. 5–4). Inactivation is a fundamental process of most channels that regulates the duration of the ionic signal and provides greater sensitivity to changing stimuli. It is important to examine the dynamic properties in studies of transduction because the steady-state response may have no relation to the dynamic response.[46] This applies to studies of pharmacologic agents as well. We have found that the inactivation mechanism is sensitive to cytoskeletal integrity. Mechanical or chemical disruption eliminates inactivation (Table 5–1).

In mammalian cells, the decline in activity with time is inactivation, not adaptation,[16] as suggested for amphibian and bacterial MSC.[45,47] This conclusion is based on two lines of evidence. First, the activation mechanism is more robust than the inactivation, so that activation can be separated from inactivation. Inactivating channels do not respond to an increase in stimulus intensity once they are inactivated (see Fig. 5–4A). However, noninactivating channels respond to the same stimulus with an increased Po.

Second, membrane capacitance will change as the membrane area or thickness changes. Using the relation between area change and tension, we can relate the change in capacitance to the area by $\Delta C / C = 2 \Delta A / A$, where ΔC is the change in capacitance, and C is the total capacitance. Using a phase lock amplifier, patch capacitance (C_p) could be tracked while measuring channel current.[16] This allowed correlation of the change in membrane area (change in patch capacitance: ΔC_p) in response to pressure with channel activity. The average patch current decreased, whereas patch area continued to increase (see Fig. 5–4B).

The kinetics of the phasic channel response is sensitive to voltage and to the membrane environment. Figure 5–4B and C compares the phasic response in chick cardiocytes and rat astrocytes. The channels in both systems show a voltage-sensitive, phasic response to pressure, are cation selective, sensitive to the same range of pressures, and have nearly identical unitary conductance and inward rectification (rat astrocyte: 1.25 pA at +50 mV / 1.75 pA at −50 mV; chick heart cells: 1.1 pA at +50 mV / 1.75 pA at −50 mV). Thus, although these channels are from different species, they appear to be the same ubiquitous channel that occurs in many vertebrate systems. The one significant difference between these channels is their rate of response to similar pressure stimuli. The chick heart channels inactivate (see Fig. 5–4B) and activate (see Fig. 5–4C) nearly three times faster than those in rat astrocytes (21°C). Interestingly, the chick heart membrane also responds to the pressure stimuli about three times faster, suggesting that the difference in rates is because of the membrane–cytoskeletal relaxation time rather

TABLE 5–1   Cation-Selective Mechanosensitive Channel Inactivation is lost when the Cytoskeleton is Disrupted in Adult Rat Astrocytes

	Patches (n)	Active MSC (n)	Showing inactivation (n)
Cell-attached untreated	123	41 (33%)	17
Outside-out	42	21 (50%)	1
Cell-attached acrylamide/colchicine/ cytochalasin D	36	17 (47%)	0

MSC, Mechanosensitive channel.
From Suchyna TM, Besch SD, Sachs F: Dynamic regulation of mechanosensitive channels; capacitance used to monitor patch tension in real time. *Physical Biology* 1:1–18, 2004, with permission.

than an inherent difference in channel structure. The cytoskeleton from chick heart cells appears more robust that that of astrocytes because outside-out patch formation does not usually disrupt the inactivation mechanism in cardiomyocytes as it does in astrocytes.

MEMBRANE MODIFIERS: AMPHIPATHS, POLYVALENT CATIONS, AND PEPTIDES

MSC are particularly sensitive to agents that modify the physical properties of the bilayer. Amphiphiles are chemicals with polar and apolar regions. The physical–chemical characteristics of an amphiphile dictate how it partitions into the bilayer and determine its effect on membrane spontaneous curvature, thickness, and stiffness.[48] Exogenous amphiphiles may produce complex phase separations in association with, or separate from, the endogenous components. In addition to modifying membrane mechanical properties, exogenous amphiphiles can show distinct interactions with integral membrane proteins.

Amphipath activity is determined by shape (conical or cylindrical), charge, and dimensions of the hydrophobic region. If the amphipath has a hydrophobic:hydrophilic area ratio $\neq 1$, it will be approximately conical, and its insertion into a bilayer will create an area difference between the interior and exterior, causing a change in curvature and a torque on integral proteins.[48] An example of this is lysophosphatidylcholine (LPC), a product of phospholipase A_2 (PLA_2) cleavage of phosphatidyl choline. PLA_2 removes one of the acyl chains, leaving an amphiphile with a head group area larger than the remaining single acyl chain.

Cytoplasmic and extracellular forms of PLA_2 can produce LPC on either the inner leaflet or outer membrane leaflet. LPC insertion into the outer monolayer activates the K^+-selective MSC TREK and TRAAK[49] (see Chapter 2) and the bacterial channel MscL,[48,50] but it has no effect when inserted into the inner leaflet. Thus, activation of these channels appears to require crenators (Fig. 5–5),[51] or an outward bending force.

For small amphiphiles that can traverse the bilayer, head group charge will affect which leaflet the amphiphiles favors. Biologic membranes normally are negatively charged on the inside; therefore, small anionic amphiphiles will tend to partition into the outer leaflet (see Fig. 5–5, crenator; e.g., trinitrophenol and salicylate). Cationic amphiphiles tend to partition into the inner leaflet (see Fig. 5–5, cup-former; e.g., chlorpromazine and tetracaine).

The dimensions of the hydrophobic moiety will affect the distribution of acyl chains in the hydrophobic interior. Amphiphiles with shorter hydrophobic regions will tend to decrease the average membrane thickness as the interior chains lose their ordering. This can produce changes in the bending and surface shear moduli. In addition, thickness changes can produce hydrophobic mismatch at the interface between the bilayer and integral proteins. This may drive protein conformational changes[48] to reduce the membrane–protein association energy. TREK and TRAAK, which are sensitive to the sign of curvature, also have significant sensitivity to the acyl chain length on LPC.[49]

Among the polyvalent cations, gadolinium ions (Gd^{3+}) are potent blockers of MSC.[52,53] In contrast to amphiphiles, polyvalent cations appear to exert their effect primarily by interaction with the lipid head groups. These effects include dehydration of the lipid surface, ordering of membrane lipids, and changes in the transmembrane dipole potential.[54] The trivalent structure of the lanthanides makes them particularly adept at condensing phospholipid head groups,

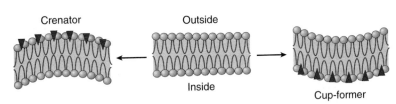

■ **Figure 5–5** Differential effects of anionic and cationic amphiphiles. *(From Kim Y, Bang H, Gnatenco C, et al: Synergistic interaction and the role of C-terminus in the activation of TRAAK K⁺ channels by pressure, free fatty acids and alkali. Pflügers Arch 442:64–72, 2001, with permission.)*

decreasing membrane area, and increasing curvature. Exposure of the outer surface of lipid vesicles to Gd^{3+} causes cup formation. However, the bonding may have large effects on the line tension about the channels[13] inhibiting channel activation. Polyvalent cations also shift the internal electric field of the membrane, causing significant effects on voltage-sensitive channel domains. This may explain the variable effects of Gd^{3+} on different channels.

The membrane modifiers discussed earlier also modify the gating behaviour of MSC in the patch in a variety of ways (Fig. 5–6). Gd^{3+} completely inhibits channel activity, whereas Ca^{2+} *increases* the rate of both activation and inactivation. The Ca^{2+} effect on inactivation may be caused by a shift in the membrane dipole, because the inactivation mechanism is known to be voltage sensitive.[16] External application of LPC increases channel Po and decreases channel conductance.

Surprisingly, all the agents that modify MSC gating have no effect on ΔC_p. This suggests that they have no significant effect on the membrane elasticity. However, they do reduce the total patch capacitance and increase the total patch resistance.

These results suggest that the agents are affecting the patch-sealing region. Gd^{3+} is greater than 10-fold more effective at reducing total patch capacitance than Ca^{2+}; it makes the membrane stick more tightly to the glass.[16] It may be that the area change that occurs during mechanical stress of a patch is too small to measure. Furthermore, outside-out patches do not form as "drumlike" patches, but as floppy bulbs. (Note that the changes in C_p and R_p have different time constants, suggesting the patch is not homogeneous.)

The small peptide inhibitor GsMTx-4, having a +5 charged and hydrophobic surface, may have both polyvalent ion and amphiphilic molecule characteristics. It does not interact with MSC in a lock and key fashion, and it acts as a gating modifier rather than a pore blocker.[55]

The lack of a "specific" peptide–peptide interaction was demonstrated when an enantiomeric (all D-amino acid) form of the peptide showed the same potency for MSC inhibition as the L-amino acid form. This is surprising because GsMTx-4 is ~10 times more potent than Gd^{3+}, with a K_D of 200 to 500 nM. Furthermore, GsMTx-4 appears to interact closely with the channel because, during inhibition, residual channel inward currents are reduced, whereas outward currents are unaffected. This suggests that a charged portion of the peptide is within a Debye length (~10Å) of the pore. However, unlike Gd^{3+}, which is somewhat promiscuous, GsMTx-4 appears to be selective for MSC_{CAT}[55] and has been shown to be ineffective at micromolar concentrations on many other channel types,[44,56,57] including some MSC such as TREK and TRAAK. Specificity may arise because GsMTx-4 is attracted to the MSC_{CAT}-lipid interface that has a unique curvature or distribution, or both, of charged lipids. Interestingly, whereas 5 µM GsMTx-4 completely

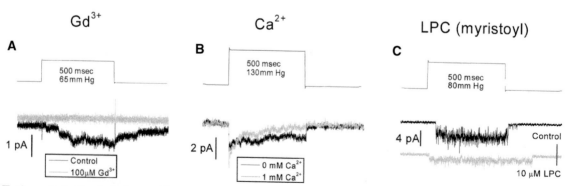

■ **Figure 5–6** Chemicals that modify membranes have varying effects on MSC_{CAT} gating. For each modifier (A–C), data include: pressure stimulus, average patch currents in the presence (gray) and absence (black) of the modifier. Gd^{3+} and Ca^{2+} records are average current records, whereas the lysophosphatidylcholine (LPC) traces show single-channel records to emphasize the changes in conductance and gating properties.

inhibits channels in outside-out patches, it has no effect on C_p, unlike the agents shown in Figure 5–6. This suggests a different mode of action.

GsMTx-4 may prove useful as an antiarrhythmic agent[56] and in treatment and prevention of congestive heart failure.[44] Because the D-peptide is effective, it could be a better drug by reducing immunogenicity and susceptibility to degradation.[58]

Summary

MSC exist in a complex mechanical environment where the properties of the individual components are not easily tractable. We cannot predict the effect of an intervention on MSC activity unless we know the effect on the environment. For structures as complex and elaborate as the cell cortex, no dependable material properties are known to enable useful analytic models. Nonetheless, it is not hard to visualize trends and to remain wary of the interpretation of data.

For example, if an agent produces a decrease in MSC current, the inhibition could arise from a block of the pore, a change in the channel gating properties, a change in properties of the local lipids, or changes to the cytoskeleton. The variety of inputs to MSC suggests that Mother Nature has not remained ignorant of this fact. She may have provided amphipathic second messengers that are to be received and interpreted by MSC. We do not know whether much of the mechanosensitivity of MSC seen in patches is nonphysiologic. Perhaps the primary role of the channels has evolved to be amphipath receptors, and the mechanosensitivity, because of activation by far-field tension, is just a global version of what is usually handled locally.

The physiologic role of the MSC is likely to be resolved in the near future using specific peptide reagents applied to tissues and whole animals. Once that is done, however, we must not lose sight of the multifarious ways in which nature can modulate that activity through the cytoskeleton, the ECM, and second messengers.

References

1. Gillespie PG, Walker RG: Molecular basis of mechanosensory transduction. Nature 413:194–202, 2001.
2. Sachs F, Morris CE: Mechanosensitive ion channels in nonspecialized cells. Rev Physiol Bioch P 132:1–78, 1998.
3. Evans EA, Hochmuth RM: Mechanical properties of membranes. Curr Top Membr Trans 10:1–64, 1978.
4. Hamill OP, Martinac B: Molecular basis of mechanotransduction in living cells. Physiol Rev 81:685–740, 2001.
5. Petrov AG: The Lyotropic State of Matter. Amsterdam, Gordon and Breach Science Publishers, 1999.
6. Evans E, Yeung A: Hidden dynamics in rapid changes of bilayer shape. Chem Phys Lipids 73:39–56, 1994.
7. Rawicz W, Olbrich KC, McIntosh T, et al: Effect of chain length and unsaturation on elasticity of lipid bilayers. Biophys J 79:328–339, 2000.
8. Olbrich K, Rawicz W, Needham D, Evans E: Water permeability and mechanical strength of polyunsaturated lipid bilayers. Biophys J 79:321–327, 2000.
9. Hill WG, Zeidel ML: Reconstituting the barrier properties of a water-tight epithelial membrane by design of leaflet-specific liposomes. J Biol Chem 275:30176–30185, 2000.
10. Alonso MA, Millan J: The role of lipid rafts in signalling and membrane trafficking in T lymphocytes. J Cell Sci 114:3957–3965, 2001.
11. Anderson RG: The caveolae membrane system. Annu Rev Biochem 67:199–225, 1998.
12. Kohl P, Cooper PJ, Holloway H: Effects of acute ventricular volume manipulation on in situ cardiomyocyte cell membrane configuration. Prog Biophys Mol Biol 82:221–227, 2003.
13. Markin VS, Sachs F: Thermodynamics of mechanosensitivity: Lipid shape, membrane deformation and anesthesia. Biophysical J 86:370A, 2004.
14. Franco-Obregon A, Lansman JB: Changes in mechanosensitive channel gating following mechanical stimulation in skeletal muscle myotubes from the mdx mouse. J Physiol 539:391–407, 2002.
15. Morris CE: Mechanoprotection of the plasma membrane in neurons and other non-erythroid cells by the spectrin-based membrane skeleton. Cell Mol Biol Lett 6:703–720, 2001.
16. Suchyna TM, Besch SD, Sachs F: Dynamic regulation of mechanosensitive channels; capacitance used to monitor patch tension in real time. Physical Biology 1:1–18, 2004.
17. Masuda T, Fujimaki N, Ozawa E, Ishikawa H: Confocal laser microscopy of dystrophin localization in guinea pig skeletal muscle fibers. J Cell Biol 119:543–548, 1992.
18. Discher DE, Mohandes N, Evans EA: Molecular maps of red cell deformation: Hidden elasticity and in situ connectivity. Science 266:1032–1036, 1994.
19. Mukhopadhyay R, Lim HWG, Wortis M: Echinocyte shapes: Bending, stretching, and shear determine spicule shape and spacing. Biophys J 82:1756–1772, 2002.
20. Sheetz MP: Cell control by membrane-cytoskeleton adhesion. Nat Rev Mol Cell Biol 2:392–396, 2001.
21. Dai J, Sheetz MP: Membrane tether formation from blebbing cells. Biophys J 77:3363–3370, 1999.
22. Raucher D, Stauffer T, Chen W, et al: Phosphatidylinositol 4,5-bisphosphate functions as a second messenger that regulates cytoskeleton-plasma membrane adhesion. Cell 100:221–228, 2000.
23. Hall A: Rho GTPases and the actin cytoskeleton. Science 279:509–514, 1998.
24. Togo T, Krasieva TB, Steinhardt RA: A decrease in membrane tension precedes successful cell-membrane repair. Mol Biol Cell 11:4339–4346, 2000.
25. Sechi AS, Wehland J: The actin cytoskeleton and plasma membrane connection: PtdIns(4,5)P(2) influences cytoskeletal pro-

tein activity at the plasma membrane. J Cell Sci 113(pt 21):3685–3695, 2000.

26. Roper K, Gregory SL, Brown NH: The 'spectraplakins': cytoskeletal giants with characteristics of both spectrin and plakin families. J Cell Sci 115:4215–4225, 2002.

27. Bretscher A, Edwards K, Fehon RG: ERM proteins and merlin: Integrators at the cell cortex. Nat Rev Mol Cell Biol 3:586–599, 2002.

28. Ervasti JM: Costameres: The Achilles' heel of Herculean muscle. J Biol Chem 278:13591–13594, 2003.

29. Porter GA, Dmytrenko GM, Winkelmann JC, Bloch RJ: Dystrophin colocalizes with beta-spectrin in distinct subsarcolemmal domains in mammalian skeletal muscle. J Cell Biol 117:997–1005, 1992.

30. Rybakova IN, Patel JR, Ervasti JM: The dystrophin complex forms a mechanically strong link between the sarcolemma and costameric actin. J Cell Biol 150:1209–1214, 2000.

31. Pasternak C, Wong S, Elson EL: Mechanical function of dystrophin in muscle cells. J Cell Biol 128:355–361, 1995.

32. Stevenson S, Rothery S, Cullen MJ, Severs NJ: Dystrophin is not a specific component of the cardiac costamere. Circ Res 80:269–280, 1997.

33. Muntoni F, Torelli S, Ferlini A. Dystrophin and mutations: One gene, several proteins, multiple phenotypes. Lancet Neurol 2:731–740, 2003.

34. Tskhovrebova L, Trinick J: Titin: Properties and family relationships. Nat Rev Mol Cell Biol 4:679–689, 2003.

35. Furukawa T, Ono Y, Tsuchiya H, et al: Specific interaction of the potassium channel beta-subunit minK with the sarcomeric protein T-cap suggests a T-tubule-myofibril linking system. J Mol Biol 313:775–784, 2001.

36. Vandenberg JI, Rees SA, Wright AR, Powell T: Cell swelling and ion transport pathways in cardiac myocytes. Cardiovasc Res 32:85–97, 1996.

37. Brette F, Orchard C: T-tubule function in mammalian cardiac myocytes. Circ Res 92:1182–1192, 2003.

38. Morris CE, Horn R: Failure to elicit neuronal macroscopic mechanosensitive currents anticipated by single-channel studies. Science 251:1246–1249, 1991.

39. Zhang Y, Hamill OP: On the discrepancy between whole-cell and membrane patch mechanosensitivity in Xenopus oocytes. J Physiol (Lond) 523(pt 1):101–115, 2000.

40. Zhang Y, Gao F, Popov VL, et al: Mechanically gated channel activity in cytoskeleton-deficient plasma membrane blebs and vesicles from Xenopus oocytes. J Physiol 523(pt 1):117–130, 2000.

41. Zeng T, Bett GCL, Sachs F: Stretch-activated whole-cell currents in adult rat cardiac myocytes. Am J Physiol Heart Circ Physiol 278:H548–H557, 2000.

42. Salmon AH, Mays JL, Dalton GR, et al: Effect of streptomycin on wall-stress-induced arrhythmias in the working rat heart. Cardiovasc Res 34:493–503, 1997.

43. Tatsukawa Y, Kiyosue T, Arita M: Mechanical stretch increases intracellular calcium concentration in cultured ventricular cells from neonatal rats. Heart Vessels 12:128–135, 1997.

44. Suchyna TM, Johnson JH, Clemo HF, et al: Identification of a peptide toxin from Grammostola spatulata spider venom that blocks stretch activated channels. J Gen Physiol 115:583–598, 2000.

45. Hamill OP, McBride DW Jr: Rapid adaptation of single mechanosensitive channels in Xenopus oocytes. Proc Natl Acad Sci USA 89:7462–7466, 1992.

46. Sachs F, Qin F, Palade P: Models of Ca2+ release channel adaptation [letter]. Science 267:2010–2011, 1995.

47. Koprowski P, Kubalski A: Voltage-independent adaptation of mechanosensitive channels in *Escherichia coli* protoplasts. J Membr Biol 164:253–262, 1998.

48. Perozo E, Kloda A, Cortes DM, Martinac B: Physical principles underlying the transduction of bilayer deformation forces during mechanosensitive channel gating. Nat Struct Biol 9:696–703, 2002.

49. Maingret F, Patel AJ, Lesage F, et al: Lysophospholipids open the two-pore domain mechano-gated K(+) channels TREK-1 and TRAAK. J Biol Chem 275:10128–10133, 2000.

50. Martinac B, Adler J, Kung C: Mechanosensitive ion channels of *E. coli* activated by amphipaths. Nature 348:261–263, 1990.

51. Kim Y, Bang H, Gnatenco C, et al: Synergistic interaction and the role of C-terminus in the activation of TRAAK K+ channels by pressure, free fatty acids and alkali. Pflügers Arch 442:64–72, 2001.

52. Bode F, Katchman A, Woosley RL, Franz MR: Gadolinium decreases stretch-induced vulnerability to atrial fibrillation. Circulation 101:2200–2205, 2000.

53. Caldwell RA, Clemo HF, Baumgarten CM: Using gadolinium to identify stretch-activated channels: Technical considerations. Am J Physiol 275:C619–C621, 1998.

54. Ermakov YA, Averbakh AZ, Yusipovich AI, Sukharev S: Dipole potentials indicate restructuring of the membrane interface induced by gadolinium and beryllium ions. Biophys J 80:1851–1862, 2001.

55. Suchyna TM, Tape SE, Koeppe RE, et al: Bilayer-dependent inhibition of mechanosensitive channels by neuroactive peptide enantiomers. Nature 430:235–240, 2004.

56. Bode F, Sachs F, Franz MR: Tarantula peptide inhibits atrial fibrillation: A peptide from spider venom can prevent the heartbeat from losing its rhythm. Nature 409:35–36, 2001.

57. Ruta V, MacKinnon R: Localization of the voltage-sensor toxin receptor on KvAP. Biochemistry 43:10071–10079, 2004.

58. Gottlieb PA, Suchyna TM, Ostrow L, Sachs F: Mechanosensitive ion channels as drug targets. Curr Drug Targets CNS Neurol Disord 3:287–295, 2004.

CHAPTER 6

The Response of Cardiac Muscle to Stretch: The Role of Calcium

• • • •

John Jeremy Rice and Donald M. Bers

Mammalian muscle is characterized by a biphasic force response to stretch. In isolated myocardium, stretch induces an immediate increase in twitch force (immediate force response [IFR]), followed by a slowly developing second phase (slow force response [SFR]) as first described by Parmley and Chuck.[1] The IFR is the result of a length-dependent increase in myofilament Ca^{2+} sensitivity of cardiac muscle. Whereas the increase in Ca^{2+} sensitivity is well characterized and generally accepted as the cellular basis of the Frank–Starling mechanism, the underlying mechanisms of the length dependence remains controversial. After the immediate increase in force, SFR is characterized by a gradual increase in force that saturates over a time course of minutes. This increase is probably involved in the classic Anrep effect, because it is assumed to correspond to the secondary increase in developed pressure found in whole heart. The increase in force is paralleled by an increase in the Ca^{2+} transient amplitude,[2] but the source of the increase is still under debate. Several mechanisms have been suggested to contribute to the SFR, including changes in transmembrane Ca^{2+} influx and changes in sarcoplasmic reticulum (SR) Ca^{2+} uptake or release. These mechanisms are reviewed in this chapter.

IMMEDIATE FORCE RESPONSE

Length-Dependent Changes in Ca^{2+} Sensitivity

Changing cardiac muscle length has an immediate effect on myofilament force production as a function of activator Ca^{2+} that is commonly assumed to be the cellular basis of the Frank–Starling law of the heart. A typical quantification of a Force-Ca^{2+} (F-Ca) relation that describes developed force as a function of steady-state activator Ca^{2+} concentration is shown in Figure 6–1. The length-dependent changes in the F-Ca functions can be separated into two main categories: changes in plateau or maximal force and changes in the Ca^{2+} sensitivity. The changes in plateau force at high Ca^{2+} are most likely the result of sarcomere geometry in that length changes the overlap of thick and thin filaments; however, not all evidence supports this view. The most classical data from Gordon and colleagues[3] in skeletal muscle shows an ascending limb of the length–tension relation up to a sarcomere length (SL) of 2.0 μm after which no further increase is found in maximally activated force. In contrast, cardiac muscle can show an increase in maximal force up to SLs in the range of 2.2 to 2.3 μm[4,5] (see Fig. 6–1*A*). This inconsistency has been noted previously.[6,7] Conceivably, the thin filament length is longer in cardiac muscle, extending the ascending limb up to longer SL than in skeletal muscle. Although there is no anatomic confirmation of such a systematic difference in thin filament lengths in cardiac muscle compared with skeletal muscle, greater variability is reported in cardiac muscle that may contribute to a longer plateau region.[7] The greater variability may result from a lack of nebulin that acts like a template for the thin filament in skeletal but not cardiac muscle. Although anatomic evidence may be lacking, the observation that force[5,8] and adenosine triphosphatase (ATPase) rate[9] of maximally activated cardiac muscle is a linear function of the change in SL is strongly suggestive of a simple linear relation between SL and the number of recruitable crossbridges as set by the overlap of thick and thin filaments.

The second main length-dependent change is an increase in Ca^{2+} sensitivity that is shown by the

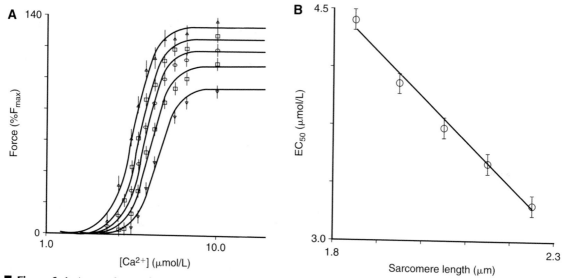

■ **Figure 6–1** Average force-Ca^{2+} (F-Ca) relations from pooled data in skinned rat cardiac trabeculae (n = 10) at five sarcomere lengths (SL = 1.85, 1.95, 2.05, 2.15, and 2.25 μm). *A,* Force measurements were made with SL controlled at each length to the values shown during steady-state activation at varying Ca^{2+} concentration. Force is normalized to maximum force measured at SL = 1.9 μm (trace not shown). Data are fitted to a modified single Hill relationship:

$$F = F_{max}[Ca^{2+}]^{n_H} / (EC_{50}^{n_H} + [Ca^{2+}]^{n_H})$$

Increases in SL induced a significant increase in maximum Ca^{2+}-saturated force (F_{MAX}: mean values = 49.1, 56.8, 60.6, 65.3, and 72.9) and Ca^{2+} sensitivity (EC$_{50}$); however, the level of cooperativity as assessed by the Hill coefficient (n_H: mean values = 7.4, 7.2, 7.3, 7.0, and 6.9) was not affected by SL. Force measurements were made with SL controlled during steady-state activation (see Reference 8 for details). *B,* Ca^{2+} sensitivity as indexed by the EC$_{50}$ parameter (Ca^{2+} at half-maximal tension), plotted as function of SL. EC$_{50}$ is a linear, inverse function of SL. Data are presented as mean ± SE. *(Reproduced from Dobesh DP, Konhilas JP, de Tombe PP: Cooperative activation in cardiac muscle: Impact of sarcomere length. Am J Physiol Heart Circ Physiol 282:H1055–H1062, 2002, with permission.)*

leftward shift of the F-Ca traces in Figure 6–1*A.* The source of this length sensitivity is still under debate. An attractive hypothesis suggests that length changes the lattice spacing of the thick and thin filaments as a result of the isovolumetric properties of heart cell.[10] This change in actin and myosin lattice spacing then modulates the crossbridge attachment or detachment rates, or both, to change the developed force. In contrast, some recent estimates of myofilament lattice spacing by synchrotron X-ray diffraction suggest that the changes in lattice spacing occurring over the physiologic range cannot account for length-dependent changes in Ca^{2+} sensitivity in cardiac muscle.[11] However, using similar methods, other researchers found that the fraction of weakly bound crossbridges is dependent on lattice spacing.[12] If one assumes a con-

stant rate of turnover from the weakly bound to the force-generating strongly bound state, then this evidence supports a mechanism for lattice spacing to modulate force. It should be noted that all the X-ray diffraction studies cited above are somewhat unphysiologic because lattice spacing is measured under relaxed conditions that may not correspond to activated conditions where attached crossbridges may also modify the lattice spacing. More work is required to better quantify the effects of lattice spacing on activated, force-producing muscle.

If the lattice spacing hypothesis is found not to account for the length-dependent Ca^{2+} sensitivity, then few other possibilities exist. Some authors suggest that titin may play a role[13]; this protein is situated between the thick filament and the Z-disk, and hence its length will be modulated by the SL. Another possibility is that the SL-dependent Ca^{2+} sensitivity may result from interplay of cooperative mechanisms (discussed below) and the number of recruitable crossbridges as set by length-dependent sarcomere overlap.[14]

Although the basis of length-dependent changes in Ca^{2+} sensitivity is not fully understood, the question is closely tied with why cardiac muscle shows such a steep dependence on activator $[Ca^{2+}]$ at each length. Specifically, the single regulatory binding site on troponin should predict a Hill coefficient of 1, whereas Hill coefficients up to the range of 7 to 8 have been reported (such as those in Fig. 6–1 from Reference 8).

To account for the large Hill coefficient, researchers have described several types of cooperative mechanisms that could account for the steep dependence (see Reference 14 for review). Attached crossbridges have been shown to increase the Ca^{2+} affinity of troponin. Hence, this is feedback from crossbridge formation (actin-myosin binding) to Ca^{2+} binding of troponin C (specifically, binding to the single low-affinity regulatory site on troponin, rather than the two high-affinity Ca^{2+}-Mg^{2+} sites, which are not thought to be affected by crossbridge binding). Another type of cooperativity among the regulatory proteins is thought to arise from nearest neighbor interactions produced by the overlap of adjacent tropomyosin units along the thin filament. A third proposed type of cooperative interaction is between neighboring crossbridges—that is, the binding of one crossbridge may increase the binding rate of neighboring crossbridges by holding the regulatory proteins in a more permissive conformation. Alternatively, the binding of one crossbridge may pull binding sites on a compliant thin filament into register with myosin heads that have an inherently different characteristic distance in their repeating structure.

Effects on the Ca^{2+} Transient

Although the underlying cooperative mechanisms that bring about steep F-Ca relations are under debate, the exact mechanisms may not be important to understand the effects of length-dependent changes in the Ca^{2+} transients. The Ca^{2+} binding affinity of regulatory proteins appears to be modulated by the number of attached or force-generating crossbridges instead of length itself.[2,15] Hence, the Ca^{2+} affinity of troponin should change in accord with the number of attached crossbridges that can be modulated by cooperative thin filament activation, sarcomere geometry, or the interaction of the two.

The change in Ca^{2+} buffering strength can produce secondary effects on the intracellular Ca^{2+} transient, as shown in Figure 6–2 and reported in other studies.[2,16,17] However, the effects on the Ca^{2+} transient tend to be rather small, and sometimes no change is reported.[18,19] These observations suggest that the changes in force, secondary to length modulation, are unlikely to produce large perturbations in intracellular Ca^{2+} concentration that could be proarrhythmic by activating Ca^{2+}-dependent inward currents (e.g., through Na^+-Ca^{2+} exchange [NCX]). For example, one would not expect the amount of Ca^{2+} released by the myofilaments to trigger delayed afterdepolarizations as seen in some pathologic conditions such as heart failure.[20] This can also be appreciated by considering that the local submembrane $[Ca^{2+}]$ that Ca^{2+}-activated currents sense is increased more dramatically by SR Ca^{2+} release or L-type Ca^{2+} current influx than would be expected by $[Ca^{2+}]$ changes in the myofilament matrix (see Chapter 22).

SLOW FORCE RESPONSE

After the immediate increase in force, there is an SFR in a staircase-like fashion that eventually reaches a plateau. The increase in force is closely mirrored by an increase in the Ca^{2+} transient amplitude.[2] A similar response is shown in Figure 6–2, and further results in that study demonstrate that there are no slow time-dependent changes in Ca^{2+} sensitivity at the level of the myofilaments. Moreover, studies have shown that the length changes during the diastolic period alone are sufficient to generate SFR,[16,21] again suggesting mechanisms other than the myofilaments themselves. In contrast, some researchers have proposed enhanced myofilament Ca^{2+} responsiveness related to intracellular alkalinization,[22] although these results may be artifacts of the experimental preparation (see "Roles of Angiotensin II and Endothelin-1"). The origin of the SFR in terms of a mechanism that mostly increases the amplitude of the Ca^{2+} transient is discussed in the following, although alternative mechanisms are also discussed.

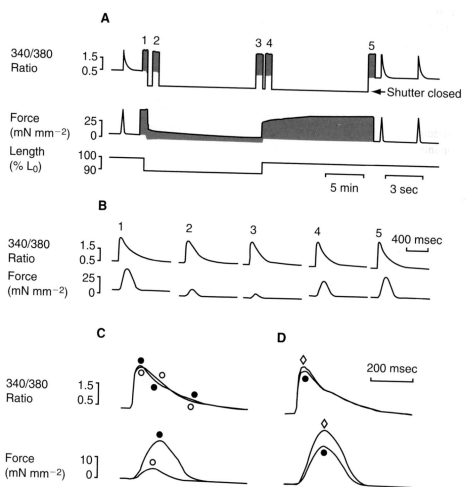

■ **Figure 6–2** Records of the changes in fura-2 fluorescence ratio and force produced by shortening a rat trabecula by 10% for 15 minutes. A, Chart records of 340:380 nm fluorescence ratio and force, with a representation of the length change from the initial length (L_0). A shutter in the excitation light pathway was opened only for discrete 48-sec recording periods (labeled 1–5) to avoid photobleaching of fura-2. The shutter was closed also during the adjustment of muscle length using a micromanipulator. Traces were scanned digitally from the original records (filtered at 15 Hz). Note the slow changes in twitch force after the changes in muscle length. B, Mean records (from 16 twitches) of fluorescence ratio and Force measured during periods 1 to 5 in A. Unfiltered records. C, Overlaid traces of the fluorescence ratio and Force averaged during periods 3 (closed circles) and 4 (open circles) to illustrate the rapid effects of the length increase. Resting forces have been subtracted from these traces. D, Similar overlaid traces averaged during periods 4 (open circles) and 5 (open diamonds) to illustrate the delayed effects of the length increase (24°C, 1 mM external Ca^{2+}, 0.33 Hz stimulation rate). (Reproduced from Kentish JC, Wrzosek A: Changes in force and cytosolic Ca^{2+} concentration after length changes in isolated rat ventricular trabeculae. J Physiol 506[pt 2]:431–444, 1998, with permission.)

Stretch-Induced Changes in Sarcolemmal Ionic Influx

The primary source of Ca^{2+} influx in cardiac cells is through L-type channels, but these have not shown sensitivity to stretch in numerous species (i.e., rat[23] and

rabbit[24]) and have even been shown to decrease in response to membrane stretch[25] (see Chapter 4 for a more detailed discussion). Ca^{2+} influx through L-type channels occurs throughout the whole action potential; therefore, prolonged action potential duration (APD) is another possible mechanism to increase Ca^{2+}

influx, SR load, and the Ca^{2+} transient. However, the story is complicated because changes in the Ca^{2+} transient can also affect APD.[27] Although a complete treatment of stretch-induced changes in APD is beyond the scope of this chapter, it is sufficient to say that APD changes are often but not always reported with SFR.

For example, studies in which guinea pig myocytes were axially stretched with carbon fibers also showed that increasing SL by approximately 10% prolonged the APD_{90} (APD at 90% repolarization) by 16%.[28] This effect could be blocked by 40 μM streptomycin, a blocker of stretch-activated channels (SAC), suggesting a role for stretch-sensing membrane currents. However, pretreatment with 5 μM bis-(aminophenoxy) ethane-tetraacetic, membrane permanent acetomethoxy ester form (BAPTA-AM) to buffer $[Ca^{2+}]_i$ also blocked the change in APD; therefore, the results are hard to interpret given the inherent interdependency between the Ca^{2+} transient and APD. In this study,[28] the prolongation occurs throughout the repolarization phase. In other studies using similar methods in guinea pig, axial membrane stretch between glass tools produced first an acceleration of repolarization followed by a slowing to produce a longer APD_{90}.[25] This effect was attributed to a stretch-sensitive, cation-nonspecific current with a reversal of −5 mV that could be blocked by 30 μM streptomycin.

Note, however, that other reports show little change in APD in isolated rabbit trabeculae,[29] isolated sheep Purkinje fibers,[30] and Langendorff perfused canine hearts.[31] Hence, APD changes do not appear to be a prerequisite for the SFR in all species, tissues, or both.

Role of Stretch-Activated Channels

There is some evidence that SAC are the source of increased intracellular Ca^{2+}. A Ca^{2+} influx that often led to waves of Ca^{2+}-induced Ca^{2+} release (CICR) could be produced by mechanical prodding or pulling on neighboring cells in tissue-cultured heart cells[32] (see Chapter 1). The researchers attributed the effect to Ca^{2+}-permeable SAC because the response was blocked by removing extracellular Ca^{2+} or by adding gadolinium ions (Gd^{3+}). Other evidence for the roles of SAC shows that SFR is reduced by 80% in rat myocytes by

using streptomycin.[33] However, another study in rabbit myocytes showed little effect of Gd^{3+} on the SFR[29] (although free $[Gd^{3+}]$ may have been less than expected because of interactions with the bicarbonate buffer[34]). Although we have focused on the role of SAC on the SFR, Gd^{3+}-sensitive ion channels do not appear to be necessary for transduction of mechanical stretch into the hypertrophic gene expression,[35] suggesting the existence of other stretch-sensing mechanisms (see Chapter 7).

Although some early reports[32] indicated Ca^{2+} influx through SAC, most reports[25,36] have shown cation-nonselective SAC in which inward current is mostly carried by Na^+. SAC permeable to Na^+ will increase intracellular $[Na^+]$, or perhaps the local subsarcolemmal $[Na^+]$. For example, studies with fluorescent imaging and electron probe analysis show stretch-induced hotspots with $[Na^+]$ greater than 24 mM that appeared close to the surface membrane and T-tubules.[25] Increasing intracellular Na^+ has a secondary effect of increasing intracellular Ca^{2+} through the NCX. NCX is the primary Ca^{2+} extrusion pathway from the cell, and increasing intracellular Na^+ will thermodynamically limit Ca^{2+} efflux and can even favor Ca^{2+} entry through NCX in its reverse mode. The 3:1 stoichiometry generally assumed for this transporter will generate a cubic dependence on intracellular and extracellular $[Na^+]$; hence, a small increase in intracellular $[Na^+]$ can bias the exchanger to lessen the forward mode and increase the reverse mode that brings in Ca^{2+}.

Roles of Angiotensin II and Endothelin-1

An alternative method thought to increase intracellular Na^+ is activation of the Na^+-H^+ exchanger (NHE) by cellular signaling mechanisms. A stretch-dependent release of angiotensin II (Ang II) was first shown in neonatal rat myocytes[37] causing induction of immediate-early genes and protein synthesis related to hypertrophy. Later work in isolated feline and rat cardiac muscle showed stretch-induced autocrine/paracrine release of Ang II and endothelin-1 (ET-1) can activate Na^+ influx through this pathway that is followed by increased $[Ca^{2+}]$ through the NCX.[22,38]

The initial reports demonstrated a stretch-dependent intracellular alkalinization that could be blocked by either the angiotensin receptor type 1 (AT_1) antagonist losartan or the endothelin receptor A antagonist BQ123. However, SFR was not blocked with losartan or BQ123 according to later studies with ferret papillary muscle by Calaghan and White[39] and rabbit ventricular trabeculae by von Lewinski and colleagues.[29] The study of Calaghan and White suggests another mechanism of action in that blockage of endothelin receptor B receptors reduced SFR by 50% and removal of the endocardial endothelium completely removed SFR. The authors suggest endocardial epithelium as the source of ET-1 instead of the ventricular myocytes themselves in the case of rat and cat cardiac muscle. The study of von Lewinski and colleagues[29] also proposed that autocrine/paracrine angiotensin and endothelin release is more important for mediating SFR in rat and cat cardiac muscle than in rabbit and ferret.

The dependence of SFR on the activation of NCX in its reverse mode was first demonstrated by Perez and coworkers[40] based on studies with KB-R7943, a pharmacologic blocker of reverse-mode NCX. The activation of the NCX reverse mode would lead to cellular Ca^{2+} gain (increasing force) coupled to outward transport of Na^+ (which depends on $[Na^+]_i$). Such an interpretation is consistent with the results of von Lewinski and colleagues[29] in which SFR also was blocked by KB-R7943. However, KB-R7943 is not an ideal agent, affecting other transport systems such as K^+, Na^+, and Ca^{2+} channels, and Ca^{2+} transients, even in NCX-knockout heart tubes.[41]

Although some reports suggest a role for enhanced myofilament Ca^{2+} responsiveness because of intracellular alkalinization,[22] the importance of this mechanism recently has been challenged. The primary issue is the use of unphysiologic, bicarbonate-free buffers.[42] Using CO_2/HCO_3^- buffered medium, Alvarez and coworkers[38] demonstrated a stretch-induced NHE activation with consecutive increases in intracellular Na^+, intracellular Ca^{2+}, and twitch force without changes in pH in rat trabeculae at room temperature. Presumably in CO_2/HCO_3^- solutions, $Na-HCO_3^-$ cotransport and $Cl-HCO_3^-$ exchange counteract NHE activation, preventing significant alkalinization. Another study showed similar results in rabbit myocardium and suggested pH changes are not a prerequisite for the SFR.[29]

The exact role of Ang II and AT_1 receptors is further complicated because any contribution to SFR may be small compared with a much larger role in hypertrophic signaling. Ang II induces immediate early genes, late genes, and growth factor genes that are fully blocked by an AT_1 receptor antagonist, but not by an AT_2 receptor antagonist.[37] Ang II activation of the G protein–coupled receptor AT_1 rapidly increased kinase activity of mitogen-activated protein kinases and 90-kD S6 kinase.[43] This study also showed a critical role for Ca^{2+} in this pathway, as chelating intracellular Ca^{2+} by BAPTA-AM completely abolished Ang II–induced activation of these kinases (see Chapter 7 for more information on gene regulation).

Effects on Diastolic Ca^{2+} Concentration

Assuming SFR results from increased Ca^{2+} influx or decreased Ca efflux from the cell, one could predict an increase in diastolic $[Ca^{2+}]_i$. However, the effects of stretch on diastolic $[Ca^{2+}]_i$ have been mixed. Some have reported an increase, whereas others have not. For example, diastolic $[Ca^{2+}]_i$ tended to increase in guinea pig ventricular cells[13,19] but not in rat trabeculae.[23,26] These differences may be attributed to difference in species. The diastolic $[Ca^{2+}]_i$ may be more strongly determined by a leak from SR in rat given the high spark rate in this species[44] coupled with faster uptake by the SR Ca ATPase (SERCA) pumps into SR. The greater level of diastolic Ca^{2+} cycling could potentially mask a small sarcolemmal Ca^{2+} influx to produce a smaller perturbation in diastolic $[Ca^{2+}]_i$ in rat compared with other species.

Effect of Altered Myofilament Buffering

One might conjecture that the increased buffering strength of the myofilaments during IFR may have a secondary effect to increase SR load in SFR. Such a mechanism would require the increased amount of Ca^{2+} bound to troponin during IFR to be sequestered into SR to increase the load. However, this does not appear to occur. Steele and Smith[19] showed no change in SR load as assessed by rapid cooling contractures after blocking force generation with 2,3-butanedione monoxime. Hence, the modulations of troponin Ca^{2+} binding had no effect on SR load. Other results from mathematical modeling of SFR in rat atria also pointed to little effect of altered troponin Ca^{2+} affinity on either the Ca^{2+} transient or the APD,[45] although altered buffering played other roles and was required in conjunction with SAC to best reproduce all length effects in this study.

Stretch-Induced Changes in Sarcoplasmic Reticulum Ca^{2+} Release and Uptake

If SFR is the result of an increased Ca^{2+} transient, then a change in SR release is expected, because SR is the source of most of the Ca^{2+} in the transient. One plausible mechanism is that SR Ca^{2+} load increases during SFR. Such a result has been reported for rabbit ventricle.[29,46] An alternative is that Ca^{2+} loading of SR does not change, but a greater fraction of SR is released. However, the limited data do not point to this mechanism. In rat ventricle, the fraction of release was 32% to 35% and independent of length, and, interestingly, the loading capacity of the SR is greater when the muscle operates at a shorter diastolic length.[47] These features are counter to the SFR where greater release is found for long, not short, diastolic length.

Although a functional SR is required to generate the Ca^{2+} transient, the role of SR appears to be as an accomplice rather than the primary culprit in inducing SFR. Inhibition of SR release by ryanodine[46] or caffeine[48] has no effect on the relative magnitude of SFR. Another possibility to load SR is to increase uptake through the SERCA pump. However, disruption of the CICR system by blocking both release by ryanodine and uptake by cyclopiazonic acid, a blocker of the SERCA pump, still had little effect on SFR.[26,46] These results should not be overinterpreted to say that SR has no role; that is, although SR Ca^{2+} is not required to see SFR, the effective removal of SR does change the time course of SFR[26] and could amplify any change in diastolic $[Ca^{2+}]_i$ or Ca^{2+} influx.

Role of Nitric Oxide

Another signaling pathway implicated in SFR is nitric oxide (NO), which affects many aspects of excitation–contraction (E-C) coupling, including interactions with Ca^{2+}-handling proteins (L-type channel and the ryanodine receptors [RYR]), contractile myofilaments, and respiratory complexes (see References 49 and 50 for reviews). Although a full description of these effects is beyond the scope of this chapter, several aspects related to SFR are discussed.

Direct measurement of NO production in the beating rabbit and rat heart using a porphyrinic microsensor demonstrated that NO concentrations fluctuate in the submicromolar range with the cardiac cycle.[51] Although this beat-to-beat regulation suggests a physiologic role for NO, the story is somewhat complicated because NO has several sources from distinct nitric oxide synthases (NOS), produces downstream interaction that occur through multiple second messenger pathways, and may produce opposing or biphasic effects on E-C coupling.[50] Specifically, NOS1 is localized to the SR (affecting RYR and SERCA pumps), and NOS3 is found in sarcolemmal caveolae compartmentalized with cell-surface receptors and the L-type channels. Electron micrographic evidence suggests caveolae become incorporated into membranes under stretch.[52] A third type, NOS2, appears to be induced by inflammation or cytokines and may be important in pathologic conditions such as heart failure, but it is not present in healthy tissue and is independent of Ca^{2+}; hence, NOS2 is not considered in more detail in this chapter.

NOS1 is localized to the SR. There is evidence of downstream regulation by protein thiol nitrosylation (S-nitrosylation) on RYR that increases their open probability.[53] The RYR channel was proposed to be the end effector of stretch-induced NO activation of phosphatidylinositol 3 kinase–stimulated pathway causing phosphorylation of both Akt protein kinase and the endothelial isoform of NOS3 to produce NO.[54] Akt (also known as protein kinase B) activation has been shown to reduce cardiomyocyte death and to induce cardiac hypertrophy, as well as regulate metabolic substrate utilization and cardiomyocyte function.[55] One end effect of this signaling cascade is increased Ca^{2+} sparks and electrically stimulated Ca^{2+} transients. However, as suggested by others,[56] changing RYR properties alone may have little effect on sustained changes in the Ca^{2+} transient, such as those in SFR. Specifically, changing RYR release properties alone produces only transient changes in the Ca^{2+} transient, given negative feedback mechanisms such as Ca^{2+}-mediated inactivation of L-type channels.[57] An alternative possibility exists that SR uptake is modified by NO, possibly by reacting with regulatory thiols of SERCA,[58] or by inhibition of phosphorylation of phospholamban, to decreasing SERCA uptake.[59]

NOS3 is localized to the caveolae of the sarcolemma and the T-tubules where it is typically attached to and inactivated by caveolin-3, a scaffold protein. After an agonist-induced increase in Ca^{2+}, Ca^{2+}-calmodulin causes NOS3 dissociation from caveolin-3. Another downstream target of NOS3-derived NO is activation of guanylyl cyclase that produces cyclic guanosine monophosphate (cGMP), which activates protein kinase G (PKG) and other signaling cascades. Other effects are cGMP independent, and are mediated by S-nitrosylation. One such target is the L-type channel that shows a 60% increase in current under stimulation with S-nitrosoglutathione, a naturally occurring S-nitrosothiol that induces S-nitrosylation.[60] In contrast, PKG phosphorylation has the opposite effect to decrease L-type current, thus illustrating the complexity of NO signaling. Moreover, the localization of L-type channels with RYR is suggestive of possible cross talk between NO signals produced by NOS3 and NOS1 in junctional space of the diad.[50] Additional research is required to sort out the complexities in NO signaling.

Summary

Mammalian muscle is characterized by a biphasic force response to stretch. In the first phase, stretch induces an immediate increase in twitch force that is the result of a length-dependent increase in Ca^{2+} sensitivity of cardiac muscle that is generally accepted as the cellular basis of the Frank–Starling mechanism. Considerable controversy exists over which cooperative mechanisms in Ca^{2+} activation produce the steep F-Ca^{2+} relations. Moreover, there is no consensus as to what is the molecular sensor of muscle length that brings about the increased Ca^{2+} sensitivity.

After the immediate increase in force, the second phase is characterized by a slow increase in force that saturates over a time course of minutes. The increase in force is most often reported to be secondary to an increase in Ca^{2+} release, but the source of greater release is controversial. Although direct stretch modulation of typical Ca^{2+}-handling mechanisms has not been completely ruled out, the stretch sensitivity is most often attributed to specialized mechanisms. Specifically, the proposed mechanisms include Ca^{2+} influx through SAC, or Na^+ influx through SAC that leads to a secondary increase in $[Ca^{2+}]$ through the NCX. Another proposed mechanism is Na^+ influx through the NHE that is activated by stretch-induced autocrine/paracrine release of Ang II and ET-1. Alternatively, NO may act on one or more targets including the L-type channels, RYR, or the SERCA pumps directly to increase Ca^{2+} cycling. Further work is required to elucidate the exact contribution of these, or perhaps other mechanisms, to SFR. Considerable differences are reported across tissues and species, suggesting that multiple mechanisms could be responsible for the SFR. The possibility exists that some changes in Ca^{2+} may not be related to SFR per se, but instead are epiphenomena of calcium's role in inducing gene expression or other cellular signals.

References

1. Parmley WW, Chuck L: Length-dependent changes in myocardial contractile state. Am J Physiol 224:1195–1199, 1973.
2. Allen DG, Kurihara S: The effects of muscle length on intracellular calcium transients in mammalian cardiac muscle. J Physiol 327:79–94, 1982.
3. Gordon AM, Huxley AF, Julian FJ: The variation in isometric tension with sarcomere length in vertebrate muscle fibres. J Physiol (Lond) 184:170–192, 1966.
4. ter Keurs HE, Rijnsburger WH, van Heuningen R, Nagelsmit MJ: Tension development and sarcomere length in rat cardiac trabeculae. Evidence of length-dependent activation. Circ Res 46:703–714, 1980.
5. Stuyvers BD, McCulloch AD, Guo J, et al: Effect of stimulation rate, sarcomere length and Ca^{2+} on force generation by mouse cardiac muscle. J Physiol 544(pt 3):817–830, 2002.
6. Allen DG, Kentish JC: The cellular basis of the length-tension relation in cardiac muscle. J Mol Cell Cardiol 17:821–840, 1985.
7. Robinson TF, Winegrad S: The measurement and dynamic implications of thin filament lengths in heart muscle. J Physiol 286:607–619, 1979.
8. Dobesh DP, Konhilas JP, de Tombe PP: Cooperative activation in cardiac muscle: Impact of sarcomere length. Am J Physiol Heart Circ Physiol 282:H1055–H1062, 2002.

9. Wannenburg T, Heijne GH, Geerdink JH, et al: Cross-bridge kinetics in rat myocardium: Effect of sarcomere length and calcium activation. Am J Physiol Heart Circ Physiol 279: H779–H790, 2000.

10. McDonald KS, Moss RL: Osmotic compression of single cardiac myocytes eliminates the reduction in Ca^{2+} sensitivity of tension at short sarcomere length. Circ Res 77:199–205, 1995.

11. Konhilas JP, Irving TC, de Tombe PP: Length-dependent activation in three striated muscle types of the rat. J Physiol 544(pt 1):225–236, 2002.

12. Martyn DA, Adhikari BB, Regnier M, et al: Response of equatorial x-ray reflections and stiffness to altered sarcomere length and myofilament lattice spacing in relaxed skinned cardiac muscle. Biophys J 86:1002–1011, 2004.

13. Le Guennec JY, White E, Gannier F, et al: Stretch-induced increase of resting intracellular calcium concentration in single guinea-pig ventricular myocytes. Exp Physiol 76:975–978, 1991.

14. Rice JJ, De Tombe PP: Approaches to modeling crossbridges and calcium-dependent activation in cardiac muscle. Prog Biophys Mol Biol 85:179–195, 2004.

15. Bremel RD, Weber A: Cooperation within actin filament in vertebrate skeletal muscle. Nature New Biol 238:97–101, 1972.

16. Allen DG, Nichols CG, Smith GL: The effects of changes in muscle length during diastole on the calcium transient in ferret ventricular muscle. J Physiol 406:359–370, 1988.

17. Janssen PM, de Tombe PP: Uncontrolled sarcomere shortening increases intracellular Ca^{2+} transient in rat cardiac trabeculae. Am J Physiol 272(4 pt 2):H1892–H1897, 1997.

18. Saeki Y, Kurihara S, Hongo K, Tanaka E: Tension and intracellular calcium transients of activated ferret ventricular muscle in response to step length changes. Adv Exp Med Biol 332: 639–648, 1993.

19. Steele DS, Smith GL: Effects of 2,3-butanedione monoxime on sarcoplasmic reticulum of saponin-treated rat cardiac muscle. Am J Physiol 265(5 pt 2):H1493–H1500, 1993.

20. Pogwizd SM, Bers DM: Cellular basis of triggered arrhythmias in heart failure. Trends Cardiovasc Med 14:61–66, 2004.

21. Nichols CG: The influence of 'diastolic' length on the contractility of isolated cat papillary muscle. J Physiol 361:269–279, 1985.

22. Cingolani HE, Alvarez BV, Ennis IL, Camilion de Hurtado MC: Stretch-induced alkalinization of feline papillary muscle: An autocrine-paracrine system. Circ Res 83:775–780, 1998.

23. Hongo K, White E, Le Guennec JY, Orchard CH: Changes in Ca^{2+}i, [Na+]i and Ca^{2+} current in isolated rat ventricular myocytes following an increase in cell length. J Physiol 491(pt 3):609–619, 1996.

24. Kentish JC, Davey R, Largen P: Isoprenaline reverses the slow force responses to a length change in isolated rabbit papillary muscle. Pflugers Arch 421:519–521, 1992.

25. Isenberg G, Kazanski V, Kondratev D, et al: Differential effects of stretch and compression on membrane currents and [Na+]c in ventricular myocytes. Prog Biophys Mol Biol 82(1-3):43–56, 2003.

26. Kentish JC, Wrzosek A: Changes in force and cytosolic Ca^{2+} concentration after length changes in isolated rat ventricular trabeculae. J Physiol 506(pt 2):431–444, 1998.

27. duBell WH, Boyett MR, Spurgeon HA, et al: The cytosolic calcium transient modulates the action potential of rat ventricular myocytes. J Physiol 436:347–369, 1991.

28. Belus A, White E: Streptomycin and intracellular calcium modulate the response of single guinea-pig ventricular myocytes to axial stretch. J Physiol 546(pt 2):501–509, 2003.

29. von Lewinski D, Stumme B, Maier LS, et al: Stretch-dependent slow force response in isolated rabbit myocardium is Na+ dependent. Cardiovasc Res 57:1052–1061, 2003.

30. Dominguez G, Fozzard HA: Effect of stretch on conduction velocity and cable properties of cardiac Purkinje fibers. Am J Physiol 237:C119–C124, 1979.

31. Calkins H, Maughan WL, Kass DA, et al: Electrophysiological effect of volume load in isolated canine hearts. Am J Physiol 256(6 pt 2):H1697–H1706, 1989.

32. Sigurdson W, Ruknudin A, Sachs F: Calcium imaging of mechanically induced fluxes in tissue-cultured chick heart: Role of stretch-activated ion channels. Am J Physiol 262(4 pt 2):H1110–H1115, 1992.

33. Calaghan SC, White E: Signaling pathways which underlie the slow inotropic response to myocardial stretch. J Physiol 544P:23S, 2002.

34. Caldwell RA, Clemo HF, Baumgarten CM: Using gadolinium to identify stretch-activated channels: Technical considerations. Am J Physiol 275(2 pt 1):C619–C621, 1998.

35. Sadoshima J, Takahashi T, Jahn L, Izumo S: Roles of mechanosensitive ion channels, cytoskeleton, and contractile activity in stretch-induced immediate-early gene expression and hypertrophy of cardiac myocytes. Proc Natl Acad Sci USA 89: 9905–9909, 1992.

36. Naruse K, Sokabe M: Involvement of stretch-activated ion channels in Ca^{2+} mobilization to mechanical stretch in endothelial cells. Am J Physiol 264(4 pt 1):C1037–C1044, 1993.

37. Sadoshima J, Izumo S: Molecular characterization of angiotensin II–induced hypertrophy of cardiac myocytes and hyperplasia of cardiac fibroblasts. Critical role of the AT1 receptor subtype. Circ Res 73:413–423, 1993.

38. Alvarez BV, Perez NG, Ennis IL, et al: Mechanisms underlying the increase in force and Ca^{2+} transient that follow stretch of cardiac muscle: A possible explanation of the Anrep effect. Circ Res 85:716–722, 1999.

39. Calaghan SC, White E: Contribution of angiotensin II, endothelin 1 and the endothelium to the slow inotropic response to stretch in ferret papillary muscle. Pflugers Arch 441:514–520, 2001.

40. Perez NG, de Hurtado MC, Cingolani HE: Reverse mode of the Na+-Ca^{2+} exchange after myocardial stretch: Underlying mechanism of the slow force response. Circ Res 88:376–382, 2001.

41. Reuter H, Henderson SA, Han T, et al: Knockout mice for pharmacological screening: Testing the specificity of Na+-Ca^{2+} exchange inhibitors. Circ Res 91:90–92, 2002.

42. Mattiazzi A, Perez NG, Vila-Petroff MG, et al: Dissociation between positive inotropic and alkalinizing effects of angiotensin II in feline myocardium. Am J Physiol 272(3 pt 2): H1131–H1136, 1997.

43. Sadoshima J, Qiu Z, Morgan JP, Izumo S: Angiotensin II and other hypertrophic stimuli mediated by G protein-coupled receptors activate tyrosine kinase, mitogen-activated protein kinase, and 90-kD S6 kinase in cardiac myocytes. The critical role of Ca^{2+}-dependent signaling. Circ Res 76:1–15, 1995.

44. Satoh H, Blatter LA, Bers DM: Effects of Ca^{2+}i, SR Ca^{2+} load, and rest on Ca^{2+} spark frequency in ventricular myocytes. Am J Physiol 272(2 pt 2):H657–H668, 1997.

45. Tavi P, Han C, Weckstrom M: Mechanisms of stretch-induced changes in Ca²⁺i in rat atrial myocytes: Role of increased troponin C affinity and stretch-activated ion channels. Circ Res 83:1165–1177, 1998.

46. Bluhm WF, Lew WY: Sarcoplasmic reticulum in cardiac length-dependent activation in rabbits. Am J Physiol 269(3 pt 2): H965–H972, 1995.

47. Gamble J, Taylor PB, Kenno KA: Myocardial stretch alters twitch characteristics and Ca²⁺ loading of sarcoplasmic reticulum in rat ventricular muscle. Cardiovasc Res 26:865–870, 1992.

48. Chuck LH, Parmley WW: Caffeine reversal of length-dependent changes in myocardial contractile state in the cat. Circ Res 47:592–598, 1980.

49. Hare JM: Nitric oxide and excitation-contraction coupling. J Mol Cell Cardiol 35:719–729, 2003.

50. Ziolo MT, Bers DM: The real estate of NOS signaling: Location, location, location. Circ Res 92:1279–1281, 2003.

51. Kanai AJ, Mesaros S, Finkel MS, et al: Beta-adrenergic regulation of constitutive nitric oxide synthase in cardiac myocytes. Am J Physiol 273(4 pt 1):C1371–C1377, 1997.

52. Kohl P, Cooper PJ, Holloway H: Effects of acute ventricular volume manipulation on in situ cardiomyocyte cell membrane configuration. Prog Biophys Mol Biol 82(1-3):221–227, 2003.

53. Stoyanovsky D, Murphy T, Anno PR, et al: Nitric oxide activates skeletal and cardiac ryanodine receptors. Cell Calcium 21:19–29, 1997.

54. Petroff MG, Kim SH, Pepe S, et al: Endogenous nitric oxide mechanisms mediate the stretch dependence of Ca²⁺ release in cardiomyocytes. Nat Cell Biol 3:867–873, 2001.

55. Matsui T, Nagoshi T, Rosenzweig A: Akt and PI 3-kinase signaling in cardiomyocyte hypertrophy and survival. Cell Cycle 2:220–223, 2003.

56. Calaghan SC, Belus A, White E: Do stretch-induced changes in intracellular calcium modify the electrical activity of cardiac muscle? Prog Biophys Mol Biol 82(1-3):81–95, 2003.

57. Trafford AW, Diaz ME, Sibbring GC, Eisner DA: Modulation of CICR has no maintained effect on systolic Ca²⁺: Simultaneous measurements of sarcoplasmic reticulum and sarcolemmal Ca2+ fluxes in rat ventricular myocytes. J Physiol 522(pt 2):259–270, 2000.

58. Wawrzynow A, Collins JH: Chemical modification of the Ca(2+)-ATPase of rabbit skeletal muscle sarcoplasmic reticulum: Identification of sites labeled with aryl isothiocyanates and thiol-directed conformational probes. Biochim Biophys Acta 1203:60–70, 1993.

59. Stojanovic MO, Ziolo MT, Wahler GM, Wolska BM: Anti-adrenergic effects of nitric oxide donor SIN-1 in rat cardiac myocytes. Am J Physiol Cell Physiol 281:C342–C349, 2001.

60. Campbell DL, Stamler JS, Strauss HC: Redox modulation of L-type calcium channels in ferret ventricular myocytes. Dual mechanism regulation by nitric oxide and S-nitrosothiols. J Gen Physiol 108:277–293, 1996.

CHAPTER 7

Stretch Effects on Second Messengers and Early Gene Expression

•   •   •   •

Toru Suzuki and Tsutomu Yamazaki

The heart responds to hemodynamic overload by hypertrophic adaptation. Because pathologic hypertrophy and decompensation by the maladaptive heart lead to heart failure, much effort has been directed to understand how pressure stimuli are transduced. To date, the cardiac mechano-chemical receptor, if one exists, has yet to be identified. To this end, we have used an in vitro system of cardiomyocyte stretching to understand the signal transduction processes. Cultured cardiomyocytes stretched on silicone rubber dishes show activation of second-messenger components such as protein kinase C (PKC), Raf-1 kinase, and mitogen-activated protein kinases (MAPK) that are followed by an increase in protein synthesis. Interestingly, angiotensin II (Ang II) type 1 receptor antagonists attenuate increased protein synthesis, induction of MAPK activity, and *c-fos* gene expression induced by the stretching of cardiomyocytes. This suggests involvement of the cardiac renin-angiotensin system in pressure overload hypertrophy. Ang II–induced signaling pathways differ between cardiac myocytes and cardiac fibroblasts. Whereas Ang II activates MAPK through a pathway including the $G_{\beta\gamma}$ subunit of G_i protein, Src, Shc, Grb2, and Ras in cardiac fibroblasts, G_q and PKC activation are necessary in cardiac myocytes. Mechanical stretch also enhances endothelin (ET)-1 release from cardiomyocytes and activates the Na^+-H^+ exchanger. Furthermore, norepinephrine (NE) activates Raf-1 kinase and MAPK and increases amino acid uptake in cardiomyocytes. β-Adrenoreceptor (AR) and α_1-AR stimulation are involved in NE-induced MAPK activation. (Note that not only PKC activation but also protein kinase A [PKA] activation increases the activity of Raf-1 kinase and MAPK in cardiac myocytes). Finally, β-AR–induced activation of MAPK is dependent on both G_s/cyclic adenosine monophosphate (cAMP)/PKA and G_i/Src/Ras signaling pathways, and phosphorylation of β-AR is critical to cross talk between these signaling pathways. Thus, the cellular signalling pathways invoked by mechanical stretch have a fundamental role in mechanical transduction in the heart.

MECHANICAL OVERLOAD AND CARDIAC HYPERTROPHY

Mechanical overload causes adaptive changes in the cardiomyocytes. These changes include protein expression (e.g., myosin heavy chain) and increased cell size.[1] AR are activated in cardiac hypertrophy induced by hemodynamic overload. Laboratory experiments first showed that mechanical overload of papillary muscles accelerated protein synthesis.[2] Subsequently, increased aortic pressure was shown to increase protein synthesis in beating perfused hearts.[3] It was then shown that no hypertrophic changes occurred in papillary muscles where a cut tendon released the tension. In contrast, the neighboring uncut papillary muscles showed marked changes.[4] Similar results in culture showed that stretching cardiomyocytes induced protein synthesis and specific gene expression in the absence of neural or systemic humoral factors.[5,6] These data suggest that mechanical stretch per se induces hypertrophic changes.

Protein kinase cascades are candidates for the molecular mechanisms by which external overload evokes cardiac hypertrophy.[7] Mechanical stretch of cardiomyocytes activates second messengers such as phosphatidylinositol, PKC, Raf-1 kinase, and extracellular signal-regulated protein kinase (ERK). These proteins are involved in re-expression of a number of genes including atrial natriuretic peptide, skeletal α-actin and β-myosin heavy chain followed by increased protein synthesis.[8–10]

Involvement of the Renin-Angiotensin System in Cardiac Hypertrophy

Much evidence suggests that the cardiac renin-angiotensin system is linked to formation of pressure overload–induced hypertrophy. The renin-angiotensin system is activated in experimental left ventricular (LV) hypertrophy by hemodynamic overload.[11–14] LV mass increases induced by abdominal aortic constriction can be completely prevented by angiotensin-converting enzyme inhibitors. This occurs without changes in afterload or plasma renin activity.[15] Notably, a local renin-angiotensin system (e.g., renin, angiotensinogen, angiotensin-converting enzyme, and Ang II receptors) is present in the heart. All components are found at both the messenger RNA (mRNA) and protein levels.[14] In fact, an in vitro study has shown that mechanical stretch induces secretion of Ang II from cardiac myocytes of neonatal rats.[16]

To gain insight into the role of Ang II in mechanical stress–induced cardiac hypertrophy, cardiac myocytes were stretched in the absence or presence of Ang II inhibitors: saralasin (an antagonist of Ang II type 1 and 2 receptors), candesartan (an Ang II type 1 receptor–specific antagonist), and PD123319 (an Ang II type 2 receptor–specific antagonist).[17] Stretching control cells rapidly increased activities of Raf-1 kinase and MAPK. Both saralasin and candesartan partially inhibited the stretch-induced increase in the activities of both kinases, whereas PD123319 did not show inhibitory effects. Stretching increased amino acid incorporation in cardiomyocytes, which also was partially diminished by pretreatment with saralasin or candesartan. Culture medium conditioned by stretched cardiomyocytes increased MAPK activity in unstretched cardiac myocytes. This increase was completely suppressed by saralasin or candesartan. Taken collectively, the data suggest that the locally activated renin-angiotensin system plays a vital role in pressure overload cardiac hypertrophy. Ang II may act to promote the growth of cardiomyocytes by an autocrine mechanism.

To further assess the requirement of Ang II, heart cells from Ang II type 1a receptor knockout mice were stretched.[18] When cardiac myocytes were stretched by 20% for 10 minutes, ERK was strongly activated in both knockouts and wild types. However, basal and stimulated levels of ERK were greater in cardiomyocytes of knockout mice than in those of wild type mice. A broad-spectrum tyrosine kinase inhibitor and selective inhibitors of epidermal growth factor receptor suppressed stretch-induced activation of ERK in knockouts, but not in the wild type. The epidermal growth factor receptor was phosphorylated at tyrosine residues. Thus, mechanical stretch can evoke hypertrophic responses in cardiac myocytes lacking the Ang II type 1 receptor signaling pathway, possibly through tyrosine kinase activation.

Ang II induces hypertrophy without an increase in vascular resistance or cardiac afterload.[11] We examined Ang II–evoked signal transduction pathways leading to activation of MAPK in cardiac myocytes by using a variety of inhibitors.[19] Inhibition of PKC with calphostin C, or down-regulation of PKC by pretreatment with a phorbol ester for 24 hours, abolished Ang II–induced activation of Raf-1 kinase and MAPK. In contrast, pretreatment with tyrosine kinase inhibitors, genistein and tyrphostin, did not attenuate Ang II–induced activation of MAPK. Overexpression of c-src tyrosine kinase (CSK), which inhibits the function of Src family tyrosine kinases, had no effect on Ang II–induced activation of MAPK. However, pretreatment with manumycin, a Ras farnesyltransferase inhibitor, or overexpression of a dominant-negative construct against Ras inhibited insulin-induced MAPK activation. None of the inhibitors affected Ang II–induced activation of MAPK. On the contrary, overexpression of dominant-negative (DN) Raf-1 kinase completely suppressed MAPK activation by Ang II. These results, together with previous data,[10] indicate that Ang II induces cardiomyocyte hypertrophy through the PKC–Raf-1 kinase–MAPK cascade.

Ang II also evokes a variety of signals and induces proliferation of cardiac fibroblasts.[20] Unlike in cardiac myocytes, Ang II–induced MAPK activation is suppressed by tyrosine kinase inhibitors, but it is not affected by PKC down-regulation in cardiac fibroblasts[21] (Fig. 7–1). Inhibition of tyrosine kinases, but not PKC, abolished Ang II–induced MAPK activation

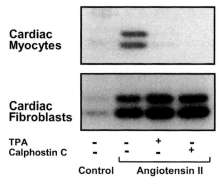

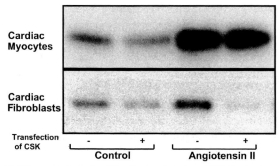

Figure 7–1 Involvement of protein kinase C (PKC) in angiotensin II (Ang II)–induced extracellular signal-regulated protein kinase (ERK) activation. Note that neither 12-0-tetradecanoylphorbol-13-acetate (TPA) nor calphostin C affect Ang II–induced ERK activation in cardiac fibroblasts, in contrast to cardiomyocytes.

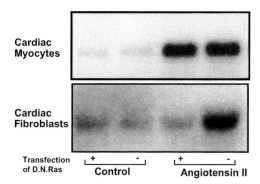

Figure 7–3 Role of Ras in Ang II–induced ERK activation. Note that transfection of a dominant negative (DN) construct against Ras inhibits ERK activation in cardiac fibroblasts, in contrast to cardiomyocytes.

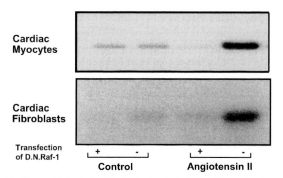

Figure 7–4 Role of Raf-1 in Ang II–induced ERK activation. Note that transfection of a dominant negative (DN) construct against Raf-1 inhibits ERK activation in cardiac fibroblasts, in contrast to cardiomyocytes.

in cardiac fibroblasts. Overexpression of CSK, DN Ras, or DN Raf-1 completely suppressed the activation of MAPK in cardiac fibroblasts (Figs. 7–2 to 7–4). Ang II rapidly induced phosphorylation of Shc and the association of Shc with Grb2 adapter protein in cardiac fibroblasts, but not in cardiac myocytes. This suggests that Ang II–evoked signal transduction pathways differ among cell types. In cardiac fibroblasts, Ang II activates MAPK through a pathway including G_i proteins, tyrosine kinases including Src family tyrosine kinases, Shc, Grb2, Ras, and Raf-1 kinase. In contrast, in cardiac myocytes, G_q and PKC are important (Fig. 7–5).

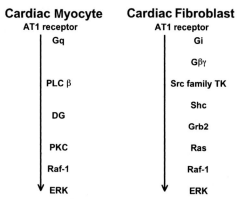

Figure 7–2 Role of Src in Ang II–induced ERK activation. Note that transfection of c-src tyrosine kinase (CSK) inhibits ERK activation in cardiac fibroblasts, but not cardiomyocytes.

Figure 7–5 Different Ang II signaling pathways in cardiac fibroblasts as compared with cardiac myocytes. AT1, angiotensin receptor type 1; PKC, protein kinase C; PLC, phospholipase C; TK, tyrosine kinase.

Role of Endothelin in Mechanical Stretch-Induced Hypertrophic Responses

The vasoactive peptide, ET-1, is involved in mechanical stretch-induced hypertrophic responses.[22] In cardiomyocytes, pretreatment with BQ123, an antagonist selective for the ET-1 receptor A (ET$_A$) subtype, diminished stretch-induced activation of MAPK and the increase in phenylalanine uptake; however, an ET$_B$-specific antagonist, BQ788, had no effect.

ET-1 was constitutively secreted from cardiomyocytes, and a significant increase in ET-1 concentration appeared in the culture medium of cells stretched for only 10 minutes. After 24 hours of stretching, ET-1 concentration increased threefold compared with unstretched myocytes. ET-1 mRNA levels were also increased at only 30 minutes after stretch. Moreover, ET-1 and Ang II synergistically activated Raf-1 kinase and MAPK in cardiac myocytes. Thus, ET-1, in addition to Ang II, modulates mechanical stress–induced cardiac hypertrophy.

Role of Ion Channels in Cardiac Hypertrophy

Activation of mechanosensitive ion channels has been proposed as a mechanism linking load and protein synthesis in cardiac hypertrophy.[23] Many cells rapidly respond to environmental stimuli using ion channels; mechanosensitive ion channels have been observed with single-channel recordings in more than 30 cell types of prokaryotes, plants, fungi, and all animals.[24] When cardiomyocytes are exposed to a Na$^+$ ionophore, c-fos expression is induced, possibly through increased Ca^{2+} uptake by the Na$^+$-Ca^{2+} exchange.[25] However, the expression of fetal-type genes is not induced by Na$^+$ increase (unpublished data). The Na$^+$-H$^+$ exchanger mediates mechanical stretch-induced hypertrophic responses such as activation of Raf-1 kinase and MAPK.[26,27]

To determine whether mechanosensitive ion channels and exchangers are involved in stretch-induced hypertrophic responses, cardiomyocytes were stretched after pretreatment with relatively nonspecific inhibitors of stretch-sensitive ion transporters: gadolinium ions (Gd^{3+}) and streptomycin for cation nonselective stretch-activated channels, glibenclamide for adenosine triphosphate–sensitive K$^+$ channels, CsCl for hyperpolarization-activated inward channels, and HOE 694 for the Na$^+$-H$^+$ exchanger.[27] Gd^{3+}, streptomycin, glibenclamide, and CsCl did not show any inhibitory effects on MAPK activation by mechanical stretch. HOE 694, however, markedly diminished the stretch-induced activation of Raf-1 kinase and MAPK and attenuated stretch-induced increases in phenylalanine incorporation.

Furthermore, HOE 694, in combination with an Ang II type 1 receptor antagonist (candesartan) and an ET$_A$ antagonist (BQ123), almost completely suppressed mechanical stretch-induced MAPK activation.

The Na$^+$-H$^+$ exchanger and the autocrine release of vasoactive peptides such as Ang II and ET-1 represent at least two different signaling pathways by which mechanical stretch can activate MAPK, leading to hypertrophy.

Rho Family Small Guanosine Triphosphate–Binding Proteins in Mechanical Stretch-Evoked Hypertrophy

To further elucidate how mechanical stretch induces hypertrophic responses, the role of the Rho family small guanosine triphosphate–binding proteins (G proteins) was examined.[28]

Treatment of neonatal rat cardiomyocytes with C3 exoenzyme, which inhibits Rho functions, suppressed stretch-induced activation of MAPK. Overexpression of the Rho guanosine diphosphate dissociation inhibitor (Rho-GDI), DN mutant of RhoA (DN RhoA), or DN Rac1 significantly inhibited stretch-induced activation of MAPK.

In contrast, overexpression of DN Ras had no effect on stretch-induced activation of MAPK. The promoter activity of skeletal α-actin and c-fos genes was increased by stretch, and these increases were completely inhibited by either cotransfection of Rho-GDI or pretreatment with C3 exoenzyme. Mechanical stretch-induced phenylalanine uptake was also suppressed by pretreatment with C3 exoenzyme. However, overexpression of Rho-GDI or DN RhoA did not affect

Ang II–induced activation of MAPK. MAPK also were activated by conditioned culture media from stretched control cardiomyocytes. However, pretreatment by C3 exoenzyme inhibited this activity. The Rho family of small G proteins appears to be critically involved in stretch-induced hypertrophic responses, including the release of Ang II.

NOREPINEPHRINE-INDUCED SIGNAL TRANSDUCTION PATHWAYS IN CARDIOMYOCYTES

Cardiac hypertrophy is often associated with an increase in intracardiac sympathetic nerve activity and with increased plasma catecholamines. Treatment of cardiac myocytes with catecholamines not only changes properties such as beating rate and contractility, but also induces typical hypertrophic responses. There are two major receptor subtypes of AR: α and β. AR agonists such as NE (α and β), phenylephrine (PHE; α), and isoproterenol (ISO; β) have been reported to induce hypertrophy. Prolonged infusion of subpressor doses of NE increases the mass of the myocardium and the thickness of the LV wall, suggesting that NE has direct hypertrophic effects without affecting afterload.[11]

Although NE induces cardiac hypertrophy by activating PKA and PKC through β- and α_1-AR, respectively, PKA has been reported to inhibit cell growth in other cell types. To discover the molecular mechanism of NE-induced hypertrophic responses and the effects of PKA and PKC on the activities of Raf-1 kinase and MAPK and on protein synthesis rates, we used cultured cardiomyocytes of neonatal rats. NE-induced activation of MAPK was partially inhibited by either an α_1-AR blocker, prazosin, or a β-AR blocker, propranolol. Simultaneous application of both inhibitors produced a complete block. A β-AR agonist, ISO, and an α_1-AR agonist, PHE, increased the activities of Raf 1 kinase and MAPK, and accelerated phenylalanine incorporation into proteins suggestive of increased protein synthesis. Furthermore, ISO and PHE synergistically activated these kinases and protein synthesis.[29,30]

Inhibitors for cAMP and PKA abolished ISO-evoked MAPK activation, suggesting that G_s protein

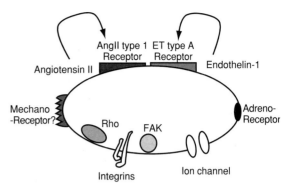

■ **Figure 7–6** Selected cell-signaling processes involved in cardiac mechano-chemical induction.

is involved in this activation.[31] Inhibition of G_i protein by pertussis toxin also suppressed ISO-induced MAPK activation. Overexpression of the $G_{\beta\gamma}$ subunit-binding domain of the β-AR kinase 1, which inhibits functions of $G_{\beta\gamma}$, also inhibited ISO-induced MAPK activation.

Overexpression of DN Ras, DN Raf-1 kinase, or β-AR mutant which lacks phosphorylation sites by PKA abolished ISO-stimulated MAPK activation. ISO-induced increase in protein synthesis was also suppressed by inhibitors for PKA, G_i, and tyrosine kinases including Src or Ras. These results suggest that ISO induces MAPK activation and cardiomyocyte hypertrophy through two different G proteins, G_s and G_i. β_2-AR mutant lacking phosphorylation sites for PKA when introduced into cardiac myocytes showed that inhibition of β_2-AR phosphorylation inhibits ISO-induced activation of MAPK. In summary, cAMP-dependent PKA activation through G_s, phosphorylates β-AR, leading to coupling of the receptor to G_i from G_s. Activation of G_i stimulates MAPK through $G_{\beta\gamma}$, the Src family of tyrosine kinases, Ras, and Raf-1 kinase (Fig. 7–6).

Role of Extracellular Matrix and Cytoskeleton

Mechanical stress is coupled to cells from the extracellular matrix (ECM).[32] Transmembrane ECM receptors, such as the integrins, are candidates for mechanoreceptors. The large extracellular domain of the integrin receptor complex binds to various ECM proteins, whereas the cytoplasmic domain interacts with the cytoskeleton.[32] Integrins, which are heterodimeric proteins composed of α and β subunits, can transmit signals through the cytoskeleton. They also can alter the cell's biochemical properties through tyrosine phosphorylation of proteins using, for example, the integrin-linked, focal adhesion kinase pp125FAK.[33] In addition, cytoskeleton proteins can potentially regulate plasma membrane proteins and stimulate second messenger systems. In this regard, pp125FAK has been reported to exhibit ECM-dependent phosphorylation of tyrosine and to physically associate with nonreceptor protein kinases through their Src homology 2 domains.[34] Integrins that are mechanically stressed probably serve as mechanical transducers.

Signaling Factors Involved in Mechanical Overload Cardiac Hypertrophy

In rat hearts pressure overloaded by aortic banding, mRNA levels of tumor growth factor (TGF)-β are increased.[25] However, because the increase is only seen 12 hours after binding, it is unlikely that TGF-β is the transducer for mechanical stress. Aldosterone also has been suggested to affect cardiac hypertrophy, independent of blood pressure.[35] When aldosterone is coinfused peripherally, intracerebroventricular infusion of mineralocorticoid receptor antagonists blocks blood pressure increase, but not cardiac hypertrophy or fibrosis. The role of kinins in cardiac hypertrophy also needs be addressed in the near future.

Summary

Mechanical stretch-induced Ang II and ET-1 can produce cardiac hypertrophy. The Na^+-H^+ exchanger is directly activated by mechanical stretch and can induce hypertrophic responses independently of autocrine release of Ang II and ET-1. The hypertrophic response is, in turn, modulated by activation of Rho family G proteins. The Ang II–induced signal transduction pathways that lead to MAPK activation diverge among cell types. Acting through signaling pathways, Ang II evokes cardiac myocyte hypertrophy and fibroblast proliferation (see Figs. 7–5 and 7–6).

NE activates the MAPK cascade, which is followed by an increase in protein synthesis through both α_1- and β-AR. The β-AR–evoked signal transduction pathways leading to MAPK activation are different among cell types. In cardiac myocytes, ISO activates MAPK through the pathway consisting of TGF-β–AR phosphorylation by G_s/cAMP-dependent PKA, $G_{\beta\gamma}$ subunits derived from G_i, Src, the formation of Shc-Grb2-Sos complex, Ras, and Raf-1 kinase. Further understanding of the signal transduction system will contribute to new therapeutic strategies for cardiovascular diseases.

References

1. Morgan HE, Gordon EE, Kita Y, et al: Biochemical mechanisms of cardiac hypertrophy. Annu Rev Physiol 49:533–543, 1987.
2. Peterson MB, Lesch M: Protein synthesis and amino acid transport in isolated rabbit right ventricular muscle. Circ Res 31:317–327, 1972.
3. Kira Y, Kochel PJ, Gordon EE, et al: Aortic perfusion pressure as a determinant of cardiac protein synthesis. Am J Physiol 246:C247–258, 1984.
4. Cooper G, Kent RL, Uboh CE, et al: Hemodynamic versus adrenergic control of cat right ventricular hypertrophy. J Clin Invest 75:1403–1414, 1985.
5. Komuro I, Kaida T, Shibazaki Y, et al: Stretching cardiac myocytes stimulates proto-oncogene expression. J Biol Chem 265:3595–3598, 1990.
6. Komuro I, Katoh Y, Kaida T, et al: Mechanical loading stimulates cell hypertrophy and specific gene expression in cultured rat cardiac myocytes. J Biol Chem 266:1265–1268, 1991.
7. Yamazaki T, Komuro I, Yazaki Y: Molecular mechanism of cardiac cellular hypertrophy by mechanical stress. J Mol Cell Cardiol 27:133–140, 1995.
8. Sadoshima J, Izumo S: Mechanical stretch rapidly activates multiple signal transduction pathways in cardiac myocytes: Potential involvement of an autocrine/paracrine mechanism. EMBO J 12:1681–1692, 1993.
9. Yamazaki T, Tobe K, Hoh E, et al: Mechanical loading activates mitogen-activated protein kinase and S6 peptide kinase in cultured rat cardiac myocytes. J Biol Chem 268:12069–12076, 1993.
10. Yamazaki T, Komuro I, Kudoh S, et al: Mechanical stress activates protein kinase cascade of phosphorylation in neonatal rat cardiac myocytes. J Clin Invest 96:438–446, 1995.
11. Baker KM, Booz GW, Dostal DE: Cardiac actions of angiotensin II: Role of an intracardiac renin-angiotensin system. Annu Rev Physiol 54:227–241, 1992.
12. Schunkert H, Dzau VJ, Tang SS, et al: Increased rat cardiac angiotensin converting enzyme activity and mRNA expression in pressure overload left ventricular hypertrophy: Effect on coronary resistance, contractility, and relaxation. J Clin Invest 86:1913–1920, 1990.

13. Shiojima I, Komuro I, Yamazaki T, et al: Molecular aspects of the control of myocardial relaxation. In Lorell BH, Grossman W (eds): Diastolic Relaxation of the Heart. Boston, Kluwer Academic Publishers. 1994, pp 25–32.

14. Suzuki J, Matsubara H, Urakami M, et al: Rat angiotensin II (type 1A) receptor mRNA regulation and subtype expression in myocardial growth and hypertrophy. Circ Res 73:439–447, 1993.

15. Baker KM, Chernin MI, Wixon SK, et al: Renin-angiotensin system involvement in pressure-overload cardiac hypertrophy in rats. Am J Physiol 259:H324–332, 1990.

16. Sadoshima J, Xu Y, Slayter HS, et al: Autocrine release of angiotensin II mediates stretch-induced hypertrophy of cardiac myocytes in vitro. Cell 75:977–984, 1993.

17. Yamazaki T, Komuro I, Kudoh S, et al: Angiotensin II partly mediates mechanical stress-induced cardiac hypertrophy. Circ Res 77:258–265, 1995.

18. Kudoh S, Komuro I, Hiroi Y, et al: Mechanical stretch induces hypertrophic responses in cardiac myocytes of angiotensin II type 1a receptor knockout mice. J Biol Chem 273:24037–24043, 1998.

19. Zou Y, Komuro I, Yamazaki T, et al: Protein kinase C, but not tyrosine kinases or Ras, plays a critical role in angiotensin II-induced activation of Raf-1 kinase and extracellular signal-regulated protein kinases in cardiac myocytes. J Biol Chem 271:33592–33597, 1996.

20. Schorb W, Booz GW, Dostal DE, et al: Angiotensin II is mitogenic in neonatal rat cardiac fibroblasts. Circ Res 72:1245–1254, 1993.

21. Zou Y, Komuro I, Yamazaki T, et al: Cell type-specific angiotensin II-evoked signal transduction pathways. Critical roles of Gbg subunit, Src family, and Ras in cardiac fibroblasts. Circ Res 82:337–345, 1998.

22. Yamazaki T, Komuro I, Kudoh S, et al: Endothelin-1 is involved in mechanical stress-induced cardiomyocyte hypertrophy. J Biol Chem 271:3221–3228, 1996.

23. Kent RL, Hoober K, Cooper G IV: Load responsiveness of protein synthesis in adult mammalian myocardium: Role of cardiac deformation linked to sodium influx. Circ Res 64:74–85, 1989.

24. Morris CE: Mechanosensitive ion channels. J Membr Biol 113:93–107, 1990.

25. Komuro I, Katoh Y, Hoh E, et al: Mechanisms of cardiac hypertrophy and injury: Possible role of protein kinase C activation. Jpn Circ J 55:1149–1157, 1991.

26. Takewaki S, Kuro-o M, Hiroi Y, et al: Activation of Na+-H+ antiporter (NHE-1) gene expression during growth, hypertrophy and proliferation of the rabbit cardiovascular system. J Mol Cell Cardiol 27:729–742, 1995.

27. Yamazaki T, Komuro I, Kudoh S, et al: Role of ion channels and exchangers in mechanical stretch-induced cardiomyocyte hypertrophy. Circ Res 82:430–437, 1998.

28. Aikawa R, Komuro I, Yamazaki T, et al: Rho family small G proteins play critical roles in mechanical stress-induced hypertrophic responses in cardiac myocytes. Circ Res 84:458–466, 1999.

29. Yamazaki T, Komuro I, Zou Y, et al: Protein kinase A and protein kinase C synergistically activate the Raf-1 kinase/mitogen-activated protein kinase cascade in neonatal rat cardiomyocytes. J Mol Cell Cardiol 29:2491–2501, 1997.

30. Yamazaki T, Komuro I, Zou Y, et al: Norepinephrine induces the raf-1 kinase/mitogen-activated protein kinase cascade through both alpha 1- and beta-adrenoceptors. Circulation 95:1260–1268, 1997.

31. Zou Y, Komuro I, Yamazaki T, et al: Both Bs and Gi are critically involved in isoproterenol-induced cardiomyocyte hypertrophy. J Biol Chem 274:9760–9770, 1999.

32. Juliano RL, Haskill S: Signal transduction from the extracellular matrix. J Cell Biol 120:577–585, 1993.

33. Hynes RO. Integrins: Versatility, modulation and signaling in cell adhesion. Cell 69:11–25, 1992.

34. Schaller MD, Hildebrand JD, Shammon JD, et al: Autophosphorylation of the focal adhesion kinase, pp125FAK, directs SH2-dependent binding of pp60Src. Mol Cell Biol 14:1680–1688, 1994.

35. Young M, Head G, Funder J: Determinants of cardiac fibrosis in experimental hypermineralocorticoid states. Am J Physiol 269:E657–E662, 1995.

EFFECTS OF MECHANO-ELECTRIC FEEDBACK ON CARDIAC CELLULAR ELECTROPHYSIOLOGY

•   •   •   •

CHAPTER 8

Mechanical Modulation of Sinoatrial Node Pacemaking

• • • •

Patricia J. Cooper and Peter Kohl

It is well known that when venous inflow to the heart increases, the venous pressure rises and the output of the heart becomes larger. At the same time the heart beats more frequently and the increase in the rate of the pulse may be very considerable.[1]

This observation by Francis A. Bainbridge of the positive chronotropic response of the heart to stretch has given rise to numerous studies into the mechanisms and relevance of venous return–induced changes in heart rate. This chapter reviews these studies and presents evidence beyond the original nervous reflex theory toward mechanically modulated intrinsic cardiac mechanisms and mechano-electric feedback (MEF).

The Bainbridge Reflex

The studies by Bainbridge[1] used volume loading through injection of fluids into the jugular vein of anesthetized dogs to increase venous return. Arterial and venous pressures, respiration, and pulse rate were monitored. This study showed that an increase in venous pressure could increase cardiac beating rate (BR) in the absence of changes in arterial pressure. This was attributed to a vagal response and is now referred to as the Bainbridge reflex.

Several investigators have repeated Bainbridge's experiments, and the majority did observe tachycardia with increased venous return, although some found little change or the opposite response, as reviewed in detail elsewhere.[2]

The relevance of the Bainbridge reflex for human physiology is still a subject of contention. Its principal applicability, however, has been confirmed in a study where passive elevation of the legs of human volunteers

in supine position increased BR. This is caused by an increase in venous return (autotransfusion), as witnessed by an increase in central venous pressure, in the absence of changes in arterial pressure (an important difference to standard tilt-table studies where both venous return and arterial pressure are increased, resulting in the opposite effect).[3]

Interestingly, an equivalent response—stretch-induced increase in BR—has been subsequently observed in isolated hearts[4] and isolated sinoatrial node (SAN) tissue,[5] suggesting that the Bainbridge effect may be determined, at least in part, at the level of the SAN pacemaker.

Physiologic Stimuli

Changes in venous return to the atria not only affect the volume available for rapid ventricular filling and atrial contraction, but also diastolic atrial dimensions. Increased right atrial filling distends the atrial wall, including the SAN.

The majority of atrial filling is, as in the ventricles, caused by a shift in atrioventricular border position. In contrast to ventricular filling, this is an active process, caused by ventricular contraction. This pulls the atrioventricular border toward the cardiac apex, thereby distending the atria, which fill with blood from the *venae cavae* (i.e., the heart is a combined pressure and suction pump). The extent of atrial filling depends crucially on the available venous blood volume–venous return.

Mechanisms that affect venous return include interventions that cause undulation in venous pressure, which, in the presence of competent semilunar valves in the venous vasculature, direct blood flow toward the heart. Such pressure changes are caused by arterial pulse wave effects on neighboring veins, skeletal muscle activity, and respiratory fluctuations in the thoraco-abdominal pressure gradient.

The latter may be involved in the non-neuronal component of respiratory sinus arrhythmia (RSA).[6] During inspiration, the thoraco-abdominal pressure gradient favors venous return to the heart, whereas the opposite prevails during expiration. These respiratory-induced fluctuations in venous return may promote matching changes in SAN stretch and BR: an increase during inspiration and a decrease during expiration. Whereas this non-neuronal component of RSA plays little, if any, role in healthy subjects at rest (<1%), it may account for up to a third of RSA during heavy exercise (for further details, see Chapter 19).

Thus, mechanical stimuli affect SAN pacemaking. To discuss potential mechanisms of this cardiac MEF, the next section briefly reviews SAN electrophysiology.

THE SINOATRIAL NODE

Sinoatrial Node Pacemaker Electrophysiology

The SAN is the site of initiation of primary pacemaker activity in the mammalian heart.[7] Other regions of the heart that may spontaneously generate rhythmic action potentials (AP), such as the atrioventricular node and Purkinje fibers, do so at lower intrinsic rates and therefore will not determine normal cardiac BR. The SAN is located at the junction of the superior vena cava with the right atrium, extending in parallel with the *crista terminalis* toward the inferior vena cava. The precise location of the SAN differs from species to species; Figure 8–1*A* illustrates rabbit SAN location.

Pacemaker cells are characterized by the absence of a stable resting membrane potential (see Fig. 8–1*B, left*). Instead, they display spontaneous diastolic depolarization, from their maximum diastolic potential (MDP) toward threshold for AP generation. In situ, cells in the SAN center show the least negative MDP and the fastest rate of diastolic depolarization, and, despite having the slowest rate of AP upstroke, they set BR.[8]

The cycle of spontaneous electrical activity in SAN cells is brought about by the finely balanced interac-

tion of a number of ion-handling processes that are highly interdependent and both time- and voltage-modulated. Figure 8–2 depicts major contributors to central SAN pacemaking, beginning with repolarization from a preceding AP.

Outward (i.e., hyperpolarizing) K^+ currents (including, in varying amounts in different species, rapidly, I_{Kr}, and slowly, I_{Ks}, activating components of the delayed rectifier potassium current) drive the membrane potential toward the MDP. As the SAN cell membrane becomes more negative, these channels progressively inactivate, whereas the hyperpolarization-activated inward (i.e., depolarizing) current, I_f, is activated. Also, with the increasingly negative membrane potential, the inward sodium and calcium background currents, $I_{b,Na}$ and $I_{b,Ca}$, reach their maximum (determined by the difference in actual membrane potential and reversal potential of these currents). Together, these currents force a change in net membrane current from outward to inward (see I_{Cell}), thereby turning the direction of membrane potential dynamics from hyperpolarizing to depolarizing.

Progressive diastolic depolarization causes activation of the inward transient Ca^{2+} current, $I_{Ca,T}$. This increases intracellular Ca^{2+} concentration in a confined submembrane space, which, through regional Ca^{2+}-induced Ca^{2+} release, may cause local Ca^{2+} discharge events from the sarcoplasmic reticulum (SR). Increased submembrane Ca^{2+} may then activate additional inward current through the Na^+-Ca^{2+} exchanger, I_{NaCa}.[11,12]

The above inward currents eventually drive the SAN membrane potential toward threshold for activation of the long-lasting Ca^{2+} current, $I_{Ca,L}$, and global release of Ca^{2+} from the SR.[13] The rapid depolarization to maximum systolic potential (MSP) is carried chiefly by $I_{Ca,L}$ in primary SAN pacemaker cells (although the fast sodium current, I_{Na}, may contribute to peripheral SAN activity and underlie pacemaking in fast-beating species, such as mice[14]).

Depolarization to MSP causes inactivation of potential-sensitive inward currents, reduces the driving force for depolarizing background currents, and reactivates I_{Kr} and I_{Ks}, as well as the transient, I_{to}, and sustained, I_{sus}, outward currents. This causes membrane repolarization, until the subsequent SAN cycle begins.

The relative contribution of individual currents varies with location in the SAN and among species.[15]

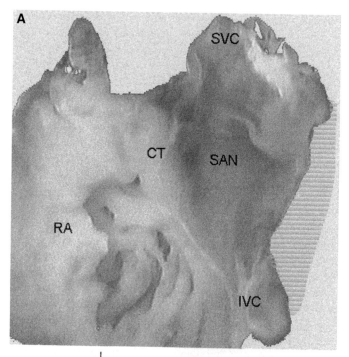

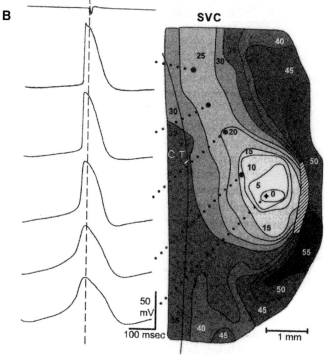

■ Figure 8–1 Rabbit sinoatrial node (SAN) and in situ pacemaker cell activity. *A,* Endocardial view of the SAN, located between the superior and inferior vena cava (SVC and IVC, respectively), and bordered by the *crista terminalis* (CT); RA, right auriculum. *B,* Single SAN cell trans-membrane potentials *(left)* and SAN spatial activation pattern *(right),* measured with microelectrode impalements; the *cross* (at 0 msec) indicates the leading pacemaker site in the SAN center. *(From Bleeker WK, Mackaay AJC, Masson-Pévet M, et al: Functional and morphological organization of the rabbit sinus node. Circ Res 46:11–22, 1980, with permission.)*

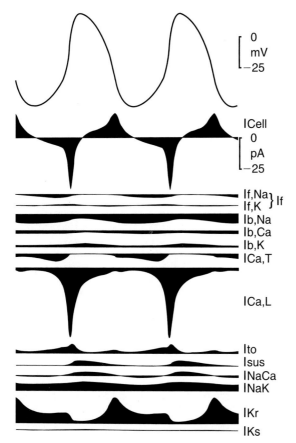

Figure 8–2 Mathematical model of SAN action potential (AP) and contributing ionic currents. *Top,* SAN AP, based on a rabbit central SAN cell model.[9] *Bottom,* Contributing ionic currents, computed using *COR*.[10] Each current is scaled to the same extent, illustrating the large magnitude of $I_{Ca,L}$ and I_{Kr} in this model.

SAN beating frequency is modulated by the autonomic nervous system, circulating hormones (see References 15 and 16 for reviews), and electrotonic interaction with surrounding atrial muscle.

Pacemaker Architecture and Conduction Pathways

SAN pacemaker excitation drives global atrial and ventricular activity through electrotonic interaction. Central SAN cells synchronize their activity through gap junctions, formed predominantly by Connexin 45,[17] that allow exchange of electrical and chemical information among neighboring cells (see Chapter 11). The extent of direct coupling among adjacent cells and effects from surrounding tissue dictate how stable the pacemaking site is and how fast and securely the electrical signal is propagated.[8,15]

The electrotonic interaction between the atrium and nodal cells has an essential influence on SAN pacemaking. Peripheral SAN cells have, after isolation, a greater intrinsic BR than central SAN cells. Their activity is suppressed, in situ, by the electrotonic effects from surrounding atrial tissue whose stable resting potential counteracts depolarization in peripheral SAN.[18] This can be illustrated by cutting the SAN free from atrial tissue, which causes a shift of the leading pacemaker site from SAN center to its periphery and an overall increase in BR.[19]

The central SAN is protected from atrial electrotonic inactivation by distance and low levels of intercellular coupling. An indication of the limited electrical coupling is the low conduction velocity in central SAN (2 to 8 cm/sec; see Reference 8). As the wave front moves toward the SAN periphery, it speeds up (20 to 80 cm/sec; see Fig. 8–1B for a map of SAN excitation[8]), because of increased connectivity among adjacent cells. Excitation finally invades atrial muscle, predominantly through the *crista terminalis* where cellular coupling is about one order of magnitude greater than in the node.[20]

Gap junctions in the SAN are not restricted to a single-cell type: pacemaker cells can be electrically connected to the extensive network of SAN fibroblasts (through Connexin 45).[17] The functional significance of this heterogeneous cell coupling in native SAN currently is unknown, but it is interesting, in the context of MEF, to note that cardiac fibroblasts are mechanosensitive cells.[21,22]

SINOATRIAL NODE MECHANICAL STIMULATION

As highlighted previously, the heart appears to be inherently able to respond to an increase in venous return with earlier initiation of the subsequent contraction. Investigations into underlying mechanisms have used a range of experimental models, from human volunteers to isolated SAN cells, each with its own advantages and limitations.

The Heart In Vivo

In vivo investigations offer the most relevant but least reproducible model system.[23] The experimental evidence resulting from this type of research was highlighted in the beginning of this chapter. Historically, it gave rise to the concept of a stretch-induced increase in cardiac BR.

For the study of underlying mechanisms, in vivo models need to be combined with lower order experimental tools that offer more control and less variability.

Isolated Heart or Atrium

Isolated organ preparations allow near-physiologic application of stretch, for example, through intra-atrial volume control, potentially in the presence of preserved vagal innervation.[24] An increase in right atrial pressure by 8 to 20 mm Hg has been found to increase BR in this type of preparation and has established the concept of an intracardiac BR response to stretch.[4,24]

Isolated Sinoatrial Node Tissue

SAN tissue strips provide a simple source for multiple SAN preparations that allow stable simultaneous recordings of electrophysiologic and mechanical parameters (either of these parameters allow identification of BR).[5,25] Stretch is usually applied uniaxially, often in parallel to the *crista terminalis* (through attachment of mechanical probes to the *venae cavae*).

In his pioneering study, Deck[5] used a photographic iris to apply concentric stretch to isolated SAN preparations, which may be more representative of in vitro mechanics. Using microelectrode recordings, he observed that the stretch-induced increase in BR is accompanied by a decrease in MSP and MDP (Fig. 8–3).

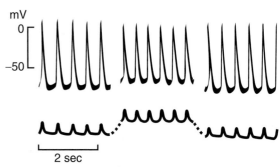

■ **Figure 8–3** Effect of stretch on cat isolated SAN pacemaking. *Top,* AP recording illustrating a stretch-induced reduction in maximum diastolic potential, decreased AP amplitude, and increased in beating rate. *Bottom,* Mechanical activity with contractions pointing upward; the shift in passive tension indicates stretch timing. *(From Deck KA: Dehnungseffekte am spontanschlagenden, isolierten Sinusknoten. Pflügers Arch 280:120–130, 1964, with permission.)*

The potential contribution of intracardiac neuronal pathways ("intramural reflex") to this response was ruled out in a thorough study by Wilson and Bolter.[24] Still, native tissue preparations have one major drawback: because of the visco-elastic properties of cardiac tissue, there is always a difference in both the timing and the extent of the external "command" mechanical intervention and its in situ equivalent at the cellular level. It is, therefore, difficult to grade, maintain, and repeat mechanical stimulation of SAN cells in native tissue. This can be overcome by using isolated cells.

Isolated Sinoatrial Node Pacemaker Cells

Cell Swelling

Isolation of spontaneously beating, Ca^{2+}-tolerant, SAN cells and maintenance of stable electrophysiologic AP recordings is no minor task. Additional mechanical stimulation therefore has initially been attempted by osmotic challenges and cell inflation, which require no additional probes and do not cause significant lateral translocation of the cell membrane under the recording electrode.

Hagiwara and colleagues[26] identified a swelling-activated Cl^- channel, $I_{Cl,Swell}$, in rabbit SAN cells, whose electrophysiologic properties, together with a cell volume–related increase in $I_{Ca,L}$ open probability, could underlie the stretch-induced increase in cardiac BR.

Subsequent research by Lei and Kohl,[27] however, showed that hyposmotic swelling actually reduces BR of spontaneously active SAN cells (Fig. 8–4A). Pharmacologic block of $I_{Cl,Swell}$ reduced BR further (in swollen cells only), reconfirming that this current indeed has a positive chronotropic effect. This does not, however, dominate the pacemaker response to swelling. Cell swelling, therefore, is not a suitable model for the study of mechanisms involved in the positive chronotropic response of the SAN to stretch.

In fact, cell swelling and stretch cause different micro-mechanical changes: swelling increases SAN cell diameter but not length, whereas stretch increases length and (because cell volume is understood to remain constant) reduces cell diameter. In addition, cell volume–controlled ion channels usually activate with a marked lag-time (≥ 1 minute compared with cell volume dynamics), suggesting the presence of intermediary reaction steps in their response to a mechanical event (for more details, see Chapter 3).

Cell Stretch

A number of experimental approaches have been deployed to stretch cardiac myocytes, including suction pipettes attached to opposite cell ends, glass probes or cantilevers for local deformation, and magnetic beads (although the latter do not currently allow

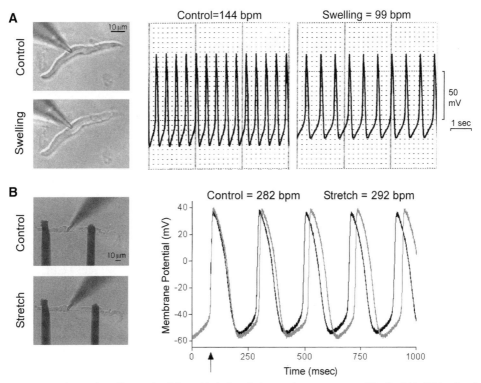

■ **Figure 8–4** Comparison of swelling and axial stretch induced changes in spontaneous BR of rabbit SAN cells. *A,* Swelling, induced by perfusion with 75% hyposmotic solution, causes a 32% increase in cell area *(inset)* and slowing of SAN cell BR.[27] *B,* Axial stretch by 7% of cell length *(inset)* increases spontaneous BR in SAN cells *(gray trace:* control; *black trace:* stretch).[29] *(From Lei M, Kohl P: Swelling-induced decrease in spontaneous pacemaker activity of rabbit isolated sino-atrial node cells. Acta Physiol Scand 164:1–12, 1998; and Cooper PJ, Lei M, Cheng L-X, et al: Axial stretch increases spontaneous pacemaker activity in rabbit isolated sinoatrial node cells. J Appl Physiol 89:2099–2104, 2000, with permission.)*

application of axial stretch, but rather cause "centrifu-gal" membrane deformation that is, perhaps, more akin to cell swelling). Attachment of probes can be by negative pressure, various tissue glues, or electrostatic surface interactions. The carbon fiber technique, in particular, allows application of reasonably homogeneous cell distension, judging by the consistency of sarcomere lengthening established in ventricular myocytes.[28]

Using this technique, Cooper and colleagues[29] applied axial stretch to single, spontaneously beating SAN cells. AP were recorded before, during, and after application of stretch (increasing cell length by 5% to 10% of control; see Fig. 8–4B). Stretch results in an instantaneous and reversible increase in BR by about 5%, combined with a reduction in MDP and MSP, as observed by Deck[5] in the intact node. This, together with the isolated heart and SAN tissue experiments described previously, confirms that at least part of the Bainbridge effect is intrinsic to the heart and encoded at the level of individual SAN pacemaker cells.

Magnitude of the Sinoatrial Node Stretch Response

The stretch-induced increase in BR of single rabbit SAN cells (5%; see Reference 29) is significantly smaller than that observed in multicellular preparations (often 15% to 40%; see References 4 and 5). Although the observed increase in whole animal experiments is variable, it tends to exceed 10% of control BR.

This difference in the magnitude of SAN responses to stretch may occur for several reasons. Thus, isolation of single pacemaker cells from SAN tissue involves digestion of the extracellular matrix and may therefore remove or uncouple essential elements of the mechano-electrical transduction system (it is also conceivable that some of the removed components may normally protect a mechanosensitive pathway from activation, thereby potentially yielding false-positive findings in isolated cells). Also, intercellular interaction of SAN cells in situ may reinforce the dynamic response to a stimulus. In this context, the nature of SAN histoarchitecture may confer additional mechanosensitivity through stretch-activated fibroblasts[21] electrically coupled to pacemaker cells.[17]

There are major discrepancies in the amount of stretch that can be reversibly applied to single SAN cells (5% to 8% increase in cell length) and SAN/right atrial tissue preparations. Tissue preparations have been successfully stretched an order of magnitude more than isolated cells.[25] The extent of actual SAN pacemaker cell stretch in situ remains unknown, even though Kamiyama and colleagues[30] note that the peripheral SAN region is more distensible than the central SAN, presumably because of the greater connective tissue content of the center.

In situ stretch is a three-dimensional event for each cell that, given that SAN tissue behaves largely like an incompressible body, must involve positive *and* negative strain. This is further affected by the anatomic constraints placed on the heart in situ (e.g., by the pericardium), which affect the interrelation of venous return, atrial filling, and transmural pressure (see Chapter 23). For example, it has been known since 1915 that the increase in BR produced by venous return is more pronounced when the pericardium is intact,[31] suggesting a possible contribution of lateral tissue compression to the BR increase.

Stretch modality is another important determinant of the SAN response. Concentric stretch of isolated SAN tissue has a greater effect on BR (+16 %) than uniaxial stretch (+9 %).[5] Also, fast stretch is more efficient in increasing BR than slow distension, and stretch timed to occur during the electrical diastole has a greater effect than during systole.[25,32,33]

INTRINSIC MECHANISMS OF THE SINOATRIAL NODE RESPONSE TO STRETCH

Current Evidence

The observation that axial stretch of isolated SAN cells leads to an instantaneous and reversible increase in BR was followed up by the identification of a stretch-induced whole-cell current with a reversal potential near −11 mV and a conductivity of 6 nS/pF.[29] The amplitude and current-voltage characteristics of this current are compatible with activation of cation nonselective stretch-activated channels (SAC_{CAT}). Implementation of a matching ion current, $I_{SAC,CAT}$, in quantitative mathematical models of SAN pacemaker activity confirmed that this electrophysiologic mechanism would be sufficient to cause the changes in BR observed in isolated cells.[29]

To what extent can this activation of $I_{SAC,CAT}$ be reconciled with preexisting observations? The contribution of $I_{SAC,CAT}$ to pacemaking depends not only on its mechanosensitive open probability, expressed through the effective whole-cell conductance $G_{SAC,CAT}$, but on the effective driving force for ions to pass the channel. This is largely determined by the voltage difference between the current's reversal potential, $E_{SAC,CAT}$, and the actual membrane potential, E_M, according to $I_{SAC,CAT} = G_{SAC,CAT} (E_{SAC,CAT} - E_M)$.

This voltage dependence of the current helps to explain why stretch during diastole is more efficient in increasing BR than during systole or maintained distension.[25] SAC_{CAT} activation at an E_M negative to $E_{SAC,CAT}$ will produce depolarization. If this coincides with the spontaneous diastolic depolarization of SAN cells, the threshold for subsequent AP activation will be reached faster, thereby increasing BR.

This model also is in keeping with the general observation that the positive chronotropic response of the SAN to stretch is enhanced by reduction in background BR of the preparation[22,34] (reflected even in the 1882 study of Sewall and Donaldson,[35] who found that the effect of stretch on SAN BR is greatly enhanced by vagal stimulation). The rationale is that a reduction in BR predominantly prolongs the diastolic interval, the phase during which SAC_{CAT} activation will have its most pronounced positive chronotropic effect.

More precisely, SAC_{CAT} activation at membrane potentials that are different from, but moving toward, $E_{SAC,CAT}$ will have a positive chronotropic effect by enhancing the prevailing change in voltage ($\uparrow \Delta V$; e.g., during spontaneous diastolic depolarization; Fig. 8–5), whereas SAC_{CAT} activation during all other times will have the opposite effect ($\downarrow \Delta V$) and may be negatively chronotropic.

This suggests that the actual shape of the SAN AP will have a major effect on stretch-induced changes in BR. Figure 8–5 compares how the SAN AP, recorded from rabbit (see Fig. 8–5A) and mouse (see Fig. 8–5B), relate to $E_{SAC,CAT}$ (at −11 mV).

As indicated previously, electrical diastole is characterized by $\uparrow \Delta V$ effects. During systole, both $\uparrow \Delta V$ and $\downarrow \Delta V$ effects can be observed, although with species-dependent differences in their relative duration. In rabbit, systolic $\uparrow \Delta V$ and $\downarrow \Delta V$ effects are of roughly equal duration, whereas in mouse, SAN systole is dominated by effects of $\downarrow \Delta V$.

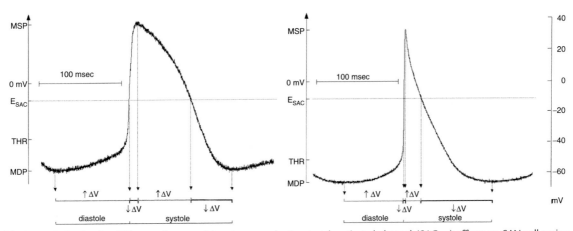

■ **Figure 8–5** Species differences in potential cation nonselective stretch-activated channel (SAC_{CAT}) effects on SAN cell action potential (AP). Membrane potential recordings illustrate the interrelation of cell electrophysiologic parameters (maximum systolic potential [MSP]; maximum diastolic potential [MDP]; threshold [THR] for activation of AP), and E_{SAC}. Electrical diastole, systole, and time periods during which SAC_{CAT} activation would cause either positive ($\uparrow \Delta V$) or negative ($\downarrow \Delta V$) chronotropic effects are labeled. A, Rabbit SAN cell. B, Mouse SAN cell.

The actual net charge transfer by SAC_{CAT} activation can be approximated by taking into account the potential difference between E_M and $E_{SAC,CAT}$ (driving force for $I_{SAC,CAT}$) during $\uparrow\Delta V$ and $\downarrow\Delta V$ phases. This is illustrated in Table 8–1, where both the relative duration of these phases and the product of time and driving force (area between E_M and $E_{SAC,CAT}$ in Fig. 8–5) are listed.

The data suggest that murine SAN is a model where stretch, depending on the actual $\uparrow\Delta V$:$\downarrow\Delta V$ ratio of the leading pacemaker, may have little effect on BR, or may even cause a negative chronotropic response (if, as in the given example, the ratio is <1.0). These responses have been observed in isolated murine SAN tissue, where uniaxial stretch by 40% to 80% caused either an increase in BR (8%), no change (8%), or a reduction (84%, n = 25; all changes were fully reversible; authors' observation).

Although it is intriguing that a majority of stretch-induced changes in SAN activity can be mathematically reproduced solely on the basis of SAC_{CAT} activation, there are additional direct and indirect effects of stretch. These include effects on other ion-transporting systems and second messengers. An influx of Na^+ through $I_{SAC,CAT}$, for example, may lead to a local (submembrane) increase in Na^+ concentration, thereby reducing the ability of the Na^+-Ca^{2+} exchanger to extrude Ca^{2+} (or, potentially, activating reverse mode Na^+-Ca^{2+} exchange). This would increase intracellular Ca^{2+} levels[36] and affect pacemaking. (Stretch effects on ion channels that are not customarily considered to be SAC are discussed in more detail in Chapter 4.)

Furthermore, stretch causes release of nitric oxide (NO),[37] which enhances SR Ca^{2+} release,[38] probably through S-nitrosylation of the ryanodine-sensitive SR Ca^{2+} release channel. There is constitutive NO synthase in SAN cells.[39] Because block of SR Ca^{2+} release by ryanodine reduces the heart's positive chronotropic response to stretch,[25] it is possible that NO-mediated effects on ryanodine-sensitive SR Ca^{2+} release contribute to the SAN response to stretch.

Future Investigations

Effects of NO on the SAN stretch response have not yet been addressed directly. The mechanism that links stretch and NO release is unknown. In cardiac myocytes in situ, stretch promotes integration of caveolae (the location of endothelial NO synthase[40]) into the sarcolemma.[41] The relevance of this effect, and its presence in SAN, are unknown.

Another possible mechanism of the positive chronotropic response to stretch—direct electrotonic interaction of SAN pacemaker cells with mechanosensitive[21,22] cardiac fibroblasts[17]—has only been assessed in mathematical models,[42] but not yet in direct experiments.

To reintegrate findings at the (sub)cellular level with tissue and organ function, selective pharmacologic tools are ideally required to modulate the transduction of a mechanical event into an electrophysiologically relevant signal in situ. Although gadolinium ions (Gd^{3+}) are potent blockers of $I_{SAC,CAT}$, their use is limited by nonselectivity[43,44] and precipitation in physiologic buffers.[45] In experiments on rabbit SAN strips, Gd^{3+} had no effect on the stretch-induced increase in BR.[25] The aminoglycoside antibiotic streptomycin has been shown to efficiently block SAC_{CAT} in isolated cardiomyocytes at concentrations less than 50 μM[36,46] (at greater concentrations, streptomycin also affects $I_{Ca,L}$[47]). Unfortunately, streptomycin appears to be ineffective in blocking SAC_{CAT} if applied to SAN tissue preparations through coronary circulation or bath superfusion (Fig. 8–6). Sung and colleagues[48] also saw no effect of 200 μM streptomycin on the stretch-induced slowing of conduction velocity in isolated whole-heart preparations, suggesting that its utility may be restricted to isolated cells.

More recently, a peptide (GsMTx-4), isolated from the venom of the Chilean tarantula *Grammostola*

TABLE 8–1   Species Dependence of Cation Nonselective Stretch-Activated Channel Effects on Sinoatrial Node Electrophysiology

Species	$T_{\uparrow\Delta V}$: $T_{\downarrow\Delta V}$	$\Delta Q_{\uparrow\Delta V}$: $\Delta Q_{\downarrow\Delta V}$
Rabbit SAN	70.8 : 29.2	72.7 : 27.3
Mouse SAN	46.4 : 53.6	47.5 : 52.5

Relation of duration, T, and net charge transport capacity, ΔQ, of positive ($\uparrow\Delta V$) and negative ($\downarrow\Delta V$) chronotropic effects. SAN, Sinoatrial node.

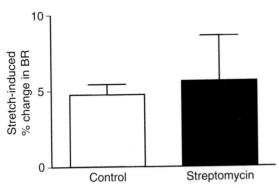

Figure 8–6 Lack of streptomycin effect on stretch-induced BR acceleration in guinea pig isolated SAN. Stretch of SAN tissue by, on average, 50% to 55% of resting length (using <5 mN applied force) causes a BR increase of 4.8% to 5.2% (n = 6). This response is not abolished by application of 40 μM streptomycin. Greater concentrations (200 μM) slow control SAN BR, in keeping with an effect of streptomycin on $I_{Ca,L}$, still without affecting the BR response to stretch. This suggests that, in contrast to L-type Ca^{2+} channels, SAC_{CAT} may be protected in situ from streptomycin action, perhaps by extracellular components that are lost in the process of cell isolation.

spatulata, has been identified as a potent SAC_{CAT} blocker.[49] It is highly specific (100 nM range) and has no reported side effects on any other cardiac ion-handling mechanism (see Chapter 42). This peptide has been shown to inhibit atrial arrhythmogenesis in isolated hearts during pressure overload,[50] and, in pilot experiments, blocked the SAN BR response to stretch (authors' unpublished data).

Summary

The stretch-induced increase in SAN BR has been observed in many different cardiac preparations, in the presence and absence of sympathetic and parasympathetic control pathways, and in using a multitude of methods to apply the mechanical stimulus. Studies dating back to the 1880s show that this response is observed in amphibians and mammals, including humans. The magnitude of the SAN response to stretch depends on a large variety of conditions, including background BR, modalities of mechanical stimulation, and pacemaker AP shape. Although the exact cellular mechanisms of this expression of cardiac MEF require further investigation, it appears that SAC_{CAT} play a key role.

References

1. Bainbridge FA: The influence of venous filling upon the rate of the heart. J Physiol 50:65–84, 1915.
2. Hakumäki MO: Seventy years of the Bainbridge reflex. Acta Physiol Scand 130:177–185, 1987.
3. Donald DE, Shepherd JT: Reflexes from the heart and lungs: Physiological curiosities or important regulatory mechanisms. Cardiovasc Res 12:449–469, 1978.
4. Blinks JR: Positive chronotropic effect of increasing right atrial pressure in the isolated mammalian heart. Am J Physiol 186:299–303, 1956.
5. Deck KA: Dehnungseffekte am spontanschlagenden, isolierten Sinusknoten. Pflügers Arch 280:120–130, 1964.
6. Kohl P, Hunter P, Noble D: Stretch-induced changes in heart rate and rhythm: Clinical observations, experiments and mathematical models. Prog Biophys Mol Biol 71:91–138, 1999.
7. Keith A, Flack MW: The form and nature of the muscular connections between the primary divisions of the vertebrate heart. J Anat Physiol 41:172–189, 1907.
8. Bleeker WK, Mackaay AJC, Masson-Pévet M, et al: Functional and morphological organization of the rabbit sinus node. Circ Res 46:11–22, 1980.
9. Garny A, Kohl P, Noble D: Cellular Open Resource (COR): A public CellML based environment for modeling biological function. Int J Bifur Chaos 13:3579–3590, 2003.
10. Garny A, Kohl P, Hunter PJ, et al: One-dimensional rabbit sinoatrial node models: Benefits and limitations. J Cardiovasc Electrophysiol 14:S121–S132, 2003.
11. Kimura J, Noma A, Iriswara H: Na-Ca exchange current in mammalian heart cells. Nature 319:596–597, 1986.
12. Bogdanov KY, Vinogradova TM, Lakatta EG: Sinoatrial nodal cell ryanodine receptor and Na^+-Ca^{2+} exchanger: Molecular partners in pacemaker regulation. Circ Res 88:1254–1258, 2001.
13. Hüser J, Blatter LA, Lipsius SL: Intracellular Ca^{2+} release contributes to automaticity in cat atrial pacemaker cells. J Physiol 524:415–422, 2000.
14. Mangoni ME, Nargeot J: Properties of the hyperpolarization-activated current (I_f) in isolated mouse sino-atrial cells. Cardiovasc Res 52:51–64, 2001.
15. Boyett MR, Honjo H, Kodama I: The sinoatrial node, a heterogeneous pacemaker structure. Cardiovasc Res 47:658–687, 2000.
16. Beaulieu P, Lambert C: Peptidic regulation of heart rate and interactions with the autonomic nervous system. Cardiovasc Res 37:578–585, 1998.
17. Camelliti P, Green CR, LeGrice I, et al: Fibroblast network in rabbit sinoatrial node: Structural and functional identification of homogeneous and heterogeneous cell coupling. Circ Res 94:828–835, 2004.
18. Garny A, Noble D, Kohl P: Dimensionality in cardiac modelling. Prog Biophys Mol Biol 87:47–66, 2005.
19. Kirchhof CJHJ, Bonke FIM, Allessie MA, et al: The influence of the atrial myocardium on impulse formation in the rabbit sinus node. Pflügers Arch 410:198–203, 1987.
20. Verheule S, van Kempen MJA, Postma S, et al: (2001) Gap junctions in the rabbit sinoatrial node. Am J Physiol 280:H2103–H2115, 2001.

21. Stockbridge LL, French AS: Stretch-activated cation channels in human fibroblasts. Biophys J 54:187–190, 1988.
22. Kohl P, Kamkin AG, Kiseleva IS, et al: Mechanosensitive fibroblasts in the sino-atrial node region of rat heart: Interaction with cardiomyocytes and possible role. Exp Physiol 79:943–956, 1994.
23. Hearse DJ, Sutherland FJ: Experimental models for the study of cardiovascular function and disease. Pharmacol Res 41:597–603, 2000.
24. Wilson SJ, Bolter CP: Do cardiac neurons play a role in the intrinsic control of heart rate in the rat? Exp Physiol 87:675–682, 2002.
25. Arai A, Kodama I, Toyama J: Roles of Cl⁻ channels and Ca²⁺ mobilization in stretch-induced increase of SA node pacemaker activity. Am J Physiol 270:H1726–H1735, 1996.
26. Hagiwara N, Masuda H, Shoda M, et al: Stretch-activated anion currents of rabbit cardiac myocytes. J Physiol 456:285–302, 1992.
27. Lei M, Kohl P: Swelling-induced decrease in spontaneous pacemaker activity of rabbit isolated sino-atrial node cells. Acta Physiol Scand 164:1–12, 1998.
28. Le Guennec J-Y, Peineau N, Argibay JA, et al: A new method of attachment of isolated mammalian ventricular myocytes for tension recording: Length dependence of passive and active tension. J Mol Cell Cardiol 22:1083–1093, 1990.
29. Cooper PJ, Lei M, Cheng L-X, et al: Axial stretch increases spontaneous pacemaker activity in rabbit isolated sinoatrial node cells. J Appl Physiol 89:2099–2104, 2000.
30. Kamiyama A, Niimura I, Sugi H: Length-dependent changes of pacemaker frequency in the isolated rabbit sinoatrial node. Jap J Physiol 34:153–165, 1984.
31. Kuno Y: The significance of the pericardium. J Physiol 50:1–46, 1915.
32. Brooks CM, Lu H-H, Lange G, et al: Effects of localized stretch of the sinoatrial node region of the dog heart. Am J Physiol 211:1197–1202, 1996.
33. Lange G, Lu H-H, Chang A, et al: Effect of stretch on the isolated cat sinoatrial node. Am J Physiol 211:1192–1196, 1966.
34. Barrett CJ, Bolter CP, Wilson SJ: The intrinsic rate response of the isolated right atrium of the rat, Rattus norvegicus. Comp Biochem Physiol A 120:391–397, 1998.
35. Sewall H, Donaldson F: On the influence of variations of intracardiac pressure upon the inhibitory action of the vagus nerve. J Physiol 3:358–368, 1882.
36. Gannier F, White E, Lacampagne A, et al: Streptomycin reverses a large stretch induced increase in [Ca²⁺]ᵢ in isolated guinea pig ventricular myocytes. Cardiovasc Res 28:1193–1198, 1994.

37. Pinsky DJ, Patton S, Mesaros S, et al: Mechanical transduction of nitric oxide synthesis in the beating heart. Circ Res 81:372–379, 1997.
38. Vila-Petroff MG, Kim SH, Pepe S, et al: Endogenous nitric oxide mechanisms mediate the stretch dependence of Ca²⁺ release in cardiomyocytes. Nat Cell Biol 3:867–873, 2001.
39. Han X, Kobzik L, Severson D, et al: Characteristics of nitric oxide-mediated cholinergic modulation of calcium current in rabbit sino-atrial node. J Physiol 509:741–754, 1998.
40. Feron O, Belhassen L, Kobzik L, et al: Endothelial nitric oxide synthase targeting to caveolae: Specific interactions with caveolin isoforms in cardiac myocytes and endothelial cells. J Biol Chem 271:22810–22814, 1996.
41. Kohl P, Cooper PJ, Holloway H: Effects of acute ventricular volume manipulation on in situ cardiomyocyte cell membrane configuration. Prog Biophys Mol Biol 82:221–227, 2003.
42. Kohl P, Noble D: Mechanosensitive connective tissue: Potential influence on heart rhythm. Cardiovasc Res 32:62–68, 1996.
43. Lacampagne A, Gannier F, Argibay J, et al: The stretch-activated ion channel blocker gadolinium also blocks L-type calcium channels in isolated ventricular myocytes of the guinea-pig. Biochim Biophys Acta 1191:205–208, 1994.
44. Pascarel C, Hongo K, Cazorla O, et al: Different effects of gadolinium on I(KR), I(KS) and I(K1) in guinea-pig isolated ventricular myocytes. Br J Pharmacol 124:356–360, 1998.
45. Caldwell RA, Clemo HF, Baumgarten CM: Using gadolinium to identify stretch-activated channels: Technical considerations. Am J Physiol 275:C619–C621, 1998.
46. Belus A, White E: Streptomycin and intracellular calcium modulate the response of single guinea-pig ventricular myocytes to axial stretch. J Physiol 546:501–509, 2003.
47. Belus A, White E: Effects of streptomycin sulphate on Iᴄₐₗ, I_Kr and I_Ks in guinea-pig ventricular myocytes. Eur J Pharmacol 445:171–178, 2002.
48. Sung D, Mills RW, Schettler J, et al: Ventricular filling slows epicardial conduction and increases action potential duration in an optical mapping study of the isolated rabbit heart. J Cardiovasc Electrophysiol 14:739–749, 2003.
49. Suchyna TM, Johnson JH, Hamer K, et al: Identification of a peptide toxin from Grammostola spatulata spider venom that blocks cation-selective stretch-activated channels. J Gen Physiol 115:583–598, 2000.
50. Bode F, Sachs F, Franz MR: Tarantula peptide inhibits atrial fibrillation. Nature 409:35–36, 2001.

CHAPTER 9

Temporal Modulation of Mechano-Electric Feedback in Cardiac Muscle

• • • •

Ed White

MECHANICAL INFLUENCES DURING THE NORMAL CARDIAC CYCLE

The normal heart is under constantly changing mechanical influences. During diastolic filling, the atria and ventricles are distended. During the isovolumic phase of systole, there is an increase in ventricular pressure, and during the ejection phase, there is muscle shortening. Both muscle lengthening and shortening are important mechanical stimuli. Under conditions of increased cardiac output, such as exercise, there is increased diastolic filling and an increased ejection fraction (i.e., increased muscle lengthening and shortening). In diseased states, there often is significant mechanical and electrical remodeling (see Chapters 24–32), which, in the specific context of this chapter, includes increased diastolic load but depressed systolic ejection.

The pressure–volume relations of the cardiac chambers can be related to electrical activity, the electrocardiogram (ECG). However, both wall stress[1] and strain[2,3] vary across the thickness of the ventricular wall, and the effect of a mechanical stimulus on an individual myocyte is influenced by the orientation of the ventricular muscle sheets. These also vary across the ventricular wall.[4,5] These factors are difficult to characterize experimentally, but they have been predicted in a model of the pig heart by Hunter's group (see Chapter 41). Figure 9–1 shows how the strain may vary at different points within the left ventricle during the cardiac cycle.

In addition to this mechanical heterogeneity, there is electrical heterogeneity. The action potential duration (APD) of the subendocardial myocardium is typically reported to be longer than that of the subepicardial myocardium. These differences are thought to contribute to the transmural staggering of ventricular depolarization and repolarization.[6] Despite (or because of) this complicated system, the normal heart is mechanically effective and electrically stable. Mechano-electric feedback (MEF) is part of this normal functioning.

Because the mechanical stimuli on the heart change throughout the cardiac cycle, it seems reasonable to suppose that their effects on electrical activity will vary in time. The principle purpose of this chapter is to summarize the available information on how the nature of MEF changes throughout the cardiac cycle.

DIASTOLIC STIMULI

Transient diastolic stretch can produce transient depolarizations. The amplitude of these often is proportional to the amplitude of the stretch. They are more readily triggered by quick stretches than slow stretches. If sufficiently large, the depolarizations are suprathreshold and provoke action potentials. Clear examples of this phenomenon have been shown in rabbit[7] (Fig. 9–2) and canine[8] ventricles. In these experiments, a fluid-filled balloon was placed in the left ventricle, and its volume was increased to stretch the ventricular muscle. Changes in electrical activity are monitored by recording of monophasic action potentials (MAP). MAP do not measure the transmembrane potential of cells, but they do accurately reflect changes in the local transmembrane potential from the recording region, and thus are useful to show changes in resting polarization and action potential shape. The ability to trigger such stretch-induced excitations has been used to investigate the mechanisms of production

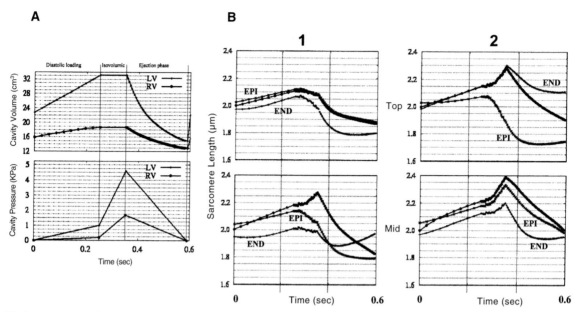

■ **Figure 9–1** *A*, Changes in left (LV) and right (RV) ventricular volume and pressure during the first 0.6 sec of a cardiac cycle in a computer model of the porcine heart. *B*, Simulated changes in sarcomere length in response to the changes in volume and pressures given in *A. 1* and *2* correspond to different positions on the LV free wall; sarcomere lengths are calculated at equatorial regions toward the base and mid-line of the chamber at positions *1* and *2*, for points within the subepicardium (EPI), subendocardium (END), and mid-myocardium (unlabeled). It is apparent that a great deal of strain inhomogeneity is predicted throughout the cardiac cycle (see Chapter 41). *(From Stevens C, Hunter PJ: Sarcomere length changes in a 3D mathematical model of the pig ventricles. Prog Biophys Mol Biol 82:229–241, 2003, with permission.)*

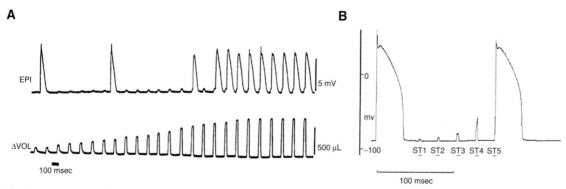

■ **Figure 9–2** Diastolic stretch: stretch-activated channels (SAC). *A*, Monophasic action potentials recorded from the epicardial surface of a rabbit, quiescent left ventricle *(top trace)*. Increases in ventricular volume *(bottom trace)* below a threshold volume cause visible transient depolarizations. Above this threshold increases in volume trigger action potentials. *B*, The experimental observations shown in *A* can be modeled by activation of nonspecific cationic SAC with the properties of those reported in the literature. ST1 to ST5 represent transient and increasing activation of SAC, which evokes increasing levels of membrane depolarization until, at ST5, an action potential is triggered. *(A, From Franz MR, Cima R, Wang D, et al: Electrophysiological effects of myocardial stretch and mechanical determinants of stretch-activated arrhythmias. Circulation 86:968–978, 1992, with permission; B, from Kohl P, Day K, Noble D: Cellular mechanisms of cardiac mechano-electric feedback in a mathematical model. Can J Cardiol 14:111–119, 1998, with permission.)*

and the conditions that potentiate them. For example, it has been shown that they are more easily triggered in diseased tissue than in healthy tissue (e.g., see Reference 9).

In resting single cardiac myocytes, stretch has been shown to provoke large increases in resting Ca^{2+} (see References 10 and 11) thought to be associated with a stretch-induced action potential that fails to fully repolarize (as a consequence of a stable membrane potential existing at depolarized potentials in these cells[12,13]). The mechanism for all these depolarizing effects is thought to be the opening of stretch-activated channels (SAC; see later in this chapter and also Fig. 9–2).

SYSTOLIC STIMULI

Brief systolic stretches of frog ventricle[14] that produced transient repolarizations, when applied early to the action potential plateau, had little effect at mid-

repolarization. They lengthened the final phase of repolarization when applied late in the action potential. Stretch throughout systole shortened the APD in frog ventricle strips, but not the APD of cat papillary muscle.[15] Early repolarization and late depolarization have been reported in rabbit hearts[16] (see Fig. 9–3) and are referred to as a "crossover" effect. Effects late in systole can resemble early afterdepolarizations in form and can develop into extrasystoles.[17] Changing the mode of contraction of the canine left ventricle from isovolumic (at high volume) to systolic ejection abolished these late depolarizations.[18,19]

MECHANISMS

Stretch-Activated Channels

The importance of this "crossover" effect is that it (and the diastolic depolarization mentioned earlier)

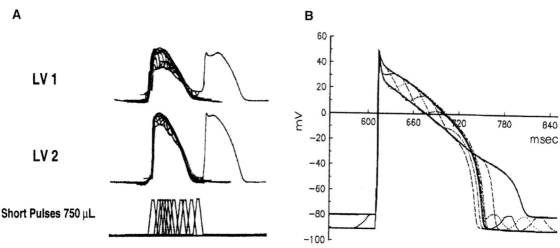

■ **Figure 9–3** Systolic stretch: stretch-activated channels (SAC). *A,* Monophasic action potentials (MAP) recorded from two sites on a rabbit left ventricle *(top and middle traces).* Transient increases in ventricular volume *(bottom trace)* during systole caused repolarization early in the MAP plateau and depolarization later. There is an intermediate "crossover" effect. The envelope of effect of the transient dilations described a MAP with a reduced amplitude and longer overall time course, this conformed well with the effect of a sustained stretch (not shown). *B,* The experimental observations shown in *A* can be modeled by activation of nonspecific cationic SAC with a reversal potential of −20 mV. The *heavy line* showing early repolarization and late depolarization represents the effect of steady-state (sustained) activation. *Thin lines* represent the effect of transient activations of 50 msec in total, every 20 msec throughout the action potential. The transient activations cause responses that conform to the steady-state waveform early in the action potential but deviate when activation occurs late in systole. *(From Zabel M, Koller BS, Sachs F, Franz MR: Stretch-induced voltage changes in the isolated beating heart: Importance of timing of stretch and implications for stretch-activated ion channels. Cardiovasc Res 32:120–130, 1996, with permission.)*

can be explained by a stretch-activated conductance that generates an outward (repolarizing) current at positive membrane potentials, a reversal potential at mid-repolarization levels (typically in the region of −30 to 0 mV), and inward (depolarizing) current at more negative potentials. The apparent reversal potential of this conductance suggests a nonspecific cation conductance. Single-channel recordings from nonspecific cationic SAC (see Chapter 1) that would fit this role were first reported in the mammalian heart by Craelius and colleagues in 1988.[20] Figure 9–4 shows an example of how whole-cell stretch-activated currents can be measured in single adult cardiac myocytes.

Simulations using the OXSOFT HEART (Oxsoft Ltd, Oxford, UK) model have investigated the effect of

SAC activation on a ventricular action potential with a high plateau phase (as found in humans and most mammals used experimentally but not in the adult rat and mouse). The model includes the properties of membrane channels and exchangers and of Ca^{2+} handling processes (of a guinea pig ventricular myocyte). Incorporating cationic SAC, with the properties found in experimental studies, can produce results similar to those seen experimentally[16,21] (see Figs. 9–2 and 9–3).

A class of K^+-selective SAC also has been reported (e.g., see References 22 and 23). During diastole, the membrane potential is quite close to the reversal potential of such channels, and they would be expected to generate little current when open. By contrast, during systole, their activation would be predicted to shorten APD, and stretch has been reported to shorten

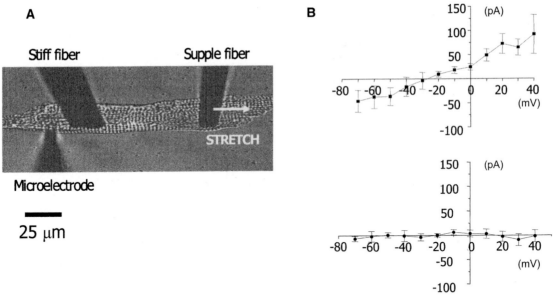

■ **Figure 9–4** Stretch-activated currents in single cardiac myocytes. *A,* A technique for stretching single cardiac myocytes. Carbon fibers are attached to the upper surface of the myocytes close to either end. The stiff fiber acts as an anchor, whereas the supple fiber is used to stretch the myocytes and is bent when the myocyte contracts. Bending of the supple fiber allows systolic shortening and the calculation of tension developed during these auxotonic contractions. Electrical activity is recorded through a microelectrode or patch pipette that is placed behind the stiff fiber to protect the site of impalement. Increased sarcomere length between the fibers is used as the index of stretch. *B,* Current–voltage (IV) curve for stretch-activated currents recorded in single guinea pig ventricular myocytes using the technique in A. Myocytes are action potential clamped; that is, the imposed voltage clamp waveform is that of the action potential previously recorded from the same cell under current clamp conditions. Axial stretch increased sarcomere length by approximately 8%. *Top panel,* IV relation in control solution (n = 10 cells); a stretch-induced current with a reversal potential close to −30 mV was recorded. *Bottom panel,* No stretch-activated currents were recorded in the presence (40 μM) of the stretch-activated channel blocker streptomycin (n = 8 cells). *(From Belus A, White E: Streptomycin and intracellular calcium modulate the response of single guinea-pig ventricular myocytes to axial stretch. J Physiol 546:501–509, 2003, with permission.)*

the late APD in some studies (for a review of this topic, see Reference 24).

Other Membrane Channels

Of course, stretch may also influence currents that normally flow during the action potential or are induced by other types of stimuli. One such channel that is not specifically mechanosensitive, but that is reported to be mechanically modulated, is the K^+ current activated by low levels of intracellular adenosine triphosphate (I_{K-ATP}).[25] By contrast, voltage clamp experiments have provided little evidence to support direct effects of axial stretch (as opposed to cell inflation) on the L-type Ca^{2+} current.[26,27] There may be an effect of stretch on the inward rectifier (I_{K1})[28,29] (see Chapter 4).

Notably, any SAC-induced changes in action potential configuration would affect the profile of current flowing through other channels during the action potential. This could occur through voltage-dependent changes in the driving force or activation or inactivation of voltage-sensitive but mechanically insensitive channels. Mechanically induced changes in Ca^{2+} may also influence any Ca^{2+}-dependent properties of channels and exchangers (see later). Such changes are complicated to assess experimentally, because to measure currents a preparation must be voltage clamped, but voltage clamping removes the stimulus—altered membrane potential. Models such as the one described earlier can address the interdependence of membrane potential, intracellular ion concentration, and electrogenic exchangers and ion channels.

Ca^{2+}

The introduction of this chapter noted that after the isovolumic phase of systole, there is ejection caused by muscle shortening. Changing the loading conditions on papillary muscles (at close to L_{max}, the length at which maximum force is produced) from "isometric" (force production rather than muscle shortening) to "isotonic" (muscle shortening rather than force production) was found to lengthen the action potential.[30] This effect was more prominent when the release of the muscle was close to peak force, which corresponds

to the rapid phase of action potential repolarization. A similar delay in the declining phase of the intracellular calcium transient is caused by release of stretched muscle (e.g., see Reference 31). These phenomena were related by the study of Lab and colleagues[32] (Fig. 9–5), which showed that the response of the Ca^{2+} transient to muscle release was faster than that of the action potential. This sequence of events supports the hypothesis that abrupt shortening of the muscle causes a rapid release of the Ca^{2+} bound to troponin C (TnC) into the cytoplasm. Some of this "extra" Ca^{2+} is extruded from the cell through the electrogenic Na^+-Ca^{2+} exchange, which extrudes one Ca^{2+} in exchange for the entry of three Na^+. This generates an inward depolarizing current responsible for the prolongation of the action potential. The study by Janvier and Boyett[33] (see Fig. 9–5) supports this hypothesis. Studies have shown some abbreviation of the early decrease in the Ca^{2+} transient on stretch, but these effects typically have less impact than the effects on release.[31] The study of Kohl and colleagues[21] predicted that because of changes in the Ca^{2+} affinity of TnC, a stretch throughout systole will lengthen the APD, whereas a stretch late in the action potential will shorten it through Ca^{2+} homeostasis: the interactions of free Ca^{2+}, sarcoplasmic reticulum Ca^{2+} release, and Ca^{2+}-activated currents.

However, it is worth noting that the changes in mechanical state that have been shown to produce changes in the cytosolic intracellular Ca^{2+} transient and the action potential are quite large, often from isometric at L_{max} to free shortening, and Franz and colleagues[18] and Hansen[19] have reported that changing from isovolumic to an ejecting mode of contraction flattened the late depolarizations in canine ventricle MAP. The observations in these two studies are consistent with ejection-associated muscle shortening causing the inactivation of depolarizing cationic SAC rather than the activation of depolarizing Ca^{2+}-dependent currents.

Another important point to bear in mind is that it is the subsarcolemmal Ca^{2+} (and, in the case of the Na^+-Ca^{2+} exchanger, Na^+), rather than bulk cytosolic ion concentrations, that will affect the sarcolemmal exchangers and ion channels. Stretch-induced increases in ion concentrations in this subsarcolemmal "fuzzy space," around the inner surface of open ion channels, may be greater than cytosolic changes.[34] If SAC and

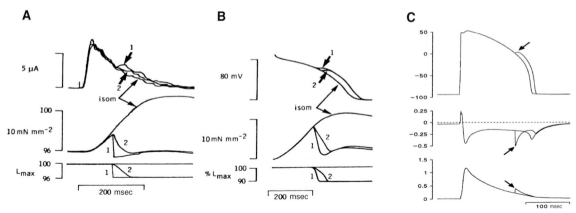

■ Figure 9–5 Systolic release: Na⁺-Ca²⁺ exchange. Intracellular calcium transients measured with aequorin *(A, top panel)* and action potentials *(B, top panel)*; tension *(middle panels)* and muscle length *(bottom panels)* in papillary muscle (of ferret *[A]* and cat *[B]*). Superimposed traces under isometric conditions (isom) and during a fast¹ or slower² release of the muscle during the development of tension. Release causes a lengthening of the intracellular Ca²⁺ transient and the action potential. The effects are faster if the release is fast. *C,* Modeling of the basic effect in *A* and *B* with the OXSOFT HEART model of the guinea pig ventricular myocyte. The affinity of TnC for Ca²⁺ is reduced at the *arrow* to simulate the effect of muscle release; there is a transient increase in intracellular Ca²⁺ *(bottom trace)* that generates extra inward Na⁺-Ca²⁺ exchange current *(middle trace)*, which prolongs the action potential *(top trace)*. *(A, From Lab M, Allen D, Orchard CH: The effect of shortening on myoplasmic calcium concentration and on action potential in mammalian ventricular muscle. Circ Res 55:825–829, 1984, with permission; B, from Janvier NC, Boyett MR: The role of Na-Ca exchange current in the cardiac action potential. Cardiovasc Res 32:69–84, 1996, with permission.)*

exchanger molecules are co-localized, then Na⁺-Ca²⁺ exchange current could be influenced by the entry of Na⁺ and Ca²⁺ through SAC that experimental techniques based on the measurement of cytosolic ion concentrations may not detect. By contrast, other changes, such as the liberation of Ca²⁺ from the myofilaments, will be greatest and will appear first in the cytosol.

IMPLICATIONS FOR TIMING OF STIMULUS

If the above discussion describes the "normal" influences of MEF, it also can be appreciated how these effects might be disrupted. For example, an area of weakened, stunned, or damaged tissue may be stretched during systole by the healthy neighboring tissue (e.g., see Reference 35). The balance between Ca²⁺-activated currents and SAC will be different between the healthy and weakened tissue. This is expected to lead to a relative shortening of the APD in the stretched region, with an increased dispersion of the APD and the associated risk for re-entry and arrhythmia.[36]

Commotio cordis is an example where the timing of an acute mechanical stimulus has been shown to be important (see Chapters 15 and 29). *Commotio cordis* describes the triggering of (sometimes fatal) arrhythmias by sudden chest impact over the heart, in the absence of obvious cardiac damage. The typical subject is a juvenile athlete. Using a porcine model, it has been shown that there is a vulnerable period for the triggering of ventricular fibrillation: 10 to 30 msec before the peak of the T wave in the ECG (i.e., ventricular repolarization). Outside this period impact could cause ST-segment elevation and transient heart block.[37] Interestingly, these researchers found the triggering of fibrillation and ST-elevation by chest wall impact (but not heart block) was significantly reduced by treatment with glibenclamide. On the basis of this result, the authors concluded activation of I_{K-ATP} is an important cellular mechanism in these effects.[38] Interestingly, the effect of glibenclamide on other cationic SAC is unknown, and K⁺-channel activation on its own may not explain the triggering of dysrhythmia during ventricular repolarization (see References 39 and 40). Conversely, it may be that the ability of a chest thump, or a more controllable equivalent, to correct electrical dysfunction is influenced by its timing (see Chapter 33).

SUSTAINED STIMULI

The Early Response

Increased dilation of the ventricles causes a greater (and in cases such as exercise, a faster) stretch of the myocardium in diastole. This leads to a greater muscle shortening during systole because of the Frank–Starling mechanism. The discussion to this point suggests that mechanosensitive influences on electrical activity from SAC will be depolarization in diastole and early action potential repolarization. During the late plateau, there will be conflicting effects of SAC carrying nonspecific cationic currents (depolarization) and those carrying K^+ currents (repolarization). But as the ventricle ejects, these may be outweighed by a depolarizing effect of Ca^{2+}-activated currents caused by muscle shortening. This analysis also predicts a crossover effect on the action potential. However, little is known about the time-dependent properties of cardiac SAC (see Chapter 1). For example, do SAC or the membrane/cytoskeleton adapt during a lengthy sustained stretch (see Chapter 5)? Also, it is known that intracellular Ca^{2+} changes in the minutes after stretch (see later); therefore, the effect predicted above may not be a stable response.

Indeed, many multicellular and whole-heart studies have applied a sustained stimulus throughout systole and diastole. Details of the specific interventions and responses are discussed in various other chapters of this textbook. To broadly summarize, the effects of sustained stretch on APD (see Reference 24), shortening (in situ human ventricle),[41] unchanged (canine ventricle),[42] crossover (in guinea pig atria),[43] and lengthening (in rabbit ventricle)[44] can all occur. Indeed, there can even be a difference in the response to stretch within a given preparation.[45]

In single myocyte studies, stretching by flexible carbon fibers increases diastolic sarcomere length, but also allows greater systolic shortening. The results include both APD shortening at 20 to 25°C[46] and lengthening at 37°C.[26] Using a different stretching technique, Kamkin and colleagues[27] have reported crossover

effects. Sinusoidal stretch in frog myocytes caused little change in APD.[47] Interestingly, sinusoidal *compression* elicited currents that increased and decreased in phase with the compressing stimulus,[48] thus suggesting SAC activity may indeed fluctuate through the cardiac cycle.

It is possible that the variety of reported effects of mechanical stimulation on the APD is caused by the impact SAC and shortening-dependent Ca^{2+}-activated currents have directly on membrane potential (as determined by the mechanical and electrical state of a given preparation). These effects are then modulated by intracellular ion concentrations (principally Na^+ and Ca^{2+}, as well as voltage-dependent channels and electrogenic exchangers.

The "Slow" Response

The discussion to date has centered on the response that typically occurs within the first minute after mechanical stimulation. When a sustained stretch is maintained over 10 to 15 minutes, there is a secondary increase in force and the amplitude of the intracellular Ca^{2+} transient (see Reference 49). Initial work suggested these slow changes in intracellular Ca^{2+} were dependent on diastolic stretch rather than systolic stretch.[50] Later work concluded that it is the proportion of each cycle under stretch, rather than any specific phase, that is important.[51] One might expect this slow increase in intracellular Ca^{2+} to influence electrical activity. Interestingly, Allen[52] reported that in papillary muscles, stretch caused initial APD shortening, followed by a slow lengthening of APD. Tavi and colleagues[53] also reported a slow increase in developed pressure and a lengthening of the APD with sustained stretch. However, von Lewinski and colleagues[54] found no correlation between the slow increase in force and APD.

Conclusions

When considering experimental data pertinent to MEF, the complex electrical and mechanical interactions in the heart (discussed only briefly in this chapter) should be borne in mind. This is because technical limitations require the integration of findings from studies performed on very different preparations (e.g., membrane patches to in situ whole hearts) using different mechanical stimuli (e.g., membrane deforming pressure, uniaxial stretch, whole ventricle dilation). In addition, most studies have applied what has been termed here a sustained mechanical stimulus—a stimulus that remains in place through several successive diastolic and systolic periods. This type of stimulus, often enforced by technical considerations, does simulate some but not all of the situations under which mechanical stimuli occur. Despite these problems, real progress in understanding the cellular mechanisms that underpin mechanical stimulation in the heart is being made. The studies that have been able to precisely coordinate the mechanical stimulus with a given phase of the cardiac cycle have provided elegant demonstrations and compelling evidence for cellular mechanisms of MEF.

With specific reference to the temporal effects of mechanical stimulation, the outcome of an intervention will be influenced by its timing within the cardiac cycle. The leading candidates for the mechanisms responsible for these time-dependent effects during diastole are SAC. During systole, shortening-dependent Ca^{2+}-activated currents, SAC, and consequent effects on voltage-sensitive processes are implicated. The challenge is to define the relative importance of these mechanisms under a given set of experimental conditions and relate that knowledge to observed effects on APD.

ACKNOWLEDGMENT

I thank Dr. Rachel Stones for comments on this manuscript.

References

1. Novak VP, Yin FC, Humphrey JD: Regional mechanical properties of passive myocardium. J Biomech 27:403–412, 1994.
2. Mazhari R, Omens JH, Pavelec BS, et al: Transmural distribution of three-dimensional systolic strains in stunned myocardium. Circulation 104:336–341, 2001.
3. Stevens C, Hunter PJ: Sarcomere length changes in a 3D mathematical model of the pig ventricles. Prog Biophys Mol Biol 82:229–241, 2003.
4. Streeter DD, Spotnitz HM, Patel DP, et al: Fiber orientation in the canine left ventricle during diastole and systole. Circ Res 24:339–347, 1969.
5. Bovendeerd PH, Huyghe JM, Arts T, et al: Influence of endocardial-epicardial crossover of muscle fibers on left ventricular wall mechanics. J Biomech 27:941–951, 1994.
6. Antzelevitch C, Fish J: Electrical heterogeneity within the ventricular wall. Basic Res Cardiol 96:517–527, 2001.
7. Franz MR, Cima R, Wang D, et al: Electrophysiological effects of myocardial stretch and mechanical determinants of stretch-activated arrhythmias. Circulation 86:968–978, 1992.
8. Stacy GP, Jobe RL, Taylor K, Hansen DE: Stretch-induced depolarisations as a trigger of arrhythmias in isolated canine left ventricles. Am J Physiol 263:H613–H621, 1992.
9. Wang Z, Taylor LK, Denny WD, Hansen DE: Initiation of ventricular extrasystoles by myocardial stretch in chronically dilated and failing canine left ventricle. Circulation 90:2022–2031, 1994.
10. Gannier F, White E, Lacampagne A, et al: Streptomycin reverses a large stretch-induced increase in $[Ca^{2+}]_i$ in isolated guinea-pig ventricular myocytes. Cardiovasc Res 28:1193–1198, 1994.
11. Gannier F, White E, Garnier D, Le Guennec J-Y: A possible mechanism for large, stretch-induced increases in $[Ca^{2+}]_i$ in isolated guinea-pig ventricular myocytes. Cardiovasc Res 32:158–167, 1996.
12. Calaghan SC, White E: The role of calcium in the response of cardiac muscle to stretch. Prog Biophys Mol Biol 71:59–90, 1999.
13. Gadsby D, Cranefield P: Two levels of resting potential in cardiac Purkinje fibres. J Gen Physiol 70:725–746, 1977.
14. Lab MJ: Mechanically dependent changes in action potentials recorded from the intact frog ventricle. Circ Res 42:519–528, 1978.
15. Lab MJ: Transient depolarisations and action potential alterations following mechanical changes in isolated myocardium. Cardiovasc Res 14:624–637, 1980.
16. Zabel M, Koller BS, Sachs F, Franz MR: Stretch-induced voltage changes in the isolated beating heart: Importance of timing of stretch and implications for stretch-activated ion channels. Cardiovasc Res 32:120–130, 1996.
17. Levine JH, Guarnieri T, Kadish AH, et al: Changes in myocardial repolarization in patients undergoing balloon valvuloplasty for congenital pulmonary stenosis: Evidence for contraction-excitation feedback in humans. Circulation 77:70–77, 1988.
18. Franz, MR, Burkhoff D, Yue DT, Sagawa K: Mechanically induced action potential changes and arrhythmia in isolated and in situ canine hearts. Cardiovas Res 23:213–231, 1989.
19. Hansen DE: Mechanoelectric feedback effects of altered preload, afterload, and ventricular shortening. Am J Physiol 264:H423–H432, 1993.
20. Craelius W, Chen V, El-Sherif N: Stretch activated ion channels in ventricular myocytes. Biosci Rep 8:407–414, 1988.
21. Kohl P, Day K, Noble D: Cellular mechanisms of cardiac mechano-electric feedback in a mathematical model. Can J Cardiol 14:111–119, 1998.
22. Kim D: A mechanosensitive K^+ channel in heart cells: Activation by arachidonic acid. J Gen Physiol 100:1021–1040, 1992.
23. Niu W, Sachs F: Dynamic properties of stretch-activated K^+ channels in adult rat atrial myocytes. Prog Biophys Mol Biol 82:121–136, 2003.
24. Cazorla O, Pascarel C, Brette F, Le Guennec J-Y: Modulation of ion channels and membrane receptor activities by mechanical interventions in cardiomyocytes: Possible mechanisms for mechanosensitivity. Prog Biophys Mol Biol 71:29–59, 1999.
25. Van Wagoner DR: Mechanosensitive gating of atrial ATP-sensitive potassium channels. Circ Res 72:973–983, 1993.
26. Belus A, White E: Streptomycin and intracellular calcium modulate the response of single guinea-pig ventricular myocytes to axial stretch. J Physiol 546:501–509, 2003.
27. Kamkin A, Kiseleva I, Isenberg G: Stretch-activated currents in ventricular myocytes: Amplitudes and arrhythmogenesis

effect increase with hypertrophy. Cardiovasc Res 48:409–420, 2000.

28. Sasaki N, Mitsuiye T, Noma A: Effects of mechanical stretch on membrane currents of single ventricular myocytes of guinea-pig heart. Jpn J Physiol 42:957–970, 1992.

29. Isenberg G, Kazanski V, Kondratev D, et al: Differential effects of stretch and compression on membrane currents and $[Na+]c$ in ventricular myocytes. Prog Biophys Mol Biol 82:43–56, 2003.

30. Hennekes R, Kaufmann R, Lab M: The dependence of cardiac membrane excitation and contractile ability on active muscle shortening (cat papillary muscle). Pflugers Arch 392:22–28, 1981.

31. Allen DG, Kurihara S: The effects of muscle length on intracellular calcium transients in mammalian cardiac muscle. J Physiol 327:79–94, 1982.

32. Lab M, Allen D, Orchard CH: The effect of shortening on myoplasmic calcium concentration and on action potential in mammalian ventricular muscle. Circ Res 55:825–829, 1984.

33. Janvier NC, Boyett MR: The role of Na-Ca exchange current in the cardiac action potential. Cardiovasc Res 32:69–84, 1996.

34. Bers BM: Cardiac excitation-contraction coupling. Nature 415:198–205, 2002.

35. Moulton MJ, Downing SW, Creswell LL, et al: Mechanical dysfunction in the border zone of an ovine model of left ventricular aneurysm. Ann Thorac Surg 60:986–998, 1995.

36. Babuty D, Lab MJ: Mechanoelectric contributions to sudden cardiac death. Cardiovasc Res 50:270–279, 2001.

37. Link MS, Wang PJ, Pandian NG, et al: An experimental model of sudden death due to low-energy chest-wall impact (commotio cordis). N Engl J Med 338:1805–1811, 1998.

38. Link MS, Wang PJ, Vanderbrink BA, et al: Selective activation of the K+(ATP) channel is a mechanism by which sudden death is produced by low-energy chest-wall impact (commotio cordis). Circulation 100:413–418, 1999.

39. Kohl P, Nesbitt A, Cooper PJ, Lei M: Sudden cardiac death by *Commotio cordis*: Role of mechano-electric feedback. Cardiovasc Res 50:280–289, 2001.

40. Garny AG, Kohl P: Mechanical induction of arrhythmias during ventricular repolarization: Modeling cellular mechanisms and their interaction in two dimensions. Ann N Y Acad Sci 1015:133–143, 2004.

41. Taggart P, Sutton PM, Treasure T, et al: Monophasic action potentials at discontinuation of cardiopulmonary bypass:

Evidence for contraction-excitation feedback in man. Circulation 77:1266–1275, 1988.

42. Calkins H, Maughan WL, Kass DA, et al: Electrophysiological effect of volume load in isolatedcanine hearts. Am J Physiol 256:H1697–H1706, 1989.

43. Nazir SA, Lab MJ: Mechanoelectric feedback in the atrium of isolated guinea-pig heart. Cardiovasc Res 32:112–119, 1996.

44. Sung S, Mills RW, Schettler J, et al: Ventricular filling slows epicardial conduction and increases action potential duration in an optical mapping study of the isolated rabbit heart. J Cardiovasc Electrophysiol 14:1–11, 2003.

45. Babuty D, Lab MJ: Heterogeneous changes of monophasic action potential induced by sustained stretch in atrium. Cardiovasc Electrophysiol 12:323–329, 2001.

46. White E, Le Guennec J-Y, Nigretto JM, et al: The effects increasing cell length on auxotonic contractions, membrane potential and intracellular calcium transients in single guinea-pig ventricular myocytes. Exp Physiol 78:65–78, 1993.

47. Reimer TL, Tung L: Stretch-induced excitation and action potential changes in single cardiac cells. Prog Biophys Mol Biol 82:97–110, 2003.

48. Bett GCL, Sachs F: Whole-cell mechanosensitive currents in rat ventricular myocytes activated by direct stimulation. J Membr Biol 173:255–263, 2000.

49. Calaghan SC, Belus A, White E: Do stretch-induced changes in intracellular calcium modify the electrical activity of cardiac muscle? Prog Biophys Mol Biol 82:81–95, 2003.

50. Allen DG, Nichols CG, Smith GL: The effects of changes in muscle length during diastole on the calcium transient in ferret ventricular muscle. J Physiol 406:359–370, 1988.

51. Hongo K, White E, Orchard CH: The effect of stretch on contraction and the Ca^{2+} transient in ferret ventricular muscles during acidosis and hypoxia. Am J Physiol 269:C690–C697, 1995.

52. Allen DG: On the relationship between action potential duration and tension in cat papillary muscle. Cardiovasc Res 11:210–218, 1977.

53. Tavi P, Han C, Weckstrom M: Mechanisms of stretch-induced changes in $[Ca^{2+}]_i$ in rat atrial myocytes: Role of increase troponin C affinity and stretch-activated ion channels. Circ Res 83:1165–1177, 1998.

54. von Lewinski D, Stumme B, Maier LS, et al: Stretch-dependent slow force response in isolated rabbit myocardium is Na+ dependent. Cardiovasc Res 57:1052–1061, 2003.

CHAPTER 10

Cardiac Fibroblasts:
Origin, Organization, and Function

• • • •

Thomas K. Borg

Classical histology of most organs including the heart describes the connective tissue as consisting of cellular and acellular components. The acellular components include the extracellular matrix (ECM) components: collagens, proteoglycans, glycoproteins, proteases and cytokines, and growth factors. For the most part, the ECM is produced by the cellular components. Cellular components can be further divided into permanent and transient cells. The permanent fraction consist of the parenchyma, which in the heart consists of the myocytes, cellular components of the vasculature and the connective tissue cells such as fibroblasts. In the heart, the transient cells include macrophages, mast cells, and lymphocytes. As our knowledge has expanded as to the lineage and function of these various cell types, it has become apparent that these designations are rather arbitrary. Within the last 10 years, there has been a dramatic increase in our knowledge of cardiac fibroblasts regarding their origin, function, and response to pathophysiologic stimuli. The purpose of this chapter is to describe these various functions of the cardiac fibroblast in the heart.

CARDIAC FIBROBLASTS

For many years the cardiac fibroblast was described as a cell of mesenchymal origin that was present in the stroma surrounding parenchyma. Frequently, these cells were recognized by the ability to make collagen, as well as other ECM components. The morphologic features of fibroblasts were quite variable and apparently were dependent on the physiologic status of the surrounding tissue. However, little was known as to the origin, turnover, and interaction with myocytes.

Initially, fibroblasts were mainly associated with the production of collagen. In early development, the mesenchymal cells formed the collagenous structures of the cardiac skeleton, valves, cordae tendonae, and the connective tissue network. The role of the fibroblast in making other ECM components such as fibronectin, proteoglycans, growth factors, and cytokines was only recently investigated.[1,2]

The primary source of ECM components is the fibroblast. Other sources include cardiac myocyte basement membrane containing laminin, collagen type IV, fluid from the systemic circulation (fibronectin, vitronectin), and transient cells such as mast cells and macrophages.[3] However, the dynamic regulation of these sources of ECM components is not well understood. Fibroblasts, clearly central to this regulation, have been termed *sentinel cells* in the stroma.[4,5] In this concept, the fibroblast can respond to a variety of local and systemic stimuli. These responses can include chemical secretion of immune modulators and growth factors, as well as the generation of mechanical force.[6]

Most of these investigations have not been done with cardiac fibroblasts, and their particular function is inferential to the heart. Investigations have shown that fibroblasts can produce growth factors such as transforming growth factor (TGF)-β that can regulate the growth of tumor epithelial cells.[6] These tumor-associated fibroblasts are critical in expression of peptide growth factors, cytokines, and chemokines. These studies clearly show that fibroblasts are capable of regulating their extracellular environment and the surrounding parenchyma.[4-6]

The characteristics of this dynamic interaction between different cell types are just beginning to be understood in the heart. Investigations into the permanent cellular components of the heart have shown that the heart is composed primarily of myocytes, fibroblasts, and endothelial cells, with minor contributions of smooth muscle cells. Cardiac myocytes make up the largest volume of the heart, but cardiac fibroblasts represent approximately 70% to 80% of the cells by number.[2] Most studies have taken a reductionist approach and have focused on the molecular, biochemical, and cellular biology of the cardiac myocyte. Few studies have focused on the fibroblasts and their interaction with cardiac myocytes to regulate cardiac function. In part, this paucity of investigations arises from the lack of specific markers for cardiac fibroblasts.

ORIGIN OF THE FIBROBLASTS IN THE HEART

The source of mesenchymal cells that form the fibroblast populations in the heart are believed to be derived from two principal sources: the proepicardial organ and the result of epithelial–mesenchymal transformation during the formation of cardiac valves.[7] Few studies have examined other sources, such as the developing bone marrow or differentiation from the vascular wall, as potential contributors to the fibroblast lineage. Examination of the embryonic heart for fibroblasts, collagen deposition, or both, indicates that these cells are few in number, because there is little connective tissue in the heart at this time.[8] Most of the connective tissue is involved with the formation of the cardiac skeleton and the various valvular structures.

Cossu and Bianco[9] have defined the mesoangioblast as a progenitor of mesodermal tissues. These multipotent progenitors have the ability to differentiate into a variety of both vascular and mesodermal tissues.[10–12] The term *mesoangioblasts* means that these bone marrow–derived cells have the ability to be a common progenitor of either the endothelial cells or mesodermal cells (fibroblasts). The origin of these progenitors in the bone marrow is the hematopoietic stem cell.[12] Analysis of mesoangioblasts by lineage markers indicates that they have early endothelial markers, Flk1, CD34, and VE cadherin, as well as α-smooth muscle actin.[9] These data indicate there is a likely progression from the mesoangioblast to the vascular wall where these cells serve as the precursors of pericytes and fibroblasts.

Although the precise lineage of the fibroblast remains to be defined, there are indications that a progenitor population may lie within the vascular wall.[10,11] These cells in the vascular wall have the potential to form a variety of cells including fibroblasts, smooth muscle cells, and endothelial cells. However, little is known concerning the stimulus that drives these progenitors into the various differentiated cell types.

Studies on collagen deposition in neonates and sedentary adults indicate high rates during neonatal growth, followed by low to zero rates in adults.[13] However, collagen deposition in models of cardiac hypertrophy and failure, as well as infarction models, show a dramatic up-regulation of collagen content.[14] Initial studies by Weber[15] have divided this pattern into two groups: reparative fibrosis, which occurs dispersed through the myocardium, and reactive fibrosis, which occurs initially with capillaries and spreads to the myocardium. It was believed that these groups were two distinct processes arising from separate signals. In both cases, the number of fibroblasts appeared to increase, but it is not known whether they were derived from existing populations or from progenitor cells. Investigations using a variety of probes to mark dividing cell populations indicated that only some fibroblasts were labeled.[14] Most data indicated that the label was greatest near the vessels. These data have been interpreted to mean that only some fibroblasts have the ability to divide.

In studies on collagen deposition in tumors, the collagen-producing cells appeared to arise from the pericytes associated with the vasculature. In response to systemic signals from platelet-derived growth factor, pericytes migrated away from the vessel wall and into the interstitial space where they began producing collagen.[16] Recent studies have indicated that cells associated with the intima of vessels, as well as pericytes, have the ability to form fibroblasts or smooth muscle cells.[10,11] Furthermore, it has been shown that the mononuclear cells derived from the bone marrow have the ability to contribute to this intimal population.[12] These data suggest that fibroblasts can arise from a stem cell population of the bone marrow.

Critical to the investigations on fibroblasts has been the lack of specific markers that denote different stages in cell lineage or are definitive for mature fibroblasts.

Vimentin has been used to mark fibroblast in vivo, but this label tends to have a nonspecific expression in vitro. Studies using the calcium binding protein, fibroblast specific protein-1, have not proven specificity.[17] More promising is the recent work by Goldsmith and colleagues,[18] which has shown that the collagen receptor, discoidin domain receptor 2 (DDR2), is a specific marker for cardiac fibroblasts. In this seminal study, DDR2 was only found on fibroblasts and not endothelial, smooth muscle, or cardiac myocyte cells. Originally defined as collagen receptor on mesenchymal cells, DDR2 has been shown to be present on leukocytes, as well as in tumors. Recent evidence has shown that DDR2 is positive on bone marrow–derived cells that home to the heart after infarction. However, some caution is warranted because DDR2 staining has not been confirmed in healthy and pathologic tissues other than in the heart.

The discoidin domain receptors, DDR1 and DDR2, represent a relatively new family of collagen-specific receptor tyrosine kinases.[19] Receptor tyrosine kinases are a family of proteins involved in the conversion of extracellular stimuli into cellular response.[20] These receptors mediate a variety of cell functions including growth, migration, morphology, and differentiation. Whereas the tissue distribution of DDR1 and DDR2 varies and can be mutually exclusive,[21] DDR2 expression has been detected in both rat and mouse heart.[22]

Studies are just beginning to elucidate the functional role of DDR2. Temporal expression of DDR2 in dermal fibroblasts was found to remain constant during development, despite increases in collagen expression.[23] Stimulation of DDR2 by collagen type I revealed that this receptor is capable of up-regulating the expression of matrix metalloproteinase 1,[19] an enzyme involved in the degradation of collagen types I, II, III, VII, and X.[22] Expression of DDR2 has been shown to be specific for cardiac fibroblasts, and DDR2 was not detected on myocytes, endothelial cells, or smooth muscle cells.[18]

ORGANIZATION OF FIBROBLASTS

The three-dimensional collagen network composed of the epimysium, perimysium, and endomysium begins to form late in fetal development and is primarily laid

down during neonatal development.[24] Fibroblasts lie within the connective tissue network and are integral in the formation of this network.[18,24] During the formation of this network, specific attachments of the collagen are made to the myocytes involving integrins.[25] In this arrangement, the fibroblasts, together with the collagenous network, surround groups of cardiac myocytes in a lamellar organization.[18,26]

With the advent of confocal microscopy, the three-dimensional organization of fibroblasts can now be appreciated. Recent studies have shown that fibroblasts lie within the connective tissue network and show a variety of contacts with each other and the components of the ECM.[18,24] Fibroblasts are connected to the ECM through integrins and other receptors, such as those of the DDR family. Connexins 40, 43, and 45 have been shown to be involved in these connections and to provide electrical contact. In addition, other cell–cell molecules such as cadherins may also be important in forming links. Recent studies indicate that cadherins serve as cell–cell contacts. Fibroblasts appear to have cell–cell contact between other fibroblasts and with myocytes.[24] Western blot analysis of fibroblast membrane proteins indicated the presence of cadherin 11 and N-cadherin (Fig. 10–1). Although the

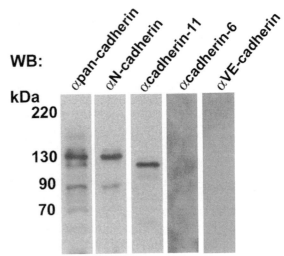

■ **Figure 10–1** Western blot for cadherins on membrane proteins extracted from cardiac fibroblasts. Specific antibodies show the presence of N-cadherin and cadherin 11 on the fibroblasts but not cadherin 6 or VE cadherins. Pan-cadherin, control.

functional aspects of this organization of cardiac fibroblasts are not fully understood, important implications in the electrical, mechanical, and chemical signaling are apparent.

EXTRACELLULAR MATRIX, SIGNALING, AND THE FIBROBLAST

The regulation of components of the ECM is a dynamic interaction among a specific cell surface receptor, ECM components or their degraded products, and the cellular response. This interaction is a key component in development and response to pathophysiologic stimuli.[27] Some ECM components are usually large molecular weight components such as collagens, glycoproteins, or proteoglycans; whereas other smaller molecular weight components such as growth factors, proteases, or cytokines may be latent and require activation. This degradation of large molecular weight components or the removal of latency usually requires proteolytic activity. These components, which are released or activated, have been termed *matrikines*. Numerous examples include the activation of growth factors such as TGF-β, fragmentation of fibronectin, or the small oligosaccharide fragments of proteoglycans.[6,28]

The perception of ECM components, whether as whole components or matrikines, usually involves specific receptors on the cell surface. These are usually transmembrane receptors that heterodimerize or aggregate to activate signaling by the cytoplasmic face.[25] Several classes of receptors are specific for ECM components, including integrins,[25] growth factors,[29] and cytokines.[30] The dynamic interaction among the ECM, membrane receptors, and gene expression has long been recognized as a fundamental factor in growth and development, as well as in response to disease signals.[31] Signaling can be both outside-in and inside-out.[25,32]

Because of this dynamic interaction, it has been virtually impossible to separate chemical and mechanical signaling.[32] Most types of chemical signaling from the ECM generate a cellular response of migration, cytoskeletal reorganization, or contraction that causes an increase in mechanical force.[33] Key to understanding the role of this generated mechanical force is the under-standing that to deliver mechanical strain, cells must be attached to either each other through cell–cell contact, connected to ECM components, or both. This critical aspect is apparent in the heart where the fibroblasts form a syncytial network within the connective tissue network. They are interconnected through connexins and to the collagen by integrins and DDR2 receptors.[33] Signaling pathways involving growth factors and cytokines, mechanical force, and electrical activity are integrally involved with connexin expression, emphasizing the dynamic nature of these contacts.[33] Generation of force by increased expression and assembly of actin, such as in a myofibroblast, results in increased mechanical strain on the collagen network. This force is "delivered" to the myocytes, which are encased in this collagen network (Fig. 10–2). The force generation by cardiac fibroblasts and its effect on myocytes is not well investigated but is potentially important.

This interaction of cardiac fibroblasts with the ECM is analogous to the in vitro investigations of fibroblasts within collagen gels. The contraction of the collagen gel can be blocked by a variety of reagents aimed at either the outside or the inside of the cells. A wide variety of investigations has clearly shown that the arrangement and density of the ECM influences the mechanical tension developed.[34–37] This complex process again involves the dynamic function of individual ECM components, specific receptors, and cellular responses.

ROLE OF FIBROBLASTS FOR CARDIAC MECHANO-ELECTRIC FEEDBACK

The overall electrical activity of the heart is generated in cardiomyocytes. Therefore, mechano-electric feedback (MEF) is, in its ultimate consequence and expression, a mechanically induced change in cardiomyocyte electrophysiology. Any role of fibroblasts in this process would therefore require them to somehow alter cardiomyocyte electrical behavior. This could be achieved either passively—for example, through changing the mechanical environment in which cardiomyocyte-based MEF responses occur (see earlier for mechanically-induced changes in fibroblast activity that have the potential to affect myocardial mechanical properties)—or actively. Active fibroblast-mediated MEF effects require that

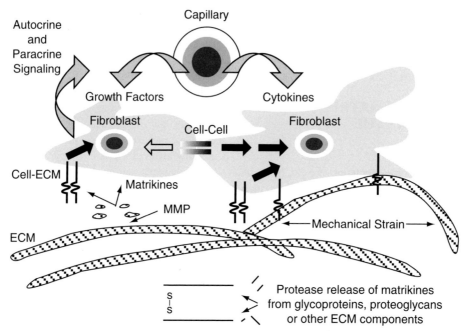

■ **Figure 10–2** Schematic representation of the dynamic interaction among components of the acellular extracellular matrix (ECM) and the cardiac fibroblasts. MMP, matrix metalloproteinases; s-s, fibronectin disulfide bond. (See color insert.)

(1) fibroblasts are able to translate a mechanical stimulus into an electrophysiologically relevant signal, which (2) can be communicated to cardiomyocytes (Fig. 10–3). What is the evidence for any of this?

Fibroblasts as Mechano-Electrical Transducers

Fibroblasts have been shown to contain stretch-activated ion channels.[38–40] The first evidence for mechano-electrical transduction by cardiac fibroblasts in situ was found in the 1990s in the sinoatrial region of frog[41] and rat heart.[38] Fibroblast MEF has subsequently been confirmed in human atrial tissue[42] (see Reference 43 for a review of this topic).

Fibroblast/Cardiomyocyte Electrical Coupling

Cardiac fibroblasts have exceedingly high membrane resistances (in the GΩ range), which makes them ideal

long-distance conductors; however, it also complicates in situ electrophysiologic identification of fibroblasts that are electrically coupled to adjacent cardiomyocytes, because they will mimic the cardiomyocyte action potential shape, as confirmed in isolated cell pairs.[44]

In cell cultures, fibroblast cardiomyocyte electrical coupling is common, to the extent that distant cardiomyocytes, interconnected only by fibroblasts, beat synchronously.[45] Such coupling can bridge distances of about 300 μm.[46] Whether this in vitro behavior is representative of healthy cardiac tissue remains a topic of debate.[47]

Until recently, the histologic substrate underlying electrical coupling of cardiac fibroblasts and myocytes remained unknown,[48] but connexin45 has emerged as a strong contender to support functional heterologous cell interaction in mammalian cardiac tissue.[49]

Thus, the emerging evidence strongly supports a role for fibroblasts in cardiac MEF, through slow (proliferation, gene expression, matrix protein turnover, and so on), intermediate (paracrine effects on cardiomyocytes), and fast (direct electrical coupling) mechanisms.

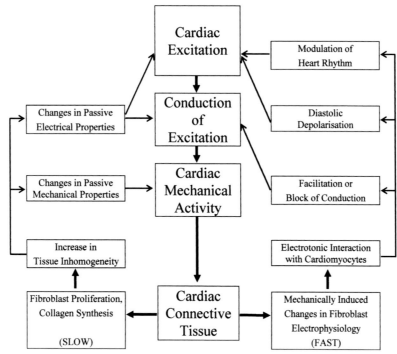

■ **Figure 10–3** Schematic representation of possible relevance of fibroblasts for cardiac mechano-electric feedback, including slow/passive *(left)* and fast/active *(right)* mechanisms. *(Modified from Kohl P, Noble D: Mechanosensitive connective tissue: Potential influence on heart rhythm. Cardiovasc Res 32:62–68, 1996, with permission.)*

Summary

The cellular and acellular components of the ECM in the heart are qualitatively similar but quantitatively different from other organs. There is a dynamic relationship in the heart between these components that is essential for normal growth and development, as well as for the response to pathophysiologic signals, including electrical and mechanical stress and strain (see Fig. 10–1). The complex signaling occurs from the outside-in, as well as from the inside-out, and is in all likelihood of direct relevance for cardiac MEF. Understanding the complexity of this dynamic interaction is both a challenge and a hope for therapy.

Acknowledgments

I apologize to the authors of numerous citations that have been omitted because of space limitations. I offer special thanks to Drs. Wayne Carver, Edie Goldsmith, and Robert Price for their abundant comments. Dr. Ron Heimark was helpful with the Western blot for cadherins. Support was received from the following sources: HL-37669, HL-72160, HL-68038, and the COBRE NIH grant P20 RR16434.

References

1. Harvey RP, Rosenthal N (eds): Heart Development. New York, Academic Press, 1999.
2. Manabe I, Sindo T, Nagai R: Gene expression in fibroblasts and fibrosis. Circ Res 91:1103–1113, 2002.
3. Janicki JS, Brower GL, Gardner JD, et al: The dynamic interaction between matrix metalloproteinase activity and adverse myocardial remodeling. Heart Fail Rev 9:33–42, 2004.
4. Smith RS, Smith TJ, Blieden TM, Phipps RP: Fibroblasts as sentinel cells. Am J Path 151:317–322, 1997.
5. Silzle T, Randolph GJ, Kreutz M, Kunz-Schughart LA: The fibroblast: Sentinel cell and local immune modulator in tumor tissue. Int J Cancer 108:173–180, 2004.
6. Schor SL, Schor AM: Tumour-stroma interactions. Phenotypic and genetic alterations in mammary stroma: Implications for tumour progression. Breast Cancer Res 3:373–379, 2001.
7. Perez-Pomares JM, Carmona R, Gonzalez-Iriarte M, et al: Origin of coronary endothelial cells from epicardial mesothelium in avian embryos. Int J Dev Biol 46:1005–1013, 2002.

8. Borg TK, Gay R, Johnson LD: Changes in the distribution of fibronectin and collagen during development of the neonatal heart. Coll Relat Res 2:211–218, 1982.

9. Cossu G, Bianco P: Mesoangioblasts-vascular progenitors for extravascular mesodermal tissues. Curr Opin Genet Dev 13:537–542, 2003.

10. Satore S, Chiavegato A, Faggin E, et al: Contribution of adventitial fibroblasts to neointima formation and vascular remodeling. Circ Res 89:1111–1121, 2001.

11. Kinnaird T, Stablile E, Burnett MS, et al: Marrow derived stromal cells express genes encoding a broad spectrum of arteriogenic cytokines and promote in vitro and in vivo arteriogenesis through paracrine mechanisms. Circ Res 94:1–8, 2004.

12. Abe R, Donnelly SC, Peng T, et al: Peripheral blood fibrocytes: Differentiation pathway and migration to wound sites. J Immunol 166:7556–7562, 2001.

13. Kusachi S, Ninomiya Y: Myocardial infarction and cardiac fibrogenesis. In Razzaque MS (ed): Fibrogenesis: Cellular and Molecular Basis. New York, Eurekah Press, 2003.

14. Bing OHL, Ngo HQ, Humphries DE, et al: Localization of α1(1) collagen mRNA in myocardium from the spontaneously hypertensive rat during the transition from compensated hypertrophy to failure. J Mol Cell Cardiol 29:2335–2344, 1997.

15. Weber KT: Cardiac interstitium in health and disease: The fibrillar collagen network. J Am Coll Cardiol 13:1637–1652, 1989

16. Sundberg C, Branting M, Gerdin B, Rubin K: Tumor cell and connective tissue cell interactions in human colorectal adenocarcinoma. Transfer of platelet-derived growth factor-AB/BB to stromal cells. Am J Pathol 151:479–492, 1997.

17. Strutz F, Okada H, Lo CW, et al: Identification and characterization of a fibroblast marker: FSP1. J Cell Biol 130:393–405, 1995.

18. Goldsmith EC, Hoffman A, Morales MO, et al: Organization of fibroblasts in the heart. Dev Dyn 230:787–794, 2004.

19. Vogel W, Gish GD, Alves F, Pawson T: The discoidin domain receptor tyrosine kinases are activated by collagen. Mol Cell 1:13–23, 1997.

20. Schlessinger J: Direct binding and activation of receptor tyrosine kinases by collagen. Cell 91:869–872, 1997.

21. Alves F, Vogel W, Mossie K, et al: Distinct structural characteristics of discoidin I subfamily receptor tyrosine kinases and complementary expression in human cancer. Oncogene 10:609–618, 1995.

22. Lai C, Lemke G: Structure and expression of the Tyro 10 receptor tyrosine kinase. Oncogene 9:877–883, 1994.

23. Chin GS, Lee S, Hsu M, et al: Discoidin domain receptors and their ligand, collagen, are temporally regulated in fetal rat fibroblasts in vitro. Plast Reconstr Surg 107:769–776, 2001.

24. Borg TK, Caulfield JB: The collagen matrix of the heart. Fed Proc 40:2037–2041, 1981.

25. Ross RS, Borg TK: Integrins and the myocardium. Circ Res 88:1112–1119, 2001.

26. LeGrice IJ, Hunter PJ, Smaill BH: Laminar structure of the heart: A mathematical model. Am J Physiol 272(5 Pt 2):H2466–H2476, 1997.

27. Eckes B, Zigrino P, Kessler D, et al: Fibroblast-matrix interactions in wound healing and fibrosis. Matrix Biol 19:325–332, 2000.

28. Labat, RJ: Fibronectin in malignancy. Semin Cancer Biol 12:187–195, 2003.

29. Werner S, Grose R: Regulation of wound healing by growth factors and cytokines. Physiol Rev 83:835–870, 2003.

30. Atamas SP, White B: The role of chemokines in scleroderma. Curr Opin Rheumatol 15:772–777, 2003.

31. Bissell MJ, Hall HG, Perry G: How does the ECM direct gene expression? J Theor Biol 99:31–68, 1982.

32. Sussman MA, McCulloch A, Borg TK: Dance band on the Titanic: Biomechanical signaling in cardiac hypertrophy. Circ Res 91:888–898, 2002.

33. deMali Kam, Wennerberg K, Burridge K: Integrin signaling to actin cytoskeleton. Curr Opin Cell Biol 15:572–582, 2003.

34. Saffitz JE, Kleber AG: Effects of mechanical forces and mediators of hypertrophy on remodeling of gap junctions in the heart. Circ Res 94:585–591, 2004.

35. Ehrlich HP, Gabbiani G, Meda P: Cell coupling, CX43, expression and fibroblast populated collagen lattice contraction. J Cell Physiol 184:86–92, 2000.

36. Grinnell F: Fibroblast-collagen matrix contraction: Growth factor signaling and mechanical loading. Trends Cell Biol 10:362–365, 2000.

37. Borg KT, Burgess W, Terracio L, Borg TK: Expression of metalloproteases by cardiac myocytes and fibroblasts in vitro. Cardiac Pathol 6:261–269, 1997.

38. Kohl P, Kamkin AG, Kiseleva IS, Noble D: Mechanosensitive fibroblasts in the sino-atrial node region of rat heart: Interaction with cardiomyocytes and possible role. Exp Physiol 79:943–956, 1994.

39. Stockbridge LL, French AS: Stretch-activated cation channels in human fibroblasts. Biophys J 54:187–190, 1988.

40. Kamkin A, Kiseleva I, Isenberg G: Activation and inactivation of a non-selective cation conductance by local mechanical deformation of acutely isolated cardiac fibroblasts. Cardiovasc Res 57:793–803, 2003.

41. Kohl P, Kamkin AG, Kiseleva IS, Streubel T: Mechanosensitive cells in the atrium of frog heart. Exp Physiol 77:213–216, 1992.

42. Kamkin A, Kiseleva I, Wagner KD, et al: Mechanically induced potentials in fibroblasts from human right atrium. Exp Physiol 84:347–356, 1999.

43. Kohl P, Noble D: Mechanosensitive connective tissue: Potential influence on heart rhythm. Cardiovasc Res 32:62–68, 1996.

44. Rook MB, Jongsma HJ, De Jonge B: Single channel currents of homo- and heterologous gap junctions between cardiac fibroblasts and myocytes. Pflugers Arch 414:95–98, 1989.

45. Goshima K, Tonomura Y: Synchronized beating of embryonic mouse myocardial cells mediated by FL cells in monolayer culture. Exp Cell Res 56:387–392, 1969.

46. Gaudesius G, Miragoli M, Thomas SP, Rohr S: Coupling of cardiac electrical activity over extended distances by fibroblasts of cardiac origin. Circ Res 93:421–428, 2003.

47. Kohl P: Heterogeneous cell coupling in the heart: An electrophysiological role for fibroblasts. Circ Res 93:381–383, 2003.

48. De Mazière AMGL, van Ginneken ACD, Wilders R, et al: Spatial and functional relationship between myocytes and fibroblasts in the rabbit sinoatrial node. J Mol Cell Cardiol 24:567–578, 1992.

49. Camelliti P, Green CR, LeGrice I, Kohl P: Fibroblast network in rabbit sino-atrial node: Structural and functional identification of homo- and heterologous cell coupling. Circ Res 94:828–835, 2004

CHAPTER 11

Effects of Mechanical Signals on Ventricular Gap Junction Remodeling

• • • •

André G. Kléber and Jeffrey E. Saffitz

Integration of cells into tissue involves binding to the extracellular matrix, cell-to-cell adhesion, and functional cell-to-cell communication. The functions of cell–matrix and cell-to-cell adhesion are not only to anchor cells, but to determine the architecture and the passive mechanical properties of tissues. Cell–matrix interactions are also important for signaling in development and homeostasis in adult tissues.

The transition from normal heart function to cardiac hypertrophy and failure is associated with changes in gene expression and in phenotype. In addition to intrinsic genetic diseases leading to cardiac failure, the upstream external stimuli leading to hypertrophy include chronically increased sympathetic tone and mechanical overload. The downstream changes in cellular function occur at all levels, including metabolism, electromechanical coupling, the contractile apparatus, and electrical function.

Changes in electrical function are accompanied by tachyarrhythmias, which are a major cause of sudden death in the setting of cardiac hypertrophy and failure. Remodeling of gap junctions is a major component of the changes that affect altered electrical function in hypertrophied or failing hearts. The questions regarding how adhesion and electrical junctions interact and how mechanical signaling may affect gap junction expression have been addressed only recently. However, there is a large body of literature on the role of cellular adhesion molecules as transmitters of signals from the extracellular to the intracellular space. This chapter provides an overview of the field.

INTERACTIONS BETWEEN CELL-TO-CELL ADHERENS AND GAP JUNCTIONS

Mechanical junctions between cells are composed of clusters of adhesion molecules that connect the membranes of adjacent cells. In addition, they form a continuum with the cytoskeleton of the intracellular space.[1] Extracellular binding is Ca^{2+}-dependent, and intracellular binding to the cytoskeleton is achieved through linker proteins that form a submembranous scaffold.

As shown schematically in Figure 11–1, the two types of adhesion junctions in heart are *fascia adherens* and *desmosomes*. The main adhesion molecules that span the membranes in intercalated disks are the *N-cadherins* (fascia adherens junctions) and the *desmogleins* and *desmocollins* (desmosomes). The major linker proteins include members of the catenin and plakin families. In *fascia adherens junctions* of cardiac myocytes, N-cadherins are linked to the actin in sarcomeres by both β-catenin and γ-catenin (plakoglobin). In desmosomes, the desmosomal cadherins are associated with intracellular *desmoplakin* and *plakoglobin*, which in turn bind to desmin, the intermediate filament protein of the myocyte cytoskeleton.[1]

As shown in ultrastructural analyses of intercalated disks in dog ventricular myocardium, gap junction plaques exhibit a close spatial relationship with fascia adherens junctions.[2,3] At the ends of ventricular myocytes, in the so-called terminal intercalated disks, large ribbon-like gap junctions oriented perpendicularly to the long cell axis alternate with interdigitated fascia adherens junctions.

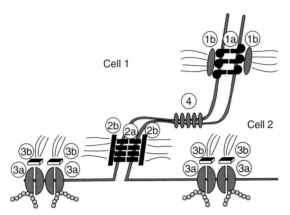

■ **Figure 11–1** The cell membranes of two adjacent cardiomyocytes are connected by fascia adherens junctions *(1)*, desmosomes *(2)*, and gap junctions *(4)*. The surface membranes are connected to extracellular matrix proteins through cell adherens molecules *(3)*. Fascia adherens junctions consist of the transmembrane-spanning Ca^{2+}-dependent adherens proteins (N-cadherins, *1a*) that are anchored in a submembranous scaffold *(1b)* consisting of several proteins (plakoglobin, catenins). The submembranous complex binds to the microfilaments of the cytoskeleton (actin). Desmosomes are formed by the transmembrane-spanning proteins desmocollin and desmoglein *(2a)* and are anchored in a submembranous scaffold of plakoglobin and desmoplakin *(2b)*. The latter proteins are bound to intermediate filaments (desmin). Gap junctions *(4)* consist of clustered gap junction channels each formed by two juxtaposed hemi-channels (each formed by six connexin proteins). The extracellular matrix is connected to integrin *(3a)* through fibronectin. Intracellularly, integrins bind to cytoskeletal proteins through a number of intermediate proteins *(3b)* that cluster integrin molecules and can induce intracellular signals when activated by extracellular mechanical stimuli. (See color insert.)

That gap junctions are oriented in parallel to the long axis of the contractile apparatus[2] is generally interpreted as reflecting mechanical protection of the gap junction plaque (consisting of channels clustered at high density) against contraction.[3]

A number of studies in cardiac and noncardiac tissues suggest some degree of regulatory interaction between the number of channels clustered in the gap junction plaque and the function and integrity of adhesion junctions. For example, epidermal CA3/7 carcinoma cells have fewer gap *and* adherens junctions than normal mouse epidermal cells of the same type (3PC).[4] Tumor promoters such as phorbol esters

and benzoyl peroxide diminish both connexin and E-cadherin expression in 3PC and CA3/7 cells. This indicates that dysregulation of cell growth in tumours is associated with diminished cell-to-cell adhesion and communication.[4]

In the heart, evidence for a close interaction between regulation of cell-to-cell adhesion and functional cell-to-cell coupling can be derived from the following sources: (1) the formation of cell-to-cell junctions during experimental cell apposition; (2) experiments involving mechanical stretch of cardiac myocytes; and (3) rare human diseases caused by mutations in linker proteins at fascia adherens junctions, desmosomes, or both.

Neoformation of adherens and gap junctions has been studied in cell culture in which dissociated adult rat ventricular myocytes were observed during neoformation of cell-to-cell coupling.[5–8] Disaggregated myocytes start to lose their typical rodlike shape and remodel intracellular architecture within 24 hours after seeding.[9] During this process of dedifferentiation, the membrane regions corresponding to former intercalated disks become smooth and unstructured. Reformation of intercalated disks with increasing age in culture (culture days 3 to 4) is characterized by initial formation of intercellular fibrillar structures and subsequent appearance of subsarcolemmal plaques. These nascent adhesion junctions subsequently differentiate to intercalated disks. Immunohistochemical analysis at this early stage shows positive signals for N-cadherin, β-catenin, and plakoglobin, but only minor amounts of connexin. Gap junctions containing connexin43 (Cx43) become evident only when complete adherens junctions have formed. The new gap junctions are located adjacent to the adherens junctions after 6 to 12 days in culture.

Several studies have suggested an important role for β-catenin in assembly or maintenance, or both, of adherence and gap junctions and in regulating connexin expression. β-catenin acts as a transcription factor in early embryonic development and is also a component of the submembranous scaffolding complex of adherens junctions, as described previously (see Fig. 11–1). Ai and colleagues[10] used immunohistochemical and biochemical approaches to show that Cx43 and β-catenin co-localize in cardiac myocytes, and that Cx43/β-catenin complexes can be immunoprecipitated from Triton X100–soluble lysates, suggesting co-localization in the membranous compartment. More recently, Wu and colleagues[11] showed a consistent temporal sequence in the reappearance of α-catenin, β-catenin, and Cx43 into the membrane. First, immunoreactive signals for α-catenin, β-catenin, and Cx43 were redistributed to intracellular loci by culturing neonatal rat cardiac myocytes under low Ca^{2+} conditions. Then, addition of Ca^{2+} at physiologic concentration led to appearance of α-catenin and β-catenin in the cell surface membrane within 10 minutes at sites of cell–cell contact. Cx43 was observed at the cell surface only after these catenin proteins accumulated at apparent junctions.

Exposure of neonatal rat myocytes grown on a collagen substrate to pulsatile stretch has been shown to induce rapid and marked up-regulation of Cx43, N-cadherin,[12] plakoglobin, and desmoplakin.[13] This further suggests a close relation between regulation of gap junctions and adhesion junctions by signals mediated by mechanical forces. However, the exact mechanisms of the signaling pathways remain to be determined.[14]

CLINICAL MANIFESTATION OF DEFECTS IN GENES CODING FOR ADHERENS JUNCTION PROTEINS

A fascinating new facet of interaction between expression of adhesion and gap junctions has become evident from the analysis of familial cardiomyopathies caused by mutations in plakoglobin and desmoplakin (see Fig. 11–1). Naxos disease is a cardiocutaneous syndrome that includes woolly hair, palmoplantar keratoderma, and arrhythmogenic right ventricular cardiomyopathy.[15] It is caused by a recessive mutation characterized by a deletion of nucleotides 2157 and 2158 in the plakoglobin gene.[16] This defect leads to premature termination of translation and a truncation of the C-terminus of plakoglobin with a loss of 56 amino acids.[16]

At the level of the heart, the disease produces a progressive loss of right ventricular myocardium and concomitant replacement by fat and connective tissue. Life-threatening ventricular arrhythmias and sudden cardiac death are the resulting clinical manifestations.[17,18] Although alterations in the right ventricle dominate the pathologic findings, involvement of the left ventricle also has been observed. Because of the plakoglobin mutation, it is postulated that this defect interferes with the linkage between the intercellular adhesion molecules and the cytoskeleton. The extent to which this potential defect in mechanical cell-to-cell coupling may lead to altered regulation of connexin expression, and resulting arrhythmias, has not yet been elucidated.

Carvajal syndrome, described in 1998 by Dr. Luis Carvajal-Huerta,[19] is a second type of cardiocutaneous syndrome. It is caused by a recessive mutation in the desmoplakin gene consisting of a single nucleotide deletion producing a premature stop codon with a truncation of the desmoplakin protein.[20] Clinically, Carvajal syndrome is manifested by woolly hair, palmoplantar keratoderma, and dilated cardiomyopathy. The cardiomyopathy is characterized by markedly reduced left ventricle function. The electrocardiogram exhibits low-voltage, pathologic QRS complexes; polymorphic ventricular premature beats; and/or runs of ventricular tachycardia.[21] The cardiac pathoanatomic findings involve both ventricles and do not include fibrofatty replacement. In agreement with the defined genetic defect, analysis of palm skin from patients has shown abnormal distribution of desmoplakin.[20] In the heart, a recent immunohistochemical analysis reported diminished expression of desmoplakin, plakoglobin, and Cx43 at the level of the intercalated disks.[22] These observations, made in rare genetic defects, support the findings made in experiments on neoformation of cell-to-cell contacts and mechanical stretch, suggesting interactions in the regulation of both gap and adhesion junctions. However, the underlying molecular mechanisms remain to be determined. In the setting of common forms of heart failure, no links between remodeling of adherens and gap junctions currently have been reported.[23]

MEDIATORS OF HYPERTROPHY AND MECHANICAL STRETCH REMODEL GAP JUNCTIONS

The amount of connexin expression at gap junctions depends on the balance of connexin synthesis, channel assembly, and connexin degradation. The turnover of connexins in the junctional plaques is rapid with half-lives of one to a few hours.[24–27] New connexons assembled in the endoplasmic reticulum and the Golgi complex travel in vesicles to the plasma membrane where they are added to the periphery of existing junctional plaques. Steady state is maintained by continuous movement of protein from the periphery to the center, where protein is removed[28] and subsequently degraded through lysosomal and proteasomal pathways.[26,27] This continuous trafficking has been associated with phosphorylation of specific amino acids in the C-terminus of connexin proteins.[29,30]

Connexin phosphorylation in its totality and integrity has not been fully elucidated. However, it has been shown that specific phosphorylation sites are responsive to typical molecules involved in signaling cascades.[29,30] Enzymes that phosphorylate connexins at serine residues include mitogen-activated protein kinases (MAPK),[31] protein kinase C,[32] protein kinase A,[33] and casein kinase. Tyrosine phosphorylation occurs in cells that express activated tyrosine kinases and usually causes a decrease in junctional conductance.[34–37]

Information about transcriptional regulation of connexin expression is scarce, and it relates to transcription factors that are also involved in cell fate determination during early development. Nkx2.5 is a homeodomain transcription factor involved in fate determination of embryonic cells to procardiomyocytes during early development.[38] It has been shown to regulate Cx40 gene expression during this embryonic stage.[39] In adult cardiomyocytes, Nkx2.5 reduced Cx43 expression,[40] a change that may be responsible for atrioventricular nodal conduction disturbances and bradycardia.[41] Wnt1, another important factor involved in embryonic development, induces Cx43 expression, probably through pathways involving β-catenin as a transcription factor.[10] Further studies are needed to define the exact role of transcriptional regulation of connexin expression in adult cardiomyocytes.[42]

Cardiac hypertrophy and failure are associated with changes in electrical function caused by disturbances of impulse initiation and propagation leading to an increased propensity for tachyarrhythmias. Electrical propagation velocity first increases in hypertrophied ventricles, but then decreases as hypertrophy becomes more severe.[43–45] Decrements in conduction velocity and conduction block may be related to discontinuities in extracellular resistance caused by interstitial fibrosis[46–48] and an increase in intercellular resistance caused by decreased connexin expression.[49–51] In patients with chronic ischemic heart disease, Cx43 expression in the gap junctions of the ventricular myocardium is reduced.[52]

These and other results suggest that reduced gap junction channel protein levels occur as a general rule in chronic myocardial disease states, such as healed myocardial infarction,[49–51] chronic hibernation,[52] and end-stage aortic stenosis.[53] In the setting of hypertrophy and failure, the signaling mechanisms leading to connexin down-regulation have not yet been fully defined. An important role may be played by c-Jun activated N-terminal kinase (JNK). Indeed, a rapid and massive decrease of Cx43 expression (up to 90%) was consistently observed with activation of JNK in cultured cardiac myocytes or in vivo.[54]

In contrast to the findings observed in advanced stages of heart failure, compensatory *myocardial hypertrophy* leads to increased connexin levels, increased number of gap junctions, and enhanced intercellular coupling. With respect to mediators of myocardial hypertrophy, cyclic adenosine monophosphate (cAMP) and angiotensin II (Ang II) have been shown to up-regulate gap junctions.

Exposure of cultured neonatal rat ventricular myocytes to a membrane-permeable form of cAMP for 24 hours increases the tissue content of Cx43 approximately twofold and increases the number of gap junctions interconnecting cells.[55] These changes are associated with a significant increase in electrical propagation velocity.[55] Cultured neonatal rat ventricular myocytes exposed for 24 hours to Ang II exhibit a twofold increase in Cx43 content and an increase in the number of gap junctions interconnecting cells.[56]

Numerous studies have characterized changes in cardiac myocytes subjected to mechanical load in vitro. Early studies demonstrated that brief intervals of static stretch of neonatal rat myocytes induced features of the hypertrophic response including increases in proto-oncogene and contractile protein expression (see Chapter 7).

More recent experiments in which myocytes have been subjected to pulsatile stretch have demonstrated activation of numerous signal transduction pathways including all three members of the MAPK family, focal adhesion kinase (FAK), and the JAK/STAT pathway.[57,58] Mechanical stretch of cultured neonatal rat ventricles induces release of growth-promoting factors including Ang II, endothelin I, vascular endothelial growth factor (VEGF), and transforming growth factor-β (TGF-β).[59–63] Shyu and colleagues[60] reported a threefold increase in Ang II in the culture media of rat neonatal myocytes stretched for 1 hour. Seko and colleagues[61] demonstrated that 5 minutes of pulsatile stretch is sufficient to induce rapid secretion of VEGF and increased expression of both VEGF and VEGF receptor mRNA in cultured cardiac myocytes.

Recent experiments carried out in our laboratories indicate that a number of the signaling pathways mentioned previously also exert an effect on connexin expression in gap junctions. Stretching monolayers of neonatal rat ventricular myocytes to 110% of resting cell length at a frequency of 3 Hz produced marked up-regulation of Cx43 after only 1 hour.[12] A further increase occurred after 6 hours of stretch. The increase in gap junctional Cx43 was accompanied by a significant increase in electrical propagation velocity,[12] suggesting that the change in conduction velocity was related mainly to enhanced electrical coupling.[12]

VEGF and TGF-β are both known to be synthesized and secreted by cardiac myocytes in response to pulsatile stretch.[61] These same molecules, when added to the culture medium, also up-regulate Cx43.[64] Thus, addition of either exogenous TGF-β (10 ng/mL) or VEGF (100 ng/mL) to unstretched neonatal rat ventricular myocytes for 1 hour increases Cx43 expression by as much as ~1.8-fold, an amount comparable to that observed in cells subjected to pulsatile stretch for 1 hour. A close association between stretch-induced Cx43 up-regulation and VEGF or TGF-β is suggested by the observation that the stretch-induced effect is blocked by either anti-VEGF or anti–TGF-β antibodies.[64] Anti-VEGF antibodies also block the stretch-induced increase in electrical propagation velocity. Complementary results, confirming the involvement of VEGF or TGF-β, include the observation of stretch-induced VEGF release into the culture medium.[64] Up-regulation of Cx43 expression stimu-

lated by exogenous TGF-β was blocked by anti-VEGF antibody, but VEGF stimulation of Cx43 expression was not blocked by anti–TGF-β antibody. This confirmed that TGF-β was acting upstream of VEGF. In similar studies on Ang II, Shyu and colleagues[60] showed that up-regulation of Cx43 after several hours of stretch could be blocked by addition of the angiotensin receptor type 1 antagonist losartan. It is likely that multiple chemical signals released from cells in response to stretch, in addition to those described previously, may act on connexin regulation through complex interacting signaling pathways.

INTEGRIN SIGNALING AND ITS POTENTIAL ROLE IN STRETCH-ACTIVATED UP-REGULATION OF CONNEXIN43

Interactions between integrins and extracellular matrix proteins are known to play a pivotal role in stretch-activated changes of cardiac myocyte structure and function. Overexpression of β_1 integrins, by itself, can induce a hypertrophic response in neonatal rat ventricular myocytes in vitro and can enhance the effects of α_1-adrenergic stimulation.[65] Inhibition of β_1-integrin function and signaling reduces the hypertrophic response.[65] FAK, a primary mediator of integrin signaling, may also play a role in the hypertrophic and adhesive responses of neonatal rat ventricular myocytes in culture.[66–69] FAK is also activated by VEGF[66] and translocates to costameres in cardiac myocytes subjected to stretch.[70] Future research hopefully will shed light on the exact nature of the extracellular stimuli, which may exert multiple and concerted actions. The resulting complex intracellular signaling reactions, by which mechanical stimulation leads to altered cell–cell communication at gap junctions, may change at different times during the evolution of a cardiac disease.

Summary

Recent experimental work has shown that the application of mechanical stretch to cardiac tissue rapidly up-regulates gap and adherence junctions. Although the effect appears to be mediated by integrin signaling, the full pathways of regulation that involve TGF-β and

VEGF remain unknown. Several lines of evidence exist for a close relation between the regulation of adherence junction and gap junction protein. Thus, neoformation of cell-to-cell junctions in culture is characterized first by the formation of adherence junctions, whereas gap junctions are only introduced into the junctional membrane at a later stage. In the Carvajal syndrome, a disease involving a defect in the desmoplakin gene, a change in gap junction expression is observed. This corroborates the experimental findings of a close association between adherence and gap junction regulation. Further research will be needed to elucidate the exact mechanisms of connexin regulation after a change in mechanical stress on the myocardium. These findings may be particularly important to understand the remodeling of cell-to-cell coupling in cardiac failure.

References

1. Gumbiner BM: Cell adhesion: The molecular basis of tissue architecture and morphogenesis. Cell 84:345–357, 1996.
2. Fawcett DW, McNutt NS: The ultrastructure of the cat myocardium. I. Ventricular papillary muscle. J Cell Biol 42:1–45, 1969.
3. Hoyt RH, Cohen ML, Saffitz JE: Distribution and three-dimensional structure of intercellular junctions in canine myocardium. Circ Res 64:563–574, 1989.
4. Jansen LA, Mesnil M, Jongen WM: Inhibition of gap junctional intercellular communication and delocalization of the cell adhesion molecule E-cadherin by tumor promoters. Carcinogenesis 17:1527–1531, 1996.
5. Hertig CM, Butz S, Koch S, et al: N-cadherin in adult rat cardiomyocytes in culture. II. Spatio-temporal appearance of proteins involved in cell-cell contact and communication. Formation of two distinct N-cadherin/catenin complexes. J Cell Sci 109:11–20, 1996.
6. Hertig CM, Eppenberger-Eberhardt M, Koch S, Eppenberger HM: N-cadherin in adult rat cardiomyocytes in culture. I. Functional role of N-cadherin and impairment of cell-cell contact by a truncated N-cadherin mutant. J Cell Sci 109:1–10, 1996.
7. Kostin S, Hein S, Bauer EP, Schaper J: Spatiotemporal development and distribution of intercellular junctions in adult rat cardiomyocytes in culture. Circ Res 85:154–167, 1999.
8. Zuppinger C, Schaub MC, Eppenberger HM: Dynamics of early contact formation in cultured adult rat cardiomyocytes studied by N-cadherin fused to green fluorescent protein. J Mol Cell Cardiol 32:539–555, 2000.
9. Lipp P, Huser J, Pott L, Niggli E: Spatially non-uniform Ca^{2+} signals induced by the reduction of transverse tubules in citrate-loaded guinea-pig ventricular myocytes in culture. J Physiol 497:589–597, 1996.
10. Ai Z, Fischer A, Spray DC, et al: Wnt-1 regulation of connexin43 in cardiac myocytes. J Clin Invest 105:161–171, 2000.
11. Wu JC, Tsai RY, Chung TH: Role of catenins in the development of gap junctions in rat cardiomyocytes. J Cell Biochem 88:823–835, 2003.
12. Zhuang J, Yamada KA, Saffitz JE, Kleber AG: Pulsatile stretch remodels cell-to-cell communication in cultured myocytes. Circ Res 87:316–322, 2000.
13. Yamada K, Cole EB, Green KG, et al: Coordinated regulation of intercellular junction proteins in cardiac myocytes. Circulation 106:II-309, 2002.
14. Gopalan SM, Flaim C, Bhatia SN, et al: Anisotropic stretch-induced hypertrophy in neonatal ventricular myocytes micropatterned on deformable elastomers. Biotechnol Bioeng 81:578–587, 2003.
15. Protonotarios N, Tsatsopoulou A, Patsourakos P, et al: Cardiac abnormalities in familial palmoplantar keratosis. Br Heart J 56:321–326, 1986.
16. McKoy G, Protonotarios N, Crosby A, et al: Identification of a deletion in plakoglobin in arrhythmogenic right ventricular cardiomyopathy with palmoplantar keratoderma and woolly hair (Naxos disease). Lancet 355:2119–2124, 2000.
17. Marcus FI, Fontaine GH, Guiraudon G, et al: Right ventricular dysplasia: A report of 24 adult cases. Circulation 65:384–398, 1982.
18. Thiene G, Nava A, Corrado D, et al: Right ventricular cardiomyopathy and sudden death in young people. N Engl J Med 318:129–133, 1988.
19. Carvajal-Huerta L: Epidermolytic palmoplantar keratoderma with woolly hair and dilated cardiomyopathy. J Am Acad Dermatol 39:418–421, 1998.
20. Norgett EE, Hatsell SJ, Carvajal-Huerta L, et al: Recessive mutation in desmoplakin disrupts desmoplakin-intermediate filament interactions and causes dilated cardiomyopathy, woolly hair and keratoderma. Hum Mol Genet 9:2761–2766, 2000.
21. Duran M, Avellan F, Carvajal L: Miocardiopatia dilatada en las displasias del ectodermo. Observaciones electroechocardiograficas en la hiperqueratosis palmpplantar con perlo lanoso. Rev Esp Cardiol 53:1296–1300, 2000.
22. Kaplan SR, Gard JJ, Carvajal-Huerta L, et al: Structural and molecular pathology of the heart in Carvajal syndrome. Cardiovasc Pathol 13:26–32, 2004.
23. Hein S, Kostin S, Heling A, et al: The role of the cytoskeleton in heart failure. Cardiovasc Res 45:273–278, 2000.
24. Darrow BJ, Laing JG, Lampe PD, et al: Expression of multiple connexins in cultured neonatal rat ventricular myocytes. Circ Res 76:381–387, 1995.
25. Laird DW, Puranam KL, Revel JP: Turnover and phosphorylation dynamics of connexin43 gap junction protein in cultured cardiac myocytes. Biochem J 273:67–72, 1991.
26. Laing JG, Tadros PN, Westphale EM, Beyer EC: Degradation of connexin43 gap junctions involves both the proteasome and the lysosome. Exp Cell Res 236:482–492, 1997.
27. Beardslee MA, Laing JG, Beyer EC, Saffitz JE: Rapid turnover of connexin43 in the adult rat heart. Circ Res 83:629–635, 1998.
28. Gaietta G, Deerinck TJ, Adams SR, et al: Multicolor and electron microscopic imaging of connexin trafficking. Science 296:503–507, 2002.
29. Goodenough DA, Goliger JA, Paul DL: Connexins, connexons, and intercellular communication. Annu Rev Biochem 65:475–502, 1996.
30. Lampe PD, Lau AF: Regulation of gap junctions by phosphorylation of connexins. Arch Biochem Biophys 384:205–215, 2000.
31. Lau AF, Kurata WE, Kanemitsu MY, et al: Regulation of connexin43 function by activated tyrosine protein kinases. J Bioenerg Biomembr 28:359–368, 1996.

32. Lampe PD, TenBroek EM, Burt JM, et al: Phosphorylation of connexin43 on serine368 by protein kinase C regulates gap junctional communication. J Cell Biol 149:1503–1512, 2000.

33. TenBroek EM, Lampe PD, Solan JL, et al: Ser364 of connexin43 and the upregulation of gap junction assembly by cAMP. J Cell Biol 155:1307–1318, 2001.

34. Crow DS, Beyer EC, Paul DL, et al: Phosphorylation of connexin43 gap junction protein in uninfected and Rous sarcoma virus-transformed mammalian fibroblasts. Mol Cell Biol 10:1754–1763, 1990.

35. Giepmans BN, Hengeveld T, Postma FR, Moolenaar WH: Interaction of c-Src with gap junction protein connexin-43. Role in the regulation of cell-cell communication. J Biol Chem 276:8544–8549, 2001.

36. Lin R, Warn-Cramer BJ, Kurata WE, Lau AF: v-Src phosphorylation of connexin 43 on Tyr247 and Tyr265 disrupts gap junctional communication. J Cell Biol 154:815–827, 2001.

37. Toyofuku T, Yabuki M, Otsu K, et al: Functional role of c-Src in gap junctions of the cardiomyopathic heart. Circ Res 85:672–681, 1999.

38. Moorman A, Webb S, Brown NA, et al: Development of the heart: (1) Formation of the cardiac chambers and arterial trunks. Heart 89:806–814, 2003.

39. Bruneau BG, Nemer G, Schmitt JP, et al: A murine model of Holt-Oram syndrome defines roles of the T-box transcription factor Tbx5 in cardiogenesis and disease. Cell 106:709–721, 2001.

40. Kasahara H, Ueyama T, Wakimoto H, et al: Nkx2.5 homeoprotein regulates expression of gap junction protein connexin 43 and sarcomere organization in postnatal cardiomyocytes. J Mol Cell Cardiol 35:243–256, 2003.

41. Wakimoto H, Kasahara H, Maguire CT, et al: Cardiac electrophysiological phenotypes in postnatal expression of Nkx2.5 transgenic mice. Genesis 37:144–150, 2003.

42. Akazawa H, Komuro I: Too much Csx/Nkx2-5 is as bad as too little? J Mol Cell Cardiol 35:227–229, 2003.

43. McIntyre H, Fry CH: Abnormal action potential conduction in isolated human hypertrophied left ventricular myocardium. J Cardiovasc Electrophysiol 8:887–894, 1997.

44. Winterton SJ, Turner MA, O'Gorman DJ, et al: Hypertrophy causes delayed conduction in human and guinea pig myocardium: Accentuation during ischaemic perfusion. Cardiovasc Res 28:47–54, 1994.

45. Cooklin M, Wallis WR, Sheridan DJ, Fry CH: Changes in cell-to-cell electrical coupling associated with left ventricular hypertrophy. Circ Res 80:765–771, 1997.

46. Spach MS, Dolber PC: Relating extracellular potentials and their derivatives to anisotropic propagation at a microscopic level in human cardiac muscle. Evidence for electrical uncoupling of side-to-side fiber connections with increasing age. Circ Res 58:356–371, 1986.

47. Spach MS, Josephson ME: Initiating reentry: The role of nonuniform anisotropy in small circuits. J Cardiovasc Electrophysiol 5:182–209, 1994.

48. Peters NS, Coromilas J, Severs NJ, Wit AL: Disturbed connexin43 gap junction distribution correlates with the location of reentrant circuits in the epicardial border zone of healing canine infarcts that cause ventricular tachycardia. Circulation 95:988–996, 1997.

49. Luke RA, Saffitz JE: Remodeling of ventricular conduction pathways in healed canine infarct border zones. J Clin Invest 87:1594–1602, 1991.

50. Peters NS: New insights into myocardial arrhythmogenesis: Distribution of gap-junctional coupling in normal, ischaemic and hypertrophied human hearts. Clin Sci (Lond) 90:447–452, 1996.

51. Smith JH, Green CR, Peters NS, et al: Altered patterns of gap junction distribution in ischemic heart disease. An immunohistochemical study of human myocardium using laser scanning confocal microscopy. Am J Pathol 139:801–821, 1991.

52. Kaprielian RR, Gunning M, Dupont E, et al: Downregulation of immunodetectable connexin43 and decreased gap junction size in the pathogenesis of chronic hibernation in the human left ventricle. Circulation 97:651–660, 1998.

53. Peters NS, Green CR, Poole-Wilson PA, Severs NJ: Reduced content of connexin43 gap junctions in ventricular myocardium from hypertrophied and ischemic human hearts. Circulation 88:864–875, 1993.

54. Petrich BG, Gong X, Lerner DL, et al: c-Jun N-terminal kinase activation mediates downregulation of connexin43 in cardiomyocytes. Circ Res 91:640–647, 2002.

55. Darrow BJ, Fast VG, Kleber AG, et al: Functional and structural assessment of intercellular communication. Increased conduction velocity and enhanced connexin expression in dibutyryl cAMP-treated cultured cardiac myocytes. Circ Res 79: 174–183, 1996.

56. Dodge SM, Beardslee MA, Darrow BJ, et al: Effects of angiotensin II on expression of the gap junction channel protein connexin43 in neonatal rat ventricular myocytes. J Am Coll Cardiol 32:800–807, 1998.

57. Ruwhof C, van der Laarse A: Mechanical stress-induced cardiac hypertrophy: Mechanisms and signal transduction pathways. Cardiovasc Res 47:23–37, 2000.

58. Seko Y, Takahashi N, Tobe K, et al: Pulsatile stretch activates mitogen-activated protein kinase (MAPK) family members and focal adhesion kinase (p125(FAK)) in cultured rat cardiac myocytes. Biochem Biophys Res Commun 259:8–14, 1999.

59. Sadoshima J, Izumo S: Mechanical stretch rapidly activates multiple signal transduction pathways in cardiac myocytes: Potential involvement of an autocrine/paracrine mechanism. EMBO J 12:1681–1692, 1993.

60. Shyu KG, Chen CC, Wang BW, Kuan P: Angiotensin II receptor antagonist blocks the expression of connexin43 induced by cyclical mechanical stretch in cultured neonatal rat cardiac myocytes. J Mol Cell Cardiol 33:691–698, 2001.

61. Seko Y, Takahashi N, Shibuya M, Yazaki Y: Pulsatile stretch stimulates vascular endothelial growth factor (VEGF) secretion by cultured rat cardiac myocytes. Biochem Biophys Res Commun 254:462–465, 1999.

62. Ruwhof C, van Wamel AE, Egas JM, van der Laarse A: Cyclic stretch induces the release of growth promoting factors from cultured neonatal cardiomyocytes and cardiac fibroblasts. Mol Cell Biochem 208:89–98, 2000.

63. Sadoshima J, Xu Y, Slayter HS, Izumo S: Autocrine release of angiotensin II mediates stretch-induced hypertrophy of cardiac myocytes in vitro. Cell 75:977–984, 1993.

64. Pimentel RC, Yamada KA, Kleber AG, Saffitz JE: Autocrine regulation of myocyte Cx43 expression by VEGF. Circ Res 90:671–677, 2002.

65. Ross RS, Pham C, Shai SY, et al: Beta1 integrins participate in the hypertrophic response of rat ventricular myocytes. Circ Res 82:1160–1172, 1998.

66. Takahashi N, Seko Y, Noiri E, et al: Vascular endothelial growth factor induces activation and subcellular translocation of focal

adhesion kinase (p125FAK) in cultured rat cardiac myocytes. Circ Res 84:1194–1202, 1999.

67. Pham CG, Harpf AE, Keller RS, et al: Striated muscle-specific beta(1D)-integrin and FAK are involved in cardiac myocyte hypertrophic response pathway. Am J Physiol Heart Circ Physiol 279:H2916–H2926, 2000.

68. Taylor JM, Rovin JD, Parsons JT: A role for focal adhesion kinase in phenylephrine-induced hypertrophy of rat ventricular cardiomyocytes. J Biol Chem 275:19250–19257, 2000.

69. Eble DM, Strait JB, Govindarajan G, et al: Endothelin-induced cardiac myocyte hypertrophy: Role for focal adhesion kinase. Am J Physiol Heart Circ Physiol 278:H1695–H1707, 2000.

70. Torsoni AS, Constancio SS, Nadruz W Jr, et al: Focal adhesion kinase is activated and mediates the early hypertrophic response to stretch in cardiac myocytes. Circ Res 93:140–147, 2003.

EXPERIMENTAL MANIFESTATIONS OF MECHANO-ELECTRIC FEEDBACK IN THE HEART

• • • •

CHAPTER 12

Regional Stretch Effects in Pathologic Myocardium

• • • •

Max J. Lab

There is a pathophysiologic enigma concerning the relations between sudden arrhythmic death during myocardial pathology and the diversity of their cardiac correlates. Electrophysiologic correlates (Fig. 12–1A, *left*) include late potentials, QT dispersion, and alternans, and mechanical/hemodynamic indices include ejection fraction and blood pressure. Nonlinear dynamics ("chaos") and heart rate variability also provide indices, as do psychosocial factors and autonomic imbalance. Explanatory mechanisms in more focussed experimental observations in regional ischemia are also diverse and include extracellular potassium ($[K^+]_o$) accumulation (see Fig. 12–1A, *right*).

Numerous studies have provided various explanations for these diverse observations. Ideally, however, a single hypothesis is preferable.

THE ASSERTION

A unified hypothesis for mechano-electric feedback (MEF) is emerging (see Fig. 12–1B; see previous reviews[1,2] that discuss mechanisms of MEF, including stretch-activated channels[3]). This chapter focuses on three characteristic observations—and departs from familiar explanations—contending that a major contributor is regional variation in cardiac load. This presentation uses experiments from our laboratory, and mainly centers on $[K^+]_o$, pathologic amplification of MEF, and alternans.

Requirements to Support Assertion

For the previous assertion, we need the etiologic factors to produce mechanical changes, and through MEF, link to $[K^+]_o$, as well as electrical correlates of lethal arrhythmias. Can the diverse electrophysiologic factors relating to arrhythmias relate to mechano-electric mechanisms at the cellular level?

BRIEF METHODOLOGY

Basic Model and Electrical Measurements

Studies on MEF center on heart preparations with a mechanical input (e.g., changes in length, force, pressure) that produce an electrophysiologic change (e.g., membrane current, action potential). This chapter draws on our studies of intact heart during acute regional ischemia.

In most experiments described in this chapter, large mammals were premedicated with ketamine or azaperone, then deeply anesthetized (5% halothane in 1:1 nitrous oxide and oxygen) and their hearts exposed.

The recordings (Fig. 12–2A) were from (1) prospective ischemic regions; (2) border regions; (3) remote (control) regions; or all three simultaneously. Epicardial suction and strain gauge electrodes[4] were used to record simultaneous monophasic action potentials (MAP) and segment length (see Fig. 12–2B) from the left ventricular epicardium. (The time course of repolarization of the MAP is comparable with that seen with microelectrodes). Snaring a branch of the left anterior descending coronary artery created acute regional ischemia and systolic bulging (dyskinesia).

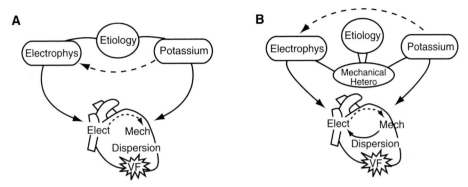

■ **Figure 12–1** Etiologic factors, arrhythmic mechanisms, and potassium in relation to mechano-electric feedback (MEF)/ transduction. *A,* Conforming situation. Etiologic factors produce both electrophysiologic (electrophys) arrhythmic mechanisms and potassium accumulation. Potassium changes produce electrophysiologic changes *(dashed arrow)*. Electrical changes (Elect) can compromise mechanical function (Mech). The electrical "Dispersion," in the diagrammatic heart, is conducive to ventricular fibrillation (VF). *B,* The proposed MEF hypothesis for arrhythmias. The etiologic factors produce mechanical heterogeneity (Hetero). This produces the electrophysiologic arrhythmic symptoms, as well as the potassium changes. MEF produces electrical dispersion, which predisposes to VF. *(Modified from Lab MJ: Mechanoelectric transduction/feedback: Prevalence and pathophysiology. In Zipes DP, Jalife J (eds): Cardiac Electrophysiology from Cell to Bedside, 4th ed. Philadelphia, WB Saunders, 2004, pp 242–253, with permission.)*

Mechanical Measurements

Ventricular and arterial pressures were monitored. We measured end-diastolic length (that coinciding with action potential upstroke) and maximum length excursion (end-diastolic length *minus* the greatest deviation from this value). In the control area, this had a positive value indicating shortening during systole; in the ischemic area, it was negative, indicating systolic lengthening. The integral of pressure and length for each beat gives an index of regional work.

Potassium Study

To measure $[K^+]_o$, a flexible polyvinyl chloride–valinomycin electrode (patterned after Reference 5) was inserted mid-myocardially in the proposed ischemic

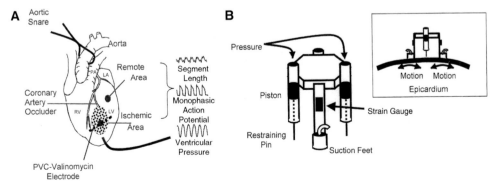

■ **Figure 12–2** Diagrams of experimental setup *(A)* and tripodal recording device *(B)*. Three faces of the hexagonal recording device platform have suction feet attached, which incorporate strain gauges to record motion when sucked onto the epicardium. One of the feet can record a monophasic action potential (or a separate suction electrode may be used). The other three platform faces have pressure-operated pistons driving the restraining pins into the myocardium. *Inset,* Diagram of device on epicardium.

region. Thereafter, regional dyskinesia was curtailed with a restraining device (see Fig. 12–2B) positioned over the proposed ischemic region using suction. The device consisted of three pins (outer diameter ~0.25 mm), at the apices of a triangle, driven into the myocardium during diastole, before the artery was occluded.

Protocols for All Presented Studies

[K+]o Study

The following protocol was used for the $[K^+]_o$ study: (1) Record control regional electromechanical signals. (2) Affix the device to later restrain the affected area. (3) Scrutinize the electrical records for evidence of damage; and if minimal, (4) record preischemic signals. (5) Occlude the selected branch of the coronary artery and record changes in $[K^+]_o$ and electromechanical signals. (6) Reperfuse the area to reattain control values. (7) Restrain area repeating protocol (5).

"Amplification" Study

The following protocol was used for the amplification study: snare aorta (with or without coronary occlusion).

Alternans Study

The following protocol was used for the alternans study: Increase pacing rate to determine the pacing threshold for pulsus alternans; ligate the selected coronary artery and apply 10- to 15-sec burst pacing at the cycle length required to produce alternans at 5-min intervals after the coronary tie to a total of 30 min.

Alternans Simulation

The following protocol was used for the alternans simulation: Place pneumatically driven snare around the proximal aorta and activate on alternate beats during steady-state right atrial pacing at between 450- and 500-msec cycle length to produce beat-to-beat fluctuation in peak intraventricular pressure that is qualitatively similar to that seen during pacing-induced pulsus alternans.

MECHANO-ELECTRIC FEEDBACK AND $[K^+]_o$ IN ISCHEMIA

Can MEF provide an alternative mechanism for the well-known changes in the action potential and accumulation of $[K^+]_o$ in ischemic areas? Acute regional ischemia increases regional $[K^+]_o$ with a defined time course, which contributes to arrhythmogenesis.[4] For example, the action potential duration changes, which have been described in the current experimental model (see Reference 5), increase $[K^+]_o$. This accumulation results from altered transport or a reduction in extracellular space, or both. The precise mechanisms by which this accumulation occurs have yet to be finally elucidated. It seems that none of the currently proposed mechanisms for this accumulation, also implicated in lethal arrhythmia, are entirely satisfactory. These mechanisms include partial inhibition of Na^+–K^+ pump, cellular loss of anions as a consequence of intracellular metabolic acidification, and opening of ATP-sensitive K^+ channels.[6]

The question is: Does the regional dyskinesia (stretch during systole, "bulging") observed in the acutely ischemic area open mechanosensitive channels to contribute to $[K^+]_o$ accumulation? To test this hypothesis, an experimental model must be used in which regional ischemia reliably produces dyskinesia (stretch during systole),[7] and then the model must be manipulated to test the hypothesis.

Results and Discussion

We had to ensure that pin insertion did significantly restrain and reduce segment length excursion. The tripodal strain gauge system incorporated in the restraining device to monitor segment motion[4] produced pressure/length loops. These were normal, inscribing an "upright" roughly rectangular clockwise loop, with shortening during systole (active contraction). The restraining device reduced systolic shortening and reduced the inscribed area (Fig. 12–3A). In regional ischemia, it also, clearly, reduced the passive (segment is noncontractile) systolic stretch observed in the now clockwise loops (not shown).

Acute regional ischemia reduces action potential duration in a time-dependent manner (e.g., see Figs. 12–4 and 12–5).[8] In the current "K^+" series of six exper-

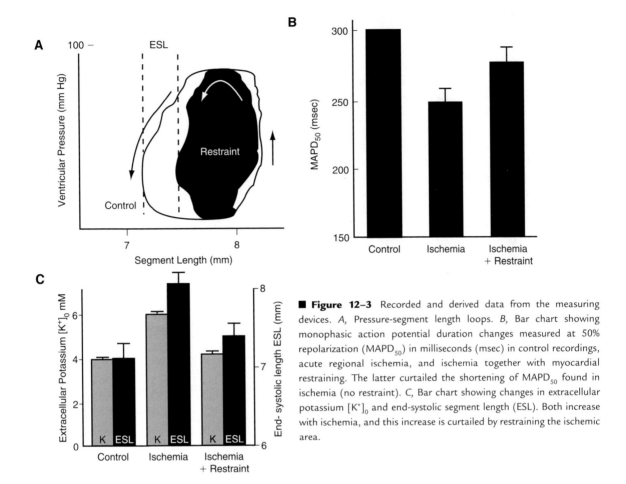

■ Figure 12–3 Recorded and derived data from the measuring devices. *A,* Pressure-segment length loops. *B,* Bar chart showing monophasic action potential duration changes measured at 50% repolarization (MAPD$_{50}$) in milliseconds (msec) in control recordings, acute regional ischemia, and ischemia together with myocardial restraining. The latter curtailed the shortening of MAPD$_{50}$ found in ischemia (no restraint). *C,* Bar chart showing changes in extracellular potassium [K$^+$]$_0$ and end-systolic segment length (ESL). Both increase with ischemia, and this increase is curtailed by restraining the ischemic area.

iments (see Fig. 12–3*B*), 10 minutes of mechanically unrestrained ischemia reduced the MAP duration (MAPD) by 55 ± 8 msec, measured at 50% repolarization (MAPD$_{50}$). After reperfusion and recovery, mechanical restraints reduced the MAPD$_{50}$ by 25 ± 9 msec in a subsequent period of 10 minutes of ischemia.

Ischemia with the area unrestrained produced clear dyskinetic, systolic, bulging of the affected region.[8] End-systolic length increased from 7.0 ± 0.2 mm to 8.0 ± 0.3 mm (~1 mm; see Fig. 12–3*C*). Correspondingly, [K$^+$]$_0$ increased from 3.8 ± 0.1 to 5.7 ± 0.2 mM. After recovery and repeated transient ischemia, restraining of the ischemic area curtailed the increase in end-systolic

length to 0.25 mm (7.0 ± 0.2 to 7.25 ± 0.2 mm). With the restraint, [K$^+$]$_0$ increased less than with no restraint (see Fig. 12–3*C*; from 3.8 ± 0.1 to 4.7 ± 0.4 mM). Shorter ischemia (2 minutes) produced comparable results. All the above effects were fully reversible (on reperfusion, removal of restraint, or both).

Comments

These observations are not yet published; therefore, they should be interpreted with caution. A reviewer's comments might include the following:

1. The K$^+$ electrode is large with respect to the region being measured. The damage on its insertion will influence the recordings. **Reply:** These electrodes have previously been used in pig ventricles,[5] and similar ones have been used in rat. There appeared to be no objections to the interpretation of results.

2. "Myocardial preconditioning" may confound the interpretation (for review, see Reference 9). Preconditioning with a transient episode of ischemia reduces damage from a second episode. The changes in the second episode of ischemia may relate to preconditioning, not mechanical restraint. **Reply:** In some experiments, the ischemic and restraint episodes were reversed, with no effect on the outcome.

3. Pin insertion itself, not the restraint, alters [K$^+$]$_o$. **Reply:** Direct measurements show that pin insertion does not significantly affect [K$^+$]$_o$.

4. Pin insertion produces unacceptable damage to the area, confounding interpretation. **Reply:** The pins produced minimal myocardial damage, as assessed by scrutinizing the epicardial electrogram from the restrained area, which showed no changes in the ST segment, T wave, or action potential duration; there also was no effect on cardiovascular pressures.

5. Correlation does not imply causality. There could be residual collateral or retrograde perfusion during the ischemia. Stretching could increase intramural tension and compromise residual perfusion. Curtailing stretch allows more perfusion compared with "unrestrained" ischemia, explaining the improvement. **Reply:** There is little or no collateral circulation in this preparation: The coronary arteries are end-arteries. There is little chance of improved perfusion.

A plausible explanation could be related to stretch of the ischemic area opening stretch-sensitive K$_{ATP}$ channels[10] (see Chapter 2), which increases K$^+$ efflux. These results provide a potential therapeutic avenue in ischemic arrhythmias, perhaps even explaining why blockers of K$_{ATP}$ channels are antiarrhythmic.[11]

Interestingly, clinical hypokalemia can be arrhythmogenic[12] and, experimentally, low K$^+$ enhances mechanically induced arrhythmias, as reviewed elsewhere.[1,2]

MECHANO-ELECTRIC FEEDBACK, ELECTROPHYSIOLOGY, AND REGIONAL ISCHEMIA

Regional Amplification of Mechano-Electric Feedback

MEF, induced by aortic occlusion in the intact heart in situ, shortens the action potential duration during normal coronary perfusion (see Fig. 12–4A, top traces). During regional ischemia, aortic occlusion shortens the action potential (see Fig. 12–4A, bottom traces). However, the net effect is enhanced compared with control, particularly after 10 minutes of ischemia (see Fig. 12–4B). Also, it varies over the first 30 minutes of ischemia,[8] with an initial increase peaking at 10 minutes, and then decaying to virtually zero at 30 minutes. The enhanced contribution of MEF compared with control is in keeping with other studies conducted in the context of heart failure (as reviewed in References 1 and 2). The increased expression of MEF corresponds in time with the occurrence of phase IA arrhythmias and with the increase in arrhythmias after acute regional ischemia in this pig model.[13]

Does ischemia change the expression or sensitivity of MEF, or are the effects simply related to altered passive mechanical properties?

Although there are compliance changes, their nature and time course are different from that of the action potential duration changes seen in the experiments of Horner and colleagues.[8] There is an immediate decrease in stiffness with coronary occlusion, followed by a progressive monotonic stiffening over the next 2 hours. In the experiments of Horner and colleagues, action potential responses are biphasic, despite the systolic stretches in control and the ischemia being comparable. Thus, the variation in the expression of MEF cannot be easily attributed to changes in loading conditions.

The potentiation of MEF by ischemia could also be explained by: (1) sympathetic stimulation, which increases early in ischemia[14] (β agonists can modulate load-induced changes in electrical restitution and arrhythmia, as reviewed in References 1 and 2); (2) cell swelling, seen in acute ischemia, which could activate mechanosensitive channels (see Chapter 3)[15]; (3) changes

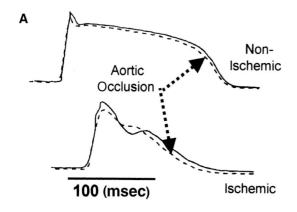

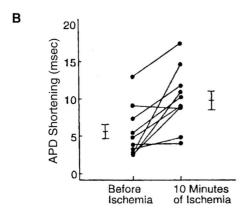

■ **Figure 12–4** Effects of aortic occlusion on action potential with and without ischemia. *A,* Action potentials. Aortic occlusion reduced action potential durations (APD) *(dashed lines)* in the control nonischemic situation *(top traces)* and under ischemic conditions *(bottom traces).* However, the effect was greater during ischemia as illustrated in *B. B,* APD shortening produced by aortic occlusion was greater after 10 minutes of ischemia than before. *(A, Modified from Horner SM, Lab MJ, Murphy CF, et al: Mechanically induced changes in action potential duration and left ventricular segment length in acute regional ischaemia in the in situ porcine heart. Cardiovasc Res 28:528–534, 1994, with permission.)*

in intracellular calcium handling[16] (see Chapters 6 and 22, respectively); or (4) changes in $[K^+]_o$, as described earlier in the chapter.

The conduction velocity in ischemic myocardium may be reduced, delaying activation and repolarization (compare timing of upstrokes in Fig. 12–4*A*).

Nonetheless, ischemic myocardium usually repolarizes before nonischemic myocardium, and this dispersion is proarrhythmic. The enhanced shortening of the ischemic action potential by MEF would increase electrical dispersion and would be deleterious. In addition, action potential duration and refractory period shorten heterogeneously in this preparation, and the decreased conduction velocity promotes re-entry.

Heterogeneous Alternans

Alternans describes alternate beat-to-beat changes in derived measures from myocardium, at a steady heart rate. It may be electrical, mechanical, or both simultaneously. Electromechanical alternans may be discordant in the relation between systolic pressure and action potential duration (small pressure/long action potential; e.g., see Fig. 12–5*A*), or concordant (small pressure/short action potential; e.g., see Fig. 12–5*B*). In addition, when comparing one region of the ventricular wall with another, alternans may be in phase (e.g., both regions big/small/big) or out of phase (e.g., one region big/small/big, the other small/big/small; see Fig. 12–5). There is also beat-to-beat regional heterogeneity.

In this preparation, rapid atrial pacing of normal heart induced global pulsus alternans in all experiments, with a persistent discordant relation (see Fig. 12–5*A*). Ventricular wall motion showed a highly heterogeneous regional contraction pattern.[17]

Acute regional ischemia produced characteristic changes in the morphology of the MAP—reduction of action potential duration (see Figs. 12–4*A* and 12–5*B*) and a failure of regional contraction, with systolic bulging or dyskinesia.[4] Pressure-length loops (See Fig. 12–3*A*), indices of regional work: were either reduced or showed "negative" work: Instead of a clockwise loop, as in perfused myocardium (see Fig. 12–3*A*), the loop was counterclockwise.

The control areas always showed a discordant relation between peak systolic pressure and action potential duration (see Fig. 12–5*A*), whereas the ischemic areas could initially display concordant alternans, but after 10 minutes they became discordant (see Fig. 12–5*B*). After 20 minutes, the MAP degenerated or showed no alternans.[18,19]

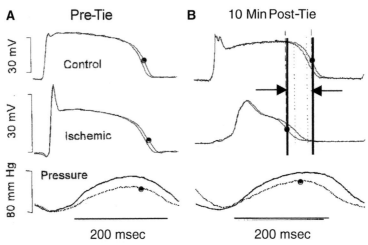

■ **Figure 12–5** Electromechanical relations during alternans before and after regional ischemia. *Top traces* are control areas remote from ischemic area, *middle traces* are from ischemic or denoted ischemic area, and *bottom traces* intraventricular pressures. *A,* Before ischemia (pre-tie). Control and denoted ischemic areas show discordant electromechanical relations—longer action potentials with small pressure. *B,* After ischemia (post-tie). Control area still shows discordant electromechanical relationship *(right vertical line),* but ischemic area now shows a concordant electromechanical relationship *(left vertical line)*—short action potential with small pressure. *(Modified from Murphy CF, Lab MJ, Horner SM, et al: Regional electromechanical alternans in anesthetized pig hearts: Modulation by mechanoelectric feedback. Am J Physiol 267:H1726–H1735, 1994, with permission.)*

Simulating pulsus alternans using a pneumatically driven snare programmed to occlude the aorta on alternate beats (during steady-state pacing without evidence of alternans), control areas faithfully simulated discordant alternans. Alternate beat occlusion produced an alternate shortening and lengthening of MAPD on clamped and unclamped beats, respectively.[17] In the ischemic areas, alternate beat occlusion either produced no discernible action potential alternans, or a concordant alternans that was out of phase with the simultaneous discordant alternans in the control area: a regional beat-to-beat dispersion of repolarization comparable with that found in spontaneous or pacing-induced alternans.[19]

MECHANO-ELECTRIC FEEDBACK AND ARRHYTHMIC MECHANISMS

Electrophysiologic Heterogeneity

The previous results show that MEF can induce electrophysiologic heterogeneity, dispersion of repolariza-

tion, and excitability/refractoriness (Fig. 12–6, *left*). Dispersion of repolarization promotes abnormal current flow between areas of myocardium that are at different membrane potentials. This current can initiate abnormal depolarizations, particularly in pathologic hearts.[20]

Spatial electrophysiologic heterogeneity and re-entry is a crucial aspect of arrhythmic pathology. The major factors involved in re-entry are reductions in conduction velocity and refractory period and increased excitability. As reviewed previously,[1,2] mechanical changes can induce changes in myocardial refractoriness and excitability, with some studies being less convincing. The latter may be related to where the recordings were taken—that is, heterogeneity of the expression of MEF. Fully activated (refractory) cells recover full excitability over time, which is termed *electrical restitution.* There are changes in the restitution curve (supernormality and steepening) that could theoretically produce fibrillation (and chaos), and mechanical load can produce analogous changes, through mechano-electric transduction or MEF.[1,2]

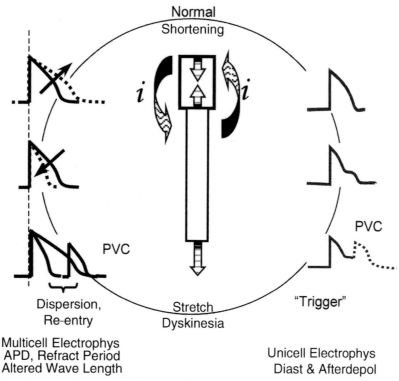

■ **Figure 12–6** Generalized arrhythmic mechanisms invoking mechano-electric changes and heterogeneity. Two myocardial segments are diagrammed in the center. The normal segments *(top)* contracts normally if loaded with a normal segment in series. It produces a normal action potential (at 2 o'clock). If a normal segment contracts against a weaker (e.g., ischemic) segment *(bottom)*, it shortens more and produces a prolonged *(dotted line)* action potential (superimposed at 10 o'clock). In the case of the weaker stretched segment, the action potential (and refractory period) abbreviates *(dotted line at 9 o'clock)*. The stretched segment may also trigger an afterdepolarization (at 3 o'clock) and premature ventricular beats (PVC). This would be a unicellular (unicell) event influencing the electrophysiology (Electrophys) close to diastole (Diast). The repolarization times are dispersed and produce current flow between the segments *(top center, curved arrows and i)*. Dispersion also depicted in the superimposed action potentials (at 8 o'clock). Dispersion of refractory periods will promote changes in wavelength and re-entry *(bottom left)*, with attendant PVC. These are multicellular (multicell) events. *(From Lab MJ: Mechanoelectric transduction/feedback: Prevalence and pathophysiology. In Zipes DP, Jalife J (eds): Cardiac Electrophysiology from Cell to Bedside, 4th ed. Philadelphia, WB Saunders, 2004, pp 242–253, with permission.)*

Electrophysiologic Alternans

Electrophysiologic alternans, in experimental and clinical ischemia,[19,21,22] can precede ventricular fibrillation, and cardiac failure can modulate or produce electromechanical alternans.[24] Importantly, mechano-electric alternans, as demonstrated previously, can be heterogeneous[17,18]; MEF would be heterogeneous and proarrhythmic.

Triggered Afterdepolarizations

Triggered afterdepolarizations are a well-recognized way of producing arrhythmias. Mechanically induced afterdepolarizations (see Fig. 12–6, *right*), which have been described in several preparations of myocardium, appear able to reach threshold to initiate premature beats. This "hump" on the action potential has been described as an early afterdepolarization, but a more appropriate term in a mechano-electric context might be "mechanically activated depolarization" or "stretch-induced depolarization."

Cell Mechanisms

Is there some commonality between the well-established diverse causes and mechanisms for arrhythmias? Stretch-activated channels, as reviewed by Hu and Sachs,[3] appear to be a major mechanism for mechano-electric transduction. Stretch opens the channels moving the membrane potential toward the relevant equilibrium potential. This alters the electrophysiology. In addition, we[23] and Tavi in Weckstrom's group[25] have shown a form of mechano-electric coupling that involves myofibrils and intracellular calcium during systole.

Changes in intracellular calcium may have a pivotal role in the generation of arrhythmias. This is a component of MEF, as reviewed by Calaghan and White.[26] Importantly, calcium alternans features in both mechanical[27] and electrical alternans. It is likely that calcium changes underlie the proarrhythmic electrophysiologic changes relayed by MEF.

MECHANO-ELECTRIC FEEDBACK CORRELATES AND ARRHYTHMIA

The experiments described previously fit into the context of arrhythmic mechanism, but do they have any context in patient populations? This is summarized in Table 12–1. The clinical correlations, which are some possible consequences of the MEF arrhythmic mechanisms, have been reviewed.[1,2]

In keeping with the observations reviewed and presented previously, "MEF begets MEF." Pathologic situations appear to amplify MEF, and one could predict an increased likelihood of mechanically induced arrhythmia in these situations.

CONCLUSION: IS THE ASSERTION VALID?

It is tenable that there are indeed multiple contributors to arrhythmic mechanisms and clinical correlations with sudden arrhythmic death. However, the essence of the presented assertion proposes that many clinical and electrophysiologic correlates of lethal arrhythmias

TABLE 12–1   Mechano-Electric Feedback Measures, Procedures, and Clinical Correlations

Measures	MEF	Clinical Correlation	Pathology/Comment
Mechanical	Increased force/length alters electrophysiology	Dyskinesia, arrhythmia,[28,29] poor ejection	Patchy remodeling
Systemic load	Peripheral vasodilators nitroprusside	Good for arrhythmia (ACE inhibitors)	Reduce wall stress/strain
	Aortic occlusion	Hypertension, aortic stenosis	Related to arrhythmia
Electrophysiology	ME alternans in experimental ischemia	ME alternans, in clinical ischaemia	Heralds VF
	Can produce EAD and U-wave[30,31]	Abnormal U wave[32] (also low K+)[12]	EAD, arrhythmia
ANS	β agonists/blockers modify MEF [33-35]	β-Blockers reduce arrhythmic death	Load changes/ANS coexist
	Bretylium tosylate curtails ME arrhythmia[36]	Similarly bretylium tosylate (acute)	Depletes catecholamines
Hypokalemia	Low K+ enhances MEF arrhythmia	Diuretic therapy, low K+, are arrhythmogenic	Patients need K+ supplements
Chronic load	Stretch alters early genes, action potential[37]	Chronic stretch, hypertrophy, remodeling	ME heterogeneity

ACE, angiotensin-converting enzyme; ANS, autonomic nervous system; EAD, early afterdepolarization; ME, mechano-electric; MEF, mechano-electric feedback.

have their equivalent in MEF or coupling—that is, they are accompanied by pathologic mechanical changes, which would produce electrical changes. At one extreme, this would be ischemically induced dyskinesia or infarction, with gross mechano-electric dispersion. At the other end, remodeling, with patchy mechano-electric coupling, could produce less mechano-electric dispersion, but nonetheless a potentially grave one. Moreover, there is an extensive reach for interaction with other apparently unrelated clinical correlates, for example, electrolyte and autonomic imbalances. The altered stress and strain could summon afterdepolarizations, electrical dispersion, and changes in wavelength and re-entry, all of which play a part in arrhythmic mechanisms. In addition, MEF, perhaps acting as a homeostatic feedback control system in the normal situation,[1,2] is amplified in cardiac pathology. The feedback is now a destabilizing mechanism. The tentative argument is that the common factor in many of the known arrhythmic mechanisms and clinical correlates or risk factors in arrhythmic death is a patchy but lethal expression of MEF.

References

1. Lab MJ: Mechanosensitivity as an integrative system in heart: An audit. Prog Biophys Mol Biol 71:7–27, 1999.
2. Lab MJ: Mechanoelectric transduction/feedback: Prevalence and pathophysiology. In Zipes DP, Jalife J (eds): Cardiac Electrophysiology from Cell to Bedside, 4th ed. Philadelphia, WB Saunders, 2004, pp 242–253.
3. Hu H, Sachs F: Stretch-activated ion channels in the heart. J Mol Cell Cardiol 29:1511–1523, 1997.
4. Kleber AG: Resting membrane potential, extracellular potassium activity, and intracellular sodium activity during acute global ischemia in isolated perfused guinea pig hearts. Circ Res 52:442–450, 1983.
5. Hill JL, Gettes LS: Effect of acute coronary artery occlusion on local myocardial extracellular K+ activity in swine. Circulation 61:768–778, 1980.
6. Wilde AA, Escande D, Schumacher CA, et al: Potassium accumulation in the globally ischemic mammalian heart. A role for the ATP-sensitive potassium channel. Circ Res 67:835–843, 1990.
7. Lab MJ, Woollard KV: Monophasic action potentials, electrocardiograms and mechanical performance in normal and ischaemic epicardial segments of the pig ventricle in situ. Cardiovasc Res 12:555–565, 1978.
8. Horner SM, Lab MJ, Murphy CF, et al: Mechanically induced changes in action potential duration and left ventricular segment length in acute regional ischaemia in the in situ porcine heart. Cardiovasc Res 28:528–534, 1994.
9. Lawson CS, Downey JM: Preconditioning: State of the art myocardial protection. Cardiovascular Res 27:542–550, 1993.
10. Van Wagoner DR, Lamorgese M: Ischemia potentiates the mechanosensitive modulation of atrial ATP-sensitive potassium channels. Ann N Y Acad Sci 723:392–395, 1994.
11. D'Alonzo AJ, Sewter JC, Darbenzio RB, Hess TA: Effects of cromakalim or glibenclamide on arrhythmias and dispersion of refractoriness in chronically infarcted dogs. Naunyn Schmiedebergs Arch Pharmacol 352:222–228, 1995.
12. Podrid PJ: Potassium and ventricular arrhythmias. Am J Cardiol 65:33E–44E, 1990.
13. Dilly SG, Lab MJ: Changes in monophasic action potential duration during the first hour of regional myocardial ischaemia in the anaesthetised pig. Cardiovasc Res 21:908–915, 1987.
14. Sakai K, Abiko Y: Acute changes of myocardial norepinephrine and glycogen phosphorylase in ischemic and non-ischemic areas after coronary ligation in dogs. Jpn Circ J 45:1250–1255, 1981.
15. Clemo HF, Stambler BS, Baumgarten CM: Persistent activation of a swelling-activated cation current in ventricular myocytes from dogs with tachycardia-induced congestive heart failure. Circ Res 83:147–157, 1998.
16. Steenbergen C, Murphy E, Levy L, London RE: Elevation in cytosolic free calcium concentration early in myocardial ischemia in perfused rat heart. Circ Res 60:700–707, 1987.
17. Murphy CF, Lab MJ, Horner SM, et al: Regional electromechanical alternans in anesthetized pig hearts: Modulation by mechanoelectric feedback. Am J Physiol 267:H1726–H1735, 1994.
18. Murphy CF, Horner SM, Dick DJ, et al: Electrical alternans and the onset of rate-induced pulsus alternans during acute regional ischaemia in the anaesthetised pig heart. Cardiovasc Res 32:138–147, 1996.
19. Dilly SG, Lab MJ: Electrophysiological alternans and restitution during acute regional ischaemia in myocardium of anaesthetized pig. J Physiol (Lond) 402:315–333, 1988.
20. Janse MJ, van Capelle FJ, Morsink H, et al: Flow of "injury" current and patterns of excitation during early ventricular arrhythmias in acute regional myocardial ischemia in isolated porcine and canine hearts. Evidence for two different arrhythmogenic mechanisms. Circ Res 47:151–165, 1980.
21. Janse MJ, Kleber AG, Capucci A, et al: Electrophysiological basis for arrhythmias caused by acute ischemia. Role of the subendocardium. J Mol Cell Cardiol 18:339–355, 1986.
22. Rosenbaum DS, Jackson LE, Smith JM, et al: Electrical alternans and vulnerability to ventricular arrhythmias. N Engl J Med 330:235–241, 1994.
23. Lab MJ, Allen DG, Orchard CH: The effects of shortening on myoplasmic calcium concentration and on the action potential in mammalian ventricular muscle. Circ Res 55:825–829, 1984.
24. Cannon RD, Schenke WH, Bonow RD, et al: Left ventricular pulsus alternans in patients with hypertrophic cardiomyopathy and severe obstruction to left ventricular outflow. Circulation 73:276–285, 1986.
25. Tavi P, Han C, Weckstrom M: Mechanisms of stretch-induced changes in [Ca2+]i in rat atrial myocytes: Role of increased troponin C affinity and stretch-activated ion channels. Circ Res 83:1165–1177, 1998.
26. Calaghan SC, White E: The role of calcium in the response of cardiac muscle to stretch. Prog Biophys Mol Biol 71:59–90, 1999.
27. Lab MJ, Lee JA: Changes in intracellular calcium during mechanical alternans in isolated ferret ventricular muscle. Circ Res 66:585–595, 1990.

28. Siogas K, Pappas S, Graekas G, et al: Segmental wall motion abnormalities alter vulnerability to ventricular ectopic beats associated with acute increases in aortic pressure in patients with underlying coronary artery disease. Heart 79:268–273, 1998.

29. Perticone F, Ceravolo R, Maio R, et al: Mechano-electric feedback and ventricular arrhythmias in heart failure. The possible role of permanent cardiac stimulation in preventing ventricular tachycardia. Cardiologia 38:247–252, 1993.

30. Lepeschkin E: Role of myocardial temperature: electrolyte and stress gradients in the genesis of the normal T-wave. In Schlant RC, Hurst JW (eds): Advances in Electrocardiography. New York, Grune & Stratton, 1976, pp 339–352.

31. Choo MC, Gibson DG: U-waves in ventricular hypertrophy: Possible demonstration of mechano-electric feedback. Br Heart J 55:428–433, 1986.

32. el Sherif N, Bekheit SS, Henkin R: Quinidine-induced long QTU interval and torsade de pointes: Role of bradycardia-dependent early afterdepolarizations. J Am Coll Cardiol 14:252–257, 1989.

33. Horner SM, Murphy CF, Coen B, et al: Sympathomimetic modulation of load-dependent changes in the action potential duration in the in situ porcine heart. Cardiovasc Res 32:148–157, 1996.

34. Lab MJ, Dick D, Harrison FG: Propranolol reduces stretch arrhythmia in isolated rabbit heart [abstract]. J Physiol (Lond) 446:539P, 1992.

35. Lab MJ: Contraction-excitation feedback in myocardium: Physiological basis and clinical relevance. Circ Res 50:757–766, 1982.

36. Dick DJ, Lab MJ, Harrison FG, et al: A possible role of endogenous catecholamines in stretch induced premature ventricular beats in the isolated rabbit heart. J Physiol 479:133P, 1994.

37. Meghji P, Nazir SA, Dick DJ, et al: Regional workload induced changes in electrophysiology and immediate early gene expression in intact in situ porcine heart. J Mol Cell Cardiol 29:3147–3155, 1997.

Mechanical Triggers and Facilitators of Cardiac Excitation and Arrhythmias

• • • •

Markus Zabel and Michael R. Franz

Early experimental work using transmembrane action potential (AP) recordings recognized that mechanical stretch shortens action potential duration (APD) in isolated cardiac tissue.[1-5] This was later confirmed in intact canine heart.[6] It was also demonstrated that mechanical stretch can elicit ventricular arrhythmias in intact frog ventricle,[7] intact pig heart,[8] and canine ventricle.[9,10] This association between mechanical and electrical effects has been termed *contraction-excitation* or *mechano-electric* feedback (MEF),[6,11] and subsequently has led to a novel research area.[12-15] At the cellular level, patch clamp studies identified stretch-activated ion channels (SAC) in myocytes from chick[16] and rabbit[17] that helped explain direct electrophysiologic effects of myocardial stretch. Because the surface ECG is too insensitive to detect electrophysiologic stretch effects, a significant amount of data have been acquired using contact electrode monophasic action potential (MAP) recordings.[18-20] Various mechanisms of arrhythmia induction and facilitation by mechanical stretch have been suggested and are reviewed in this chapter. Special emphasis is given to the effects of short, pulsatile stretch and prolonged, static mechanical stimulation.

ELECTROPHYSIOLOGIC EFFECTS OF ACUTE STRETCH

The first intracellular studies found stretch to shorten APD.[1,3] In MAP recordings from the left ventricular (LV) epicardium of the isolated canine heart,[6,21,22] acutely increased mechanical load also resulted in a decrease of APD and refractory period. Similar results were found in isolated rabbit hearts.[22] Other investiga-

tors, however, reported a lengthening of APD in response to direct myocardial stretch.[7,23] Stretch-induced electrophysiologic changes appeared to differ depending on whether acute mechanical stretch was applied in the form of increased preload or increased afterload.[6,23-25] The repolarization level at which APD was measured, as well as the mode of ventricular contraction, seemed to explain the conflicting results. Franz and colleagues[23] studied stretch-induced changes in the isovolumically beating canine ventricle and demonstrated that an increase in ventricular volume load with a simultaneous increase in ventricular pressure shortened the APD at early repolarization levels, whereas APD near complete repolarization was lengthened (Fig. 13–1).

Similar findings were reported by Hansen[24] from isolated canine hearts. Both investigators noted that the increase in overall APD under increased isovolumic load occurred in the shape of early afterdepolarizations.[23,24] These divergent results were later reconciled by the time- and voltage-dependent characteristics of SAC in direct comparison between computer simulation and experimental data.[26]

A decrease in the resting potential and AP amplitude was reported under various conditions of isovolumic load in both dog[23] and rabbit[27] studies. These findings were in line with data reported from intracellular recordings in Purkinje and ventricular muscle fibers exhibiting both a decrease in resting and AP amplitudes under stretch.[2,28] The studies by Franz and colleagues[23] and Hansen[24] also addressed the question whether preload (i.e., diastolic volume increase) or systolic outflow impedance (afterload) is more important for inducing stretch-induced electrophysiologic changes. Both studies showed that only increased preload leads

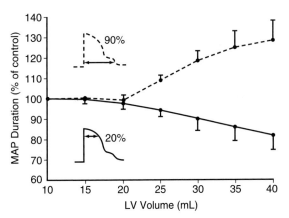

■ **Figure 13–1** Monophasic action potential (MAP) recordings were obtained from epicardium of isolated cross-perfused canine left ventricles (LV) instrumented with servo-controlled intracavity balloon. Data are average ±SD from six ventricles beating isovolumically at constant cycle length of 500 msec during seven volume loading interventions. Action potential duration (APD) responded divergently depending on the level of repolarization. Plateau duration (APD at 20% repolarization) shortened with increasing volume, whereas APD at 90% repolarization lengthened because of occurrence of afterdepolarizations (see Fig. 13–2). *(From Franz MR, Burkhoff D, Yue DT, Sagawa K: Mechanically induced action potential changes and arrhythmia in isolated and in situ canine hearts. Cardiovasc Res 23:213–223, 1989, with permission.)*

to the acute stretch-induced electrophysiologic changes described earlier. Changing the ventricular contraction mode from isovolumic to ejecting, despite increased preload, abolished early afterdepolarizations immediately[23] (Fig. 13–2).

The effects of suddenly increased afterload on MAP recordings were further demonstrated in in situ hearts of open-chest dogs. When the ascending aorta was transiently occluded with large rubber-coated hemostats, the sudden increase in LV pressure resulted in afterdepolarizations and premature beats (Fig. 13–3). In this example, the first beat after the onset of the clamp is followed by a premature depolarization that generates relatively little pressure. The beat after the compensatory pause exhibits postextrasystolic potentiation and an afterdepolarization that triggers another premature depolarization. This sequence repeats itself three times, until release of the aortic clamp.[23]

Electrophysiologic Effects of Short Transient Stretch: Importance of Timing during Systole or Diastole

Using a computer-controlled servo motor that drove intraventricular volume through a fluid-filled latex balloon inserted into the left ventricle of an intact, isolated, rabbit heart with atrioventricular block and a slow escape rhythm, Franz and colleagues[27] applied a series of volume pulses of successively increasing amplitudes. These volume pulses induced transient diastolic depolarizations that increased in parallel with an increase in pulse volume. Above a certain amplitude or threshold, each transient depolarization was associated with a premature ventricular response—that is, the preparation was "paced" by the volume pulses (Fig. 13–4).

Stretch-induced premature ventricular contractions were also reported in isolated frog,[7] pig,[8] and canine[9,10] hearts. Franz and coworkers[27] also varied the velocity with which acute stretch pulses were applied (the stretch onset ramp velocity) and found that an increased stretch velocity was an independent contributor to the induction of premature beats.

Zabel and colleagues[26] investigated the effects of short volume pulses administered at different times during systole and diastole, in comparison with longer, static stretch of the same amplitude. In this study, both repolarizing and depolarizing responses were observed with a remarkable dependence on the timing of the stretch pulse with respect to the AP phase. A short, transient stretch pulse elicited either transient depolarizations when applied during late systole or diastole, or transient repolarizations when applied during the plateau of the MAP. A stretch pulse placed toward the end of the MAP caused depolarizations that mimicked early afterdepolarizations or, if placed after the MAP, delayed afterdepolarizations. With sufficient amplitude of the stretch-induced (diastolic) depolarizations, premature ventricular contractions were caused, confirming the results of a previous study (see earlier discussion).

Stacy and colleagues[10] also confirmed these results; however, they postulated an accelerated phase 4 depolarization of Purkinje fibers as the mechanism for premature beats. In contrast to "classical" early or delayed afterdepolarizations, stretch-activated depolarizations

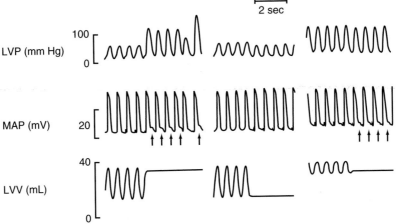

■ Figure 13–2 MAP recordings from epicardium of isolated cross-perfused canine left ventricle (same preparation as in Fig. 13–1). Left ventricular volume (LVV) and outflow impedance were controlled by an intraventricular fluid-filled balloon coupled to a servo-controlled piston pump. *Left,* Normal MAP were recorded when the LV was allowed to eject freely, but with sudden clamping of LVV at end-diastolic level, afterdepolarizations immediately occurred *(arrows). Middle,* Clamping LVV at end-systole did not cause afterdepolarizations in the MAP recording. *Right,* Small afterdepolarizations were recorded when ventricular contractions started at high diastolic volume and also had to eject against increased afterload. These afterdepolarizations increased when the volume was clamped at end-systole. LV pressure (LVP) was measured with a catheter-tip transducer inserted within the balloon. *(From Franz MR, Burkhoff D, Yue DT, Sagawa K: Mechanically induced action potential changes and arrythmia in isolated and in situ canine hearts. Cardiovasc Res 23:213–223, 1989, with permission.)*

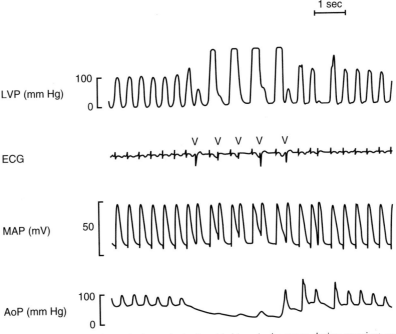

■ Figure 13–3 Afterdepolarizations and ventricular arrhythmia with bigeminal pattern during transient aortic occlusion. AoP, aortic pressure; ECG, electrocardiogram; V, ectopic ventricular beat. *(From Franz MR, Burkhoff D, Yue DT, Sagawa K: Mechanically induced action potential changes and arrhythmia in isolated and in situ canine hearts. Cardiovasc Res 23:213–223, 1989, with permission.)*

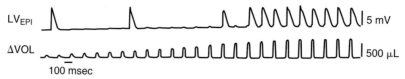

■ **Figure 13–4** Volume pulses of increasing amplitude applied to rabbit heart with intraventricular fluid-filled balloon. Note diastolic depolarizations during subthreshold pulses and ectopic beats during suprathreshold pulses. ΔVOL denotes balloon volume changes; LV$_{EPI}$, one of two epicardial MAP recordings. *(From Franz MR, Cima R, Wang D, et al: Electrophysiological effects of myocardial stretch and mechanical determinants of stretch-activated arrythmias [published erratum in Circulation 86: 1663, 1992]. Circulation 86: 968–978, 1992, with permission.)*

did not depend on the trigger of a preceding AP. The studies by Zabel and colleagues[26] and Stacy and colleagues[10] could together demonstrate that the amplitude of a stretch-activated depolarization is linearly correlated with the amplitude of the underlying stretch pulse. In addition, Zabel and colleagues[26] also found that the amplitude of a stretch-related *repolarization "dip"* during the plateau phase of the MAP exhibited a similar linear relation to the stretch pulse amplitude as the diastolic *depolarization "hump"* (Fig. 13–5). When applying the stretch pulse during early phase 3 of the MAP, the repolarizing deflection was less than during the plateau of the AP. Similarly, stretch-activated depolarizations became smaller when the pulse was moved from full repolarization levels toward a less complete repolarization level. Halfway between these opposing responses, a neutral response to stretch (stretch immunity) was found (see Fig. 13–5). Notably, the peak ventricular pressure occurs within the down-slope of the AP, and thus within the window of electrophysiologic "immunity" (see Fig. 13–5*D*).

The study by Zabel and colleagues[26] extended previous data by Lab[7] in isolated strips and whole-frog ventricles, which also demonstrated opposite electrophysiologic stretch effects dependent on the AP phase. Premature beats (excitations) were preceded by stretch-activated depolarizations in several studies in the intact beating canine[23,29] or pig heart[8] and in humans[30] involving a transient outflow tract obstruction as the acute mechanical stretch stimulus.

Validity of Monophasic Action Potential Recordings for Stretch-Induced Changes of Electrophysiology

The early studies by Lab[7] used insulated sucrose-gap or suction electrode AP recordings. Intracellular microelectrodes have a tendency to dislodge in vigorously beating tissue or during mechanical interventions. Thus, the question has been raised whether some of the stretch-induced voltage changes represent motion artifacts. Given the fragility of the glass microelectrode–cell membrane interface and technical difficulties in keeping a stable intracellular position, no "gold standard" technique is available to prove that MAP recordings are artifact-free. However, the following observations speak in favor of faithful MAP recordings in the studies by Franz[27] and Zabel[26] (see earlier). First, MAP recorded from the right ventricle (RV) never showed significant changes in response to short or sustained LV stretch pulses, despite that the RV moved passively with the LV volume interventions.[26] Second, the similarity between effects of short and long stretch pulses is of particular importance. There are no sudden mechanical perturbations of the heart during static stretch applied to the heart, yet the net effect on the MAP was almost identical to that with short stretch pulses. Third, there is no simple explanation why a motion artifact should change its polarity with different timings of the short stretch pulse.

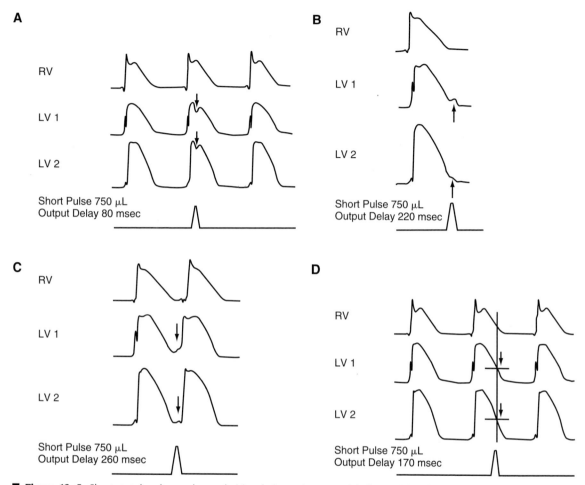

■ **Figure 13–5** Short stretch pulses evoke repolarizing during action potential plateau *(A)* and depolarizing when applied during late phase 3 *(B)* or diastole *(C)*. Minimal effects are seen when stretch pulse is given at mid-phase 3 *(D, arrows and bars)*. LV1 and LV2, monophasic action potential recordings from two left ventricular sites (all epicardial); RV, right ventricular MAP recording. *(From Zabel M, Koller BS, Sachs F, Franz MR: Stretch-induced voltage changes in the isolated beating heart: Importance of the timing of stretch and implications for stretch-activated ion channels. Cardiovasc Res 32:120–130, 1996, with permission.)*

Fourth, premature ventricular contractions emerging from a "take-off" potential—a finding confirmed in various models and species[7-10,26,27]—strongly support that these potentials are real. Mechanical behavior, such as stretch-induced ectopics, occurs regardless of whether electrical recordings are made and are in keeping with observed MEF-induced electrical phenomena. Of course, as with all techniques, stringent care must be taken to ensure stable, high-quality recordings.

Ionic Basis for Stretch-Induced Effects in Intact Heart Studies: Stretch-Activated Channels

SAC have been demonstrated in various noncardiac tissues[31-33] and subsequently in the heart.[16,34-36] The myocardium contains SAC that allow both inward and outward currents, depending on the actual membrane potential of affected cells.[16,35,36] Whole-cell recordings of cation nonselective SAC currents in the heart indicated a reversal potential in the range of -15 ± 4 mV at 35°C.[37] Characteristics of SAC from patch clamp studies were added to a heart computer model to simulate the effects of short, pulsatile stretch on the MAP. A remarkable agreement was found between the simulation and the results from the intact rabbit heart studies[26] (Fig. 13–6).

The computer model predicted that SAC activation during the diastolic resting potential should result in an inward current (i.e., depolarization), and conversely, that activation during the AP plateau should result in an outward current (i.e., repolarization). This (reversal) potential and linearity underscore the voltage independence of SAC. Deviations between the experimental data and the computer simulations occur mainly in late repolarization when the time course is most sensitive to voltage changes.[18,38]

Electrophysiologic Effects of Sustained Acute Stretch: Dispersion of Repolarization

Slowly applied and sustained stretch interventions do not trigger ventricular arrhythmias.[26,27] Sodium channel

activation is required to occur before voltage-dependent inactivation renders further depolarization futile. Zabel and colleagues[39] therefore explored the electrophysiologic effects of sustained stretch and showed that a sustained, static load of the isolated rabbit ventricle influences several electrophysiologic parameters, including repolarization and activation. APD at 90% repolarization (APD_{90}) was shortened in the volume-loaded LV. At the same time, the refractory period was shortened. Although the common effect of mechanical loading was to shorten the APD and refractoriness, we also observed lengthening of APD_{90} in some parts of the heart. The disparity of stretch effects between various locations in the ventricle, particularly between the loaded LV and the nonstretched RV, resulted in an increased dispersion of ventricular repolarization. The latter parameter is known to be arrhythmogenic in many experimental models.[40–42] The activation time—measured as the longest interval between the pacing artifact and the earliest MAP upstroke—was prolonged, particularly during premature extrastimulation. A prolongation of conduction time by stretch was also found by Dominguez and Fozzard[43] in Purkinje fibers and Calkins and colleagues[21] in the intact canine heart. Conduction time is a second arrhythmogenic parameter influenced by stretch or load. Arrhythmogenicity of sustained stretch could be demonstrated in dog models,[9,21,22] where the induction of sustained ventricular arrhythmias was facilitated by loading.

STRETCH-INDUCED ELECTROPHYSIOLOGIC CHANGES AND ATRIAL FIBRILLATION

In patients, atrial fibrillation (AF) is frequently associated with atrial dilatation generated by hemodynamic overload during various cardiac diseases.[44,45] Likewise, the success of therapeutic attempts to restore sinus rhythm is closely associated with the diameter of the atria.[46] Atrial SAC may well be involved in the pathophysiology of AF (see Chapters 16 and 17).

The hypothesis that SAC are involved was further explored by Franz and Bode.[47] These authors applied the known SAC blocker gadolinium (Gd^{3+}) in the atrial stretch model using the isolated rabbit heart.

Guinea Pig, Vr= −20 mV

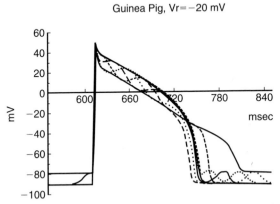

■ **Figure 13–6** Computer simulation of the effect of trapezoidal stretch pulses (20 msec increase and decrease, 10 msec plateau) on the action potential, using the program HEART (OxSoft, Oxford, UK) with integrated stretch-activated channels with a reversal potential (Vr) of −20 mV. *(From Zabel M, Koller BS, Sachs F, Franz MR: Stretch-induced voltage changes in the isolated beating heart: Importance of the timing of stretch and implications for stretch-activated ion channels. Cardiovasc Res 32:120–130, 1996, with permission.)*

Gd^{3+} decreases AF vulnerability in a dose-dependent manner. These findings were confirmed by Bode and colleagues[48] in another study where GsMTx-4, a peptide specific for blocking SAC, was applied to the isolated rabbit heart model. Again, AF could be suppressed at high mechanical loads.

SUMMARY

The electrophysiologic effects of pulsatile stretch, stretch generated by increased preload and afterload, and acute static mechanical stretch can be explained by the existence of SAC. As expected from the known characteristics of these channels, stretch generates a repolarizing response during systole, a neutral response in the middle of phase 3 near the reversal potential of SAC, and a depolarizing response during diastole. The latter response may mimic early afterdepolarizations that can induce propagated ventricular excitation. Sustained stretch increases the dispersion of ventricular excitability, refractoriness, and electrical load. This causes variations in conduction velocity, facilitating reentrant arrhythmias. There appears to be ample experimental evidence that mechanical load alters electrophysiology in a way that is likely to facilitate the induction or sustenance, or both, of ventricular and atrial arrhythmias.

References

1. Dudel J, Trautwein W: Das Aktionspotential und Mechanogramm des Herzmuskels unter dem Einfluss der Dehnung. Cardiologie 25:344, 1954.
2. Penefsky ZJ, Hoffman BF: Effects of stretch on mechanical and electrical properties of cardiac muscle. Am J Physiol 204:433, 1963.
3. Kaufmann R, Lab MJ, Hennekes R, Krause H: Autoregulation of contractility in the myocardial cell. Displacement as a controlling parameter. Pflugers Arch 332:96–116, 1972.
4. Kaufmann R, Theophile U: Automatie-foerdernde Dehnungseffekte an Purkinjefaeden, Papillarmuskeln und Vorhoftrabekeln von Rhesusaffen. Pflügers Arch 291:174–189, 1967.
5. Kaufmann RL, Lab MJ, Hennekes R, Krause H: Feedback interaction of mechanical and electrical events in the isolated mammalian ventricular myocardium (cat papillary muscle). Pflügers Arch 324:100–123, 1971.
6. Lerman BB, Burkhoff D, Yue DT, et al: Mechanoelectrical feedback: Independent role of preload and contractility in modulation of canine ventricular excitability [published erratum appears in J Clin Invest 77(6):2053, Jun 1986]. J Clin Invest 76:1843–1850, 1985.
7. Lab MJ: Mechanically dependent changes in action potentials recorded from the intact frog ventricle. Circ Res 42:519–528, 1978.
8. Dean JW, Lab MJ: Effect of changes in load on monophasic action potential and segment length of pig heart in situ. Cardiovasc Res 23:887–896, 1989.
9. Hansen DE, Craig CS, Hondeghem LM: Stretch-induced arrhythmias in the isolated canine ventricle. Evidence for the importance of mechanoelectrical feedback. Circulation 81:1094–1105, 1990.
10. Stacy GP Jr, Jobe RL, Taylor LK, Hansen DE: Stretch-induced depolarizations as a trigger of arrhythmias in isolated canine left ventricles. Am J Physiol 263:H613–H621, 1992.
11. Lab MJ: Contraction-excitation feedback in myocardium. Physiological basis and clinical relevance. Circ Res 50:757–766, 1982.
12. Franz MR: Stretch-activated arrhythmias. In Zipes DP, Jalife JW (eds): Cardiac Electrophysiology: From Cell to Bedside. New York, WB Saunders, 1994, pp 597–606.
13. Franz MR: Bridging the gap between basic and clinical electrophysiology: What can be learned from monophasic action potential recordings? J Cardiovasc Electrophysiol 5:699–710, 1994.
14. Franz MR: Mechano-electrical feedback in ventricular myocardium. Cardiovasc Res 32:15–24, 1996.
15. Kohl P, Hunter P, Noble D: Stretch-induced changes in heart rate and rhythm: Clinical observations, experiments and mathematical models. Prog Biophys Mol Biol 71:91–138, 1999.
16. Ruknudin A, Sachs F, Bustamante JO: Stretch-activated ion channels in tissue-cultured chick heart. Am J Physiol 264:H960–H972, 1993.
17. Hagiwara N, Masuda H, Shoda M, Irisawa H: Stretch-activated anion currents of rabbit cardiac myocytes. J Physiol 456:285–302, 1992.
18. Franz MR, Burkhoff D, Spurgeon H, et al: In vitro validation of a new cardiac catheter technique for recording monophasic action potentials. Eur Heart J 7:34–41, 1986.
19. Franz MR: Method and theory of monophasic action potential recording. Prog Cardiovasc Dis 33:347–368, 1991.
20. Franz MR, Chin MC, Sharkey HR, et al: A new single catheter technique for simultaneous measurement of action potential duration and refractory period in vivo. J Am Coll Cardiol 16:878–886, 1990.
21. Calkins H, Maughan WL, Kass DA, et al: Electrophysiological effect of volume load in isolated canine hearts. Am J Physiol 256:H1697–H1706, 1989.
22. Calkins H, Maughan WL, Weisman HF, et al: Effect of acute volume load on refractoriness and arrhythmia development in isolated, chronically infarcted canine hearts. Circulation 79:687–697, 1989.
23. Franz MR, Burkhoff D, Yue DT, Sagawa K: Mechanically induced action potential changes and arrhythmia in isolated and in situ canine hearts. Cardiovasc Res 23:213–223, 1989.
24. Hansen DE: Mechanoelectrical feedback effects of altering preload, afterload, and ventricular shortening. Am J Physiol 264:H423–H432, 1993.
25. Coulshed DS, Cowan JC: Contraction-excitation feedback in an ejecting whole heart model—dependence of action potential duration on left ventricular diastolic and systolic pressures. Cardiovasc Res 25:343–352, 1991.
26. Zabel M, Koller BS, Sachs F, Franz MR: Stretch-induced voltage changes in the isolated beating heart: Importance of the

timing of stretch and implications for stretch-activated ion channels. Cardiovasc Res 32:120–130, 1996.

27. Franz MR, Cima R, Wang D, et al: Electrophysiological effects of myocardial stretch and mechanical determinants of stretch-activated arrhythmias [published erratum in Circulation 86:1663, 1992]. Circulation 86:968–978, 1992.

28. Boland J, Troquet J: Intracellular action potential changes induced in both ventricles of the rat by an acute right ventricular pressure overload. Cardiovasc Res 14:735–740, 1980.

29. Benditt DG, Kriett JM, Tobler HG, et al: Electrophysiological effects of transient aortic occlusion in intact canine heart. Am J Physiol 249:H1017–H1023, 1985.

30. Levine JH, Guarnieri T, Kadish AH, et al: Changes in myocardial repolarization in patients undergoing balloon valvuloplasty for congenital pulmonary stenosis: Evidence for contraction-excitation feedback in humans. Circulation 77:70–77, 1988.

31. Yang X-C, Sachs F: Block of stretch-activated ion channels in Xenopus oocytes by gadolinium and calcium ions. Science 243:1068–1071, 1989.

32. Yang XC, Sachs F: Characterization of stretch-activated ion channels in Xenopus oocytes. J Physiol 431:103–122, 1990.

33. Naruse K, Sokabe M: Involvement of stretch-activated ion channels in Ca^{2+} mobilization to mechanical stretch in endothelial cells. Am J Physiol 264:C1037–C1044, 1993.

34. Craelius W, Chen V, El-Sherif N: Stretch activated ion channels in ventricular myocytes. Biosci Rep 8:407–414, 1988.

35. Bustamante JO, Ruknudin A, Sachs F: Stretch-activated channels in heart cells: Relevance to cardiac hypertrophy. J Cardiovasc Pharmacol 17:S110–S113, 1991.

36. Sigurdson W, Ruknudin A, Sachs F: Calcium imaging of mechanically induced fluxes in tissue-cultured chick heart: Role of stretch-activated ion channels. Am J Physiol 262:H1110–H1115, 1992.

37. Sasaki N, Mitsuiye T, Noma A: Effects of mechanical stretch on membrane currents of single ventricular myocytes of guinea-pig heart. Jap J Physiol 42:957–970, 1992.

38. Ino T, Karagueuzian HS, Hong K, et al: Relation of monophasic action potential recorded with contact electrode to underlying transmembrane action potential properties in isolated cardiac tissues: A systematic microelectrode validation study. Cardiovasc Res 22:255–264, 1988.

39. Zabel M, Portnoy S, Franz MR: Electrocardiographic indexes of dispersion of ventricular repolarization: An isolated heart validation study. J Am Coll Cardiol 25:746–752, 1995.

40. Han J, Moe GK: Nonuniform recovery of excitability in ventricular muscle. Circ Res 14:44–60, 1964.

41. Kuo CS, Munakata K, Reddy CP, Surawicz B: Characteristics and possible mechanism of ventricular arrhythmia dependent on the dispersion of action potential durations. Circulation 67:1356–1367, 1983.

42. Opthof T, Misier AR, Coronel R, et al: Dispersion of refractoriness in canine ventricular myocardium. Effects of sympathetic stimulation. Circ Res 68:1204–1215, 1991.

43. Dominguez G, Fozzard HA: Effect of stretch on conduction velocity and cable properties of cardiac Purkinje fibers. Am J Physiol 237:C119–C124, 1979.

44. Henry WL, Morganroth J, Pearlman AS, et al: Relation between echocardiographically determined left atrial size and atrial fibrillation. Circulation 53:273–279, 1976.

45. Vasan RS, Larson MG, Levy D, et al: Distribution and categorization of echocardiographic measurements in relation to reference limits: The Framingham Heart Study: Formulation of a height- and sex-specific classification and its prospective validation. Circulation 96:1863–1873, 1997.

46. Verhorst PM, Kamp O, Welling RC, et al: Transesophageal echocardiographic predictors for maintenance of sinus rhythm after electrical cardioversion of atrial fibrillation. Am J Cardiol 79:1355–1359, 1997.

47. Franz MR, Bode F: Mechano-electrical feedback underlying arrhythmias: The atrial fibrillation case. Prog Biophys Mol Biol 82:163–174, 2003.

48. Bode F, Sachs F, Franz MR: Tarantula peptide inhibits atrial fibrillation. Nature 409:35–36, 2001.

CHAPTER 14

The Effects of Wall Stretch on Ventricular Conduction and Refractoriness in the Whole Heart

• • • •

Robert W. Mills, Sanjiv M. Narayan, and Andrew D. McCulloch

Many studies have linked volume overload or increased myocardial strain (wall stretch) with atrial and ventricular arrhythmias.[1] Even though the mechanisms for these mechanical load-induced rhythm disturbances remain unclear, they generally involve either triggered activity or re-entrant conduction.[2] Although both of these mechanisms may contribute, re-entry is the predominant mechanism underlying ventricular arrhythmias associated with mechanical dysfunction.[3] Re-entry depends on the constant presence of excitable tissue ahead of the activation wave front as it propagates around an area of structural or functional conduction block. Slowed conduction or decreased refractoriness, therefore, can promote and sustain re-entry, whereas increased *dispersion* of conduction velocity and refractoriness can provide a substrate for its initiation.[4] Observations on the acute effects of myocardial strain on conduction velocity have varied widely with experimental preparations, mechanical loading conditions, and measurement techniques, whereas findings on the stretch dependence of effective refractory period have been somewhat more consistent. Given the inherent difficulties in measuring regional myocardial mechanics and conduction velocity in the whole heart without disturbing mechanical or electrical properties, many of the discrepancies between experimental reports are probably attributable to differences in experimental methods or definitions.

EFFECTS OF MYOCARDIAL STRETCH ON CONDUCTION VELOCITY

Conduction velocity is defined as the distance an activation wave front travels per unit time (although "distance" has several definitions; see later). Conduction velocity is not an intrinsic property; it is a functional variable dependent on distributed cellular properties and wave front curvature, which influence the speed of impulse wave propagation, and on tissue architecture, anisotropy, and stimulus sites, which influence conduction path. The effect of stretch on conduction velocity in vivo is further complicated by the nonlinear, viscoelastic, anisotropic, time-varying, and heterogeneous mechanical properties of the myocardium.

Factors Influencing Conduction Speed

Intracellular conduction is determined by passive membrane capacitance, longitudinal resistances, and voltage-dependent membrane conductances.[5] Membrane capacitance is a function of membrane dielectric properties and the membrane surface-to-cell volume ratio. Increasing membrane capacitance slows the initial depolarization from resting potential to threshold, thereby reducing conduction velocity. Intracellular and extracellular longitudinal resistances determine how rapidly ions travel in the direction of conduction and are affected by the effective internal and external cross-sectional areas available for ion transport.

Above threshold, the voltage-gated fast sodium current usually determines how rapidly the local membrane depolarizes (action potential phase 0), creating the electrochemical gradient that drives longitudinal ion diffusion. These conductances are influenced by channel kinetics and other regulatory processes, such as ligand gating and autonomic stimulation.[6] Altering resting membrane potential influences conduction speed in a biphasic manner,[7] and model studies suggest that this effect acts through *membrane excitability*.[8] As the resting membrane potential depolarizes, the difference between resting potential and activation threshold decreases, requiring less membrane charging, thereby increasing conduction speed. Simultaneously, sodium channel inactivation increases with resting membrane depolarization, resulting in fewer channels available to open during activation, thus slowing conduction. Ionic movement between cells, and consequently myocardial conduction speed,[7] is primarily limited under normal conditions by the resistance of the gap junctions. Gap junction open probability is sensitive to ischemia, pH, intracellular magnesium and calcium, and *trans*junctional voltage.[9] Although increased intercellular coupling speeds conduction, it also increases electrical load on depolarizing cells as downstream cells draw away charge. Activation wave front curvature similarly affects propagation speed; a convex wave front must stimulate an expanding volume of resting tissue, imposing a greater electrical load and slowing conduction.[10]

Stretch may influence these determinants of conduction speed in several ways. Changes in cell geometry may alter membrane surface area and intracellular resistance. Stretch-activated ion currents may affect conduction velocity by altering resting potential, and thus excitability. It is unknown whether acute mechanical stimuli alter gap junction permeability, but prolonged stretch in cell culture significantly up-regulates connexin43.[11]

Factors Influencing Conduction Path

Regional conduction speed is a reflection of the fastest conduction path through local myocardial architec-ture. The direction of fastest propagation follows the myocardial fiber direction because of the distribution of gap junctions within the cell,[9] with fiber conduction speed typically being 2- to 10-fold faster than in the cross-fiber direction. Tissue conduction anisotropy is a function of gap junction distribution, myocyte branching, fiber angle dispersion, the laminar sheet organization of the myofibers, and the presence of connective tissue septa within the interstitium. Within the ventricle, fiber angles follow a left-handed helix in the epicardium and smoothly transition to a right-handed helix in the endocardium. Therefore, as activation spreads transmurally, the principal axis of fastest in-plane propagation rotates and the wave front changes shape. Transverse to the fiber direction, cardiomyocytes are stacked into branching laminar sheets about four to six cells in thickness surrounded by a perimysial collagen fascia. A model reconstruction of tissue microarchitecture showed that this organization results in conduction across the sheet planes being slowed by 40% compared with cross-fiber conduction within the sheets.[12]

Strain can change conduction path by altering local fiber and sheet directions. For example, Penefsky and Hoffman[13] suggest that increased fiber conduction velocity with stretch in isolated papillary muscles may have been associated with decreased dispersion of fiber angles. Myocardial sheets exhibit significant interlaminar shearing and rotation during early relaxation,[14] which may affect transmural conduction times and intramural electrotonic coupling.

Determinants of Regional Wall Stress and Strain

In addition to exhibiting mechanical preconditioning behavior and strain softening during repeated loading cycles, myocardium is viscoelastic at rest, with a ventricular chamber asymptotic time constant for stress relaxation on the order of 1000 sec reflecting the composite viscoelastic behavior of faster relaxing myocytes and extracellular matrix.[15] Myofilament activation also causes stress and strain to vary phasically throughout the cardiac cycle.[16] In studies of the effects of mechano-electric feedback (MEF) on conduction velocity in the normal heart, diastolic mechanics are the most important determinant as electrical activation precedes systolic contraction, but may be influenced by myofilament interactions when relaxation is incomplete at high heart rates. At lower heart rates, afterload alterations have little direct influence on conduction velocity, but may significantly affect repolarization and refractoriness. Finally, cardiac geometry and fiber architecture result in significant mechanical anisotropy and heterogeneity.[16] Changes in conduction path are determined by strain, but whether cellular responses are determined primarily by stress or strain depends fundamentally on the relative compliance of the molecular mechanotransducer, such as a stretch-activated ion channel (SAC).

TABLE 14–1 Definitions of Conduction Velocity in One Dimension		
	Unstretched	**Stretched**
Cellular		$CV = \dfrac{L_0}{\Delta t(L_1)}$
Spatial	$CV = \dfrac{L_0}{\Delta t(L_0)}$	$CV = \dfrac{L_0}{\Delta t(L_0)}$
Material		$CV = \dfrac{L_1}{\Delta t(L_1)}$

CV is the conduction velocity. $\Delta t(X)$ is the conduction time measured over the interelectrode distance X. L_0 is the unstretched interelectrode distance, whereas L_1 is the stretched distance.

Measuring Conduction Velocity during Myocardial Stretch

Conduction velocity is usually calculated in one dimension as the distance between recording electrodes aligned perpendicular to the wave path divided by the interelectrode conduction time. During mechanical loading, the distance between recording sites and the number of myocytes per unit physical length can change. In the stretched state, conduction velocity may be defined as the number of cells traversed per unit time, or as the *unstretched* tissue length divided by the *stretched* segment conduction time (Table 14–1). When intercellular coupling sufficiently decreases, conduction time and, hence, velocity become more dependent on the number of intercellular connections between the recording sites. In the extreme of discontinuous propagation, if strain had no other effect, then cellular conduction velocity would not change with stretch, and the material and spatial measures would increase, because fewer speed-limiting intercellular resistances would be encountered per unit length.

In contrast, normal continuous conduction depends on the distribution of heterogeneous properties such as membrane capacitance and resistance.[5] Consequently, if stretch had no other effect, material and spatial conduction velocity would not change, and cellular velocity would decrease as conduction path length increased. Furthermore, conduction speed is dependent on the specific distribution within the

material segment measured[13]; thus, *material* conduction velocity describes MEF effects over a constant segment of tissue. However, to make appropriate comparisons of conduction velocity before and during stretch, the material definition requires that the conduction path remains the same, which may not be accurate for conduction and stretch in more than one dimension. Consequently, in studies of two- or three-dimensional conduction, a highly resolved *spatial* description is most appropriate, because this description includes both differences in conduction speed caused by changes in tissue properties and differences in conduction direction caused by changes in wave path (Fig. 14–1). In practice, to determine the two-dimensional conduction direction, the conduction time is sampled from an array of positions, from which isochrones of conduction time are generated, indicating the position of the activation wave front. Conduction velocity is calculated as the distance traveled normal to the isochrones per unit time.

Effects of Stretch on Conduction Velocity in the Heart

Early investigations into the effects of myocardial stretch on conduction speed were limited to one-dimensional propagation. In studies of ventricular and atrial strips of myocardium from various species,

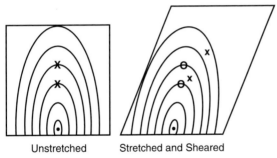

Unstretched   Stretched and Sheared

■ **Figure 14–1** Schematic of isochrones of activation caused by pacing at *solid circle*. X indicates the initial position of recording electrodes, and x indicates the electrode positions if the electrodes move with stretch, resulting in a material description of conduction velocity; but, this is only correct if the measurement remains normal to the isochrones. However, conduction velocity calculated from any position and normal to the isochrones, as from o, is an exact but spatial measure.

stretching from slack length to the length of maximal developed tension caused a proportionate increase in spatial conduction velocity, whereas material conduction velocity remained nearly unchanged, but additional stretch caused slowing of both measures.[13] Faster spatial conduction during stretch was also observed in sheep Purkinje fibers.[17,18] In canine Purkinje fibers, both spatial and material conduction velocity initially increased with stretch and then decreased; but conduction in cat trabeculae was not similarly affected.[19] Conversely, spatial conduction velocity in rat papillary muscle decreased with stretch, whereas papillary muscle from several other species showed no effect.[20] Despite the varied effects of stretch across different structures, tissue types, and species, most of these studies imply that conduction velocity may increase with stretch. However, these studies mostly concentrated on specialized structures, and after being excised, these tissues were not subject to the same multiaxial constraints as in vivo.

Other studies have focused on the effect of physiologic loading on whole-chamber activation times. In the dog heart in vivo, QRS duration correlated with acute increases in left ventricular pressure,[21] whereas left atrial dilation increased atrial activation time,[22] and ventricular volume inflation in isolated rabbit hearts increased maximal activation times.[23] In con-

trast, one study of volume load in canine ventricle in vivo reported no change in spatial conduction time,[24] whereas cellular conduction velocity increased during volume load of rat atrium.[25] These wholechamber studies indicate that stretch slows material conduction; however, possible changes in conduction path were not accounted for.

To directly study the path of propagation, more recent studies have investigated the effects of stretch on two-dimensional epicardial surface conduction. In volume-loaded left ventricle of isolated rabbit hearts after ventricular cryoablation of all but a thin epicardial layer, unloaded conduction velocities were estimated to be 76 and 26 cm/sec in the fiber and cross-fiber directions, respectively.[26] Neither graded volume load nor decrements in pacing cycle length significantly altered these values. The authors acknowledged that the cryoablation procedure stiffened the ventricle, possibly protecting the viable layer from the mechanical stimulus. Conversely, in right atrium of isolated rabbit hearts, balloon inflation caused an approximate 40% stretch in a nearly isotropic manner and caused spatial conduction velocity to decrease from 73 cm/sec to 55 cm/sec at a cycle length of 250 msec.[27] In a similar study, an atrial filling pressure of 10.3 mm Hg caused spatial conduction velocity to decrease by 3% from the control value of 65 cm/sec at a cycle length of 240 msec.[28] Atrial dilation caused a greater decrease in conduction velocity at shorter cycle lengths, increased the incidence of local functional conduction block (defined as conduction velocity <10 cm/sec), increased conduction velocity dispersion, and altered the direction of propagation. Conduction velocity returned to normal after the pressure was removed.

Electrodes require physical contact with the myocardium, possibly causing a local mechanical artifact. Sung and colleagues[29] used noncontact optical mapping during left ventricular volume loading in isolated rabbit heart, and they used a model-based analysis technique[30] that accounted for epicardial curvature and changes in conduction path, allowing comparison of conduction velocity with local fiber direction. Intraventricular pressure was increased to 30 mm Hg, which resulted in mean epicardial fiber strains on the order of 3% and mean cross-fiber strains near 1.5%; however, the distribution of these strains was regionally heterogeneous.[29] Figure 14–2 shows an example of the

A

Unloaded Loaded

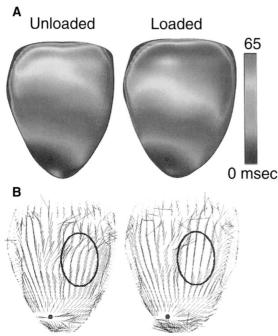

65

0 msec

B

■ **Figure 14–2** Activation time fields *(A)* and conduction velocity vector fields *(B)* before and during application of 30 mm Hg ventricular volume load in isolated rabbit heart, using methods from Sung and colleagues.[29] The *small solid circle* indicates the approximate position of pacing. The ellipses outline a region in which the apparent direction of conduction has been changed by application of load. (See color insert.)

increase in activation times caused by ventricular volume loading and the resulting velocity vector field. It also illustrates that application of stretch can alter the path of conduction. Spatial conduction velocity transverse to the fiber direction decreased on average by 16%, although spatial conduction velocity in the unloaded state near the pacing site (principally composed of epicardial conduction) was 20 cm/sec, whereas distal to the pacing site (includes the more rapidly conducting endocardium) was of the order of 60 cm/sec. Conduction velocity returned to baseline when load was removed.

These whole-chamber studies that also include changes in conduction path consistently show conduction slowing caused by stretch. The percentage slowing of spatial conduction because of stretch was not pro-portional between atrial studies in which 40% strain caused 25% slowing,[27] whereas more than 23% strain caused 3% slowing[28] at nearly the same cycle length. This may indicate that conduction slowing is stress dependent in atrial tissue, as the passive stress–strain relation of biological tissues is also nonlinear.[16] Similarly, 1.5% epicardial cross-fiber strain at 30 mm Hg caused 16% spatial conduction slowing in ventricle,[29] whereas greater than 23% strain at 9 mm Hg caused 3% spatial slowing in atrium,[28] which also implies that conduction slowing may correlate better with stress than strain.

Potential Interactions of Stretch with Factors that Influence Conduction Velocity

The effect of applied stretch on conduction velocity may be because of simple geometric or structural changes. Penefsky and Hoffman[13] postulate that increased one-dimensional spatial conduction velocity was the result of increased fiber alignment, and Deck[17] reasons that stretch may reduce specific membrane capacitance (capacitance/area), although recent data suggest an increase of capacitance with stretch.[31] Similarly, Dominguez and Fozzard[18] suggest that stretch causes membrane unfolding (as recently confirmed[32]), decreasing membrane area per unit length without altering total membrane area, which causes an apparent decrease in specific membrane capacitance. With a constant cell volume, fiber stretch will decrease cell cross-sectional area, also decreasing apparent specific membrane capacitance without changes in local membrane physical properties. However, this decrease in cell cross-sectional area would also increase longitudinal cytoplasmic resistance, thus *slowing* conduction. In canine Purkinje fibers, Rosen and colleagues[19] observe that stretch caused significant membrane unfolding and slightly increased packing of the extracellular space. These microstructural changes were accompanied by a biphasic increase then decrease in both spatial and material conduction velocity.

Stretch also has been reported to depolarize the resting membrane potential[33] and this may be sufficient to slow conduction through fast sodium channel inactivation. Cation nonselective SAC have been reported with reversal potentials ranging from −70 to 30 mV (see Chapter 1), and the resulting inward current depolarizes the resting membrane. Several of the effects of MEF in the whole heart have been seen to be blocked by nonspecific inhibitors of SAC, including gadolinium inhibition of increased cellular conduction velocity during stretch in rat atria[25]; however, Sung and colleagues[29] observed that streptomycin did not affect the slowing of spatial conduction velocity during ventricular filling. Sustained stretch may also increase (depolarize) resting membrane potential through altered cellular calcium handling.[34] Myofilament binding sensitivity to calcium increases with stretch, and prolonged stretch results in a slow increase in the calcium transient, which subsequently interacts with other currents. (Load-dependent calcium handling is covered in more detail in Chapter 6.) However, increased resting potential should lower pacing threshold, but ventricular filling has been reported to have no effect on[23,35] or to increase threshold.[26] SAC, altered calcium handling, or stretch-sensitive cellular signaling could also regulate the conductances associated with phase 0 of the action potential, thus decreasing the maximum rate of increase of membrane potential.[6]

Spear and Moore[20] suggest that stretch may increase intercellular resistance and slow conduction, and a heterogeneous or anisotropic reduction of coupling could also lead to changes in conduction path. Gap junction permeability is regulated by several rapid factors, and it has been observed to decrease within a few seconds after increases in intracellular sodium, magnesium, or especially calcium concentration.[9] Stretch may inhibit junctional conductance by increasing intracellular cation concentration through activation of SAC or altered calcium handling. Gap junctions are also subject to slower cell signaling, specifically through phosphorylation by protein kinases A and C, which have been observed to increase and decrease junctional permeability.[9] Stretch activation of these pathways could result in a decrease of intercellular conductance within 1 to 3 minutes.

Stretch may also reduce intercellular coupling by an independent mechanism. Although observed on myocyte lateral surfaces, cardiac gap junctions are primarily located in the intercalated disks along with the fascia adherens, which link the disk to the actin cytoskeleton, and desmosomes, which link to intermediate filaments.[36] Thus, most gap junctions co-localize with regions of maximum force transmission between cells and may be modulated by these stresses. Moreover, junctional complexes tend to be located transverse to the fascia adherens. Consequently, longitudinal intercellular force transmission could subject gap junctions to a high degree of shear stress, and these stresses may effectively reduce electrical coupling between cells.

Summary

Conduction speed is functionally dependent on the distribution of heterogeneous properties including membrane excitability and cellular coupling, as well as activation wave front curvature, whereas conduction path is functionally dependent on regionally heterogeneous cellular and myocardial architectures. Evidence suggests that stretch affects conduction speed in various cardiac tissue types, and that the magnitude of conduction slowing in atrial and ventricular tissue is too great to be explained by physical changes in path length alone. Conduction slowing may be caused by simple geometric and structural changes, although most of these expected changes would tend to increase conduction velocity. Conduction could also be slowed because of decreased excitability through SAC activation or length-dependent calcium handling, and may be slowed in part by increased intercellular resistance.

EFFECT OF MYOCARDIAL STRETCH ON EFFECTIVE REFRACTORY PERIOD

Determinants and Measurement of Effective Refractory Period

Effective refractory period (ERP) is the time interval after activation during which tissue is unable to activate again in response to the same stimulus; thus, it is a measure of late-repolarization membrane excitability. ERP is determined by the voltage-regulated transition of fast sodium channels from the inactivated to the resting state; thus, it is dependent on the time course of repolarization. Consequently, ERP is closely related to action potential duration (APD) and is also cycle-length dependent. One study observed that the ratio of ERP to monophasic APD at 90% repolarizaton (APD_{90}) remains nearly constant despite a 60% decrease in APD as cycle length decreases.[35] ERP is typically measured after continuous pacing at a single cycle length to minimize dynamic variations in APD and other cellular kinetics. After this stabilization period, a stimulus is delivered at a shortened time delay (coupling interval). ERP is typically defined as the longest possible coupling interval that does not elicit a propagating action potential.

Effects of Stretch on Effective Refractory Period in Whole Heart

In vivo studies of atrial MEF on ERP have varied in their mechanical loading protocols. Ravelli[4] recently reviewed the effect of stretch on ERP in atrial myocardium and attributed most variations to differences in timing and duration of stretch, as seen in model studies[37]; but some differences were attributed to homeostatic regulation in vivo or possible species differences. Despite these variations, studies have consistently shown that acute atrial stretch increases the dispersion of ERP.

Canine studies show that ERP increases when stretching isolated canine right atrium[38] or canine left ventricle in vivo through volume load.[24] These observations are consistent with most older canine studies, although ERP shortening has been observed during volume inflation of canine atrium.[22] However, in rabbit atria, increasing pressure consistently and reversibly *shortens* ERP, suggesting a possible species specificity. At a drive cycle length of 250 msec, ERP has been shown to shorten from approximately 80 to 50 msec after an increase of approximately 15 cm H_2O of atrial pressure or an increase in atrial length of 40%.[27,39–41]

Studies on the effects of stretch on left *ventricular* ERP have been more consistent across different species and experimental methods. In swine heart in vivo, an increase in afterload caused a greater decrease in ERP at the apex than at the base, thus increasing dispersion of refractoriness.[42] Similarly, in studies of isolated rabbit heart, left ventricular volume loading[23] or increased

preload[43] also decreased ERP. Increased preload decreased ERP in a manner that correlated better with increased diastolic wall stress, as estimated from end-diastolic pressure and ventricular geometry, than with increased systolic wall stress or diastolic circumference. Dilation also shortened ERP more significantly on the endocardial than epicardial surface.[35] This indicates that ERP may correlate better with cross-fiber than fiber stress or strain, because myocardial residual stress and torsion during filling allow a more uniform transmural distribution of fiber strain[16] under load at the expense of cross-fiber strain gradients.

In rabbit, ventricular stretch caused by increasing preload also caused greater shortening of ERP as the drive cycle length decreased.[26] This finding was later corroborated in isovolumically contracting rabbit ventricles.[35] Reiter and colleagues[26] suggest that this rate dependency may follow dependency on the stretch-sensitive delayed rectifier potassium current.

Those studies that also examined the effect of stretch on APD observed that MEF effects on late APD (typically APD_{90}) reflected the observed effects on ERP, either increasing[24] or decreasing[23,35,39,42] with stretch in atria and ventricles, and did not alter the ratio of ERP to late APD.[35] Several other studies have reported a decrease in late APD with stretch in various species including lamb, swine, guinea pig, rabbit, and human. However, some investigators report an *increase* in late APD during stretch in canine and other species consistent with a cation nonselective SAC, and, presumably, ERP would reflect this increase. Nilius and Boldt[44] observed a lengthening of APD_{90} with stretch in rabbit atrial trabeculae that they attributed to a decreased potassium current near resting potential. Volume loading of the left atrium in guinea pig variably affected both APD_{50} and APD_{90}, with about one-fourth of observed APD increasing during stretch.[45] In contrast, axial stretch of isolated guinea pig ventricular myocytes caused a consistent prolongation of APD_{20}, APD_{50}, and APD_{90}. Similarly, volume loading of isolated rabbit ventricle caused an increase in APD_{20} and APD_{80}.[29] These studies indicate that in some noncanine preparations, ERP may *increase* with stretch. Finally, several studies by Franz[33] also observe late APD lengthening in canine and rabbit, but see *shortening* at earlier levels of recovery. Franz suggests that depending on the stimulus strength used, MEF effects on ERP may simply reflect changes in APD at varying levels; thus, ERP could shorten during stretch reflecting shortening of early APD or lengthen with late APD. (The effect of stretch on APD is covered in more detail in Chapter 21).

Potential Interactions of Stretch with Factors that Influence Effective Refractory Period

SAC and altered calcium handling have been implicated in stretch-induced APD shortening,[4] and consequently could influence ERP. Model studies indicate that the effect of stretch can have various influences on action potential shape depending on the relative contributions of SAC and calcium handling, both of which are sensitive to timing and intensity of stretch.[37,46] Zabel and colleagues[46] have shown that including a length-dependent nonspecific cationic conductance with a reversal potential near −30 mV could reproduce several experimental observations including early APD shortening and late APD lengthening during stretch, whereas Kohl and colleagues[37] have shown that a more moderate stretch can lead to an overall shortening of APD. Kohl has further shown that stretch in a model that included sarcomere length–dependent calcium handling would produce an overall prolongation of APD if applied early or sustained throughout the action potential, but an overall shortening if applied during late repolarization.

Investigations into the mechanisms of stretch-induced ERP shortening by pharmacologic interventions have yielded inconsistent results. Streptomycin, a blocker of cationic SAC, inhibited acute stretch-induced shortening of rabbit ventricular ERP, but had no effect during sustained stretch.[35] In contrast, the more specific SAC blocker GsMTx-4 did not block stretch-induced shortening of rabbit atrial ERP, although this may have been because of resistance of the potassium-selective SAC to these compounds.[41] Zarse and colleagues[40] found that the L-type calcium channel blocker verapamil inhibited stretch-induced shortening of atrial ERP, suggesting the contribution of a length-dependent calcium handling mechanism[34]; but others have observed no effect of verapamil on rabbit ventricular ERP shortening.[35]

Increased dispersion of ERP with stretch may follow inhomogeneous stress or strain distributions. A ventricular model study that coupled physiologic fiber and cross-fiber strains to a stretch-dependent current within an action potential model predicted a near doubling of the dispersion of late APD.[47] Finally, a reduction in cellular coupling could lead to greater heterogeneity of repolarization as the electrical activity of individual cells becomes more independent.

Summary

Increased preload, afterload, or sustained load typically decreases ERP; however, ERP follows APD, and some have observed APD prolongation at all levels of recovery. How stretch effects ERP is likely a result of the balance of several competing effects including SAC that can be cation selective or K+ selective (see Chapter 2), altered calcium handling, and the timing and intensity of stretch, which could have varying levels of activation in different species and manners of stretch.

CONCLUSIONS

Recent evidence provides a basis to explain why stretch is associated with arrhythmias, particularly re-entrant forms. Both atrial and ventricular stretch slow spatial conduction, whereas atrial stretch increases conduction velocity dispersion and increases the occurrence of local functional conduction block, all of which promote re-entrant arrhythmias. These stretch effects may correlate with the application of diastolic mechanical load, but correlation with stress or strain is less clear because of regionally heterogeneous cardiac geometry, structure, and time-dependent material properties. Stretch may affect conduction velocity through reduced effective cellular coupling, cellular level geometric changes, or alterations in excitability, particularly an increase in resting membrane potential caused by the activity of SAC or altered calcium handling.

In general, atrial and ventricular stretch decrease ERP, but stretch consistently increases dispersion of ERP, both of which are associated with increased incidence of re-entrant arrhythmias. The effects of stretch on refractoriness parallel effects on APD, which may vary as a function of the relative activation of competing mechanisms, including SAC and altered calcium handling.

Acknowledgments

The authors acknowledge the research support of the National Science Foundation (BES-0086482), the National Institutes of Health (RR08605), the National Space Biomedical Research Institute (CA00216), and the American Heart Association (02651208Y).

References

1. Stevenson WG, Stevenson LW: Prevention of sudden death in heart failure. J Cardiovasc Electrophysiol 12:112–114, 2001.
2. Taggart P, Sutton PM: Cardiac mechano-electric feedback in man: Clinical relevance. Prog Biophys Mol Biol 71:139–154, 1999.
3. Kuo CS, Munakata K, Reddy CP, et al: Characteristics and possible mechanism of ventricular arrhythmia dependent on the dispersion of action potential durations. Circulation 67:1356–1367, 1983.
4. Ravelli F: Mechano-electric feedback and atrial fibrillation. Prog Biophys Mol Biol 82:137–149, 2003.
5. Kootsey JM: Electrical propagation in distributed cardiac tissue. In: Glass L, Hunter P, McCulloch AD (eds): Theory of Heart: Biomechanics, Biophysics, and Nonlinear Dynamics of Cardiac Function. New York, Springer-Verlag, 1991, pp 391–403.
6. Roden DM, Balser JR, George AL Jr, et al: Cardiac ion channels. Annu Rev Physiol 64:431–475, 2002.
7. Rohr S, Kucera JP, Kleber AG: Slow conduction in cardiac tissue. I: Effects of a reduction of excitability versus a reduction of electrical coupling on microconduction. Circ Res 83:781–794, 1998.
8. Nygren A, Giles WR: Mathematical simulation of slowing of cardiac conduction velocity by elevated extracellular [K+] in a human atrial strand. Ann Biomed Eng 28:951–957, 2000.
9. Dhein S: Cardiac Gap Junctions. New York, Karger, 1998.
10. Cabo C, Pertsov AM, Baxter WT, et al: Wave-front curvature as a cause of slow conduction and block in isolated cardiac muscle. Circ Res 75:1014–1028, 1994.
11. Zhuang J, Yamada KA, Saffitz JE, et al: Pulsatile stretch remodels cell-to-cell communication in cultured myocytes. Circ Res 87:316–322, 2000.
12. Hooks DA, Tomlinson KA, Marsden SG, et al: Cardiac microstructure: Implications for electrical propagation and defibrillation in the heart. Circ Res 91:331–338, 2002.
13. Penefsky ZJ, Hoffman BF: Effects of stretch on mechanical and electrical properties of cardiac muscle. Am J Physiol 204:433–438, 1963.
14. Ashikaga H, Criscione JC, Omens JH, et al: Transmural left ventricular mechanics underlying torsional recoil during relaxation. Am J Physiol Heart Circ Physiol 286:H640–H647, 2004.
15. Emery JL, Omens JH, McCulloch AD: Strain softening in rat left ventricular myocardium. J Biomech Eng 119:6–12, 1997.
16. McCulloch AD, Omens JH: Factors affecting the regional mechanics of the diastolic heart. In: Glass L, Hunter P, McCulloch AD (eds): Theory of Heart: Biomechanics, Biophysics, and Nonlinear Dynamics of Cardiac Function. New York, Springer-Verlag, 1991, pp 87–119.
17. Deck KA: [Changes in the resting potential and the cable properties of purkinje fibers during stretch]. Pflügers Arch Gesamte Physiol Menschen Tiere 280:131–140, 1964.
18. Dominguez G, Fozzard HA: Effect of stretch on conduction velocity and cable properties of cardiac Purkinje fibers. Am J Physiol 237:C119–C124, 1979.
19. Rosen MR, Legato MJ, Weiss RM: Developmental changes in impulse conduction in the canine heart. Am J Physiol 240:H546–H554, 1981.
20. Spear JF, Moore EN: Stretch-induced excitation and conduction disturbances in the isolated rat myocardium. J Electrocardiol 5:15–24, 1972.
21. Sideris DA, Toumanidis ST, Kostopoulos K, et al: Effect of acute ventricular pressure changes on QRS duration. J Electrocardiol 27:199–202, 1994.
22. Solti F, Vecsey T, Kekesi V, et al: The effect of atrial dilatation on the genesis of atrial arrhythmias. Cardiovasc Res 23:882–886, 1989.
23. Zabel M, Portnoy S, Franz MR: Effect of sustained load on dispersion of ventricular repolarization and conduction time in the isolated intact rabbit heart. J Cardiovasc Electrophysiol 7:9–16, 1996.
24. Zhu WX, Johnson SB, Brandt R, et al: Impact of volume loading and load reduction on ventricular refractoriness and conduction properties in canine congestive heart failure. J Am Coll Cardiol 30:825–833, 1997.
25. Tavi P, Laine M, Weckström M: Effect of gadolinium on stretch-induced changes in contraction and intracellularly recorded action- and afterpotentials of rat isolated atrium. Br J Pharmacol 118:407–413, 1996.
26. Reiter MJ, Landers M, Zetelaki Z, et al: Electrophysiological effects of acute dilatation in the isolated rabbit heart: Cycle length-dependent effects on ventricular refractoriness and conduction velocity. Circulation 96:4050–4056, 1997.
27. Chorro FJ, Egea S, Mainar L, et al: [Acute changes in wavelength of the process of auricular activation induced by stretching. Experimental study]. Rev Esp Cardiol 51:874–883, 1998.
28. Eijsbouts SC, Majidi M, van Zandvoort M, et al: Effects of acute atrial dilation on heterogeneity in conduction in the isolated rabbit heart. J Cardiovasc Electrophysiol 14:269–278, 2003.
29. Sung D, Mills RW, Schettler J, et al: Ventricular filling slows epicardial conduction and increases action potential duration in an optical mapping study of the isolated rabbit heart. J Cardiovasc Electrophysiol 14:739–749, 2003.
30. Sung D, Omens JH, McCulloch AD: Model-based analysis of optically mapped epicardial activation patterns and conduction velocity. Ann Biomed Eng 28:1085–1092, 2000.
31. Suchyna TM, Besch SR, Sachs F: Dynamic regulation of mechanosensitive channels: Capacitance used to monitor patch tension in real time. Phys Biol 1:1–18, 2004.
32. Kohl P, Cooper PJ, Holloway H: Effects of acute ventricular volume manipulation on in situ cardiomyocyte cell membrane configuration. Prog Biophys Mol Biol 82:221–227, 2003.
33. Franz MR: Mechano-electrical feedback in ventricular myocardium. Cardiovasc Res 32:15–24, 1996.
34. Calaghan SC, Belus A, White E: Do stretch-induced changes in intracellular calcium modify the electrical activity of cardiac muscle? Prog Biophys Mol Biol 82:81–95, 2003.

35. Eckardt L, Kirchhof P, Monnig G, et al: Modification of stretch-induced shortening of repolarization by streptomycin in the isolated rabbit heart. J Cardiovasc Pharmacol 36:711–721, 2000.

36. Gutstein DE, Liu FY, Meyers MB, et al: The organization of adherens junctions and desmosomes at the cardiac intercalated disc is independent of gap junctions. J Cell Sci 116:875–885, 2003.

37. Kohl P, Day K, Noble D: Cellular mechanisms of cardiac mechano-electric feedback in a mathematical model. Can J Cardiol 14:111–119, 1998.

38. Huang JL, Tai CT, Chen JT, et al: Effect of atrial dilatation on electrophysiologic properties and inducibility of atrial fibrillation. Basic Res Cardiol 98:16–24, 2003.

39. Ravelli F, Allessie M: Effects of atrial dilatation on refractory period and vulnerability to atrial fibrillation in the isolated Langendorff-perfused rabbit heart. Circulation 96:1686–1695, 1997.

40. Zarse M, Stellbrink C, Athanatou E, et al: Verapamil prevents stretch-induced shortening of atrial effective refractory period in Langendorff-perfused rabbit heart. J Cardiovasc Electrophysiol 12:85–92, 2001.

41. Bode F, Sachs F, Franz MR: Tarantula peptide inhibits atrial fibrillation. Nature 409:35–36, 2001.

42. Dean JW, Lab MJ: Regional changes in ventricular excitability during load manipulation of the in situ pig heart. J Physiol 429:387–400, 1990.

43. Halperin BD, Adler SW, Mann DE, et al: Mechanical correlates of contraction-excitation feedback during acute ventricular dilatation. Cardiovasc Res 27:1084–1087, 1993.

44. Nilius B, Boldt W: Stretching-induced changes in the action potential of the atrial myocardium. Acta Biol Med Ger 39:255–264, 1980.

45. Babuty D, Lab M: Heterogeneous changes of monophasic action potential induced by sustained stretch in atrium. J Cardiovasc Electrophysiol 12:323–329, 2001.

46. Zabel M, Koller BS, Sachs F, et al: Stretch-induced voltage changes in the isolated beating heart: Importance of the timing of stretch and implications for stretch-activated ion channels. Cardiovasc Res 32:120–130, 1996.

47. Vetter FJ, McCulloch AD: Mechanoelectric feedback in a model of the passively inflated left ventricle. Ann Biomed Eng 29:414–426, 2001.

CHAPTER 15

Ventricular Fibrillation Secondary to Nonpenetrating Chest Wall Impact (Commotio Cordis)

• • • •

Mark S. Link, Barry J. Maron, and N.A. Mark Estes III

Sudden death (or aborted sudden death) caused by nonpenetrating chest wall impact in the absence of injury to the ribs, sternum, and heart is known as commotio cordis. The Commotio Cordis Registry, in its 7-year existence, has documented more than 150 cases[1-3] and is accruing 5 to 20 new cases per year. We have developed an experimental model of commotio cordis in which anesthetized juvenile swine, struck in the chest by a baseball, develop ventricular fibrillation (VF). This model has allowed us to assess certain parameters critical to the generation of VF. Important variables include timing of impact in which only blows occurring during a narrow window of repolarization cause VF. Velocity of the impact object was also found to be critical, with baseballs moving 17.8 m/sec more likely to cause VF than velocities greater or less than 17.8 m/sec. In addition, more rigid impact objects and blows directly over the center of the chest were more likely to cause VF. Peak left ventricular pressure generated by the chest wall blow correlated with the risk for VF and best fit a Gaussian curve. Activation of the K_{ATP} channel is likely to play a role. Successful resuscitation is attainable with early defibrillation. This review focuses on the relevance of this animal model to the mechanism of those commotio cordis events occurring in the community, whereas the clinical features of commotio cordis are discussed in Chapter 29.

PREVIOUS EXPERIMENTAL MODELS

Early experimental efforts assessed relatively severe chest wall trauma, such as that typically seen with victims of motor vehicle accidents, falls from heights, and bomb blasts.[4,5] In these models, morphologic cardiac damage was typically produced. Riedinger and Kümmell[5] distinguished between "contusion" in which structural cardiac damage was present and "commotion" when the heart remained intact, although they commented on observing only two cases of true commotion. In 1934, Schlomka[6] reported his extensive experiments involving hammer strikes to the chest of various animals. In his experiments, frequent electrocardiographic (ECG) changes (generally ST-segment abnormalities) were reported, and VF was occasionally seen. Blows at the area of the heart were more likely to cause ECG abnormalities. The force of the blow was quantified only subjectively; the stronger the blow, the more likely ECG abnormalities would be produced. Most blows were of sufficient strength to cause readily evident cardiac damage. Cardiac dilation was noted in 99% of the cases (as stated in reference 7), and nearly 60% of animals observed for more than 80 days had permanent cardiac damage. Severing or blocking the vagus nerve had no effect on the ECG or survival. As a result of these experiments, Schlomka[6] distinguished between commotio cordis, which he thought was caused by coronary artery spasm, and contusio cordis, which was caused by cardiac trauma. Similarly, Bright and Beck,[8] in their experiments with direct blows in an open chest canine model, produced ECG change in all animals, including ST-segment abnormalities and VF in 2 of 25 animals. All dogs had histologic evidence of myocardial hemorrhage, and the ECG changes could be reproduced with blood injected into the myocardium. Thus, they ascribed the cardiac electrical abnormalities to myocardial contusion rather than coronary spasm.

More sophisticated experiments with grading of force began in the mid-1960s. In Louhimo's[7] series of 100 rabbits, weights were dropped equivalent to one third, one fourth, one sixth, and one eighth of the animal weight. All of the rabbits exposed to the impact of one-third their weight died, whereas the group subjected to the impact of only one-eighth their weight survived. In the animals that died, 43 of 47 had immediate ventricular tachycardia, but this did not degenerate into VF in any animal. The only instance of VF was observed in an animal with respiratory arrest. In those rabbits with ventricular tachycardia, a structural explanation for death was identified in each. Transient ventricular asystole was seen in nine animals, but was not the cause of death. On autopsy, all 51 animals that died had injuries, including 48 with sternal fractures, 19 with ruptured aorta, and 23 with cardiac rupture or contusion.

More recently, Liedtke and colleagues[9] and Cooper and colleagues,[10] using quantifiable and reproducible high energy, caused ventricular arrhythmias. In Liedtke's experimental model, a 650-joule (J) impact (equivalent to 101.4 m/sec baseball) produced nearly universal ventricular tachycardia and heart block in half of the animals. In Cooper's experimental model of impact with energies of 88 to 363 J (mean 188 J), arrhythmias from asystole to heart block, supraventricular tachycardia, and VF were produced by impact. However, similar to prior experiments, severe cardiac damage, including myocardial contusion and myocardial rupture, was found in most animals, and thus these experiments were actually models of cardiac contusion. In the early 1990s, Viano and colleagues[11] propelled baseballs 42.5 m/sec to the chest wall of swine and produced bradyarrhythmias and ventricular tachyarrhythmias; however, nearly all animals suffered severe cardiac contusions.

TUFTS EXPERIMENTAL MODEL OF COMMOTIO CORDIS

Because the focus of the previous chest wall trauma experiments was directed toward myocardial contusion, we developed an experimental model in swine that attempted to replicate the clinical scenario of commotio cordis, in which sudden cardiac death occurs in the absence of myocardial damage. In this model, a spherical object the size and weight of a baseball was propelled in free flight at velocities relevant to youth baseball to strike the chest wall of anesthetized juvenile swine directly over the anatomic position of the left ventricle (Fig. 15–1).[13]

Importance of the Timing of Impact

The release and subsequent impact could be timed relative to the cardiac cycle. The electrophysiologic outcomes of chest wall blows were dependent on the precise time in the cardiac cycle during which the impact occurred (Table 15–1). In these studies, impacts during the vulnerable portion of the T wave (10–30 msec before the T peak) triggered VF instantaneously and reproducibly (Fig. 15–2).[13,14] In 13.3 m/sec impacts during this vulnerable period, approximately 30% resulted in VF, whereas another 10% caused nonsustained polymorphic ventricular tachycardia. Chest blows near this vulnerable zone produced VF in 16% when timed −40 to −31 msec and 3% timed −9 to 0 msec before the T-wave peak. Blows during other portions of the cardiac cycle did not produce VF. Notably, monomorphic ventricular tachycardia was not observed. ST-segment elevations and transient complete heart block were frequently seen. Heart block was never permanent and usually lasted less than five beats.

Morphologic Changes

Immediately after impact, segmental and transient wall motion abnormalities were observed in the apex, a region distant from the area of precordial impact.[13] Immediate (within 60 sec) coronary angiography did not reveal any epicardial coronary artery abnormalities.[13] Myocardial bruises were rarely seen with impacts of less than 22 m/sec, but increased with greater velocity impacts to nearly 100% with impacts at 31.1 m/sec or greater.[13,16] Similarly, structural cardiac abnormalities that could trigger arrhythmias or death were not observed with impacts of 22 m/sec.

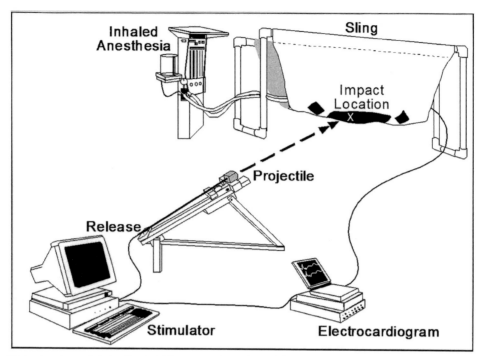

■ **Figure 15–1** Experimental design for the Tufts commotio cordis model. A swine was positioned prone in a sling and impacted with a baseball directed toward the center of the left ventricle over a distance of 1 m at 13.3 m/sec. The impact was gated to the cardiac cycle with an electrophysiologic stimulator triggering from a surface electrocardiographic input. Velocity of the baseball was measured by a chronograph (Oehler Research, Austin, TX) modified for low velocity.[12] *(From Link MS, Wang PJ, VanderBrink BA, et al: Selective activation of the K^+_{ATP} channel is a mechanism by which sudden death is produced by low-energy chest-wall impact [commotio cordis]. Circulation 100:413–418, 1999, with permission from the American Heart Association.)*

TABLE 15–1   Incidence of Ventricular Fibrillation and Nonsustained Polymorphic Ventricular Tachycardia (Excluding Impacts Resulting in Ventricular Fibrillation) with 13.3 and 17.8 m/sec[1] Impacts

	QRS	ST	−40 to −31 msec to T peak	−30 to −21 msec to T peak	−20 to −10 msec to T peak	−9 to −1 msec to T peak	T Down-Slope
VF							
Total impacts, n	58	93	74	516	384	31	47
VF induced	0	0	12	148	113	1	0
%	**0%**	**0%**	**16%**	**29%**	**29%**	**3%**	**0%**
NSPMVT							
Total impacts, n	58	93	62	368	271	30	47
NSPMVT induced	1	1	4	39	28	0	0
%	**2%**	**1%**	**6%**	**11%**	**10%**	**0%**	**0%**

Grouped according to the timing of impact in the experimental swine model.
NSPMVT, nonsustained polymorphic ventricular tachycardia; VF, ventricular fibrillation.
Reproduced from Link MS: Mechanically induced sudden death in chest wall impact. Prog Biophys Mol Biol 82:175–186, 2003, with permission.

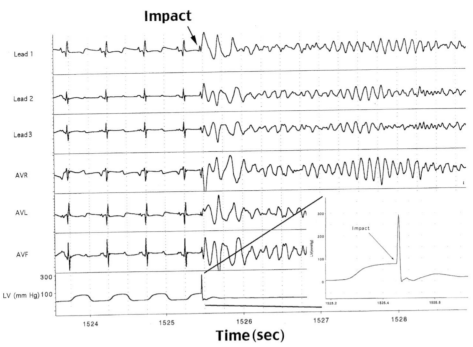

■ **Figure 15–2** Six-lead electrocardiogram from an 11-kg swine undergoing chest wall impact from an object the shape and weight of a standard baseball traveling 13.3 m/sec. After chest impact within the vulnerable zone of repolarization (10–30 msec before the T peak), ventricular fibrillation occurs instantaneously.[15] LV, left ventricular pressure. *(From Link MS, Maron BJ, VanderBrink BA, et al: Impact directly over the cardiac silhouette is necessary to produce ventricular fibrillation in an experimental model of commotio cordis. J Am Coll Cardiol 37:649–654, 2001, with permission from Journal of the American College of Cardiology.)*

Hardness of Impact Object

To assess whether the hardness of impact objects played a role in commotio cordis, we used three grades of safety baseballs, which varied in firmness from very soft to hardness just less than that of a regulation baseball. Firmer objects were more likely to cause VF, and firmness correlated linearly with the risk for VF (Fig. 15–3).[13] Impact object hardness correlated with the induction of VF not only at 13.3 m/sec, but also at 17.8 m/sec, a velocity most relevant to that causing commotio cordis in youth baseball.[17]

Location of Impact

To assess whether the location of the impact on the chest played a role in commotio cordis, we devised an

experiment in which blows were delivered to five sites on the left chest wall (including three directly over the heart) and two sites on the right chest wall. VF was only produced with impacts directly over the cardiac silhouette and was most commonly observed with impacts directly over the center of the cardiac silhouette (30%), compared with those over the base of left ventricle (13%) or over the apex (4%).[15]

Speed of Impact

In further experiments, we impacted the chest wall at a variety of velocities—that is, at 8.9, 11.1, 13.3, 17.8, 22.2, 26.9, and 31.1 m/sec. As expected, lower velocity impacts were less likely to cause VF; blows at 8.9 m/sec did not cause VF.[16] As impact velocity increased, the risk for VF increased, to nearly 70% at

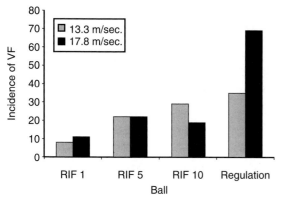

■ **Figure 15–3** Incidence of ventricular fibrillation (VF) with chest wall impacts at 13.3 *(gray bars)* and 17.8 m/sec *(black bars)* with a regulation baseball compared with softer-than-standard (safety) baseballs of three different grades of hardness.[17] Balls are arranged from softest, Reduced Impact Factor 1 (RIF 1), to hardest (regulation). Note that as the hardness of the impact object increases, the incidence of VF increases. *(From Link Link MS, Maron BJ, Wang PJ, et al: Reduced risk of sudden death from chest wall blows [commotio cordis] with safety baseballs. Pediatrics 109:873–877, 2002, with permission.)*

17.8 m/sec. Unexpectedly, at impact velocities greater than or equal to 22.2 m/sec, the likelihood of VF decreased, and cardiac structural damage occurred more commonly, including left ventricular rupture and papillary muscle tears. The mechanism for decreased vulnerability for commotio cordis at particularly high-impact velocities is unresolved, but may relate to the critical mass of myocardial tissue needed to sustain reentrant arrhythmias or possibly to critical left ventricular pressure changes produced by the blow to the chest wall.

CELLULAR MECHANISMS OF COMMOTIO CORDIS

Human and experimental data indicate that VF initiated by a chest wall blow appears to cause sudden cardiac death in commotio cordis. VF can be a primary electrical event or can be secondary to heart block, myocardial ischemia, or hemorrhage. Because human victims collapse virtually immediately after impact, and the VF produced in our animal model is also

instantaneous, we believe that commotio cordis is a primary electrical event rather than secondary to other nonelectrical factors. Other primary electrical causes of VF include the Brugada and Long QT syndromes. In these diseases, the cardiac muscle is grossly normal, but abnormal ion channels (including principally those involved in cardiac repolarization) account for electrical instability.

We propose that commotio cordis is a mechanically induced ionic channel dysfunction affecting the channels involved with repolarization.[18] In addition to an induced channel dysfunction, we suspect that the initiation of VF also requires a premature ventricular depolarization as a trigger. There is a correlate to this hypothesis in the R on T phenomenon, in which premature ventricular depolarizations that occur on the vulnerable portion of the T wave produce VF. However, R on T producing VF is present primarily in ischemic myocardial conditions.[19,20] In the setting of an acute myocardial infarction or coronary ischemia, an appropriately timed premature depolarization can trigger VF. However, in nonischemic situations (such as continuous, unsynchronized ventricular pacing), premature depolarizations during the vulnerable portion of the T wave do not generally cause VF. Greater energy T-wave shocks (1–10 J), however, do cause VF; it is thought that these global electrical stimuli may also cause channel and membrane dysfunction.[21–23]

In our hypothesis, both the channel dysfunction and the premature ventricular depolarization are produced by the blow to the chest wall. When the trigger occurs during an appropriate time window in an (induced) abnormal repolarization, VF is induced. However, initiation of a single beat by chest wall impact (such as in those cases of asynchronous pacing) is not sufficient to cause a re-entrant arrhythmia. This is shown in our experiments of impact velocity. Of 287 impacts that did not cause VF, premature ventricular depolarizations were observed in 199 (69%), including 36 of 80 (45%) at 8.8 m/sec, 63 of 86 (73%) at 11.1 m/sec, 51 of 68 (75%) at 13.3 m/sec 16 of 17 (94%) at 17.8 m/sec, and all impacts greater than or equal to 22.2 m/sec.[18] Yet, despite the premature ventricular depolarization, VF did not occur, perhaps because repolarization was incompletely altered by the blow to the chest wall.

Because of the electrical similarities between commotio cordis and myocardial ischemia, including ST-segment elevation and R on T causing VF, we hypothesized that specific ion channel activation may play a role in this phenomenon.

A likely candidate is the K_{ATP} channel, given that it is primarily responsible for the ST-segment elevation and is known to contribute to the risk for VF in the presence of myocardial ischemia.[24,25] Indeed, in our experimental model, we found that glibenclamide, a blocker of the K_{ATP} channel, reduced the magnitude of ST-segment elevation with QRS strikes and the incidence of VF after strikes at the upstroke of the T wave (Fig. 15–4),[12] suggesting that activation of this channel by chest wall impact is critical in the initiation and maintenance of VF in commotio cordis.

However, despite the reduction in VF with K_{ATP} channel blockade, premature ventricular depolarizations caused by the chest wall blow were not elimi-

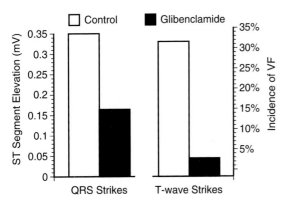

■ **Figure 15–4** Magnitude of ST-segment elevation and the incidence of VF induced by 13.3 m/sec chest wall impacts by a spherical object the size and weight of a regulation baseball in experimental model of commotio cordis. Significant differences between the control animals *(white bars)* and the animals administered glibenclamide (a blocker of the K_{ATP} channel; *black bars*) were observed with respect to the magnitude of ST-segment elevation with QRS strikes and the incidence of ventricular fibrillation with T-wave strikes.[12] *(From Link MS, Wang PJ, VanderBrink BA, et al: Selective activation of the K+ATP channel is a mechanism by which sudden death is produced by low-energy chest-wall impact [commotio cordis]. Circulation 100:413–418, 1999, with permission from the American Heart Association.)*

nated (85% of strikes in glibenclamide animals vs. 83% in control animals), again suggesting that a single ventricular depolarization is not sufficient to cause VF. We propose that glibenclamide prevented the chest blow from activating the K_{ATP} channel; thus, despite not blocking a premature ventricular depolarization, it prevented the induction of VF by preventing abnormalities in repolarization.

LEFT VENTRICULAR PRESSURE

In our experimental model, we also assessed the instantaneous left ventricular pressure increase produced by the chest blow to determine whether pressure increase mediates the electrophysiologic consequences of commotio cordis. In experiments designed to define the site of impact[15] and the velocity of impact,[16] left ventricular pressure increase created by the chest wall blow correlated with the risk for VF. In both of these studies, the peak probability of VF was seen with left ventricular pressures between 250 and 450 mm Hg (Figs. 15–5 and 15–6). Intracavitary pressures greater than 450 mm Hg and less than 250 mm Hg were less likely to be associated with development of VF. These observations suggest that it may be the rapid pressure increase immediately after the chest blow that causes VF. These rapid ventricular pressure increases could mediate channel activation through myocardial stretch, membrane deformation, or possibly by direct action on the ion channels themselves.

In addition to activation by ischemia, the K_{ATP} channel has been shown to be activated by myocardial stretch in a rat atrial model.[26]

We have shown that activation of the K_{ATP} channel is implicated in commotio cordis. Therefore, it is possible that in our model the K_{ATP} channel is activated by stretch. Other channels may be activated by myocardial stretch, and in this way underlie the genesis of ventricular arrhythmias after blows to the chest.[27–29]

Summary

Commotio cordis is an unusual, but devastating, event occurring in young people during sports-related or routine daily activities. Critical variables that

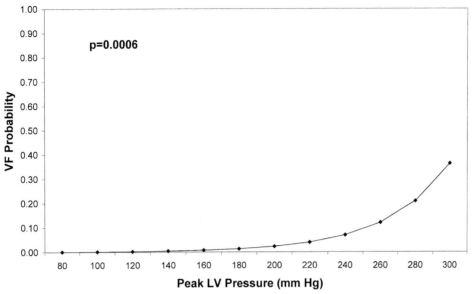

■ **Figure 15–5** Probability of VF relative to peak left ventricular (LV) pressure produced by a chest wall strike with a baseball moving 13.3 m/sec in experiment evaluating the site of impact.[16] As the peak LV pressure increases to 300 mm Hg, the probability of VF increases. *(From Link MS, Maron BJ, Wang PJ, et al: Upper and lower limits of vulnerability to sudden arrhythmic death with chest wall impact [commotio cordis]. J Am Coll Cardiol 41:99–104, 2003, with permission of Journal of the American College of Cardiology.)*

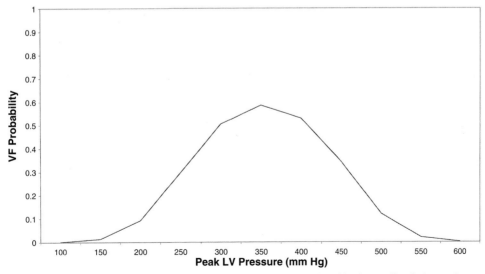

■ **Figure 15–6** Probability of VF relative to peak left ventricular (LV) pressure produced by chest wall strike in experiment evaluating the velocity of impact.[12] The probability of VF is greatest with peak LV pressures between 250 and 450 mm Hg. *(From Link MS, Wang PJ, VanderBrink BA, et al: Selective activation of the K+ATP channel is a mechanism by which sudden death is produced by low-energy chest-wall impact [commotio cordis]. Circulation 100:413–418, 1999, with permission from the American Heart Association.)*

determine the likelihood of VF occurring from a chest blow include the precise timing of the impact to a 10 to 30 msec window on the up-slope of the T wave, greater hardness of the impact object, precordial impact location of the blow, and the speed of the impact correlating to those velocities seen in youth baseball. The initiation of VF is related to the left ventricular pressure increase produced by the blow to the chest. Activation of specific cardiac ion channels, especially the K_{ATP} channel, likely occurs with this chest wall impact and produces VF and ST-segment elevation. The experimental animal model described herein simulates the human scenario of commotio cordis, offers specific insights into its mechanisms, and helps to explain why commotio cordis is a relatively rare event.

References

1. Maron BJ, Poliac LC, Kaplan JA, Mueller FO: Blunt impact to the chest leading to sudden death from cardiac arrest during sports activities. N Engl J Med 333:337–342, 1995.
2. Maron BJ, Link MS, Wang PJ, Estes III NAM: Clinical profile of commotio cordis: An under-appreciated cause of sudden death in the young during sports and other activities. J Cardiovasc Electrophysiol 10:114–120, 1999.
3. Maron BJ, Gohman TE, Kyle SB, et al: Clinical profile and spectrum of commotio cordis. JAMA 287:1142–1146, 2002.
4. Meola F: La commozione toracica. Gior Internaz Sci Med 1:923–937, 1879.
5. Riedinger F, Kümmell H: Die Verletzungen und Erkrankungen des Thorax und seines Inhaltes. In: von Bergman E, von Bruns P (eds): Handbuch der Praktischen Chirurgie, 2nd ed. Stuttgart, Ferd. Enke, 1903, pp 373–456.
6. Schlomka G: Commotio cordis und ihre Folgen. Die Einwirkung stumpfer Brustwandtraumen auf das Herz. Ergebn Inn Med Kinderheilk 47:1–91, 1934.
7. Louhimo I: Heart injury after blunt thoracic trauma. An experimental study on rabbits. Acta Chir Scand 380:7–60, 1967.
8. Bright EF, Beck CS: Nonpenetrating wounds of the heart. A clinical and experimental study. Am Heart J 10:293–321, 1935.
9. Liedtke AJ, Gault JH, Demuth WE: Electrocardiographic and hemodynamic changes following nonpenetrating chest trauma in the experimental animal. Am J Physiol 226:377–382, 1974.
10. Cooper GJ, Pearce BP, Stainer MC, Maynard RL: The biomechanical response of the thorax to nonpenetrating impact with particular reference to cardiac injuries. J Trauma 22:994–1008, 1982.
11. Viano DC, Andrzejak DV, Polley TZ, King AI: Mechanism of fatal chest injury by baseball impact: Development of an experimental model. Clin J Sports Med 2:166–171, 1992.
12. Link MS, Wang PJ, VanderBrink BA, et al: Selective activation of the K^{+}_{ATP} channel is a mechanism by which sudden death is produced by low-energy chest-wall impact (commotio cordis). Circulation 100:413–418, 1999.
13. Link MS, Wang PJ, Pandian NG, et al: An experimental model of sudden death due to low energy chest wall impact (commotio cordis). N Engl J Med 338:1805–1811, 1998.
14. Link MS, Wang PJ, VanderBrink BA, et al: Timing of chest impact is critical to the vulnerability to ventricular fibrillation and sudden death in an experimental model of commotio cordis [abstract]. Circulation 100:4612, 1999.
15. Link MS, Maron BJ, VanderBrink BA, et al: Impact directly over the cardiac silhouette is necessary to produce ventricular fibrillation in an experimental model of commotio cordis. J Am Coll Cardiol 37:649–654, 2001.
16. Link MS, Maron BJ, Wang PJ, et al: Upper and lower limits of vulnerability to sudden arrhythmic death with chest wall impact (commotio cordis). J Am Coll Cardiol 41:99–104, 2003.
17. Link MS, Maron BJ, Wang PJ, et al: Reduced risk of sudden death from chest wall blows (commotio cordis) with safety baseballs. Pediatrics 109:873–877, 2002.
18. Link MS: Mechanically induced sudden death in chest wall impact. Prog Biophys Mol Biol 82:175–186, 2003.
19. El-Sherif N, Myerburg RJ, Scherlag BJ, et al: Electrocardiographic antecedents of primary ventricular fibrillation. Br Heart J 38:415–422, 1976.
20. Naito M, Michelson EL, Kaplinsky E, et al: Role of early cycle ventricular extrasystoles in initiation of ventricular tachycardia and fibrillation: Evaluation of the R on T phenomenon during acute myocardial ischemia in a canine model. Am J Cardiol 49:317–322, 1982.
21. Wiggers CJ, Wegria R: Ventricular fibrillation due to single, localized induction and condenser shocks applied during the vulnerable phase of ventricular systole. Am J Physiol 128:500–505, 1940.
22. Hoffman BF, Gorin EF, Wax FS, et al: Vulnerability to fibrillation and the ventricular-excitability curve. Am J Physiol 167:88–94, 1951.
23. Hou CJ, Chang-Sing P, Flynn E, et al: Determination of ventricular vulnerable period and ventricular fibrillation threshold by use of T-wave shocks in patients undergoing implantation of cardioverter/defibrillators. Circulation 92:2558–2564, 1995.
24. Kubota I, Yamaki M, Shibata T, et al: Role of ATP-sensitive K^{+} channel on ECG ST segment elevation during a bout of myocardial ischemia. Circulation 88:1845–1851, 1993.
25. Kondo T, Kubota I, Tachibana H, et al: Glibenclamide attenuates peaked T wave in early phase of myocardial ischemia. Cardiovasc Res 31:683–687, 1996.
26. Van Wagoner DR: Mechanosensitive gating of atrial ATP-sensitive potassium channels. Circ Res 72:973–983, 1993.
27. Hu H, Sachs F: Stretch-activated ion channels in the heart. J Mol Cell Cardiol 29:1511–1523, 1997.
28. Niu W, Sachs F: Dynamic properties of stretch-activated K^{+} channels in adult rat atrial myocytes. Prog Biophys Mol Biol 82:121–135, 2003.
29. Kohl P, Nesbit AD, Cooper PJ, Lei M: Sudden cardiac death by commotio cordis: Role of mechano-electric feedback. Cardiovasc Res 50:280–289, 2001.

CHAPTER 16

Mechano-Electric Feedback in Atrial Fibrillation

• • • •

Michiel J. Janse

RELATION BETWEEN ELECTRICAL AND CONTRACTILE REMODELING IN ATRIAL FIBRILLATION

In 1982, Attuel and co-workers[1] described that in patients with paroxysmal atrial fibrillation, the atrial refractory period was short and no longer adapted to changes in heart rate. These findings were later confirmed by Le Heuzey and colleagues,[2] who note that in isolated atrial preparations from patients in sinus rhythm, the majority of action potentials showed a marked plateau, whereas in 97% of cells from specimens from patients with atrial fibrillation, the action potential had a triangular shape and a short duration. At that time it was thought that these changes might be causal for the development of atrial fibrillation. The landmark study of Wijffels and colleagues[3] indicates that these changes are the result, rather than the cause, of atrial fibrillation. In conscious goats, a device was implanted that could repeatedly induce atrial fibrillation by burst pacing. Initially, the arrhythmia lasted only a few seconds, but with repetitive reinitiation, the episodes of atrial fibrillation became longer until finally, after several weeks, chronic atrial fibrillation, lasting longer than 24 hours, ensued. The atrial refractory period shortened in the course of a few days by 60 msec, and the reference rate adaptation was abolished. Similar changes could be brought about by regular pacing at a rapid rate. Remarkably, when restoring sinus rate after 24 hours of rapid pacing, it took 24 hours before the atrial refractory period had returned to its original value.

Many other studies confirmed these findings.[4-7] In both dogs and humans, changes in ionic currents underlying the shortening of the atrial action potential, and thus the refractory period, were documented.[6,8] The densities of the transient outward current, I_{to}, and the L-type calcium current, $I_{Ca,L}$, were diminished, without a change in voltage- and time-dependent properties. Experiments using blockers and agonists of these currents indicated that the reduction in I_{to} had no significant effect on action potential duration, and that the major factor responsible for shortening the action potential is reduced $I_{Ca,L}$ current. Similar changes were found in human atria.[6]

It is known that after cardioversion for atrial fibrillation in patients, there is marked atrial contractile dysfunction, which, depending on the duration of atrial fibrillation, may take days to months to recover. Atrial contractile dysfunction can develop within minutes to hours of atrial fibrillation or rapid pacing.[9-11] Leistad and colleagues[11] suggest that mechanical dysfunction caused by short-lasting atrial fibrillation was because of cellular calcium overload. Nattel's group[9] was the first to measure intracellular calcium in isolated atrial myocytes subjected to rapid pacing. A 3-minute period of rapid pacing increased diastolic intracellular calcium concentration and increased the intracellular calcium transient and contractile shortening. On returning to a slow pacing rate, contractile shortening and calcium transients initially were increased, but then declined to about 60% of pretachycardia values and recovered over a period of 15 minutes. The post-tachycardia contractile dysfunction was attributed to calcium overload–induced reduced calcium release from the sarcoplasmic reticulum. Schotten and colleagues[10] measured atrial contractile function, as well as refractory periods, after 5 minutes, 3 hours, and 5 days of atrial fibrillation in goats. Even 5 minutes of atrial fibrillation significantly impaired atrial contractility; and after spontaneous cardioversion, it took 10 minutes for contractility to recover. Episodes of atrial fibrillation of longer duration were associated with more severe and longer lasting atrial dysfunction. The time courses of shortening of the refractory period and the loss of atrial contractility were identical. The calcium channel agonist BAY Y5959 increased atrial contractility to the same extent that it prolonged the refractory period. It was concluded that "electrical and contractile remodeling go hand in hand," and that both are caused by a reduction in $I_{Ca,L}$.[10] In atrial fibrillation of longer duration (months to years), electrical remodeling is completely reversible within a few days; however, contractile function takes much longer to recover. This indicates that in chronic atrial fibrillation, mechanisms other than the reduction in $I_{Ca,L}$ must play a role. Candidates are loss of atrial myocytes, altered energetics, and depressed release function of the ryanodine receptor[10] (see Chapter 17).

One consequence of reduced contractile function is that it may enhance atrial dilation, which could contribute to electrical remodeling. Electrical remodeling in the rapid atrial pacing model is different from that during atrial fibrillation induced by heart failure, caused by 5 weeks of rapid ventricular pacing.[12] In the latter, there is no change in atrial refractory period at slow rates, and there is a lengthening at rapid rates.[13] As in the rapid pacing model, $I_{Ca,L}$ was reduced, albeit to a lesser extent, but this was offset by a decrease in the delayed rectifier potassium current, I_K, and an increased inward current carried by the Na^+-Ca^{2+} exchanger.[13] In the heart failure model, the increase in atrial size is much larger than in the rapid pacing model, and it was suggested that the atrial dilation could promote atrial fibrillation by activating stretch-activated ion channels.[14] Atrial arrhythmias frequently occur when atrial size and pressure are increased. A distinction should be made between conditions in which atrial pressure is acutely increased, such as in acute myocardial infarction,[15] atrioventricular re-entrant tachycardia, and atrioventricular nodal tachycardia,[16] and those in which atrial enlargement and pressure develop slowly, such as in valvular disease, heart failure, or with age.[12,17,18] The following section focuses on the effects of acute stretch, whereas Chapter 17 concentrates on chronic stretch.

EFFECTS OF ACUTE ATRIAL STRETCH

Effects on the Refractory Period

Studies on the effects of acute atrial stretch on the atrial refractory period have produced different results. In humans and dogs, in which atrial pressure was increased by inflating a balloon catheter, by simultaneously stimulating atria and ventricles, or changing the atrioventricular interval, a shortening,[19–21] a lengthening,[16,22–25] or no change[26] has been reported. In the conscious goat, volume loading by a plasma expander did not alter the atrial effective refractory period.[27] The results of the in vivo studies have been summarized by Ravelli[28] (Table 16–1). As can be seen, moderate increases in atrial pressure caused a lengthening or no change of the refractory period, whereas greater increases in pressure shortened the refractory period. The time course of stretch also plays a role; in the studies of Calkins and colleagues, a transient increase in pressure shortened the refractory period,[19] whereas sustained stretch did not alter the refractory period.[26]

Acute stretch in isolated preparations produced more consistent results. In isolated, Langendorff-perfused hearts,[29–35] acute atrial dilation shortened the refractory period (Fig.16–1) and the duration of the monophasic action potential. Several explanations for these different results have been offered. Ravelli and Allessie[29] thought that compared with isolated hearts, less pronounced changes in atrial pressure can be produced in vivo, and that in intact animals, stretch-induced electrophysiologic changes could be partially counteracted by changes in neurohumoral changes. However, a later study from the same laboratory found no effect of atropine or propranolol on the shortening of the atrial refractory period by atrial fibrillation.[27] Satoh and Zipes[23] provided another explanation: "If the action potential of the stretched atrium shortened early in repolarization (e.g., 50% to 75% repolarization), but prolonged in the terminal portion (e.g., 90% to 100%), due to the development of a terminal 'foot,' then a relatively weak stimulus (i.e., twice diastolic threshold [which we have used]) might uncover prolonged effective refractory period, ERP), while a stimulus of higher intensity might find the ERP to be

TABLE 16–1 Summary of the Effects of Acute Stretch on Atrial Refractoriness in In Vivo Studies

Dilation Models	Species	ΔP (mm Hg)	Atrial RP	Dispersion	Atrial RP References
Simultaneous AV pacing	Dog	5	↑	----	Kaseda and Zipes (1988)[22]
	Human	3.5	↑	----	Klein et al. (1990)[16]
	Human	4	↑	↑	Chen et al. (1999)[25]
	Human	4	↔	----	Calkins et al. (1992)[26]
	Human	8 peak	↓	----	Calkins et al. (1992)[19]
	Human	7.4	↓	↑	Tse et al. (2001)[21]
SVT	Human	2.7	↑	----	Klein et al. (1990) [16]
	Human	4.5	↑	↑	Chen et al. (1998)[24]
Volume overload	Dog	≥4	↑	----	Sideris et al. (1994)[37]
	Dog	1.2	↑	↑	Satoh and Zipes (1996)[23]
	Goat	4.5	↔	----	Wijffels et al. (1997)[27]
Balloon inflation	Dog	8	↓	----	Solti et al. (1989)[20]

The parameter measured increased (↑), decreased (↓), or did not change (↔).
No data (----)
AV, atrio-ventricular; ΔP, average change in mean atrial pressure; RP, refractory period; SVT, supraventricular tachycardia.
From Ravelli F: Mechano-electric feedback and atrial fibrillation. Prog Biophys Mol Biol 82:137–149, 2003, with permission.

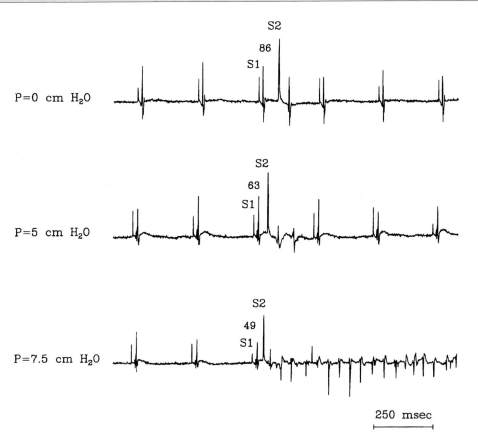

250 msec

■ **Figure 16–1** Earliest possible atrial premature beat at different atrial pressures. Unipolar electrogram was recorded from the right atrium of an isolated, Langendorff-perfused rabbit heart during regular pacing with an interval of 250 msec. At atrial pressure of 0 cm H_2O, the shortest S1-S2 interval that resulted in a premature atrial response was 86 msec. When atrial pressure was increased to 7.5 cm H_2O, a single premature stimulus with a coupling interval as short as 49 msec produced atrial fibrillation. P, intra-atrial pressure; S1, basic stimulus; S2, premature stimulus. *(From Ravelli F, Allessie MA: Effects of atrial dilatation on refractory period and vulnerability to atrial fibrillation in the isolated Langendorff-perfused rabbit heart. Circulation 96:1686–1695, 1997, with permission.)*

shortened." Indeed, in the isolated, Langendorff-perfused guinea pig heart, Nazir and Lab[31] found that stretch shortened the monophasic action potential at the 50% level of repolarization and prolonged it at the 90% level, because of the development of an early afterdepolarization. Such "crossover" effects have also been found in microelectrode studies.[32,36]

Finally, it is possible that, in vivo, atrial stretch, by volume loading for example, develops more gradually than in isolated hearts. As Nazir and Lab formulated: "atrial stretch velocity, not stretch itself, is a determinant of mechano-electric feedback."[33]

Both in studies in which stretch caused a shortening or a lengthening of the refractory period, stretch facilitated the induction of atrial fibrillation by premature stimulation[23–25,29,30,34,37]; and in only one study[26] was there no effect on inducibility. In a study in the isolated guinea pig heart, stretch caused spontaneous atrial premature beats, most likely caused by early afterdepolarizations,[31] although stretch has also been shown to induce delayed afterdepolarizations.[36] The induction of atrial fibrillation by premature electrical stimulation, or by spontaneous atrial premature beats, would be facilitated by the increased dispersion in refractoriness caused by stretch, as noted by Satoh and Zipes,[23] where the increase of the refractory period was far larger in the thin-walled portions of the atria than in the thick crista terminalis. In studies in which stretch shortened the refractory period, the resulting shortening of the wavelength of excitation favors re-entry.[38] Still, in the studies of Franz and Bode[30] and Bode and colleagues,[34] gadolinium, a blocker of stretch-activated channels, reduced the inducibility of atrial fibrillation during stretch, but it had no effect on the stretch-induced shortening of the refractory period. The authors suggest that gadolinium might have altered dispersion in refractoriness, but no evidence for this has been presented. Because gadolinium also blocks $I_{Ca,L}$ in ventricular myocytes,[39] Bode and colleagues[34] studied the effects of the calcium blocker verapamil on inducibility of atrial fibrillation during stretch, but no effect was found. A more specific blocker of stretch-activated channels, the Tarantula peptide GsMTx-4,[40] also suppressed atrial fibrillation in the rabbit model of acute dilation, without affecting the dilation-induced shortening of the refractory period.[41] It therefore seems that shortening of the refractory period does not fully explain the increased susceptibility to atrial fibrillation during stretch.

Effects on Conduction

Possibly, stretch also affects conduction. In ventricular muscle, stretch reduces conduction velocity.[42] Acute dilation prolonged interatrial conduction time, or overall conduction time in the right atrium.[20] In a recent study, Eijsbouts and colleagues[43] quantified spatial heterogeneities in atrial conduction during acute dilation of right and left atrium in the isolated rabbit heart by high-density mapping. Normalized conduction velocity (conduction time/prestretch distance) decreased by 50%. Importantly, Eijsbouts and colleagues found that acute dilation increased spatial heterogeneity in conduction: Areas of slow conduction (i.e., <20 cm/sec) increased from 6.6% to 11.5%, and areas of conduction block (apparent conduction velocity <10 cm/sec) increased from 1.6% to 6.6%. This increase in inhomogeneity favors re-entry.

Stretch applied during atrial fibrillation increases the rate and organization of waves originating from the junction of the left atrium and superior pulmonary veins. In a number of experiments, the sources of these waves were identified as rotors.[44]

Are the Effects of Stretch Only Mediated by Stretch-Activated Channels?

That blockers of stretch-activated channels reduce the vulnerability of stretched atria to atrial fibrillation, but have no effect on stretch-induced shortening of the refractory period,[30,34,41] indicates that stretch-activated channels are not the only contributors to the electrophysiologic effects of stretch. Stretch also modifies activity of other ion channels and receptors with cytoskeleton connections.

As pointed out by Boyden,[45] stretch increases the initiation and propagation of calcium waves that originate at the junction of contracting and stretched regions.[46] Such traveling calcium waves generate inward currents, delayed afterdepolarizations, and triggered activity.[47] Tavi and colleagues[36] showed that gadolinium suppressed delayed afterdepolarizations; this could be responsible for the fact that gadolinium prevented spontaneous occurrence of atrial fibrillation during stretch. Stretch increases calcium release from the sarcoplasmic reticulum through the ryanodine receptor, resulting in calcium sparks, mediated by an endogenous nitric oxide mechanism.[48]

Stretch leads to an increase in intracellular calcium,[49] most likely caused by enhancement of $I_{Ca,L}$,[50] and this eventually inhibits calcium influx[51] and activates outward potassium currents,[52] both of which shorten the action potential.

The acetylcholine-sensitive potassium channel, I_{K-ACh}, is activated by stretch through a direct effect on the channel protein/lipid bilayer,[53] and the enhanced activity of this channel also decreases atrial action potential duration.

Finally, there are mechanosensitive TREK potassium channels that also may play a role in regulating action potential duration.[54]

Effects of Calcium Antagonists

Because intracellular calcium overload appears to be an important factor leading to electrical remodeling, it is plausible to assume that blocking calcium entry might attenuate electrical remodeling. Yet, there are conflicting results that produce "more questions than answers."[55] Verapamil abolishes stretch-induced changes in the refractory period in humans.[35] Verapamil, when administered before the onset of rapid pacing or the induction of atrial fibrillation, attenuated the shortening of the atrial refractory period in goats[56] and humans.[57] Also, atrial contractile dysfunction after cessation of short-term atrial fibrillation was reduced by verapamil.[11] Remarkably, despite the effect on electrical remodeling, in the study of Tieleman and colleagues,[56] inducibility of atrial fibrillation was only slightly diminished. Clinically, there are indications that patients treated with calcium antagonists have fewer relapses of atrial fibrillation after electrical cardioversion.[58] However, after long periods of atrial fibrillation or rapid pacing, verapamil no longer has a preventive effect.[59,60] In remodeled atria, 24 hours after repeatedly induced atrial fibrillation, verapamil was actually proarrhythmic, converting paroxysmal fibrillation into sustained fibrillation.[61] Also, it shortened the fibrillatory interval.[61] Therefore, it appears that both the duration of atrial fibrillation and the moment of administration of calcium antagonists determine the outcome. Still, some experimental results are not easily explained: In dogs, verapamil increased the duration of atrial fibrillation episodes induced by burst pacing, whereas diltiazem had no effect.[62] Verapamil increased the number of re-entrant circuits, but it was unclear how this was achieved. Verapamil caused only a slight reduction in the refractory period, which was counteracted by acceleration of conduction in some regions.

There may be a role for the T-type calcium channel because mibefradil, a strong blocker of this channel, not only prevented electrical remodeling, but also reduced inducibility of atrial fibrillation,[63] in contrast to verapamil, which has little effect on inducibility.[56]

Role of Angiotensin

Mechanical stretch increases the expression of angiotensin II receptors in isolated myocytes[64]; and in patients with atrial fibrillation, the expression of angiotensin-converting enzyme (ACE) is increased.[65] The ACE inhibitor trandolapril reduces the incidence of atrial fibrillation after acute myocardial infarction in patients with left ventricular dysfunction.[66] A number of studies have attempted to unravel the mechanisms of the effects of angiotensin receptor antagonists or ACE inhibitors in atrial fibrillation, although most of these concentrated on long-term atrial fibrillation and on the effects on structural remodeling, for example, fibrosis.[67-69]

To my knowledge, only one study reported on the effects of an angiotensin II receptor antagonist (candesartan) and an ACE inhibitor (captopril) on electrical remodeling after 3 hours of rapid atrial pacing.[70] Candesartan and captopril prevented the shortening of the atrial refractory period, whereas angiotensin II infusion enhanced the shortening caused by the rapid pacing. Because angiotensin II infusion significantly increased atrial pressure, and because it has been reported that the angiotensin II receptor antagonist losartan decreases atrial pressure in patients,[71] the authors thought that the prevention of electrical remodeling might be due, at least in part, to a decrease in stretch.[70] However, no significant increase in atrial pressure was found during the 3-hour rapid atrial pacing period; therefore, in the control group, the electrical remodeling must have been caused by the rapid atrial activity itself, rather than by atrial stretch. Interestingly, when rapid atrial pacing was maintained for 7 days[69] or 5 weeks,[68] ACE inhibitors or angiotensin II receptor antagonists no longer had an effect on the atrial refractory period. The antiarrhythmic effects of these drugs in long-term atrial fibrillation, or rapid atrial pacing, appear to be largely caused by the reduction in fibrosis.

Summary

In the early phase of atrial fibrillation, or rapid atrial pacing, electrical and contractile remodeling go hand in hand. The main changes, shortening of the refractory period and loss of contractility, both are caused by a reduction in $I_{Ca,L}$. The loss of contractility may lead to atrial dilation, and it is possible that acute atrial stretch, such as may occur in acute myocardial infarction, atrioventricular re-entrant tachycardia, or atrioventricular nodal tachycardia, may contribute to electrical remodeling and promote atrial fibrillation.

Acute stretch, if sufficiently large and abrupt, shortens the atrial refractory period, causes dispersion in refractoriness, increases inhomogeneity in conduction, and causes delayed and early afterdepolarizations. These changes facilitate the induction and maintenance of atrial fibrillation (Fig. 16–2).

Blockers of stretch-activated ion channels reduce the inducibility of atrial fibrillation, but they do not affect stretch-induced shortening of the refractory

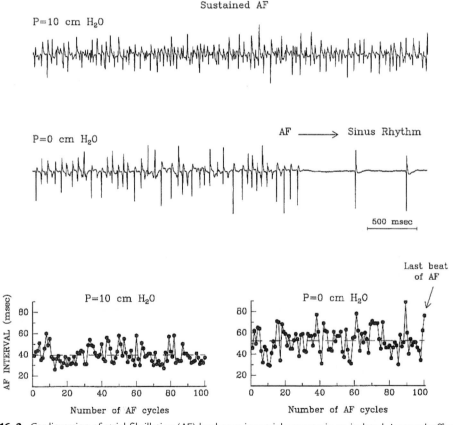

■ **Figure 16–2** Cardioversion of atrial fibrillation (AF) by decreasing atrial pressure in an isolated, Langendorff-perfused, rabbit heart. *Top,* Unipolar atrial electrogram during sustained atrial fibrillation at an atrial pressure of 10 cm H_2O. *Middle,* Same electrogram 40 sec after release of atrial stretch (pressure, 0 cm H_2O). Termination of atrial fibrillation by removal of atrial stretch was associated with slowing of fibrillation rate. *Bottom,* Beat-to-beat cycle lengths during sustained atrial fibrillation *(left)* and before termination *(right).* *(From Ravelli F, Allessie MA: Effects of atrial dilatation on refractory period and vulnerability to atrial fibrillation in the isolated Langendorff-perfused rabbit heart. Circulation 96:1686–1695, 1997, with permission.)*

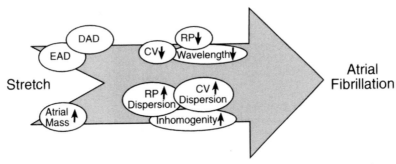

■ **Figure 16–3** Potential contribution of acute atrial stretch to atrial fibrillation development through the alteration of electrophysiologic parameters. CV, conduction velocity; DAD, delayed afterdepolarizations; EAD, early afterdepolarizations; RP, refractory period. *(From Ravelli F: Mechano-electric feedback and atrial fibrillation. Prog Biophys Mol Biol 82:137–149, 2003, with permission.)*

period. This indicates that shortening of the refractory period does not fully explain the enhanced susceptibility to atrial fibrillation during stretch, but that other factors in addition to stretch-activated channels contribute to the electrophysiologic changes during stretch. Candidates are enhanced calcium release from the sarcoplasmic reticulum, resulting in calcium sparks and waves that may generate inward currents and delayed afterdepolarizations and triggered activity, and activation of outward potassium channels, among which is I_{K-ACh}, which shortens the action potential (see Fig.16–3).

Calcium entry blockers, when given before rapid pacing or onset of atrial fibrillation, attenuate or abolish stretch-induced shortening of the refractory period. When administered after long periods of rapid pacing or atrial fibrillation, these compounds are proarrhythmic, converting paroxysmal into sustained fibrillation, and further shorten the refractory period.

Stretch increases the expression of angiotensin II receptors and ACE. ACE inhibitors and angiotensin I receptor antagonists prevent electrical remodeling caused by 3 hours of rapid pacing. It is, however, uncertain whether this is caused by a reduction of stretch. In later phases, 1 to 5 weeks of rapid pacing, these agents no longer have an effect on the refractory period, but do reduce the degree of fibrosis.

References

1. Attuel P, Childers R, Cauchemez B, et al: Failure in rate adaptation of the atrial refractory period: Its relationship to vulnerability. Int J Cardiol 2:179–197, 1982.

2. Le Heuzey J-Y, Boutjdir M, Gagey S, et al: Cellular aspects of atrial vulnerability. In: Attuel P, Coumel P, Janse MJ (eds): The Atrium in Health and Disease. Mount Kisco, NY, Futura Publishing, 1989, pp 81–94.

3. Wijffels MC, Kirchhof CJ, Dorland R, et al: Atrial fibrillation begets atrial fibrillation: A study in awake chronically instrumented goats. Circulation 92:1954–1968, 1995.

4. Morillo CA, Klein GJ, Jones DL, et al: Chronic rapid atrial pacing: Structural, functional and electrophysiological characteristics of a new model of sustained atrial fibrillation. Circulation 91:1588–1595, 1995.

5. Gaspo R, Bosch RF, Talajic M, et al: Functional mechanisms underlying tachycardia-induced atrial fibrillation in a chronic dog model. Circulation 96:4027–4035, 1997.

6. Bosch RF, Zeng X, Grammer JB, et al: Ionic mechanisms of electrical remodelling in human atrial fibrillation. Cardiovasc Res 44:121–131, 1999.

7. Daoud EG, Bogun F, Goyal R, et al: Effects of atrial fibrillation on atrial refractoriness in humans. Circulation 94:1600–1606, 1996.

8. Yue L, Feng J, Gaspo R, et al: Ionic remodeling underlying action potential changes in a canine model of atrial fibrillation. Circ Res 81:512–525, 1997.

9. Sun H, Chartier D, Leblanc N, Nattel S: Intracellular calcium changes and tachycardia-induced contractile dysfunction in canine atrial myocytes. Cardiovasc Res 49:751–761, 2001.

10. Schotten U, Duytschaever M, Ausma J, et al: Electrical and contractile remodelling during the first days of atrial fibrillation go hand in hand. Circulation 107:1433–1439, 2003.

11. Leistad E, Aksnes G, Verburg E, et al: Atrial contractile dysfunction after short-term atrial fibrillation is reduced by verapamil but increased by BAY K8644. Circulation 93:1747–1754, 1996.

12. Li D, Fareh S, Leung KT, et al: Promotion of atrial fibrillation by heart failure in dogs: Atrial remodeling of a different sort. Circulation 100:87–95, 1999.

13. Li D, Melnyk P, Feng J, et al: Effects of experimental heart failure on atrial cellular and ionic electrophysiology. Circulation 101:2631–2638, 2000.

14. Shi Y, Ducharme A, Li D, et al: Remodeling of atrial dimensions and emptying function in canine models of atrial fibrillation. Cardiovasc Res 52:217–225, 2001.

15. Cristal N, Peterburg I, Szwarcberg J: Atrial fibrillation developing in the acute phase of myocardial infarction: Prognostic implications. Chest 70:8–11, 1976.

16. Klein LS, Miles WM, Zipes DP: Effect of atrioventricular interval during pacing or reciprocating tachycardia on atrial size, pressure, and refractory period. Contraction-excitation feedback in human atrium. Circulation 82:60–68, 1990.

17. Boyden PA, Tilley LP, Pham TD, et al: Effects of left atrial enlargement on atrial transmembrane potentials and structure in dogs with mitral valve fibrosis. Am J Cardiol 49:1896–1908, 1982.

18. Manyari DE, Patterson C, Johnson D, et al: Atrial and ventricular arrhythmias in asymptomatic active elderly subjects: Correlation with left atrial size and left ventricular mass. Am Heart J 119:1069–1076, 1990.

19. Calkins H, El-Atassi R, Kalbfleisch S, et al: Effects of an acute increase in atrial pressure on atrial refractoriness in humans. Pacing Clin Electrophysiol 15:1674–1680, 1992.

20. Solti F, Vecsey T, Kekesi V, et al: The effect of atrial dilatation on the genesis of atrial arrhythmias. Cardiovasc Res 23:882–886, 1989.

21. Tse HF, Pelosi F, Oral H, et al: Effects of simultaneous atrioventricular pacing on atrial refractoriness and atrial fibrillation inducibility: Role of atrial mechanoelectrical feedback. J Cardiovasc Electrophysiol 12:43–50, 2001.

22. Kaseda S, Zipes DP: Contraction-excitation feedback in the atria: A cause of changes in refractoriness. J Am Coll Cardiol 11:1327–1336, 1988.

23. Satoh T, Zipes DP: Unequal atrial stretch in dogs increases dispersion of refractoriness conducive to developing atrial fibrillation. J Cardiovasc Electrophysiol 7:833–842, 1996.

24. Chen YJ, Chen SA, Tai CT, et al: Role of atrial electrophysiology and autonomic nervous system in patients with supraventricular tachycardia and paroxysmal atrial fibrillation. J Am Coll Cardiol 32:732–738, 1998.

25. Chen YJ, Tai CT, Chiou CW, et al: Inducibility of atrial fibrillation during atrioventricular pacing with varying intervals: Role of atrial electrophysiology and the autonomic nervous system. J Cardiovasc Electrophysiol 10:1578–1585, 1999.

26. Calkins H, El-Atassi R, Leon A, et al: Effect of the atrioventricular relationship on atrial refractoriness in humans. Pacing Clin Electrophysiol 15:771–778, 1992.

27. Wijffels MCEF, Kirchhof CJHJ, Dorland R, et al: Electrical remodeling due to atrial fibrillation in chronically instrumented goats. Roles of neurohumoral changes, ischemia, atrial stretch, and high rate of electrical activation. Circulation 96:3710–3720, 1997.

28. Ravelli F: Mechano-electric feedback and atrial fibrillation. Prog Biophys Mol Biol 82:137–149, 2003.

29. Ravelli F, Allessie MA: Effects of atrial dilatation on refractory period and vulnerability to atrial fibrillation in the isolated Langendorff-perfused rabbit heart. Circulation 96:1686–1695, 1997.

30. Franz MR, Bode F: Mechano-electrical feedback underlying arrhythmias: The atrial fibrillation case. Prog Biophys Mol Biol 82:163–174, 2003.

31. Nazir SA, Lab M: Mechanoelectric feedback in the atrium of the isolated guinea-pig heart. Cardiovasc Res 32:112–119, 1996.

32. Kamkin A, Kiseleva I, Wagner KD, et al: Mechano-electric feedback in right atrium after left ventricular infarction in rats. J Mol Cell Cardiol 32:465–477, 2000.

33. Nazir SA, Lab M: Mechanoelectric feedback and atrial arrhythmias. Cardiovasc Res 32:52–61, 1996.

34. Bode F, Katchman A, Woosley RL, et al: Gadolinium decreases stretch-induced vulnerability to atrial fibrillation. Circulation 101:2200–2208, 2000.

35. Zarse M, Stellbrink C, Athanatou F, et al: Verapamil prevents stretch-induced shortening of atrial effective refractory period in Langendorff-perfused rabbit heart. J Cardiovasc Electrophysiol 12:85–92, 2001.

36. Tavi P, Laine M, Weckstrom M: Effect of gadolinium on stretch-induced changes in contraction and intracellularly recorded action- and afterpotentials of rat isolated atrium. Br J Pharmacol 118:407–413, 1996.

37. Sideris DA, Toumanidis ST, Thodorakis M, et al: Some observations on the mechanism of pressure related atrial fibrillation. Eur Heart J 15:1585–1589, 1994.

38. Smeets JL, Allessie MA, Lammers WJ, et al: The wavelength of the cardiac impulse and reentrant arrhythmias in isolated rabbit atrium: The role of heart rate, autonomic transmitters, temperature, and potassium. Circ Res 58:96–108, 1986.

39. Lacampagne A, Gannier F, Argibay J, et al: The stretch-activated ion channel blocker gadolinium also blocks L-type calcium channels in isolated ventricular myocytes of the guinea-pig. Biochim Biophys Acta 1191:205–208, 1994.

40. Suchyna TM, Johnson JH, Hamer K, et al: Identification of a peptide toxin from Grammostola spatula spider venom that blocks cation-selective stretch activated channels. J Gen Physiol 115:583–598, 2000.

41. Bode F, Sachs F, Franz MR: Tarantula peptide inhibits atrial fibrillation. Nature 409:35–36, 2001.

42. Penefsky ZJ, Hoffman BF: Effects of stretch on mechanical and electrical properties of cardiac muscle. Am J Physiol 204:433–438, 1963.

43. Eijsbouts SCM, Majidi M, van Zandvoort M, et al: Effects of acute atrial dilatation on heterogeneity in conduction in the isolated rabbit heart. J Cardiovasc Electrophysiol 14:269–279, 2003.

44. Kalifa J, Jalife J, Zaitsev AV, et al: Intra-atrial pressure increases rate and organization of waves emanating from the superior pulmonary veins during atrial fibrillation. Circulation 108:668–673, 2003.

45. Boyden PA: It's still a BIT of a stretch. J Cardiovasc Electrophysiol 14:279–280, 2003.

46. Wakayama Y, Miura M, Sugal Y, et al: Stretch and quick release of rat cardiac trabeculae accelerates Ca^{2+} waves and triggered propagated contractions. Am J Physiol 281:H2133–H2142, 2001.

47. Ter Keurs HEDJ, Boyden PA: Ca^{2+} and arrhythmias. In: Spooner PM, Rosen MR (eds): Foundations of Arrhythmias. Basic Concepts and Clinical Arrhythmias. New York, Marcel Dekker, 2000, pp 287–317.

48. Petroff MGV, Kim SH, Pepe S, et al: Endogenous nitric oxide mechanisms mediate the stretch dependence of Ca^{2+} release in cardiomyocytes. Nat Cell Biol 3:867–873, 2001.

49. Calaghan SC, White E: The role of calcium in the response of cardiac muscle to stretch. Prog Biophys Mol Biol 71:59–90, 1999.

50. Matsuda N, Hagiwara N, Shoda M, et al: Enhancement of the L-type Ca^{2+} current by mechanical stimulation in single rabbit myocytes. Circ Res 78:650–659, 1996.

51. Sun H, Leblanc N, Nattel S: Mechanisms of inactivation of L-type calcium channels in human atrial myocytes. Am J Physiol 272:H1625–H1635, 1997.

52. Shibata EF, Drury T, Refsum H, et al: Contributions of a transient outward current to repolarization in human atrium. Am J Physiol 257:H1773–H1781, 1989.

53. Pleumsamran A, Kim D: Membrane stretch augments the cardiac muscarinic K^+ channel activity. J Membr Biol 148:287–297, 1995.

54. Terrenoire C, Lauritzen I, Lesage F, et al: A TREK-1-like potassium channel in atrial cells inhibited by beta-adrenergic stimu-

lation and activated by volatile anesthetics. Circ Res 89:336–340, 2001.

55. Zipes DP: Electrophysiological remodelling of the heart owing to rate. Circulation 95:1745–1748, 1997.

56. Tieleman RG, de Langen CDJ, van Gelder IC, et al: Verapamil reduces tachycardia-induced electrical remodeling of the atria. Circulation 95:1945–1953, 1997.

57. Goette A, Honeycutt C, Langberg JJ: Electrical remodeling in atrial fibrillation. Time course and mechanism. Circulation 94:2968–2974, 1996.

58. Daoud EG, Knight BP, Weiss R, et al: Effect of verapamil and procainamide on atrial fibrillation-induced electrical remodelling in humans. Circulation 96:1542–1550, 1997.

59. Tieleman RG, van Gelder IC, Crijns HJ, et al: Early recurrences of atrial fibrillation after electrical cardioversion: A result of fibrillation-induced electrical remodeling of the atria? J Am Coll Cardiol 31:167–173, 1998.

60. De Simone A, Stabile G, Vitale DF, et al: Pretreatment with verapamil in patients with persistent or chronic atrial fibrillation who underwent electrical cardioversion. J Am Coll Cardiol 34:810–814, 1999.

61. Duytschaever MF, Garratt CJ, Allessie MA: Profibrillatory effects of verapamil but not of digoxin in the goat model of atrial fibrillation. J Cardiovasc Electrophysiol 11:1375–1385, 2000.

62. Bénardeau A, Fareh S, Nattel S: Effects of verapamil on atrial fibrillation and its electrophysiological determinants in dogs. Cardiovasc Res 50:85–96, 2001.

63. Fareh S, Bénardeau A, Thibault B, et al: The T-type Ca²⁺ channel blocker mibefradil prevents the development of a substrate for atrial fibrillation by tachycardia-induced atrial remodelling in dogs. Circulation 100:2191–2197, 1999.

64. Kijima K, Matsubara H, Murasawa S, et al: Mechanical stretch induces enhanced expression of angiotensin II receptor subtypes in neonatal cardiac myocytes. Circ Res 79:887–897, 1996.

65. Goette A, Staack T, Rocken C, et al: Increased expression of extracellular signal-regulated kinase and angiotensin-converting enzyme in human atria during atrial fibrillation. J Am Coll Cardiol 35:1669–1677, 2000.

66. Pedersen OD, Bagger H, Kober L, et al: Trandolapril reduces the incidence of atrial fibrillation after acute myocardial infarction in patients with left ventricular dysfunction. Circulation 100:376–380, 1999.

67. Klein HU, Goette A: Blockade of atrial angiotensin II type 1 receptors. A novel antiarrhythmic strategy to prevent atrial fibrillation? J Am Coll Cardiol 41:2205–2206, 2003.

68. Kumagai K, Nakashima H, Urata H, et al: Effects of angiotensin II type 1 receptor antagonist on electrical and structural remodeling in atrial fibrillation. J Am Coll Cardiol 41:2197–2204, 2003.

69. Shinagawa K, Mitamura H, Ogawa S, et al: Effects of inhibiting Na⁺/H⁺-exchange or angiotensin-converting enzyme on atrial tachycardia-induced remodelling. Cardiovasc Res 54:438–446, 2002.

70. Nakashima H, Kumagai K, Urata H, et al: Angiotensin II antagonist prevents electrical remodeling in atrial fibrillation. Circulation 101:2612–2617, 2000.

71. Gottlieb SS, Dickstein K, Fleck E, et al: Hemodynamic and neurohormonal effects of the angiotensin II antagonist losartan in patients with congestive heart failure. Circulation 88:1602–1609, 1993.

CHAPTER 17

The Substrate of Atrial Fibrillation in Chronically Dilated Atria

• • • •

Ulrich Schotten and Maurits Allessie

ATRIAL DILATION AS A RISK FACTOR FOR ATRIAL FIBRILLATION

Ever since atrial fibrillation (AF) was first described as a clinical entity by Cushny and Edmunds in 1907,[1] it was recognized that AF has a tendency to become more stable with time. In most patients, frequency and duration of AF episodes increase until the arrhythmia becomes persistent. During the last two decades, the self-perpetuating and progressive nature of AF attracted the attention of an increasing number of researchers. They tried to understand how AF is initiated, how it is sustained, and why it eventually becomes more stable.

In 1995, two groups reported changes of the atrial electrophysiologic properties as a consequence of AF. In a dog model of prolonged rapid atrial pacing, Morillo and colleagues[2] found that the atrial refractory period was reduced by about 15%. In goats with artificially maintained AF, atrial refractoriness shortened from ~150 to ~80 msec (−45%).[3] More importantly, in both studies, a pronounced increase of the stability of AF was found. In the goat, no apparent changes of the conduction velocity occurred. The observed shortening of the refractory period resulted in a shortening of the wavelength of the atrial impulse, which might well explain increased vulnerability and stability of AF. A short wavelength favors intra-atrial conduction block in small regions, which may serve as a site for initiation of re-entry. Also, a short wavelength allows more re-entering wavelets to coexist on the available surface area of the atria, thus increasing AF stability ("atrial fibrillation begets atrial fibrillation").[3]

However, there are reasons to believe that besides the shortening of refractoriness, other factors play a role in the development of chronic AF. Already in the initial study in the goat model of AF, it was noted that the time course of the changes in atrial refractoriness did not run parallel with the increase in persistence of AF. Whereas the AF cycle length reached a new steady state within 3 to 5 days, it took an additional 1 to 2 weeks before AF became persistent.[3] This led to the hypothesis that a so-called second factor was involved in the development of persistent AF.

We recently suggested the existence of additional positive feedback loops in AF (Fig. 17–1).[4] In this scheme, atrial stretch and dilation play a crucial role. On the one hand, atrial stretch and dilation are the consequence of a loss of atrial contractility induced by AF; on the other hand, they serve as a trigger to start a deleterious structural remodeling process, which leads to atrial connective tissue formation, fibrosis, and conduction disturbances that stabilize the arrhythmia. Currently, many researchers regard atrial dilation as the most likely candidate to serve as the "second factor."

In clinical trials, a relation between atrial size and AF had been established already 50 years ago. In 1955, Fraser and Turner[5] showed that left and right atrial enlargement correlated with the incidence of AF in patients with mitral valve disease. Large prospective trials established left atrial enlargement as an independent risk factor for the development of AF.[6,7] Psaty and colleagues[8] included about 5000 participants who were all in normal sinus rhythm (SR) in the Cardiovascular Health Study. Left atrial size at baseline was strongly and independently associated with the incidence of AF during the 3-year follow-up. In a recent study,[9] left atrial size was (apart from age) the

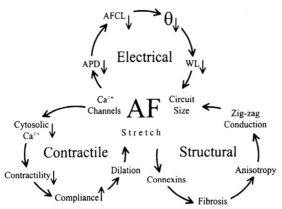

■ **Figure 17–1** Three proposed positive feedback loops of atrial remodeling on atrial fibrillation (AF). Down-regulation of the L-type calcium channels is considered to be the primary cause for electrical and contractile remodeling. The loss of atrial contractility leads to an increase in compliance of the fibrillating atria, which in turn facilitates atrial dilation. The resulting stretch acts as a stimulus for structural remodeling of the enlarged atria. The combination of electrical and structural remodeling allows intra-atrial re-entrant circuits of a smaller size, because of a reduction in wavelength (WL, shortening of refractoriness and slowing of conduction) and increased nonuniform tissue anisotropy (zigzag conduction). AFCL, atrial fibrillation cycle length; APD, action potential duration; θ, conduction velocity. *(From Allessie MA, Ausma J, Schotten U: Electrical, contractile and structural remodeling during atrial fibrillation. Cardiovasc Res 54:230–246, 2002, with permission.)*

only predictive parameter for the occurrence of AF in patients with mitral regurgitation. These data suggest that atrial dilation may be a cause of AF, and it was proposed that "interventions that maintain left atrial size may be important in the prevention of AF."[8]

However, atrial enlargement can also be a consequence of AF. In 1990, Sanfilippo and colleagues[10] performed a small but prospective echocardiographic study in patients with AF, a normal atrial size at baseline, and no evidence of other cardiac abnormalities. After an average period of 20.6 months, left and right atrial volumes were significantly increased.

None of these studies can establish a causal relation between atrial dilation and AF, but they convincingly demonstrate the mutual dependency of AF and atrial dilation.

WHY DO FIBRILLATING ATRIA DILATE?

Atrial dilation frequently occurs in patients with valve diseases, hypertension, coronary artery disease, and heart failure. In these patients, atrial dilation is mostly caused by increased mechanical load due to atrioventricular (AV) valve regurgitation or increased end-diastolic ventricular pressures. Depending on the severity of the heart disease, AF will develop in up to 50% of these patients. Once the atria fibrillate, further dilation might reflect progression of the underlying heart disease, or the dilation might be caused by AF itself. AF-related increase in atrial size is caused by several mechanisms. Two of these mechanisms, loss of atrial contractility and changes in ventricular rate, are particularly important.

We recently evaluated the effects of AF on atrial contractility, compliance, and size in goats chronically instrumented with ultrasonic piezoelectric crystals to measure the mediolateral diameter of the atrium and with a tip pressure transducer in the right atrium. After 5 days of AF, the amplitude of the pressure waves and the atrial wall excursions during AF were reduced to less than 15% of control animals, indicating that atrial contractility was nearly completely abolished. To study the effect of this loss of atrial contractility on the compliance of the fibrillating atrium, pressure and diameter were measured after unloading the atria with a fast-acting loop diuretic and after loading the atria with 1 L saline infused within 10 min (Fig. 17–2).[11] During the first days of AF, the compliance curve flattened, indicating that the compliance of the atrium increased. This caused a rightward shift of the working point (gray in Fig. 17–2), and the mean atrial diameter (D_{mean}) increased by ~10%. The mean atrial pressure (P_{mean}) did not change throughout the experiment. The changes in atrial compliance and size followed the same time course as the loss of contractility of the fibrillating atria and were fully reversible within 2 days of SR. These data suggest that atrial dilation during the first days of AF is a direct consequence of the loss of atrial contractility.

Echocardiographic studies have shown that atrial dilation during AF is a progressive process that may continue for months to years.[9] In contrast, in our

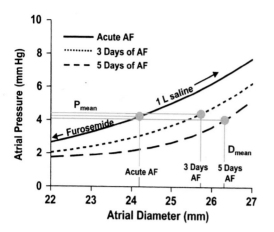

■ **Figure 17–2** Representative right atrial compliance curves during acute AF and after 3 or 5 days of AF in goat. The compliance was measured by unloading the atria with a rapidly acting loop-diuretic and loading by infusion of 1 L saline in 10 min. Because of an increase in atrial compliance at low atrial diameters (flattening of the compliance curve), the working point during AF shifted to the right. D_{mean}, mean atrial diameter; P_{mean}, mean atrial pressure. *(From Schotten U, Neuberger HR, Allessie MA: The role of atrial dilatation in the domestication of atrial fibrillation. Prog Biophys Mol Biol 82:151–162, 2003, with permission.)*

experimental studies, atrial contractile function was already almost completely abolished after a couple of days. Obviously, apart from the loss of atrial contractility, additional mechanisms are operative that cause the atria to dilate during prolonged AF. The loss of atrial contractility will transfer atrial stretch more to the passive elements of the atrial wall, which might lead to elongation of collagen fibers. Synthesis of connective tissue and cellular hypertrophy could also produce a slow increase in atrial dimensions.

An additional mechanism by which AF may induce atrial dilation is the increase in ventricular rate. In most patients, the ventricular rate during AF is greater than during SR. It has been suggested that inadequate ventricular rate response might result in reduced ventricular pump function, which might explain impaired exercise tolerance both during AF and after cardioversion. Whereas some authors have suggested that decreased exercise capacity is because of the loss of atrial systole, Van Gelder and colleagues[12] demon-

strated that reduced ventricular pump function is likely to underlie the poor exercise capacity that follows cardioversion of AF. In patients without valvular heart disease, ejection fraction and exercise capacity significantly improved between 1 week and 1 month after cardioversion, whereas the atrial systole improved by 1 week and remained unchanged thereafter. This discrepancy in time course of recovery suggests that an intrinsic left ventricular cardiomyopathy was present in these patients, but gradually subsided after cardioversion. Increased end-diastolic pressures might significantly contribute to the slow atrial dilation process during AF.

Recent experimental data support an important role of ventricular rate for the modulation of atrial size. Both high and low ventricular rates can produce significant atrial dilation (Fig. 17–3).

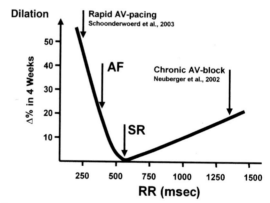

■ **Figure 17–3** Relation between RR interval and the increase in atrial dimensions in goats. Ventricular rates, both too high and too low, result in progressive atrial dilation. High ventricular rates cause a tachycardiomyopathy with ventricular dilation and increased end-diastolic pressures. Slow rates result in cyclic stretch stimuli during the long diastolic pauses. The slow atrial dilation during AF might be due in part to the fact that the RR interval during AF is shorter than during normal sinus rhythm SR. AV, atrio-ventricular. *(From Schoonderwoerd BA, Van Gelder IC, van Veldhuisen DJ, et al: Electrical remodeling and atrial dilation during atrial tachycardia are influenced by ventricular rate: Role of developing tachycardiomyopathy. J Cardiovasc Electrophysiol 12:1404–1410, 2001 and Van Gelder IC, Crijins HJ, Blanksma PK, et al: Time course of hemodynamic changes and improvement of exercise tolerance after cardioversion of chronic atrial fibrillation unassociated with cardiac value disease. Am J Cardiol 72:560–566, 1993, with permission.)*

In goats undergoing 4 weeks of rapid AV-sequential pacing at a cycle length of 250 msec, Schoonderwoerd and colleagues[13] demonstrated pronounced atrial dilation (+50%). This increase in atrial size was not because of the high atrial rate. In a control group, the AV node was ablated, and the ventricles were paced at a cycle length of 750 msec. In this group, rapid atrial pacing alone did not change atrial size throughout 4 weeks. Rather, it appeared that progressive ventricular dysfunction was the cause for atrial dilation in this model. When the ventricular rate is low, atrial dilation probably results from the accumulation of blood in the atria during the long diastolic pauses. This applies cyclic stretch stimuli to the atria. In goats with chronic AV block (cycle length, ~1200 msec), Neuberger and colleagues[14] reported atrial dilation of ~12% in 4 weeks. Regardless of whether atrial dilation was produced by too high or too low ventricular rates, the increased atrial size went together with a pronounced increase in the stability of AF in both studies.

Recently, we monitored atrial size and RR interval during 4 weeks of AF in goats. The RR interval during AF (~410 msec) was shorter than during SR (~550 msec), and the atria dilated by ~20%. It is tempting to speculate that atrial dilation during AF is at least partly caused by the greater ventricular rate, which suggests that the ventricular performance could be compromised in the goats with several weeks of AF. Notably, however, overt heart failure has never been observed in goats, even after several months of AF.

ANIMAL MODELS OF CHRONIC ATRIAL DILATION

The effect of atrial enlargement on atrial electrophysiology was repeatedly addressed during the last two decades. Primarily, the effect of *acute* atrial dilation on atrial refractoriness and conduction was investigated. These studies, however, had conflicting results. In many studies, acute atrial dilation in isolated rabbit hearts or in open-chest dogs resulted in a shortening of atrial refractoriness. Other studies described no change, or even a prolongation, of the refractory period during acute stretch. The only common finding in most of these studies was an increase in the inducibility and persistence of AF (see Chapter 16).

The first experiments on *chronic* enlargement of the atria were performed in the early 1980s by Boyden and Hoffman.[15] In eight dogs with tricuspid regurgitation and stenosis of the pulmonary artery, the right atrial volume increased by 40% during ~100 days of follow-up. Atrial arrhythmias did not occur spontaneously. However, the inducibility and the duration of artificially induced atrial tachyarrhythmias increased significantly. Atrial refractoriness was not measured, but the duration of action potentials recorded in vitro was not different compared with control animals. Histologic and ultrastructural analysis revealed cardiac hypertrophy and an increase in connective tissue content. Another study in dogs, with spontaneous mitral valve fibrosis (MVF) and left atrial enlargement, also found no change in transmembrane potentials.[16] In the MVF dogs, left atrial volume was six to eight times that of control dogs. A large amount of connective tissue was found in between the hypertrophied atrial myocytes (17 vs. 10 µm in diameter). Most MVF animals had spontaneous atrial arrhythmias, but the underlying mechanism could not be defined. The authors speculated that atrial conduction could be impaired.

To describe the chronological sequence of progressive atrial dilation and its correlation with alterations in atrial electrophysiology, we studied goats with chronic complete AV block.[14] Six goats were instrumented with modified screw-in leads with two sonomicrometer crystals attached to the tip. Two of these modified leads were placed in the right atrium, one in the anterolateral and one in the posteroseptal wall. With the ultrasound crystals the distance between the lead tips could be measured as an index of the atrial diameter. After bundle of His ablation, the ventricular heart rate decreased from about 120 to 50 beats/min. Mean atrial and end-diastolic ventricular pressures acutely increased by ~5 mm Hg, but remained constant during 4 weeks of AV block. Within the first days in AV block, the atrial diameter did not change. However, 4 weeks after the ablation, the atrial diameter was increased by ~12%. Together with atrial dilation, the duration of AF paroxysms increased from a few seconds during control to several hours (Fig. 17–4A). Because the atrial refractory period and the AF cycle length remained constant throughout 4 weeks of complete AV block, the increased persistence of AF could not be explained by a shortening of refractoriness.

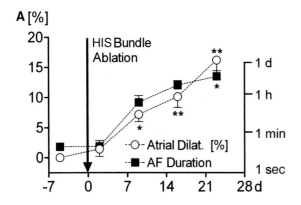

A

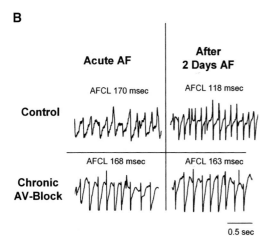

B

Figure 17–4 *A,* Relative atrial dilation and duration of induced AF episodes during control and 4 weeks of chronic complete AV block in six goats. *B,* Representative example of unipolar endocardial atrial electrograms obtained from a goat after induction of AF by burst pacing. Under control conditions (conducting AV node, *top panels*), the median AF interval and the atrial refractory period shorten as a result of 2 days of AF maintenance. During chronic complete AV block *(bottom panels),* AF maintenance for 2 days still reduces atrial refractoriness, but the AF interval remains constant. This indicates a widening of the excitable gap during electrical remodeling in the goat with AV block. *(From Van Gelder IC, Crijins HJ, Blanksma PK, et al: Time course of hemodynamic changes and improvement of exercise tolerance after cardioversion of chronic atrial fibrillation unassociated with cardiac value disease. Am J Cardiol 72:560–566, 1993, with permission.)*

Animal models of rapid pacing–induced heart failure with atrial dilation demonstrated either a prolongation of refractoriness[17,18] or no change.[19] An interesting finding in the goats with chronic AV block was that AF-induced electrical remodeling (shortening of atrial effective refractory period) was not associated with a shortening of the mean AF interval (see Fig. 17–4B). First, this demonstrates that electrical remodeling still occurs in dilated atria. Unlike reports in a dog model of heart failure,[20] the time course and the extent of tachycardia-induced electrical remodeling in AV block goats were similar to control animals, suggesting that the same mechanisms are also operating in dilated atria. Second, a shortening of the atrial effective refractory period without a concomitant shortening of atrial fibrillation cycle length means that the excitable gap during AF becomes wider. This observation may be explained by lines of conduction block resulting in macro re-entrant circuits during AF, as were described in a dog model of mitral regurgitation.[21] In dogs with cardiomyopathy and pronounced atrial dilation, AF paroxysms were prolonged, and discrete regions of slow atrial conduction were found (Fig. 17–5). The atrial myofibers were separated by thick layers of connective tissue, which may cause local conduction block during AF.[19]

Although these experimental data indicate that atrial dilation can result in impairment of atrial wave-front propagation and increased persistence of AF, in other models of atrial dilation the stability of AF was increased, but conduction disturbances were much less prominent. Verheule and colleagues[22] studied dogs with mitral valve regurgitation produced by partial mitral valve avulsion. Within 4 weeks after the operation, the left atria dilated by ~25%, whereas right atrial size remained unchanged. Sustained AF (>1 hour) was not observed in control dogs, but it was inducible in 10 of 19 dogs with mitral regurgitation. The atrial refractory period became longer in left and right atria, with the effect being more pronounced in the left atria. Although in the left atria pronounced atrial tissue fibrosis and inflammatory changes were found, no apparent conduction disturbances could be detected. The authors speculate that the already modest conduction abnormalities, which might have escaped detection in their mapping experiments, might be sufficient to produce significant increases in vulnerability for AF. Indeed, using high-resolution optical mapping, the same group recently reported that in dogs with mitral valve regurgitation, AF was more complex than in control dogs.[23] Wave fronts occupied less of the field of view, because there

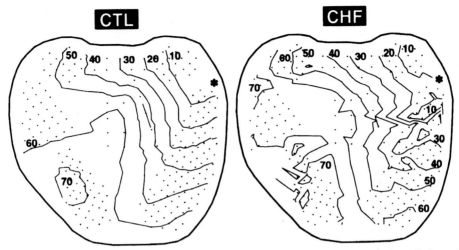

■ **Figure 17–5** Activation map in msec of the left and right atrium in dogs with tachycardiomyopathy. *Left,* Control (CTL). *Right,* A dog with congestive heart failure (CHF; rapid ventricular pacing for 6 weeks). The crowding of isochrones indicates local slowing of conduction. *(From Li D, Fareh S, Leung TK, Nattel S: Promotion of atrial fibrillation by heart failure in dogs: Atrial remodeling of a different sort. Circulation 100:87–95, 1999, with permission.)*

were large areas of slow conduction or block, and there were times when more than one wave front moved through the mapping region. Tissue discontinuities appeared to produce a decrease in the spatiotemporal organization that created a substrate for AF in this model.

CELLULAR MECHANISMS OF STRUCTURAL REMODELING IN CHRONICALLY DILATED ATRIA

Acute stretch induces various changes of the atrial electrophysiology, which are all transient and rapidly reversible. These changes include a shortening of the action potential duration, a depolarization of the resting membrane potential, the occurrence of early afterdepolarizations, and the generation of ectopic beats.[24] They are probably mediated by the activation of mechanosensitive channels. Activation might provoke stretch-induced arrhythmias through changes in excitability and refractoriness, or through the occurrence of ectopic activity.

Chronic stretch not only induces changes in shape and duration of the atrial action potential, but it also activates various intracellular signaling pathways in both cardiomyocytes and fibroblasts. This has a significant impact on atrial anatomy and structure at the microscopic and macroscopic scale. These structural changes often are irreversible.

An overview of some of the pathways probably involved in atrial connective tissue formation and structural remodeling in fibrillating atria is shown in Figure 17–6. An important step of structural remodeling of the atria caused by mechanical load is the induction of paracrine activity of the cardiomyocytes (see Chapter 7). In adult cardiomyocytes, stretch stimulates secretion of angiotensin II (Ang II), endothelin-1, and atrial natriuretic factor. These hormones activate the mitogen-activated protein kinase (MAPK) pathway, the janus kinase/signal transducers and activators of transcription pathway, and calcium calmodulin–dependent pathways.[25] Some MAPK activate extracellular signal-regulated kinases (ERK-1 and ERK-2). All these pathways are known to promote cellular hypertrophy, to stimulate fibroblast proliferation,

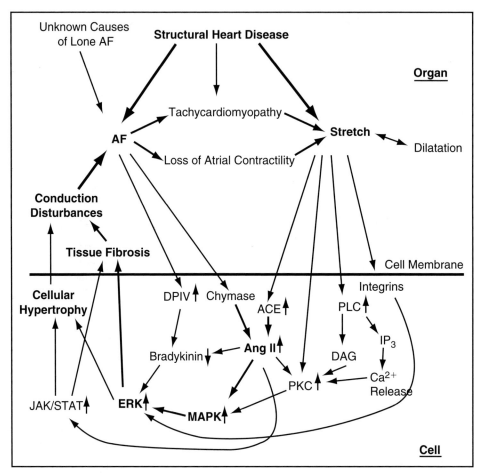

■ **Figure 17–6**   Complexity of the pathophysiologic network underlying structural remodeling caused by, or finally resulting in, AF. Blockade of a single pathway may not be sufficient to effectively and permanently prevent structural remodeling of the atria. ACE, angiotensin-converting enzyme; Ang II, angiotensin II; DAG, diacylglycerol; DPIV, dipeptidyl peptidase IV; ERK, extracellular signal-regulated kinase; IP$_3$, inositol-1,4,5-triphosphate; JAK/STAT, janus kinase/signal transducers and activators of transcription; MAPK, mitogen-activated protein kinase; PKC, protein kinase C; PLC, phospholipase C.

and to activate matrix protein synthesis leading to tissue fibrosis.[26]

Stretch can also activate ERK-1 and ERK-2 independent of Ang II by stimulation of integrins.[26] Integrins are stretch-sensitive transmembrane adhesion molecules that are anchored in the extracellular matrix. A short cytoplasmic tail binds to adaptor proteins, which interact with intracellular kinases and cytoskeleton proteins. Integrins can transfer stretch stimuli to the cytosol of the cardiomyocytes, resulting in activa-

tion of focal adhesion kinases (FAK), which in turn activate ERK. Thus, Ang II and stretch-induced activation of integrins stimulate common downstream signaling cascades. Also, Ang II up-regulates integrin expression and FAK activity, indicating close cross talk between these pathways. It has been suggested that membrane-bound metalloproteinases called ADAM (a disintegrin and metalloproteinase) interact with integrins in atrial tissue. The disintegrin activity of these enzymes loosens the tight junctions of cardiomyocytes to the surrounding extracellular matrix. In patients with chronic AF, ADAM 10 and 15 are up-regulated.[27] Progressive loss of integrins therefore might enhance sliding and slippage of cells and contribute to dilation of fibrillating atria. Whether the signaling function of integrins is altered in fibrillating or dilated atria is not known.[27]

Stretch also stimulates phospholipase C directly and through Ang II.[28] Phospholipase C generates inositol-1,4,5-triphosphate (IP$_3$) and diacylglycerol (DAG). IP$_3$-induced release of Ca^{2+} from intracellular stores and DAG stimulate protein kinase C. Protein kinase C, in turn, activates ERK.

There is increasing evidence that the renin-angiotensin system and its downstream signaling pathways are activated in atrial myocardium of patients with chronic AF. The protein expression of angiotensin-converting enzyme (ACE) and ERK-1 and -2 is up-regulated.[29] Fibroblasts seem to be the source of increased amounts of ERK in the atrial tissue of patients with AF. The Ang II type 1 receptor is down-regulated, whereas the Ang II type 2 receptor is up-regulated; both probably reflect feedback mechanisms to prevent excessive stimulation of the angiotensin system.[30] In dogs with heart failure, the amount of activated ERK could be significantly reduced by blockade of the angiotensin system.[31] Both ACE and dipeptidyl peptidase IV (DPIV), a serine protease, catalyze the release of N-terminal dipeptides; this contributes to the degradation of bradykinin. Bradykinin has cardioprotective effects, by which it diminishes the development of interstitial fibrosis. DPIV activity has been shown to be enhanced in fibrillating atrial tissue.[32] The increase in atrial ACE activity acts synergistically with increased DPIV activity to decrease atrial bradykinin levels, which further stimulates atrial connective tissue formation.[26]

HOW DOES ATRIAL DILATION PROMOTE ATRIAL FIBRILLATION?

Atrial dilation per se might promote AF because more re-entrant circuits can coexist on the atrial surface area. Because in many animal models the degree of atrial dilation is modest but AF vulnerability and stability are significantly increased, it does not seem likely that the larger mean surface area contributes much to the increased stability of AF. The consensus is that stretch-induced tissue fibrosis promotes AF in dilated atria. In fibrotic myocardium, the macroscopic conduction velocity is slowed by microscopic zigzagging circuits or depressed propagation in branching muscle bundles.[33] This electro-anatomic substrate permits multiple, small re-entrant circuits that can stabilize the arrhythmia.[34] Multiple entry and exit points, and multiple sites at which unidirectional block occurs, will shift the balance between generation and extinction of wavelets to favor the generation of new wave fronts. Also, fibrosis will tend to increase electrophysiologic dispersion.[35] Whereas the scarred matrix will transfer stretch primarily to the adjacent atrial myocardium, other regions might even become shielded by surrounding strands of connective tissue. Unequal atrial stretch has been shown to differentially affect the local refractory period depending on the degree of elongation of the atrial muscle fibers.[36] Therefore, tissue fibrosis will not only increase anisotropy in conduction but also the dispersion in refractoriness. Cellular hypertrophy increases the complexity of the substrate even more, because in hypertrophied myocytes, smaller mechanical stimuli are sufficient to activate stretch-activated channels[37] (see Chapters 3 and 28). Also, conduction transverse to the cell orientation might be slowed by cellular hypertrophy.[38]

Finally, the development of such an electro-anatomic substrate would also explain the loss of efficacy of drugs to cardiovert AF. In discontinuous tissue, the safety factor for conduction is greater than in normal tissue.[39] Thus, a greater degree of blockade of the fast sodium current is required to terminate AF. Anatomic obstacles might widen the excitable gap during AF, making drugs that prolong atrial refractoriness less effective.[40] Also, multiple sites at which unidirectional block occurs might facilitate reinduction of AF immediately after cardioversion by early premature beats.

Therefore, new experimental strategies put more focus on the prevention of structural remodeling. The ACE inhibitor enalapril has been shown to attenuate atrial fibrosis and conduction disturbances in dogs with rapid pacing–induced heart failure.[41] This observation supports the hypothesis that the activation of the renin-angiotensin system is involved in the signaling cascade leading to atrial cell growth, proliferation of fibroblasts, and atrial fibrosis. Also, in clinical trials, ACE inhibitors reduced the incidence of AF in patients with heart failure[42] or left ventricular dysfunction after myocardial infarction.[43] Although this effect could be explained by an improvement of the patients' hemodynamics, a trial with the angiotensin receptor blocker irbesartan showed that blockade of the renin-angiotensin system can reduce the recurrence rate of AF in a heterogeneous patient population with a less serious degree of heart disease.[44]

Notably, ACE-independent pathways exist in the heart that convert Ang I to Ang II. In the human heart, a considerable percentage of Ang II is formed by tissue chymase. In patients undergoing cardiac transplantation, tissue chymase even accounts for up to 75% of total cardiac Ang II–forming enzyme activity. Inhibition of cardiac chymase has been demonstrated to suppress collagen synthesis and to reduce the degree of fibrosis in humans with failing myocardium. Thus, the mechanisms finally resulting in tissue fibrosis and hypertrophy form a complex network involving parallel intracellular cascades and a variety of neurohumoral pathways. The recent finding that ACE inhibitors do not necessarily prevent atrial fibrosis in patients with chronic AF,[45] or in dogs with heart failure,[31] possibly reflects the complexity of the mechanisms that control connective tissue formation. The results also suggest that blockade of single pathways may not be sufficient to prevent, or delay, structural remodeling in dilated atria.

Summary

Numerous clinical investigations and recent experimental studies have demonstrated that AF is a progressive arrhythmia. With time, paroxysmal AF becomes persistent, and the success rate of cardioversion of persistent AF declines. Electrical remodeling (shortening of atrial refractoriness) develops within the first days of AF and contributes to the increase in stability of the arrhythmia. However, "domestication of AF" must also depend on other mechanisms because the persistence of AF continues to increase after electrical remodeling has been completed. Atrial dilation is a promising candidate to serve as such a "second factor." Loss of atrial contractility during AF enhances atrial dilation by increasing the compliance of the fibrillating atrium. Alternatively,

the increase of the ventricular rate during AF might compromise left ventricular pump function, and thus promote atrial dilation in some patients with AF. Chronic atrial stretch induces activation of numerous signaling pathways leading to cellular hypertrophy, fibroblast proliferation, and tissue fibrosis. The resulting electro-anatomic substrate in dilated atria is characterized by increased nonuniform anisotropy and macroscopic slowing of conduction, promoting re-entrant circuits in the atria. Prevention of electro-anatomic remodeling by blockade of pathways activated by chronic atrial stretch therefore has become the focus of research on future strategies for the management of AF.

References

1. Cushny AR, Edmunds CW: Paroxysmal irregularity of the heart in auricular fibrillation. Am J Med Sci 133:66–77, 1907.
2. Morillo CA, Klein GJ, Jones DL, Guiraudon CM: Chronic rapid atrial pacing. Structural, functional, and electrophysiological characteristics of a new model of sustained atrial fibrillation. Circulation 91:1588–1595, 1995.
3. Wijffels MC, Kirchhof CJ, Dorland R, Allessie MA: Atrial fibrillation begets atrial fibrillation. A study in awake chronically instrumented goats. Circulation 92:1954–1968, 1995.
4. Allessie MA, Ausma J, Schotten U: Electrical, contractile and structural remodeling during atrial fibrillation. Cardiovasc Res 54:230–246, 2002.
5. Fraser HRL, Turner RWD: Auricular fibrillation with special reference to rheumatic heart disease. Br Med J 2:1414–1418, 1955.
6. Vasan RS, Larson MG, Levy D: Distribution and categorization of echocardiographic measurements in relation to reference limits. The Framingham Heart Study. Formulation of a height- and sex-specific classification and its prospective validation. Circulation 96:1863–1873, 1997.
7. Vaziri SM, Larson MG, Benjamin EJ, Levy D: Echocardiographic predictors of nonrheumatic atrial fibrillation. The Framingham Heart Study. Circulation 89:724–730, 1994.
8. Psaty BM, Manolio TA, Kuller LH, et al: Incidence of and risk factors for atrial fibrillation in older adults. Circulation 96:2455–2461, 1997.
9. Grigioni F, Avierinos JF, Ling LH, et al: Atrial fibrillation complicating the course of degenerative mitral regurgitation: Determinants and long-term outcome. J Am Coll Cardiol 40:84–92, 2002.
10. Sanfilippo AJ, Abascal VM, Sheehan M, et al: Atrial enlargement as a consequence of atrial fibrillation. A prospective echocardiographic study. Circulation 82:792–797, 1990.
11. Schotten U, Neuberger HR, Allessie MA: The role of atrial dilatation in the domestication of atrial fibrillation. Prog Biophys Mol Biol 82:151–162, 2003.
12. Van Gelder IC, Crijns HJ, Blanksma PK, et al: Time course of hemodynamic changes and improvement of exercise tolerance after cardioversion of chronic atrial fibrillation unassociated with cardiac valve disease. Am J Cardiol 72:560–566, 1993.
13. Schoonderwoerd BA, Van Gelder IC, van Veldhuisen DJ, et al: Electrical remodeling and atrial dilation during atrial tachycardia

are influenced by ventricular rate: Role of developing tachycardiomyopathy. J Cardiovasc Electrophysiol 12:1404–1410, 2001.

14. Van Gelder IC, Crijns HJ, Blanksma PK, et al: Time course of hemodynamic changes and improvement of exercise tolerance after cardioversion of chronic atrial fibrillation unassociated with cardiac valve disease. Am J Cardiol 72:560–566, 1993,

15. Boyden PA, Hoffman BF: The effects on atrial electrophysiology and structure of surgically induced right atrial enlargement in dogs. Circ Res 49:1319–1331, 1981.

16. Boyden PA, Tilley LP, Pham TD, et al: Effects of left atrial enlargement on atrial transmembrane potentials and structure in dogs with mitral valve fibrosis. Am J Cardiol 49:1896–1908, 1982.

17. Power JM, Beacom GA, Alferness CA, et al: Effects of left atrial dilatation on the endocardial atrial defibrillation threshold: A study in an ovine model of pacing induced dilated cardiomyopathy. Pacing Clin Electrophysiol 21:1595–1600, 1998.

18. Power JM, Beacom GA, Alferness CA, et al: Susceptibility to atrial fibrillation: A study in an ovine model of pacing-induced early heart failure. J Cardiovasc Electrophysiol 9:423–435, 1998.

19. Li D, Fareh S, Leung TK, Nattel S: Promotion of atrial fibrillation by heart failure in dogs: Atrial remodeling of a different sort. Circulation 100:87–95, 1999.

20. Shinagawa K, Li D, Leung TK, Nattel S: Consequences of atrial tachycardia-induced remodeling depend on the preexisting atrial substrate. Circulation 105:251–257, 2002.

21. Cox JL, Canavan TE, Schuessler RB, et al: The surgical treatment of atrial fibrillation. II. Intraoperative electrophysiologic mapping and description of the electrophysiologic basis of atrial flutter and atrial fibrillation. J Thorac Cardiovasc Surg 101:406–426, 1991.

22. Verheule S, Wilson E, Everett T, et al: Alterations in atrial electrophysiology and tissue structure in a canine model of chronic atrial dilatation due to mitral regurgitation. Circulation 107:2615–2622, 2003.

23. Everett TH IV, Verheule S, Wilson EE, et al: Left atrial dilatation due to chronic mitral regurgitation decreases the spatiotemporal organization of atrial fibrillation in the left atrium. Am J Physiol Heart Circ Physiol 286:H2452–H2460, 2004.

24. Franz MR: Mechano-electrical feedback. Cardiovasc Res 45:263–266, 2000.

25. Ruwhof C, van der Laarse A: Mechanical stress-induced cardiac hypertrophy: Mechanisms and signal transduction pathways. Cardiovasc Res 47:23–37, 2000.

26. Goette A, Lendeckel U, Klein HU: Signal transduction systems and atrial fibrillation. Cardiovasc Res 54:247–258, 2002.

27. Arndt M, Lendeckel U, Rocken C, et al: Altered expression of ADAMs (A Disintegrin And Metalloproteinase) in fibrillating human atria. Circulation 105:720–725, 2002.

28. Sadoshima J, Izumo S: The cellular and molecular response of cardiac myocytes to mechanical stress. Annu Rev Physiol 59:551–571, 1997.

29. Goette A, Staack T, Roecken C, et al: Increased expression of extracellular signal-regulated kinase and angiotensin converting enzyme in human atria during atrial fibrillation. J Am Coll Cardiol 35:1669–1677, 2000.

30. Goette A, Arndt M, Rocken C, et al: Regulation of angiotensin II receptor subtypes during atrial fibrillation in humans. Circulation 101:2678–2681, 2000.

31. Cardin S, Li D, Thorin-Trescases N, et al: Evolution of the atrial fibrillation substrate in experimental congestive heart failure: Angiotensin-dependent and -independent pathways. Cardiovasc Res 60:315–325, 2003.

32. Lendeckel U, Arndt M, Wrenger S, et al: Expression and activity of ectopeptidases in fibrillating human atria. J Mol Cell Cardiol 33:1273–1281, 2001.

33. de Bakker JM, van Capelle FJ, Janse MJ, et al: Slow conduction in the infarcted human heart. 'Zigzag' course of activation. Circulation 88:915–926, 1993.

34. Spach MS, Josephson ME: Initiating reentry: The role of nonuniform anisotropy in small circuits. J Cardiovasc Electrophysiol 5:182–209, 1994.

35. Allessie MA, Boyden PA, Camm AJ, et al: Pathophysiology and prevention of atrial fibrillation. Circulation 103:769–777, 2001.

36. Satoh T, Zipes DP: Unequal atrial stretch in dogs increases dispersion of refractoriness conducive to developing atrial fibrillation. J Cardiovasc Electrophysiol 7:833–842, 1996.

37. Kamkin A, Kiseleva I, Isenberg G: Stretch-activated currents in ventricular myocytes: Amplitude and arrhythmogenic effects increase with hypertrophy. Cardiovasc Res 48:409–420, 2000.

38. Spach MS, Heidlage JF, Dolber PC, Barr RC: Changes in anisotropic conduction caused by remodeling cell size and the cellular distribution of gap junctions and Na(+) channels. J Electrocardiol 34(Suppl):69–76, 2001.

39. Shaw RM, Rudy Y: Ionic mechanisms of propagation in cardiac tissue. Roles of the sodium and L-type calcium currents during reduced excitability and decreased gap junction coupling. Circ Res 81:727–741, 1997.

40. Girouard SD, Pastore JM, Laurita KR, et al: Optical mapping in a new guinea pig model of ventricular tachycardia reveals mechanisms for multiple wavelengths in a single reentrant circuit. Circulation 93:603–613, 1996.

41. Li D, Shinagawa K, Pang L, et al: Effects of Angiotensin-converting enzyme inhibition on the development of the atrial fibrillation substrate in dogs with ventricular tachypacing-induced congestive heart failure. Circulation 104:2608–2614, 2001.

42. Gurlek A, Erol C, Basesme E: Antiarrhythmic effect of converting enzyme inhibitors in congestive heart failure. Int J Cardiol 43:315–318, 1994.

43. Pedersen OD, Bagger H, Kober L, Torp-Pedersen C: Trandolapril reduces the incidence of atrial fibrillation after acute myocardial infarction in patients with left ventricular dysfunction. Circulation 100:376–380, 1999.

44. Madrid AH, Bueno MG, Rebollo JM, et al: Use of irbesartan to maintain sinus rhythm in patients with long-lasting persistent atrial fibrillation: A prospective and randomized study. Circulation 106:331–336, 2002.

45. Hirayama Y, Atarashi H, Kobayashi Y, Takano T: Angiotensin-converting enzyme inhibitors are not effective at inhibiting further fibrous changes in the atria in patients with chronic atrial fibrillation. Jpn Heart J 45:93–101, 2004.

CHAPTER 18

Mechanical Versus Ischemic Preconditioning

• • • •

Michel Ovize and Karin Przyklenk

One or more brief episodes of coronary artery occlusion render the myocardium more resistant to a subsequent prolonged ischemic insult. This phenomenon has been termed *ischemic preconditioning* by Murry and colleagues.[1] Two temporal features of ischemic preconditioning have been described: the classical "early" preconditioning (as first reported by Murry and colleagues[1]) that occurs within 1 to 2 hours after the brief episodes of ischemia, and the "late" preconditioning ("second window of protection") that becomes active between 24 and 72 hours after the initial trigger stimulus.[2,3] The hallmark of ischemic preconditioning, observed in all models and species, is reduction of necrotic and apoptotic cell death by 40% to 70%, depending on the preparation that is used.[4,5] Several surrogate indices of preconditioning-induced cardioprotection, beyond reduction of myocardial cell death, also have been proposed. For example, preconditioning may be associated with an improvement in functional recovery after ischemia and reperfusion through the reduction of the amount of irreversibly injured tissue, but not through a direct effect on the contractile machinery,[6] whereas its effects on ischemia/reperfusion arrhythmias are still under debate.[7,8] Perhaps of greatest importance, several reports suggest that preconditioning may also protect the human heart.[9–11]

Several other stimuli, in addition to brief ischemia per se, have been shown to induce preconditioning, including activation of adenosine, bradykinin, opioid, adrenergic, or endothelin receptors, as well as opening of ATP-sensitive potassium (K^+_{ATP}) channels.[12] Ten years ago, our laboratory was the first to demonstrate that myocardial stretch, in the absence of ischemia, is also able to serve as a profound cardioprotective stimulus,[13] and our aim in this review is to summarize

both the evolution of and current knowledge regarding stretch-induced preconditioning.

MYOCARDIAL STRETCH DURING ISCHEMIA

The myocardium is composed of various cell types that are permanently submitted to cyclic mechanical forces. The most important cell type—the cardiomyocyte, which shortens during contraction and lengthens during relaxation—undergoes variations of approximately one third of its "resting" length during each cardiac cycle. In other words, cardiomyocytes are used to, and have adapted their physiology to, mechanical stress.

In some circumstances, abnormal mechanical strain may alter cardiomyocyte physiology, causing it to adapt. The most common response is cardiac hypertrophy. Hemodynamic overload is the predominant stimulus for cardiac hypertrophy, which is regarded as an adaptation to increased workload.[14,15] This increased mechanical loading is sensed by cardiomyocytes and is converted into a variety of intracellular biochemical and physical signals, with several reports suggesting an important role for calcium (Ca^{2+}) and calcineurin in stretch-induced gene expression.[14,16] Chronic increased workload (months to years) may eventually lead to congestive heart failure, arrhythmias, and sudden death.

A second pathologic condition that increases myocardial workload is ischemia. After cessation of coronary blood flow, contractile activity stops within seconds in the myocardial region supplied by the obstructed coronary artery. The ischemic myocardium becomes akinetic, and cardiomyocytes stop active contraction, whereas the nonischemic myocardium continues to work, and, in fact, typically exhibits compensatory hyperkinesis. During systole, increasing left ventricular (LV) pressure causes a passive deformation—that is, "bulging"—of the ischemic area, with resident cardiomyocytes undergoing excessive stretch.[17] When the ischemic period is short and does not cause irreversible damage, full recovery of myocardial structure and function is expected. If, however, the ischemia is prolonged, interstitial and intracellular edema may develop within the ischemic territory, creating additional mechanical strain.[18] Moreover, when the ischemic insult is sustained, and most of the ischemic myocardium becomes necrotic, this persistent regional stress may lead to the creation of a ventricular aneurysm.

These observations, together with the fact that preconditioning is triggered by one or more episodes of ischemia/reperfusion, prompted us to hypothesize that myocardial bulging and stretch may serve as a trigger for cardioprotection. We therefore sought to determine whether the unavoidable myocardial deformations induced by ischemia may, in themselves—that is, independently of ischemia-induced nonmechanical effects—initiate protection.

FIRST EVIDENCE THAT STRETCH PRECONDITIONS THE HEART

In the early 1990s, investigators questioned whether preconditioning was a local protection or whether it might be transported or transmitted to virgin myocardium. Specifically, Przyklenk and colleagues[19] sought to determine whether brief episodes of occlusion/reperfusion of the circumflex (CX) coronary artery may protect the remote left anterior descending (LAD)–dependent myocardium in the dog model. In that study, four episodes of 5-min CX branch occlusion reduced infarct size by 65% in the LAD bed (i.e., to a comparable extent than in situ preconditioning) in the absence of any difference of collateral blood flow. The authors concluded that preconditioning may be mediated by factor(s) activated, produced, or transported throughout the heart during brief ischemia/reperfusion.

Although the concept of "preconditioning at a distance" being mediated by a circulating factor or neuro-

transmission has been supported by several subsequent studies, another explanation to this initial observation may be proposed.[20–22] Using sonomicrometer crystals inserted within the myocardial wall, Przyklenk and colleagues[19] noticed that, during brief CX occlusion, the nonischemic LAD bed underwent a 12% increase in end-diastolic segment length (i.e., a 12% regional myocardial stretch). Accordingly, it was hypothesized that this regional stretch might serve as the trigger for the remote preconditioning-induced protection. Ovize and colleagues,[13] working in the same laboratory, tested this concept by producing myocardial stretch through an acute volume overload: Using the canine model, 500 mL/kg saline was infused over 10 min through the left atrial appendage, 10 min before 60 min of LAD occlusion and 4.5 hours of reperfusion. Acute volume overload caused a 15% increase in myocardial segment length, similar to the 19% increase observed during brief ischemia in a concurrent, preconditioned group (Fig. 18–1). Measurement of regional myocardial blood flow by radioactive microspheres demonstrated the absence of ischemia during volume overload. Interestingly, mechanical stretch proved to be as efficient as ischemic preconditioning in reducing infarct size.

One might argue that volume overload resulted in hemodilution that further led to transient hypoxia, which preconditioned the heart. However, saline infusion resulted in an increased myocardial blood flow before the prolonged coronary artery occlusion, and myocardial blood flow was comparable with control during the prolonged ischemic insult. Subsequent studies by Gysembergh and colleagues,[23] conducted in the in vivo rabbit model, confirmed cardioprotection with brief antecedent mechanical stretch, and, moreover, demonstrated that coronary venous lactate, an index of myocardial ischemia, was not increased after volume overload. In addition, they showed that volume overload through blood infusion (thereby excluding the possibility of hemodilution during saline infusion) was as effective as saline in initiating protection.

A second pivotal observation made in these studies was that gadolinium (Gd^{3+})—the archetypal blocker of stretch-activated ion channels (SAC)—despite having no significant effect on hemodynamics, contractile function, or myocardial blood flow, was able to prevent both stretch- and ischemia-induced preconditioning

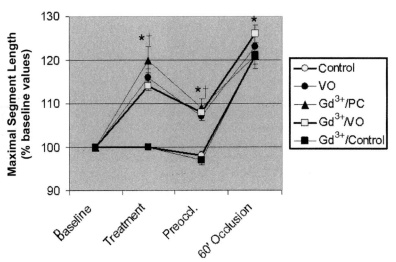

■ **Figure 18–1**　Myocardial stretch by volume overload (VO) and ischemia. Maximum segment length (expressed as percentage of baseline values) is presented for five experimental groups during the treatment (preconditioning [PC]) period and the subsequent 60 min of ischemia. Control and gadolinium (Gd^{3+})/control groups experienced no intervention before the 60-min ischemia VO and Gd^{3+}/VO groups underwent an acute volume overload (infusion of 500 mL saline over 10 min in the left atrium followed by 10 min without saline infusion). Gd^{3+} was injected intravenously at a dose of 25 μM/kg. VO, Gd^{3+}/VO, and Gd^{3+}/PC groups displayed similar degree of stretch during the treatment period. Moderate regional dilation persisted in these groups before the sustained ischemia. All hearts were similarly dilated during the 60-min ischemic insult 60 min occlusion. *, $P < 0.05$ vs. baseline; †, $P < 0.05$ vs. control. *(Modified from Ovize M, Przyklenk K, Kloner RA: Stretch preconditions the canine myocardium. Am J Physiol 266:H137–H146, 1994, with permission.)*

(Fig. 18–2). SAC have been described in various types of tissue, including cardiomyocytes.[24,25] Their physiologic role in cardiac cells remains poorly understood (see Chapters 1–4). Indirect evidence that SAC exist in the dog heart has been provided by Hansen and colleagues,[26] who induced ventricular arrhythmias by stretching the heart and, moreover, could block these stretch-induced arrhythmias using Gd^{3+}. Gd^{3+} has also been reported to inhibit other stretch-induced cardiac phenomena, including release of atrial natriuretic peptide in the rat.[27] The specificity of Gd^{3+} as a blocker of SAC has come under scrutiny, because the agent has been shown to inhibit voltage-dependent Ca^{2+} channels in some experimental preparations.[28] However, in this regard, Hansen and colleagues[26] demonstrated that stretch-induced arrhythmias were prevented by Gd^{3+}, but not by the Ca^{2+} channel blocker verapamil.

The role of volume-activated chloride currents also has been investigated in preconditioning; the rationale being that chloride (Cl^-) channels are purportedly involved in volume regulation in cardiomyocytes and may be mediators of ischemia/reperfusion injury. Diaz and colleagues[29] found that hypo-osmotic stress preconditioned isolated rabbit cardiomyocytes, and this beneficial effect was prevented by indanyloxyacetic acid 94 (IAA94) and 5-nitro-2-(3-phenylpropylamino)benzoic acid (NPPB), two blockers of Cl^- currents reportedly activated by cell swelling. Unfortunately, this observation was not confirmed by Heusch and colleagues,[30] and the potential contribution of volume-activated Cl^- channels to preconditioning remains a matter of debate. In fact, whole-cell currents activated by hypotonic swelling may be different from those activated by mechanical strain. Some of these volume-activated currents seem to depend on intracellular Ca^{2+}, adenosine triphosphate, or cyclic adenosine monophosphate (cAMP), suggesting that they might be activated through a secondary mechanism.[31]

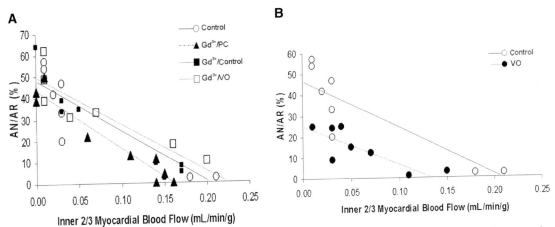

■ **Figure 18–2** Infarct size reduction after acute volume overload is prevented by gadolinium (Gd^{3+}). Infarct size is expressed as a function of regional myocardial blood flow. Area of necrosis (AN) is expressed as a function of the size of the area at risk (AR) and plotted versus the weighted inner two-thirds myocardial blood flow in the left anterior descending coronary artery bed during the 60-min coronary artery occlusion. Data points for Gd^{3+}/volume overload (VO), Gd^{3+}/preconditioning (PC), and Gd^{3+}/control lie close to the control regression line (A). In contrast, data points for VO groups are shifted downward vs. control line, indicating that they developed smaller infarcts for any level of collateral flow (B). (*Modified from Ovize M, Przyklenk K, Kloner RA: Stretch preconditions the canine myocardium. Am J Physiol 266:H137–H146, 1994, with permission.*)

STRETCH STIMULATES PRECONDITIONING-ACTIVATED SIGNALING PATHWAYS

To date, few studies have sought to elucidate the cellular mechanisms contributing to the protective effect achieved by SAC activation in myocardial preconditioning. Nonetheless, there is emerging evidence that common cellular mediators may be involved in both ischemic and stretch-induced protection. Specifically, it has been reported that phospholipases C and D are activated by ischemic preconditioning, and it is acknowledged that protein kinase C (PKC) activation is a key component of this cardioprotection.[32–34] Similarly, Komuro and colleagues demonstrated, in a primary culture of rat ventricular myocytes, that stretch activates both phospholipases C and D and increases the production of diacylglycerol, the natural activator of PKC.[35] Moreover, the PKC inhibitors staurosporine and polymyxin B blocked the infarct-sparing effect of both stretch- and ischemia-induced preconditioning in the isolated working rat heart (Fig. 18–3)

and in the in situ rabbit heart model.[32,34] These data support the concept that a mechanical challenge can activate PKC.

Downstream targets of PKC in stretch-induced preconditioned myocardium remain unclear. Takeishi and colleagues,[36] using the isolated working guinea pig heart, showed that acute mechanical stretch (through balloon inflation in the LV cavity to achieve an end-diastolic pressure of 25 mm Hg for 10–20 min) activates extracellular signal-regulated kinase (ERK)-1 and ERK-2, p90RSK (90-kDa ribosomal S6 kinase) p38, Src, and big MAP kinase (BMK)-1, but not c-Jun NH2 terminal kinase (JNK). Furthermore, mechanical stretch-induced activation of ERK-1 and -2 and p38 kinase was significantly attenuated by pretreatment with the PKC inhibitor chelerythrine. Yet, the balloon inflation within the LV cavity used to stretch the myocardium might also induce subendocardial ischemia, which, in itself, might activate ERK-1 and -2 and mitogen-activated protein kinase (MAPK). Myocardial stretch also has been achieved in anesthetized rabbits by acute constriction of the

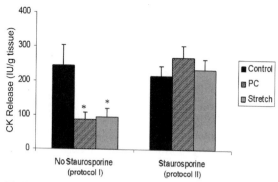

■ **Figure 18–3** The protein kinase C (PKC) inhibitor staurosporine blocks stretch-induced and ischemic preconditioning. Creatine kinase (CK) release, a surrogate end point for infarct size assessment, was measured in the coronary effluent of rat hearts submitted to either no intervention (control group), 5 min of ischemia and 10 min of reperfusion (ischemic preconditioning group [PC]), or left ventricular stretch by abruptly increasing left atrial pressure from 5 to 20 cm H_2O for 5 min (stretch group) before 30 min of ischemia and 30 min of reperfusion. Both brief ischemia and stretch reduced CK release. This protective effect was abolished by the PKC inhibitor staurosporine. *, $P < 0.05$ vs. control. (*Modified from Obadia JF, Ovize M, Abadie C, et al: Beneficial actions of preconditioning and stretch on postischemic contractile function of isolated working rat heart: Effects of staurosporine. J Cardiovasc Pharmacol 30:191–196, 1997, with permission.*)

descending thoracic aorta and a resultant increase in LV afterload. Using this latter model, Iliodromitis and colleagues[37] reported a significant infarct size limiting effect of myocardial stretch, associated with an increased phosphorylation of p38 MAPK, which was prevented by Gd^{3+}. However, in this preparation, Gd^{3+} failed to prevent ischemic preconditioning and ERK-1 and -2 phosphorylation after 20 min of ischemia. Interpretation of these data, as well as the outcome of many preconditioning studies dealing with activation of these signaling pathways, must be made with caution because of differences in experimental preparations and design, and because of the notoriously transient nature of activation of these kinases during ischemia, reperfusion, or both.[12]

STRETCH-INDUCED PRECONDITIONING SPECULATIONS AND FUTURE DIRECTIONS

Although the mechanisms of both ischemia- and stretch-induced preconditioning remain incompletely resolved, some signaling pathways seem common to both types of cardioprotection; this commonality, in turn, provides a rational foundation for speculation regarding the mechanism of stretch-induced protection. For example, several studies have indicated that Ca^{2+} may play a role in preconditioning, with transient exposure to increased extracellular Ca^{2+} mimicking ischemic preconditioning in both isolated rat hearts[38] and the in vivo canine model.[39] Bauer and colleagues[40] showed that myocardial concentrations of inositol-1,4,5-trisphosphate (IP_3), a second messenger generated "in parallel" with diacylglycerol and PKC and a crucial mediator of Ca^{2+} release from intracellular stores, was increased after brief episodes of preconditioning ischemia in the rabbit heart, whereas exogenous administration of a synthetic analogue of IP_3 mimicked preconditioning in the rabbit model.[41] It is well recognized that activation of SAC elicits an increase in intracellular Ca^{2+} concentration, and Dassouli and colleagues[42] reported that in vitro stretch causes an increase in the second messengers IP_3 and IP_4, which modulate cytosolic Ca^{2+}. These studies indirectly suggest that SAC might precondition the heart by increasing net intracellular Ca^{2+}, potentiating the release of Ca^{2+} from intracellular stores, or both.

Several studies reported a central role for ERK-1 and -2 and phosphatidylinositol-3 kinase (PI3K)-Akt pathways in myocardial hypertrophy.[43,44] The ERK-1 and -2 cascade promotes cell growth, division, and survival. During mechanotransduction, the proteins phosphorylated and activated by ERK-1 and -2 include p90RSK, which modulates apoptosis through BAD, transcription factors, and other signaling proteins. A number of biological effects that have been attributed to Akt may contribute to the protection of the ischemic myocardium. Akt leads to inhibition of BAD-triggered apoptosis through activation of p70S6 kinase, modulates carbohydrate metabolism through inhibition of glycogen synthase kinase 3, and activates endothelial nitric oxide synthase, which is important in the regulation of cardiac function.[43] In addition, Akt activates transcription factors such as nuclear factor (NF)-κB or cAMP response element-binding protein, both involved in cardioprotection.[45] Several reports have demonstrated a role for activation of ERK-1 and -2 or PI3K-Akt, specifically during the early minutes of reperfusion after a prolonged ischemic insult, in the protection afforded by ischemic preconditioning.[46,47] Jonassen and colleagues[47] reported that PD98059, an inhibitor of the ERK pathway, prevented ischemic preconditioning. Tong and colleagues[48] demonstrated that ischemic preconditioning activates PI3K, and they reported that wortmannin, an inhibitor of PI3K, attenuates the protection afforded by ischemic preconditioning.

Conclusion

The data presented in this chapter suggest—but do not prove—that acute mechanical stretch and brief ischemia may activate common prosurvival pathways and trigger myocardial preconditioning. Currently, however, there is no direct evidence to support the concept that acute mechanical stretch, in the absence of ischemia, can precondition the myocardium through activation of ERK-1 and -2 or PI3K-Akt. Furthermore, recent studies suggest that either mitochondrial K^+_{ATP} channels or the mitochondrial permeability transition pore may be end-effectors of ischemic preconditioning.[49-52] Neither of these two potential candidates for cardioprotection are known targets of myocardial stretch, although Gysembergh and colleagues[23] demonstrated that glibenclamide, a blocker of mitochondrial (as well as sarcolemmal) K^+_{ATP} channels, abolishes stretch-induced preconditioning. Therefore, further studies are required to elucidate the specific mechanisms by which acute myocardial stretch can trigger cardioprotection and to establish definitively whether common mechanisms and mediators truly underlie both stretch- and ischemia-induced preconditioning.

References

1. Murry CE, Jennings RB, Reimer KA: "Preconditioning" with ischemia: A delay of lethal cell injury in ischemic myocardium. Circulation 5:1124–1136, 1986.
2. Kuzuya T, Hoshida S, Yamashita N, et al: Delayed effects of sublethal ischemia on the acquisition of tolerance to ischemia. Circ Res 72:1293–1299, 1993.
3. Marber MS, Latchman DS, Walker JM, Yellon DM: Cardiac stress protein elevation 24 hours after brief ischemia or heat stress is associated with resistance to myocardial infarction. Circulation 88:1264–1272, 1993.
4. Ovize M, Kloner RA, Hale SH, Przyklenk K: Coronary cyclic flow variations precondition the ischemic myocardium. Circulation 85:779–789, 1992.
5. Piot CA, Padmanaban D, Ursell PC, et al: Ischemic preconditioning decreases apoptosis in rat heart in vivo. Circulation 96:1598–1604, 1997.
6. Ovize M, Przyklenk K, Kloner RA: Preconditioning does not attenuate myocardial stunning. Circulation 85:2247–2254, 1992.
7. Shiki K, Hearse DJ: "Preconditioning" of ischemic myocardium: Reperfusion-induced arrhythmias. Am J Physiol 253: H1470–H1476, 1987.
8. Ovize M, Aupetit JF, Rioufol G, et al: Preconditioning reduces infarct size but accelerates time to ventricular fibrillation in the pig heart. Am J Physiol 269:H72–H79, 1995.
9. Yellon DM, Alkhulaifi A, Pugsley WB: Preconditioning the human heart. Lancet 342:276–277, 1993.
10. Deutsch E, Berger M, Kussmaul WG, et al: Adaptation to ischemia during percutaneous transluminal angioplasty: Clinical, hemodynamic, and metabolic features. Circulation 82:2044–2051, 1990.
11. Kloner RA, Shook T, Przyklenk K, et al: "Previous angina alters in hospital outcome in TIMI 4. A clinical correlate to preconditioning?" Circulation 91:37–47, 1995.
12. Yellon DM, Downey JM: Preconditioning the myocardium: From cellular physiology to clinical cardiology. Physiol Rev 83:1113–1151, 2003.
13. Ovize M, Przyklenk K, Kloner RA: Stretch preconditions the canine myocardium. Am J Physiol 266:H137–H146, 1994.
14. Komuro I, Kaida T, Shibazaki Y, et al: Stretching cardiac myocytes stimulates protooncogene expression. J Biol Chem 265:3595–3598, 1990.
15. Sadoshima J, Izumo S: The cellular and molecular response of cardiac myocytes to mechanical stress. Annu Rev Physiol 59: 551–571, 1997.
16. Frey N, McKinsey TA, Olson EN: Decoding calcium signals involved in cardiac growth and function. Nat Med 6:1221–1227, 2000.
17. Vokonas PS, Pirzada F, Hood WB Jr: Experimental myocardial infarction: XII. Dynamic changes in segmental mechanical behavior of infarcted and non-infarcted myocardium. Am J Cardiol 37:853–859, 1976.
18. Jennings RB, Reimer KA, Hill ML: Total ischemia in dog hearts, in vitro: 2. High energy phosphate depletion and associated defects in energy metabolism, cell volume regulation, and sarcolemmal integrity. Circ Res 49:901–911, 1981.
19. Przyklenk K, Bauer B, Ovize M, et al: Regional ischemic preconditioning protects remote virgin myocardium from subsequent sustained coronary occlusion. Circulation 87:893–899, 1993.
20. Birnbaum Y, Hale SL, Kloner RA: Ischemic preconditioning at a distance. Reduction of myocardial infarct size by partial reduction of blood supply combined with rapid stimulation of the gastrocnemius muscle in the rabbit. Circulation 96: 1641–1646, 1997.
21. Pell TJ, Baxter GF, Yellon DM, Drew GM: Renal ischemia preconditions myocardium: Role for adenosine receptors and ATP-sensitive potassium channels. Am J Physiol 275:H1542–H1547, 1998.

22. Gho BCG, Schoemaker RG, van den Doel MA, et al: Myocardial protection by brief ischemia in noncardiac tissue. Circulation 94:2193–2200, 1996.

23. Gysembergh A, Margonari H, Loufoua J, et al: Stretch-induced protection shares common mechanisms with ischemic preconditioning in the rabbit heart? Am J Physiol 274:H955–H964, 1998.

24. Craelius W, Chen V, El-Sherif N: Stretch-activated ion channels in ventricular myocytes. Biosci Rep 8:407–414, 1988.

25. Guharay F, Sachs F: Stretch-activated single ion channel currents in tissue-cultured embryonic chick skeletal muscle. J Physiol Lond 352:685–701, 1984.

26. Hansen DE, Borganelli M, Stacy GP Jr, Taylor LK: Dose-dependent inhibition of stretch-induced arrhythmias by gadolinium in isolated canine ventricles. Evidence for a unique mode of antiarrhythmic action. Circ Res 69:820–831, 1991.

27. Laine M, Arjamaa O, Vuolteenaho O, et al: Block of stretch-activated atrial natriuretic peptide secretion by gadolinium in isolated rat atrium. J Physiol (Lond) 480:553–561, 1994.

28. Biagi BA, Enyart JJ: Gadolinium blocks low and high threshold calcium currents in pituitary cells. Am J Physiol 259:C515–C520, 1990.

29. Diaz RJ, Losito VA, Mao GD, et al: Chloride channel inhibition blocks the protection of ischemic preconditioning and hypo-osmotic stress in rabbit ventricular myocardium. Circ Res 84:763–775, 1999.

30. Heusch G, Liu GS, Rose J, et al: No confirmation for a causal role of volume-regulated chloride channels in ischemic preconditioning in rabbits. J Mol Cell Cardiol 32:2279–2285, 2000.

31. Hall SK, Zhang JP, Liebermann M: Cyclic AMP prevents activation of a swelling-induced chloride-sensitive conductance in chick heart cells. J Physiol (Lond) 488:359–369, 1995.

32. Obadia JF, Ovize M, Abadie C, et al: Beneficial actions of preconditioning and stretch on postischemic contractile function of isolated working rat heart: Effects of staurosporine. J Cardiovasc Pharmacol 30:191–196, 1997.

33. Cohen MV, Liu Y, Liu GS, et al: Phospholipase D plays a role in ischemic preconditioning in rabbit heart. Circulation 94:1713–1718, 1996.

34. Gysembergh A, Zakaroff A, Loufoua J, et al: Enhanced diacyl-glycerol production during the first but not during subsequent ischemia in preconditioned rabbit heart: Role of phospholipase D activation. Basic Res Cardiol 95:457–465, 2000.

35. Komuro I, Katoh Y, Kaida T, et al: Mechanical loading stimulates cell hypertrophy and specific gene expression in cultured rat cardiac myocytes. Possible role for protein kinase C. J Biol Chem 266:1265–1268, 1991.

36. Takeishi Y, Huang Q, Abe J, et al: Src and multiple MAP kinase activation in cardiac hypertrophy and congestive heart failure under chronic pressure-overload: Comparison with acute mechanical stretch. J Mol Cell Cardiol 33:1637–1648, 2001.

37. Iliodromitis EK, Gaitanaki C, Lazou A, et al: Dissociation of stress-activated protein kinase (p38-MAPK and JNKs) phosphorylation from the protective effect of preconditioning in vivo. J Mol Cell Cardiol 34:1019–1028, 2002.

38. Xu M, Wang Y, Hirai K, et al: Calcium preconditioning inhibits mitochondrial permeability transition and apoptosis. Am J Physiol 280:H899–H908, 2001.

39. Przyklenk K, Hata K, Kloner RA: Is calcium a mediator of infarct size reduction with preconditioning in rabbit myocardium? Circulation 97:692–702, 1997.

40. Bauer B, Simkhovich BZ, Kloner RA, Przyklenk K: Preconditioning-induced cardioprotection and release of the second messenger inositol(1,4,5)triphosphate are both abolished by neomycin in rabbit heart. Basic Res Cardiol 94:31–40, 1999.

41. Gysembergh A, Lemaire S, Piot C, et al: Pharmacologic manipulation of Ins(1,4,5)P3 signaling mimics preconditioning in rabbit heart. Am J Physiol 277:H2451–H2457, 1999.

42. Dassouli A, Sulpice JC, Roux S, Crozatier B: Stretch-induced inositol triphosphate and tetrakiphosphate production in rat cardiomyocytes. J Mol Cell Cardiol 25:973–982, 1993.

43. Sugden PH: Ras, Akt and mechanotransduction in the cardiac myocyte. Circ Res 93:1179–1192, 2003.

44. Armstrong SC: Protein kinase activation and myocardial ischemia/reperfusion injury. Cardiovasc Res 61:427–436, 2004.

45. Derek J, Hausenloy H, Derek M: New directions for protecting the heart against ischaemia–reperfusion injury: Targeting the reperfusion injury salvage kinase (RISK)-pathway. Cardiovasc Res 61:448–460, 2004.

46. Gao F, Gao E, Yue TL, et al: Nitric oxide mediates the antiapoptotic effect of insulin in myocardial ischemia-reperfusion. The roles of PI3-kinase, Akt, and endothelial nitric oxide synthase phosphorylation. Circulation 105:1497–1502, 2002.

47. Jonassen AK, Sack MN, Mjos OD, Yellon DM: Myocardial protection by insulin at reperfusion requires early administration and is mediated via Akt and p70s6 kinase cell-survival signalling. Circ Res 89:1191–1198, 2001.

48. Tong H, Chen W, Steenbergen C, Murphy E: Ischemic preconditioning activates phosphatidylinositol-3-kinase upstream of protein kinase C. Circ Res 87:309–315, 2000.

49. Argaud L, Gateau-Roesch O, Chalabreysse L, et al: Preconditioning delays Ca^{2+} induced mitochondrial permeability transition. Cardiovasc Res 61:115–122, 2004.

50. Piriou V, Chiari P, Gateau-Roesch O, et al: Desflurane-induced preconditioning delays mitochondrial permeability transition pore opening. Anesthesiology 100:581–588, 2004.

51. Piriou V, Chiari P, Loufoua J, et al: Prevention of isoflurane-induced preconditioning by 5-hydroxydecanoate and gadolinium: Possible involvement of mitochondrial K^+_{ATP} and stretch-activated channels. Anesthesiology 93:756–764, 2000.

52. Hausenloy DJ, Maddock HL, Baxter GF, Yellon DM: Inhibiting mitochondrial permeability transition pore opening: A new paradigm for myocardial preconditioning? Cardiovasc Res 55:534–543, 2002.

CARDIAC MECHANO-ELECTRIC FEEDBACK IN NORMAL PHYSIOLOGY

• • • •

CHAPTER 19

Non-neural Component of Respiratory Sinus Arrhythmia

• • • •

Barbara Casadei

Respiratory sinus arrhythmia (RSA) describes cyclic changes in heart rate associated with breathing.[1] Although the mechanisms involved in generating RSA are still under debate, it is widely accepted that RSA reflects fluctuations in cardiac vagal activity, and as such it can be used as an integrated measure of cardiac vagal responsiveness in conscious animal models and in humans.[2,3] This chapter describes the contribution of non-neural fluctuation of heart rate to RSA and discusses the mechanisms involved in stretch-mediated changes of sinoatrial node (SAN) activity (see Chapter 8).

RESPIRATORY SINUS ARRHYTHMIA ASSESSMENT

A precise assessment of RSA has been made possible by the application of time and frequency domain measurements of heart rate variability (HRV) to short or 24-hour electrocardiogram (ECG) recordings; these indices have been extensively used as noninvasive semi-quantitative markers of tonic cardiac vagal control in physiologic and pathologic conditions.[4] In particular, application of power spectral analysis to simultaneous short-term recordings of ECG and of a breathing signal (e.g., a nasal thermistor or a chest impedance signal) have allowed a fairly precise assessment of the frequency range and amplitude of pulse interval oscillations that are entrained by breathing. The amplitude or "spectral power" of RSA (or high-frequency power in the frequency range from 0.15–0.60 Hz) often has been expressed as a percentage of the total pulse interval variability over the time of recording (i.e., in normalized units) or as low-frequency/high-frequency (LF/HF) ratio, where LF oscillations (usually in the range from 0.04–0.15 Hz) have been taken as representing the baroreflex modulation of cardiac sympathetic outflow and the ratio as a measure of cardiac sympatho-vagal balance[5,6] (Fig. 19–1). Although several studies (e.g., see References 7 and 8) have indicated that to equate the HF oscillations of the pulse interval to cardiac vagal activity and the LF oscillation to sympathetic nerve inputs may be an oversimplification, this assumption has been found to fit the paradigm in a wide variety of experimental conditions where the spontaneous variability of the pulse interval was relatively well maintained. For example, stimuli that are known to increase sympathetic nerve discharge, such as head-up tilting, standing, and mental stress, have all been associated with a relative increase in the LF component, and hence in the LF/HF ratio. Similarly, bilateral stellectomy, β-adrenergic blockade, and muscarinic receptor stimulation cause an increase in the amplitude of the respiratory/vagal component of HRV (for a review of this topic, see Reference 6).

There are, however, some notable exceptions. For instance, patients with severe heart failure who are known to have low cardiac vagal responsiveness and increased sympathetic nerve discharge can have a relatively large HF component, when expressed in normalized units.[9–11] Similarly, other conditions characterized by a greatly reduced cardiac vagal control (e.g., severe exercise,[8] or systemic administration of muscarinic receptor blockers[7]) have shown a relative dominance of HF oscillations in the HRV power spectrum, suggesting that there might be breathing-induced heart rate oscillations that are not mediated by fluctuations in vagal efferent activity to the SAN. Indeed, a small degree of RSA is seen in patients who had a recent heart transplant and who have no functional innervation to the donor SAN (Fig. 19–2).[12–14]

A Rest

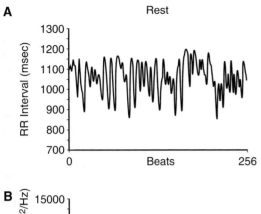

B

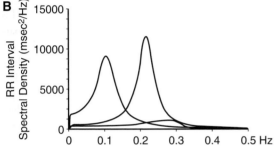

C

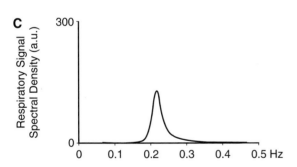

QRS Sequence

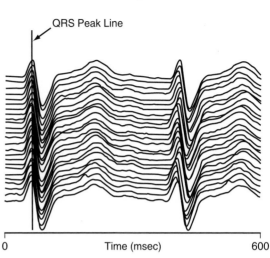

■ **Figure 19–2** Sequence of electrocardiographic QRS complexes recorded in a heart transplant patient. Note that after aligning all QRS complexes to the peak line, the QRS distance fluctuates rhythmically with breathing. *(From Bernardi L, Salvucci F, Suardi R, et al: Evidence for an intrinsic mechanism regulating heart rate variability in the transplanted and the intact heart during submaximal exercise? Cardiovasc Res 24:969–981, 1990, with permission.)*

■ **Figure 19–1** Tachogram *(A)* and spectral analysis of the RR interval variability *(B)* and of the breathing signal *(C)* at rest in a young male subject. Note that the RR interval variability comprises two main oscillations: a low-frequency peak, which is centered at approximately 0.1 Hz, and a high-frequency component, which is centered at the same frequency as breathing *(C)* and represents respiratory sinus arrhythmia. *(From Casadei B, Moon J, Caiazza A, Sleight P: Is respiratory sinus arrhythmia a good index of cardiac vagal activity during exercise? J Appl Physiol 81:556–564, 1996, with permission.)*

This indicates that non-neural mechanisms, such as rhythmic stretching of the SAN caused by changes in atrial transmural pressure with breathing, may contribute to RSA. Although the substantial reduction in

RSA (in absolute values) produced by autonomic blockade indicates that any non-neural contribution to RSA must be small in young healthy subjects at rest,[7,15,16] this may not be true in conditions in which cardiac vagal activity or responsiveness is reduced, such as in heart failure and during exercise.

NON-NEURAL RESPIRATORY SINUS ARRHYTHMIA

Non-Neural Respiratory Sinus Arrhythmia and Exercise

Spectral analysis of HRV in healthy subjects and in heart transplant recipients has shown that, despite considerable differences at rest, the amplitude of RSA during moderate and severe exercise is similar in the two groups.[17] Indeed, after the initial dramatic reduction at the beginning of exercise, the amplitude of RSA tends to remain stable and to account for most of the residual HRV, indicating either the persistence of some cardiac vagal activity or a complete vagal withdrawal in the early stages of exercise and the presence of non-neurally mediated pulse interval oscillations, driven by breathing.[8]

Studies comparing heart transplant recipients with healthy volunteers have shown that although the spectral power of the HRV decreases with increasing work rates, the non-neural component of RSA that is observed in patients with a denervated heart tends to increase in response to exercise.[14,17] Thus, in the presence of reduced HRV, the use of normalized units or of the LF/HF ratio to assess autonomic inputs to the heart grossly overestimates vagal activity.

A similar conclusion was reached by comparing the amplitude of RSA during exercise before and after ganglion blockade in young healthy volunteers.[16] These experiments have unequivocally demonstrated that non-neural mechanisms contribute to RSA, whereas pulse interval oscillations in the LF range are an entirely neurally-mediated phenomenon. Although the contribution of stretch-mediated oscillations in pulse interval is negligible at rest in young healthy subjects, during mild exercise (when vagal efferent activity to the heart is reduced) it accounts for approximately one third of the amplitude of RSA (Fig. 19–3).[16]

Non-neural Respiratory Sinus Arrhythmia in Patients with Heart Failure

Similar considerations may be applicable to patients with chronic congestive heart failure (CHF), who are known to have impaired cardiac parasympathetic responsiveness.[18] In these patients, HRV often has been used as a marker to evaluate the effect of therapeutic intervention and as a tool for risk stratification.[19–22]

Spectral analysis of the HRV in patients with CHF has shown that the absolute power in the LF range decreases with the worsening of the disease, and often it is absent in New York Heart Association (NYHA) Class IV patients.[9] Similarly, the absolute power of the HF component has been found to be significantly reduced from the early stages of the disease.[10,11] However, heart rate fluctuations in the HF range are present even in the most advanced stages of CHF, where they can account for most of the short-term HRV.[9,11] To explain this finding, it has been suggested that RSA in severe CHF might be entirely mediated by non-neural mechanisms.[9,11]

Experiments in anesthetized pigs, however, have indicated that atrial stretch (which is common in patients with CHF who have increased right atrial pressure) may suppress both neural and non-neural components of RSA,[23] suggesting that the relative contribution of non-neural mechanisms to RSA in patients with CHF may remain small, despite a reduction in the variability of the pulse interval. This hypothesis has not been confirmed by studies comparing the magnitude of non-neural RSA (recorded in the presence of complete ganglion blockade) in healthy subjects and in patients with mild CHF (NYHA Class II).[24] Non-neural RSA was similar in the two groups, but because patients with CHF had lower HRV than control subjects, the relative contribution of non-neural oscillations to RSA was greater in patients with CHF than in healthy, age-matched control subjects (15% vs. 3%) and was inversely related to HRV (as assessed by the standard deviation of the pulse interval; Fig. 19–4).

Taken together, these findings confirm that the HF power of HRV can overestimate cardiac parasympathetic responsiveness in patients with mild CHF and, indeed, whenever the HRV is significantly reduced. The strong inverse relation between contribution of non-neural mechanisms to the HF power and HRV provides a proof of principle that can be applied to virtually all pathophysiologic conditions associated with a reduction in cardiac vagal activity or responsiveness.

Mechanisms Underlying Non-neural Respiratory Sinus Arrhythmia

Non-neural heart rate fluctuations in the HF range result from periodic stretching of the SAN, secondary to changes in atrial transmural pressure with breathing.[25,26] If this were the only mechanism responsible for non-neural RSA, we would expect its amplitude to be modulated by factors that might affect the magnitude of oscillations in right atrial pressure such as tidal

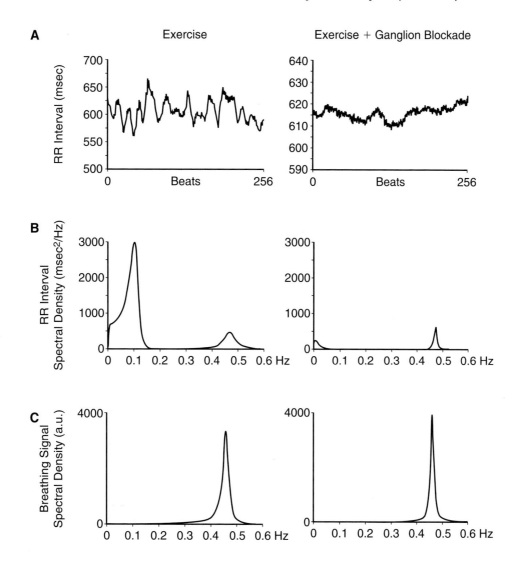

■ **Figure 19–3** Tachogram *(A)* and spectral analysis of the RR interval variability *(B)* and of the breathing signal *(C)* during mild supine exercise before and during ganglion blockade in the subject shown in Figure 19-1. Exercise caused a reduction in RR interval and its spectral density. The central frequency of the high-frequency (HF) component (on the *x* axis) shifted to the right (0.47 Hz) as a result of increased breathing rate. Note that the HF component is not much changed by ganglion blockade, indicating that during exercise a significant proportion of respiratory sinus arrhythmia is caused by non-neural mechanisms. *(From Casadei B, Moon J, Caiazza A, Sleight P: Is respiratory sinus arrhythmia a good index of cardiac vagal activity during exercise? J Appl Physiol 81:556–564, 1996, with permission.)*

volume and ventilation. This was indeed demonstrated both in heart transplant recipients[13] and in anesthetized vagotomized and β-blocked rabbits.[26] In the presence of cardiac denervation, the amplitude of non-neural RSA was found to be directly proportional to

tidal volume and ventilation and to increase with the rate of change in intrathoracic pressure. This mechanism may be responsible for the increase in the absolute magnitude of non-neural RSA that has been reported in heart transplant recipients during upright

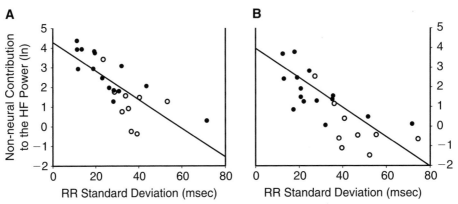

■ **Figure 19–4**   Relation between the standard deviation of the RR interval and the non-neural contribution to the high-frequency (HF) component in healthy control subjects *(open circles)* and in patients with mild chronic heart failure *(solid circles)* during spontaneous (A; r^2 = 0.53; $P < 0.0001$) and controlled breathing at 0.16 Hz (B; r^2 = 0.50; $P < 0.0001$). Note that as the RR interval variability decreases, most of the amplitude of the HF spectral component is caused by non-neural oscillations, indicating that under these conditions, respiratory sinus arrythmia ceases to be a reliable marker of cardiac vagal responsiveness. *(From El-Omar M, Kardos A, Casadei B: Mechanisms of respiratory sinus arrhythmia in patients with mild heart failure. Am J Physiol 280:H125–H131, 2001, with permission.)*

exercise.[14] Conversely, in the supine position, where fluctuations in venous return and transthoracic pressure are less affected by exercise,[27] cycloergometry did not change the amplitude of RSA in young subjects during ganglion blockade.[16]

Experiments in animals have clearly shown that non-neural mechanisms can affect heart rate and its variability.[28] Sinusoidal changes in intramural pressure of isolated atria preparations cause synchronous oscillations in heart rate.[29] Interestingly, the pressure changes required to obtain significant variations in atrial rate are quite similar to fluctuations in atrial transmural pressure that occur during respiration.

Pacemaking activity is known to be enhanced by mechanical stretch.[30] Stretch-sensitive cells have been identified in the rat SAN, and their electrophysiological characteristics suggest they may be cardiac fibroblasts, which depolarize in response to stretch.[31]

The mechanism by which stretch increases sinoatrial frequency remains unclear, but it has been suggested that an increase in length[32] or tension[33] might stimulate the pacemaker activity of SAN cells by increasing chloride permeability, mobilization of intracellular calcium (Ca^{2+}),[34] or stretch activation of cation channels. This hypothesis was confirmed by experiments showing that application of moderate longitudinal stretch to isolated SAN cells increases their spontaneous beating rate and reduces the maximum diastolic and systolic potentials.[35] Voltage clamp step protocols revealed a stretch-induced current in SAN cells that was consistent with activation of cation nonselective stretch-activated channels.[35]

Whether stretch is sensed directly by stretch-activated channels or is transduced at the channel level by a second messenger remains a matter of debate. Myocardial release of the free radical nitric oxide (NO) from the endothelial nitric oxide synthase (eNOS) has been recently implicated in the myocardial response to stretch. For instance, Pinsky and colleagues[36] have shown that NO (measured in vivo in the rabbit heart by a porphyrinic microsensor) is released in a pulsatile fashion (with a peak in diastole of 2.7 ± 0.1 µM/L), which is positively correlated with preload and enhanced by stretch. Consistent with these findings, Prendergast and colleagues[37] demonstrated that the effect of endogenous NO in isolated guinea pig working hearts became significant only in the presence of high preloads.

A causal relation between stretch and NO release in the heart also is supported by data showing that blockers of stretch-activated channels, such as gadolinium, also inhibit NO generation.[38,39]

In isolated cardiomyocytes, the slow increase in intracellular Ca^{2+} transients that is observed in response to stretch is associated with an increase in intracellular NO release and is abolished by NOS inhibition or by knockout of the eNOS gene.[40] Because stretched myocytes exhibit increased intracellular Ca^{2+} release in the absence of changes in the Ca^{2+} content of the sarcoplasmic reticulum, it was suggested that stretch-induced NO release may increase the open probability of the ryanodine receptor (RyR) Ca^{2+} release channels (by direct nitrosylation of reactive thiols on the channel protein).

In the SAN, stretch-induced NO release may contribute to the positive chronotropic response seen with an increase in right atrial filling pressure (i.e., the Bainbridge reflex[41]), and hence to the non-neural RSA, both by facilitating Ca^{2+} release through the RyR and by increasing the "pacemaker" current hyperpolarization-activated inward current (I_f).[42,43] Consistent with this idea, stretch depolarizes the maximal diastolic potential and increases the slope of spontaneous diastolic depolarization in SAN multicellular preparations without affecting action potential duration.[30,34] Moreover, stretch-mediated positive chronotropic responses are inhibited by ryanodine and thapsigargin, but not by nifedipine, suggesting that release of Ca^{2+} from intracellular stores may be an important mechanotransducer in the SAN.[34] All of the stretch-mediated changes described earlier are mimicked by the application of low-micromolar concentrations of NO donors to SAN preparations.[42,43] Taken together, these data suggest that stretch-induced modulation of I_f and RyR Ca^{2+} release channels by NO may constitute a novel mechanism involved in cardiac mechano-electric feedback in the SAN.

Conclusion

Fluctuations in heart rate, elicited by breathing-induced changes in right atrial transmural pressure, contribute to RSA. The mechanisms responsible for stretch-induced changes in the activity of the SAN are only partially elucidated and may involve stretch-activated ion channels, release of Ca^{2+} from intracellular stores, the pacemaker current I_f, and NO.

As mechanically induced heart rate oscillations are small, RSA can still be regarded as a good index of cardiac vagal responsiveness in young healthy subjects at rest. However, in situations where cardiac vagal activity is reduced (e.g., exercise and heart failure), non-neural heart rate oscillations can account for most of the residual amplitude of RSA, which therefore ceases to be a reliable marker of cardiac vagal activity.

References

1. Ludwig G: Beiträge zur Kenntniss des Einflusses der Respirationsbewegungen auf den Blutlauf im Aortensystem. Archiv der Anatomie und Physiologie 13:242–302, 1847.
2. Katona PG, Jih F: Respiratory sinus arrhythmia: A noninvasive measure of parasympathetic control. J Appl Physiol 39:801–805, 1975.
3. Eckberg DL: Human sinus arrhythmia as an index of vagal cardiac outflow. J Appl Physiol 54:961–966, 1983.
4. Task Force of the European Society of Cardiology and the North American Society of Pacing and Electrophysiology: Heart rate variability: Standards of measurement, physiological interpretation and clinical use. Circulation 93:1043–1065, 1996.
5. Pagani M, Lombardi F, Guzzetti S, et al: Power spectral analysis of heart rate and arterial pressure variabilities as a marker of sympatho-vagal interaction in man and conscious dog. Circ Res 59:178–193, 1986.
6. Malliani A, Pagani M, Lombardi F, Cerutti C: Cardiovascular neural regulation explored in the frequency domain. Circulation 84:482–492, 1991.
7. Saul JP, Berger RD, Albrecht P, et al: Transfer function analysis of the circulation: Unique insight into cardiovascular regulation. Am J Physiol 261:H1231–H1245, 1991.
8. Casadei B, Cochrane S, Johnston J, et al: Pitfalls in the interpretation of spectral analysis of the heart rate variability during exercise in humans. Acta Physiol Scand 153:125–131, 1995.
9. Mortara A, La Rovere MT, Signorini MG, et al: Can power spectral analysis of heart rate variability identify a high risk subgroup of congestive heart failure patients with excessive sympathetic activation? A pilot study before and after heart transplantation. Br Heart J 71:422–430, 1994.
10. Casolo GC, Stroder P, Sulla A, et al: Heart rate variability and functional severity of congestive heart failure secondary to coronary artery disease. Eur Heart J 16:360–367, 1995.
11. Guzzetti S, Cogliati C, Turiel M, et al: Sympathetic predominance followed by functional denervation in the progression of chronic heart failure. Eur Heart J 16:1100–1107, 1995.
12. Sands KEF, Appel ML, Lilly LS, et al: Power spectrum analysis of heart rate variability in human cardiac transplant recipients. Circulation 79:76–82, 1989.
13. Bernardi L, Keller F, Sanders M, et al: Respiratory sinus arrhythmia in the denervated human heart. J Appl Physiol 67:1447–1455, 1989.
14. Bernardi L, Salvucci F, Suardi R, et al: Evidence for an intrinsic mechanism regulating heart rate variability in the transplanted and the intact heart during submaximal exercise? Cardiovasc Res 24:969–981, 1990.
15. Akselrod S, Gordon D, Ubel FA, et al: Power spectrum analysis of heart rate fluctuations: A quantitative probe of beat-to-beat cardiovascular control. Science 213:220–222, 1981.

16. Casadei B, Moon J, Caiazza A, Sleight P: Is respiratory sinus arrhythmia a good index of cardiac vagal activity during exercise? J Appl Physiol 81:556–564, 1996.

17. Arai Y, Saul JP, Albrecht P, et al: Modulation of cardiac autonomic activity during and immediately after exercise. Am J Physiol 256:H132–H141, 1989.

18. Eckberg DL, Drabinski M, Braunwald E: Defective parasympathetic control in patients with heart disease. N Engl J Med 285:877–883, 1971.

19. Bilchick KC, Fetics B, Djoukeng R, et al: Prognostic value of heart rate variability in chronic congestive heart failure (Veterans Affairs' Survival Trial of Antiarrhythmic Therapy in Congestive Heart Failure). Am J Cardiol 90:24–28, 2002.

20. Makikallio TH, Huikuri HV, Hintze U, et al: Fractal analysis and time- and frequency-domain measures of heart rate variability as predictors of mortality in patients with heart failure. Am J Cardiol 87:178–182, 2001.

21. Nolan J, Batin PD, Andrews R, et al: Prospective study of heart rate variability and mortality in chronic heart failure: Results of the United Kingdom heart failure evaluation and assessment of risk trial (UK-Heart). Circulation 98:1510–1516, 1998.

22. Brouwer J, van Veldhuisen DJ, Man AJ, et al: Prognostic value of heart rate variability during long-term follow-up in patients with mild to moderate heart failure. J Am Coll Cardiol 28:1183–1189, 1996.

23. Horner SM, Murphy CF, Coen B, et al: Contribution to heart rate variability by mechanoelectric feedback. Stretch of the sinoatrial node reduces heart rate variability. Circulation 94:1762–1767, 1996.

24. El-Omar M, Kardos A, Casadei B: Mechanisms of respiratory sinus arrhythmia in patients with mild heart failure. Am J Physiol 280:H125–H131, 2001.

25. Bolter CP: Effect of changes in transmural pressure on contraction frequency of the isolated right atrium of the rabbit. Acta Physiol Scand 156:45–50, 1996.

26. Perlini S, Soldá PL, Piepoli M, et al: Determinants of respiratory sinus arrhythmia in the vagotomized rabbit. Am J Physiol 269:H909–H915, 1995.

27. Bevegard S, Holmgren A, Jonsson B: The effect of body position on the circulation at rest and during exercise, with special reference to the influence of stroke volume. Acta Physiol Scand 49:279–298, 1960.

28. Pathak CL: Autoregulation of chronotropic response of the heart through pacemaker stretch. Cardiology 58:45–64, 1973.

29. Blinks JR: Positive chronotropic effect of increasing right atrial pressure in the isolated mammalian heart. Am J Physiol 186:299–303, 1956.

30. Lange G, Lu HH, Chang A, Brooks CM: Effect of stretch on the isolated cat sinoatrial node. Am J Physiol 211:1192–1196, 1966.

31. Kohl P, Kamkin AG, Kiseleva IS, Noble D: Mechanosensitive fibroblasts in the sino-atrial node region of rat heart: Interaction with cardiomyocytes and possible role. Exp Physiol 79:943–956, 1994.

32. Kamiyama A, Niimura I, Sugi H: Length-dependent changes of pacemaker frequency in the isolated rabbit sinoatrial node. Jpn J Physiol 34:153–165, 1984.

33. Pathak CL: Alternative mechanism of cardiac acceleration in Bainbridge's infusion experiments. Am J Physiol 197:441–444, 1959.

34. Arai A, Kodama I, Toyama J: Roles of Cl^- channels and Ca^{2+} mobilization in stretch-induced increase of SA node pacemaker activity. Am J Physiol 270:H1726–1735, 1996.

35. Cooper PJ, Lei M, Cheng L-X, Kohl P: Cellular responses to mechanical stress: Selected contribution: Axial stretch increases spontaneous pacemaker activity in rabbit isolated sinoatrial node cells. J Appl Physiol 89:2099–2104, 2000.

36. Pinsky DJ, Patton S, Mesaros S, et al: Mechanical transduction of nitric oxide synthesis in the beating heart. Circ Res 81:372–379, 1997.

37. Prendergast BD, Sagach VF, Shah AM: Basal release of nitric oxide augments the Frank-Starling response in the isolated heart. Circulation 96:1320–1329, 1997.

38. Bannenberg GL, Gustafsson LE: Stretch-induced stimulation of lower airway nitric oxide formation in the guinea-pig: inhibition by gadolinium chloride. Pharmacol Toxicol 81:13–18, 1997.

39. Suarez J, Torres C, Sanchez L, et al: Flow stimulates nitric oxide release in guinea pig heart: Role of stretch-activated ion channels. Biochem Biophys Res Commun 261:6–9, 1999.

40. Petroff MGV, Kim SH, Pepe S, et al: Endogenous nitric oxide mechanisms mediate the stretch dependence of Ca^{2+} release in cardiomyocytes. Nat Cell Biol 3:867–873, 2001.

41. Bainbridge FA: The influence of venous filling upon the rate of the heart. J Physiol Lond 50:65–84, 1915.

42. Musialek P, Lei M, Brown HF, et al: Nitric oxide can increase heart rate by stimulating the hyperpolarization-activated inward current, I_f. Circ Res 81:60–68, 1997.

43. Musialek P, Rigg L, Terrar DA, et al: Role of cGMP-inhibited phosphodiesterase and sarcoplasmic calcium in mediating the increase in basal heart rate with nitric oxide donors. J Mol Cell Cardiol 32:1831–1840, 2000.

Is the U Wave in the Electrocardiogram a Mechano-Electric Phenomenon?

• • • •

Borys Surawicz

The U wave was first described by Einthoven in 1903[1] as a shallow, broad deflection following the T wave after an interval of 20 to 40 msec. The U wave has been of limited interest to clinicians because it has no important diagnostic significance, and its description is seldom included in the routine analysis of the electrocardiogram (ECG). The information about the characteristics of normal and abnormal U waves is contained primarily in older literature, which is not widely disseminated among contemporary clinicians. The lack of consensus about the origin of the normal U wave may also have contributed to the "neglect" of U wave analysis in clinical practice and in the electrophysiology laboratory. Yet, the exclusion of U wave from scientific scrutiny cannot be justified.

Even if the U wave is of uncertain practical significance, the mere fact that an ECG deflection has remained unexplained for 100 years since its description should provide an independent impetus for closing this gap in our knowledge.

NORMAL U WAVE IN RELATION TO T WAVE

The following points provide an analysis of the U wave in relation to the T wave:

1. U wave is a diastolic deflection, which begins usually with the second heart sound at the beginning of ventricular relaxation and ends at the third heart sound.[2]
2. U wave begins after the end of the T wave, most commonly from the isoelectric baseline, but the T-U junction may be slightly depressed or slightly elevated.

3. The duration of the QU end interval measures from 440 to 680 msec and increases with increasing RR interval[2] (Fig. 20–1).
4. U wave is usually monophasic-positive or -negative but may be biphasic—that is, positive-negative or negative-positive.
5. Within the range of heart rates from 50 to 100 beats/min, the interval from the end of the T wave to the apex of U (aU) is nearly rate independent and measures from 90 to 110 msec.[2] It has been emphasized that unlike the QT interval, the timing of aU does not change after a sudden increase in cycle length—for example, during atrial fibrillation or after a premature complex—resulting in an encroachment of T wave on the U wave.
6. Within the range of heart rates from 50 to 100 beats/min, the normal interval between the end of T and the end of U ranges from 160 to 230 msec (see Fig. 20–1).
7. Unlike the normal T wave, the ascent of U wave is either shorter than or equal to the duration of the descent (Fig. 20–2).
8. The U wave vector tends to parallel the T wave vector—that is, the U wave is normally negative in the lead aVR and occasionally in the leads III and aVF. In the leads I and aVL, U wave is usually isoelectric.
9. The amplitude of the largest U wave (usually in lead V2 or V3) ranges from 3% to 24% (average, 11%) of T wave amplitude in 98% of cases.[3] U wave amplitude seldom exceeds 0.2 mV.
10. U wave is usually better visualized in the semidirect leads—for example, precordial, esophageal, or intracoronary leads—than in the indirect leads, but the timing of the U wave is the same in all leads, and the observed increase of the U wave

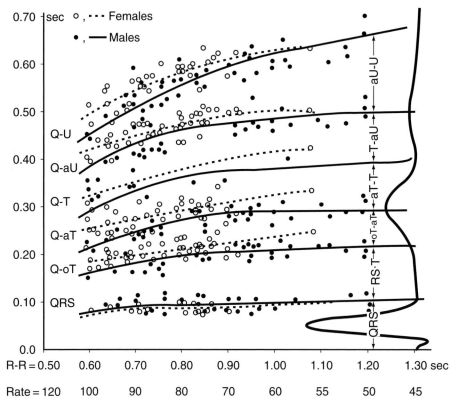

■ **Figure 20–1** Dependence of the intervals of the ventricular electrocardiogram (ECG) (ordinate) on heart rate and RR intervals (abscissa) in 100 middle-aged healthy individuals (50 males and 50 females). *Dots* mark single observations; *lines* are smoothed averages. In the case of QT interval, the end of the T wave is marked by the origin of each *arrow*, whereas the beginning of the second heart sound is marked by the *point of the arrow*. A *horizontal line* indicates that the end of T wave and the second sound coincide. *Dashed lines* represent female individuals; *solid lines* represent male individuals. *(From Lepeschkin E, Surawicz B: The duration of the Q-U interval and its components in electrocardiograms of normal persons. Am Heart J 46:9–20, 1953, with permission.)*

amplitude may be the result of the overall increase of the ECG amplitude.

11. The ease of U wave recognition depends on the heart rate. U wave amplitude is strongly rate dependent. In my study of 500 randomly selected ECG with normal QT interval,[4] U wave was discernible in more than 90% of cases when the heart rate was less than 65 beats/min, in about 66% of cases when the heart rate ranged from 65 to 80 beats/min, and in about 25% of cases when the heart rate was within 80 to 95 beats/min; the U wave was seldom detectable when the heart rate exceeded 95 beats/min. The detection of very low-

amplitude U wave during rapid rate may be facilitated by enlargement of the tracing.

12. Changes in U wave polarity occur in the absence of consistent change in the pattern of T wave or ST segment. Kishida and colleagues[5] found that the reversal from a negative to a positive U wave was associated with a decrease of T wave amplitude in 44% of patients, an increase in T wave amplitude in 35% of patients, and no change in T wave amplitude in the remaining 21% of patients. At the same time, the ST segment did not change in 52%, became elevated in 2%, and changed from depressed to isoelectric or became

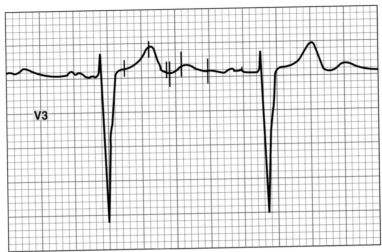

■ **Figure 20–2**   The difference between the configuration of the T wave and the U wave in a normal ECG. The consecutive *vertical lines* from left to right show the beginning, apex, and end of the T wave, followed by the beginning, apex, and end of the U wave. Note that the ascent of the T wave is longer than its descent—that is, similar to the course of repolarization of ventricular and Purkinje fibers—whereas the ascent of the U wave is shorter than its descent. The duration of the QT interval is 420 msec; the duration of the QU interval is 680 msec. *(From Surawicz B: U wave: Facts, hypotheses, misconceptions, and misnomers, J Cardiovasc Electrophysiol 9:1117–1126, 1998, with permission.)*

less depressed in the remaining 47% of patients. These observations suggest that changes in U polarity are independent of the electrophysiologic processes that control the level of the ST segment and the morphology of the T wave. Similarly, changes in the QRS duration do not affect the duration and polarity of the U wave.

THEORIES RELATING U WAVE TO VENTRICULAR REPOLARIZATION

There are two theories relating U wave genesis to ventricular repolarization: (1) repolarization of the Purkinje fibers; and (2) repolarization of some portions of ventricular myocardium. Both theories are difficult to reconcile with the characteristics of the normal U wave.

The difficulty with the concept of Purkinje fiber repolarization is the small mass of the conducting system tissue. Yan and Antzelevitch[6] found that in the isolated arterially perfused canine wedge preparation, repolarization of Purkinje fibers outlasted that of the

M cells but did not register on the ECG. Lepeschkin[7] listed several additional observations that are difficult to reconcile with the Purkinje fiber theory. First, amphibia have U wave but no Purkinje fibers. Second, configuration of the U wave does not conform to the repolarization pattern of Purkinje fibers, because the descent of the U wave tends to be longer than the ascent (see Fig. 20–2). Third, the U wave timing depends on mechanical events. When the relation between the end of T wave and the second heart sound undergoes a change, the U wave follows the second heart sound and not the T wave.[8]

I listed several additional arguments against the Purkinje fiber repolarization theory.[8] First, the interval between the end of T wave and aU is nearly constant within a wide range of heart rates at which the difference between action potential durations (APD) of Purkinje and ventricular muscle fibers increases at slower and decreases at faster heart rates.

Second, in patients with right bundle branch block, timing of U wave correlated better with the presence of right ventricular hypertrophy than with intraventricular conduction.[9] This suggests that the delayed U wave timing was caused by some factors directly related to myocardial hypertrophy rather than to the delayed activation of the Purkinje fibers.

Third, no consistent difference was found between the direction of the U wave vector in the presence of right versus left bundle branch block.[5] Kishida and colleagues[5] found no differences in the lead distribution of negative U waves among patients with hypertension who had a normal QRS duration and a pattern of either right or left bundle branch block. If the U wave was caused by Purkinje fiber repolarization, we would expect to find an opposite sequence of repolarization in right versus left bundle branch block and, consequently, a different direction of the U wave vector in patients with a right versus those with a left bundle branch block pattern. Kishida and colleagues[5] found that the average Q-Tc, Q-aUc, and Q-Uc intervals were longer in patients with a wide QRS complex. This shows that different types of intraventricular conduction disturbances contribute to the delayed appearance of the U wave. However, the average (Q-Tc, Q-aUc) intervals were not significantly different from each other, indicating that the timing of the U wave was related to the duration of the QT interval rather than to duration of the QRS interval.

Fourth, Watanabe[10] suggested that the longer duration of the T-aU interval in patients with left bundle branch block favored the Purkinje fiber repolarization theory of U wave genesis. In my opinion, however, the delayed appearance of the U wave in relation to ventricular repolarization is of no help in establishing the mechanism of the U wave because the finding could be caused by either delayed repolarization of the Purkinje fibers in the left ventricle or by delayed relaxation of the left ventricle.

Fifth, the differences between the functional refractory periods of the "His-Purkinje system" and ventricular muscle in humans reflecting the differences between APD of these structures are not sufficiently large to explain the normal duration of U wave, which lasts 160 to 230 msec. The last argument can be used also against the ventricular repolarization hypothesis, which assumes that U wave arises from repolarization delay in some portion of the ventricular myocardium such as papillary muscles[11] or the M cells.[12]

Sixth, the M cell hypothesis of the U wave originated from action potential (AP) studies in animals in vitro[12] and was supported by computer simulation;[13] however, in a later study, Sicouri and colleagues[14] reported that in the guinea pigs "the end of the T wave correlates well with repolarization of M cells." Thus, in this species, the contribution of the M cells to the U wave could be ruled out. Also, in the dog ventricular preparation, the repolarization of the M cell "was aligned with the end of the T wave."[15] It appears, therefore, that the presence of M cells does not affect the U wave, but it may be pertinent to the mechanism of QT lengthening with a notched T wave. In humans, M cells are believed to represent about 30% of ventricular mass,[16] and at a cycle length of 1000 msec, the APD in the ventricular slices in vitro averaged 439 ± 22 msec, which is close to normal duration of the QT interval. It is difficult to understand how the authors of the above study came to the conclusion that "M cells contribute importantly to the manifestation of the U wave in the ECG,"[16] when U wave at this heart rate extends for a period of 230 msec beyond the end of the T wave.[2] Moreover, it has been shown in dogs that the APD of M cells is shorter in the intact heart than in tissue slices.[17] Lazzara[18] pointed out that the delayed repolarization of ventricular fibers would be expected to prolong the T wave, or perhaps create a notched T wave, but should not create a separate deflection arising from the baseline.

Seventh, Yanowitz and colleagues[19] advanced a hypothesis that certain AP terminate after the end of T wave but do not generate deflections, because they end simultaneously and undergo cancellation. Figure 20–3 shows that Autenrieth and colleagues[20] found no evidence of the presence of "silent repolarization" on the ventricular surface in dogs because all monophasic action potentials (MAP) terminated during inscription of T wave.

Shabetai and colleagues[21] recorded simultaneously ECG and MAP with suction electrodes on the endocardial surface of the right ventricle in humans and found that MAP ended near the end of T wave before the onset of U wave. Similar findings were reported by Franz and colleagues.[22] Also, in isolated perfused rabbit hearts,[23,24] correlations between the morphology of repolarization in the ECG and in single fibers showed that the duration of AP of varying shape and duration terminated near the end of T wave, and that the dura-

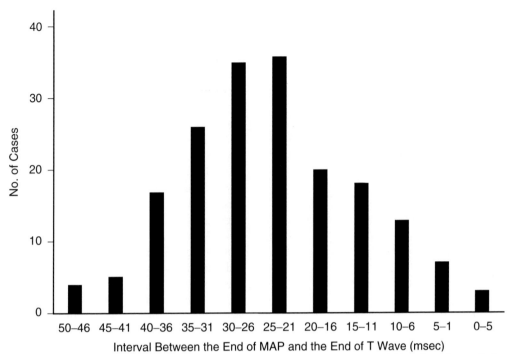

■ **Figure 20–3**   Distribution of the intervals between the end of the monophasic action potential (MAP) on the ventricular surface and the end of the T wave in 178 tracings in dogs. On the abscissa are shown intervals from the end of MAP to the end of the T wave in msec.   *(From Autenrieth G, Surawicz B, Kuo CS: Sequence of repolarization on the ventricular surface in the dog. Am Heart J 89:462–470, 1975, with permission.)*

tion of the AP roughly correlated with the duration of the QT interval in the ECG.

Thus, it can be concluded that the recordings of transmembrane AP in animal preparations and of MAP in humans indicate that under normal conditions, ventricular repolarization ends before the onset of U wave. The AP of M cells and Purkinje fibers are not sufficiently long to play roles in the genesis of U wave. Phonocardiographic recordings show that U wave is inscribed during ventricular diastole.

U WAVE AS AN AFTERPOTENTIAL DURING VENTRICULAR REPOLARIZATION

That U wave begins at the baseline after the end of T wave suggests that it represents a separate afterpo-

tential, similar to the triggered afterpotentials generated by the transient inward current and attributed to intracellular calcium overload. Such a mechanism, however, is not likely to operate under normal physiologic conditions.

The separation between T wave and U wave is clearly maintained under all circumstances in which the prolonged QT interval does not obscure the U wave. Even in the presence of acute myocardial ischemia, when ventricular repolarization assumes the shape of a MAP, the U wave does not change its shape or its relation to the QT interval (Fig. 20–4).

The early diastolic interval coincident with the inscription of the U wave encompasses the time from the closure of the semilunar valves to the opening of the atrioventricular valves and the early diastolic interval defined as the time from the opening of the mitral valve to the point of minimal left ventricular pressure.[8]

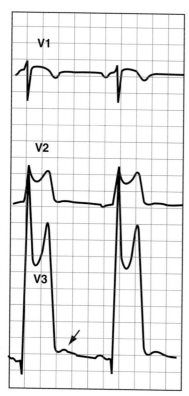

■ **Figure 20–4** Electrocardiographic pattern of acute injury in a patient with myocardial infarction of the anterior wall. *Arrow points at the U wave, which remains apart from ventricular repolarization. (From Surawicz B: U wave: Facts, hypotheses, misconceptions, and misnomers, J Cardiovasc Electrophysiol 9:1117–1126, 1998, with permission.)*

The total duration of this interval in two studies in normal subjects closely approximates the duration of the U wave.[8]

Currently, support for a mechano-electric genesis of the U wave rests mainly on the timing of the U wave at ventricular relaxation, increasing amplitude with increasing diastolic volume (slower rate), and earlier appearance of U wave in the presence of more rapid relaxation produced by β-adrenergic stimulation. Concordance of the U wave with the T wave can be explained by the sequence of relaxation paralleling the sequence of ventricular repolarization.

The timing of the U wave suggests that it may be an electrical manifestation of ventricular stretch.[25] Dudel and Trautwein[26] showed nearly 60 years ago that stretch prolongs terminal repolarization in single ventricular fibers. It can be seen in the figures illustrating their experiments that the length of the "stretched" AP is sufficient to account for the timing of the U wave, but the configuration does not explain the formation of a separate deflection after the end of ventricular repolarization.

More pertinent to the possible genesis of the U wave is the effect of stretch applied at the end of AP, as shown in Figure 20–5, which was reproduced from the study of Zabel and coworkers.[27] To produce this effect, these investigators applied stretch pulses of 50 msec in duration in the isolated perfused rabbit heart during early diastole. The amplitude of these afterdepolarizations averaged 12% ± 8% of the total MAP amplitude and almost always induced a premature ventricular complex.

Zabel and colleagues[27] postulated that stretch activates mechanosensitive ion channels that transduce changes in pressure or stretch into electrical signals through changes in membrane ion permeability. The existence of such channels in cardiac muscle has been amply demonstrated. Electrophysiologic recordings of single atrial fibroblasts indicate that mechanical compression of the cells may activate a nonselective cation conductance leading to depolarization of membrane potential.[26–28] In the study of Isenberg and colleagues[29] in single ventricular myocytes, stretch activated nonselective cation currents with a reversal potential of 0 mV. Accordingly, activation of the channel at a diastolic potential should result in an inward current, which leads to depolarization. Several different ion channels are thought to be involved in the sensing of stretch, including K+-selective, Cl−-selective, nonselective, and adenosine triphosphate–sensitive K+ channels. Some mechanosensitive channels have been cloned from nonvertebrate and vertebrate species.[28]

Di Bernardo and Murray[30] explored the hypotheses of the U wave genesis in a computer model of left ventricular repolarization, which exhibited an afterdepolarization. They investigated separately the effect of the amplitude of the afterpotential, dispersion of repolarization, and the timing of the afterpotential relative to the principal AP component on the 12-lead electrocardiogram. They found that delaying repolarization in different regions of the heart could not explain the U

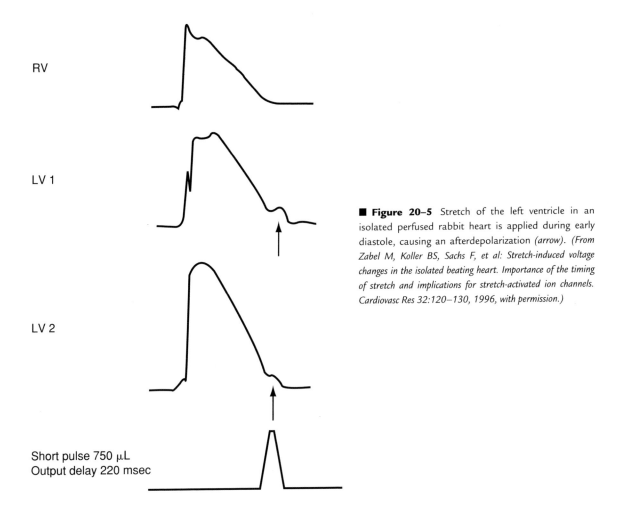

RV

LV 1

LV 2

Short pulse 750 μL
Output delay 220 msec

■ **Figure 20–5** Stretch of the left ventricle in an isolated perfused rabbit heart is applied during early diastole, causing an afterdepolarization *(arrow)*. *(From Zabel M, Koller BS, Sachs F, et al: Stretch-induced voltage changes in the isolated beating heart. Importance of the timing of stretch and implications for stretch-activated ion channels. Cardiovasc Res 32:120–130, 1996, with permission.)*

wave. However, U wave polarity and other characteristics of the U wave could be explained by the presence of afterpotentials. In their model, U wave inversion correlated with an abnormal afterpotential timing.

The concept of mechano-electric feedback championed by Lab[31] and also Lerman and coworkers[32] has been considered as a factor in the genesis of ventricular arrhythmias, but it is also applicable to the U wave as an electrical manifestation of ventricular stretch. The role of U wave in ventricular arrhythmias is uncertain. There is no evidence that potentials generating normal U wave initiate premature responses. The occurrence of most ventricular premature complexes after the T wave is probably caused by re-entry at the end of the ventricular

refractory period or by automaticity of Purkinje fibers. Arrhythmias associated with prolonged ventricular repolarization originate at the time of fusion of the T wave with the U wave, but the possible role of the U wave under such circumstances would be difficult to detect. The inscription of the U wave begins during isovolumic relaxation when the circular layers of the ventricular myocardium undergo stretching, whereas the endocardial components including the papillary muscles are believed to remain contracted.[33] Furbetta and colleagues[11] attributed U waves to repolarization of papillary muscles. To my knowledge, there are no published records of papillary muscle transmembrane AP in humans in vivo; however, in several animal species, the papillary muscle AP are usually shorter than those of Purkinje fibers.[25] The hypothesis that inverted U wave is caused by pathologic conditions of papillary muscles[11] can be dismissed because U wave inversion is readily abolished by hemodynamic changes. The possibility that the U wave is caused by late contraction of endocardial layers and papillary muscles remains a challenge to a more likely scenario that the U wave is an afterpotential caused by the stretching of the circular muscle layers— that is, a mechano-electric phenomenon. The proof of this hypothesis cannot be obtained in animal studies or by computer simulations, but requires studies of human subjects with U waves. Echocardiography is an appropriate tool to conduct such studies, because tissue Doppler imaging allows us to examine normal cardiac mechanics with an exquisite precision.[34] Equally useful may be magnetic resonance imaging.

U WAVE AS A MARKER OF CARDIAC PATHOLOGY

The U wave has been considered abnormal when its polarity is reversed or its amplitude is increased. The latter, however, may be difficult to assess in the absence of established standards for normal values of U wave amplitude. It is known that U wave amplitude is increased by inotropic interventions—for example, treatment with catecholamines, calcium and digitalis, or postextrasystolic potentiation. Digitalis and hypercalcemia do not change appreciably the temporal relation between T wave and U wave—that is, U wave begins from the baseline after the end of the T wave. After intravenous administration of adrenaline or isoproterenol, however, U wave appears earlier, resulting in U wave becoming fused with the terminal T wave portion.

Negative U wave in the standard ECG leads other than aVR (and occasionally III and aVF) occurs nearly always in the presence of myocardial ischemia, myocardial infarction, ventricular hypertrophy, or valvular regurgitation,[5] and it is usually associated with other ECG abnormalities. In the study of 488 patients by Kishida and colleagues,[5] a negative U wave was the only electrocardiographic abnormality in 5% of patients. In an additional 7% of patients, the ECG results were normal at rest and became abnormal after exercise. U wave may become transiently inverted during coronary vasospasm[35] or unstable angina pectoris.[36] An example is shown in Figure 20-6.

Several studies[37,38] found that a negative U wave in patients with left or right ventricular hypertrophy appeared usually in the left or right precordial leads, respectively. In patients with myocardial infarction, U wave tends to appear in the left precordial leads in those with anterior wall infarction and in the inferior leads in those with inferior or posterior infarction.

Early studies[39,40] showed that in patients with hypertension, the regression of U wave inversion was associated with a reduction of blood pressure. Kishida and colleagues[5] found that in patients in whom the U wave polarity changed from negative to positive in the same lead within a period of less than 1 year, the change occurred after reduction of blood pressure by medical treatment in 107 patients, and after surgical treatment of valvular or coronary heart disease or kidney transplantation in 23 patients. In 29 patients with systemic hypertension and a normal QRS duration, the change in U wave polarity occurred more than once during the follow-up period of less than 1 year. Each appearance of a negative U wave was associated with a significant increase in systolic and diastolic blood pressure without a significant change in heart rate, QRS duration, or the duration of Q-Tc, Q-aUc and Q-Uc intervals. More recently, echocardiographic studies[41] have shown that disappearance of negative U waves is an independent predictor of the reduction of left ventricular hypertrophy.

U wave inversion appears to be related to the abnormalities of diastolic ventricular function. The three conditions most frequently associated with U wave inversion—systemic hypertension, aortic or mitral valve regurgitation, and myocardial ischemia—have in common an abnormal ventricular relaxation. Fu and colleagues[42] recorded echocardiograms in patients with hypertension in whom handgrip caused inversion of the U wave associated with an increase in left ventricular dimension, which implicates stretch as a possible cause of U wave inversion. It has been shown that left ventricular relaxation is prolonged in patients with hypertension and either prolonged or incomplete in patients with myocardial ischemia. The U wave vector could be influenced by the sequence of ventricular relaxation. Asynchronous

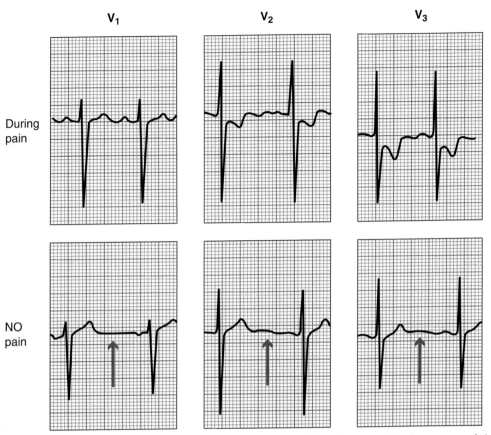

■ **Figure 20–6** Electrocardiographic leads of a 52-year-old man with unstable angina pectoris in the presence of chest pain *(top row)* and after the pain subsided *(bottom row)*. Note the change from inverted to upright U wave in the leads V₂ and V₃.

segmental early relaxation is a well-established phenomenon in patients with coronary artery disease and normal systolic function.[25] Choo and Gibson[43] have provided support for a mechano-electric mechanism of U wave inversion. They studied the relation between the ECG pattern of left ventricular hypertrophy and ventricular function using M-mode echocardiograms and apex cardiogram in hypertensive patients with and without U wave inversion and found that U wave inversion is related to a prolonged isovolumic relaxation period, delayed mitral valve opening relative to minimum cavity dimension, and reduced diastolic wall-thinning rate. The presence of U wave inversion was associated with a significant increase in transverse ventricular dimension during the period between minimum dimension and left

ventricular filling. Because the ventricular volume during this period was constant, other dimensions must have been reduced, "implying the presence of incoordinate relaxation." Thus, U wave inversion appears to be linked to a primary mechanical event, and it may represent a manifestation of a mechano-electric coupling in the presence of an abnormal sequence of ventricular relaxation.

U WAVE AND PROLONGED QT INTERVAL

To study the relation between QT interval and the U wave, it is helpful to mark the end of systole by recording the second heart sound. Hegglin[44] defined the relation between end of T wave and the second heart sound in 1000 healthy men and women and established that the end of T wave coincided with the second heart sound in more than 50% of population and was within 20 msec before or after the end of T wave in 90% (Fig. 20–7). Lepeschkin and Surawicz[2] made similar observations (see Fig. 20–1).

Lengthening of QT interval (without change in Q-Tc) results most often from the decrease in heart rate. This is associated with increased ventricular filling

and longer ejection period. Under these conditions, the relation between QT interval and U wave appearance remains unchanged—that is, the U wave begins from the baseline synchronously with the second heart sound. If, however, the increased diastolic interval occurs abruptly—for example, during atrial fibrillation or after a premature impulse—fusion between T wave and U wave may occur.[45]

The cycle length independent causes of QT interval lengthening associated with global or regional

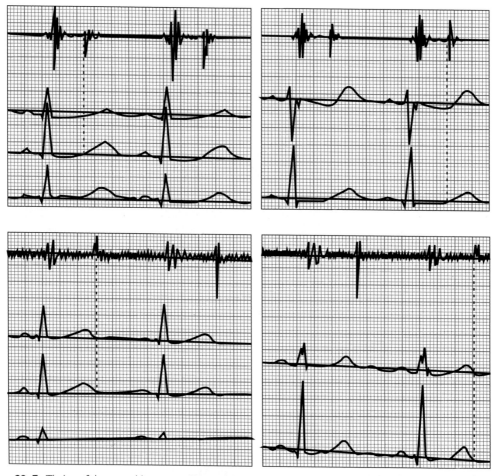

■ **Figure 20–7** Timing of the second heart sound *(vertical dashed line)* in relation to the ECG. *Top,* During hypokalemia (serum K⁺ concentration = 2.15 mEq/L). *Bottom,* After normalization of serum K concentration (3.97 mEq/L). *Top left* and *bottom left,* Leads I, II, III; *top right,* leads V_2 and V_6; *bottom right,* leads II and V6. Note that during hypokalemia, the major repolarization deflection (T+U wave) is inscribed during diastole, and after correction of hypokalemia, the second heart sound is near the T-U junction. *(From Surawicz B: U wave: Facts, hypotheses, misconceptions, and misnomers, J Cardiovasc Electrophysiol 9:1117–1126, 1998, with permission.)*

increases of ventricular APD result in fusion of T wave and U wave. As long as the QT interval is prolonged by less than 90 to 110 msec and the timing of the U wave does not change, the aU remains recognizable. With increasing duration of the QT interval, the point of T-U junction deviates progressively from the baseline. A greater than ~100-msec QT lengthening results in complete obfuscation of a normally timed U wave. In most conditions associated with lengthening of the QT interval, the duration of ventricular ejection does not lengthen proportionally or does not lengthen at all. Therefore, in most conditions associated with cycle length independent QT lengthening, a portion of the T wave is inscribed during diastole—that is, in the territory of the U wave. Figure 20–7 shows that during hypokalemia the timing of the second sound is approximately the same as when the K+ concentration is normal. This shows that the largest repolarization deflection is inscribed during diastole. It is obvious that the behavior of the U wave cannot be defined when it is obscured by the T wave.

Conclusion

The most plausible hypothesis of U wave genesis is that it is caused by a mechano-electric event generated during ventricular relaxation, but the proof of this hypothesis requires more stringent experimental confirmation. Hence, it remains impossible to answer affirmatively the question posed in the title of this chapter.

References

1. Einthoven W: Die Galvanometrische Registrierung des Mensclhlichen Electrokardiogram. Pflügers Arch 99:472–480, 1903.
2. Lepeschkin E, Surawicz B: The duration of the Q-U interval and its components in electrocardiograms of normal persons. Am Heart J 46:9–20, 1953.
3. Lepeschkin E: The U wave of the electrocardiogram. Arch Intern Med 96:600–617, 1955.
4. Surawicz B: Normal electrocardiogram: Origin and description. In: Surawicz B, Knilans TK (eds): Chou's Electrocardiography in Clinical Practice, 5th ed. Philadelphia, WB Saunders, 2001, p 24.
5. Kishida H, Cole JS, Surawicz B: Negative U wave: A highly specific but poorly understood sign of heart disease. Am J Cardiol 49:2030–2036, 1982.
6. Yan G-X, Antzelevitch C: Cellular basis for the normal T wave and the ECG manifestations of the long QT syndromes. J Electrocardiology 30(Suppl):145, 1998.
7. Lepeschkin E: Physiologic basis of the U-wave. In: Schlant RC, Hurst JW (eds): Advances in Electrocardiography. New York, Grune & Stratton, 431–447, 1972.
8. Surawicz B: U wave: Facts, hypotheses, misconceptions, and misnomers, J Cardiovasc Electrophysiol 9:1117–1126, 1998.
9. Ferrero C, Maeder M: Bloc de branche droite: Diagnostic de la hypertrophie ventriculaire droite par la chronologie de l'onde U. Schweiz Med Wochenschr 100:190–192, 1970.
10. Watanabe Y: Purkinje repolarization as a possible cause of the U wave in the electrocardiogram. Circulation 51:1030–1037, 1975.
11. Furbetta D, Bufalari A, Santucci F, Solinas P: Abnormality of the U wave and of the T-U segment of the electrocardiogram: The syndrome of the papillary muscles. Circulation 14:1129–1137, 1956.
12. Antzelevitch C, Sicouri S: Clinical relevance of cardiac arrhythmias. Role of M cells in the generation of U waves, triggered activity and torsade de pointes. J Am Coll Cardiol 23:259–277, 1994.
13. Nesterenko VV, Antzelevitch C: Simulation of the electrocardiographic U wave in heterogeneous myocardium. Effect of the local junctional resistance. In: Proceedings of Computers in Cardiology. IEEE. Los Angeles, Computer Society Press, 1992, pp 43–46.
14. Sicouri S, Quist M, Antzelevitch C: Evidence for the presence of M cells in the guinea pig ventricle. J Cardiovasc Electrophysiol 7:503–510, 1996.
15. Yan XG, Antzelevitch C: Cellular basis for the normal T wave and the electrocardiographic manifestations of the long QT syndrome. Circulation 98:1928–1936, 1998.
16. Drouin E, Charpentier F, Gauthier C, et al: Electrophysiologic characteristics of cells spanning the left ventricular wall of human heart. Evidence for presence of M cells. J Am Coll Cardiol 26:185–192, 1995.
17. Anyukhovsky EP, Sosunov EA, Rosen MR: Regional differences in electrophysiological properties of epicardium, midmyocardium, and endocardium. Circulation 94:1981–1988, 1996.
18. Lazzara R: The U wave and the M cell. J Am Coll Cardiol 26:193–194, 1995.
19. Yanowitz F, Preston JB, Abildskov JA: Functional distribution of right and left stellate innervation to the ventricles. Production of neurogenic electrocardiographic changes by unilateral alterations of sympathetic tone. Circ Res 18:416–427, 1966.
20. Autenrieth G, Surawicz B, Kuo CS: Sequence of repolarization on the ventricular surface in the dog. Am Heart J 89:462–470, 1975.
21. Shabetai R, Surawicz B, Hammill W: Monophasic action potentials in man. Circulation 38:341–350, 1968.
22. Franz MR, Bargheer K, Rafflenbeul W, et al: Monophasic action potential mapping in human subjects with normal electrocardiograms. Direct evidence of the genesis of the T wave. Circulation 75:370–386, 1987.
23. Surawicz B, Lepeschkin E, Herrlich HC, Hoffman BF: Effect of potassium and calcium deficiency on the monophasic action potential, electrocardiogram and contractile force of isolated rabbit hearts. Am J Physiol 196:1302–1308, 1959.
24. Gettes LS, Surawicz B, Shiue JC: Effect of high K, low K, and quinidine on QRS duration and ventricular action potential. Am J Physiol 203:1135–1140, 1962.
25. Surawicz B: Electrophysiologic basis of ECG and cardiac arrhythmias. Baltimore, Williams and Wilkins, 1995, pp 567, 581.

26. Dudel J, Trautwein W: Das Aktionspotential und Mechanogram des Herzmuskels unter dem Einfluss der Dehnung. Cardiologia 25:344–351, 1954.

27. Zabel M, Koller BS, Sachs F, et al: Stretch-induced voltage changes in the isolated beating heart. Importance of the timing of stretch and implications for stretch-activated ion channels. Cardiovasc Res 32:120–130, 1996.

28. Ravens U: Mechano-electric feedback and arrhythmias. Prog Biophys Mol Biol 82:255–266, 2003.

29. Isenberg G, Kazanski V, Kondratev D, et al: Differential effects of stretch and compression on membrane currents and $[Na^+]_c$ in ventricular myocytes. Prog Biophys Mol Biol 82:43–56, 2003.

30. Di Bernardo D, Murray A: Origin of the electrocardiogram of U-waves and abnormal U-wave inversion. Cardiovasc Res 53:202–208, 2002.

31. Lab MJ: Monophasic action potentials and the detection and significance of mechanoelectric feedback in vivo. Prog Cardiovasc Dis 34:29–35, 1991.

32. Lerman BB, Burkhoff D, Yue DT, et al: Mechanoelectrical feedback: Independent role of preload and contractility in modulation of canine ventricular excitability. J Clin Invest 76:1843–1850, 1985.

33. Fatenkov VN: New evidence for cardiac biomechanics. Vestn Ross Akad Med Nauk 2:44–50, 1999.

34. Oh JK, Tajik J: The return of cardiac time intervals. The phoenix is rising. J Am Coll Cardiol 42:471–474, 2003.

35. Kodama-Takahashi K, Ohshima K, Yamamoto K, et al: Occurrence of transient U-wave inversion during vasospastic anginal attack is not related to the direction of concurrent ST-segment shift. Chest 122:535–541, 2002.

36. Jaffe ND, Boden WE: Spontaneous transient, inverted U waves as initial electrocardiographic manifestation of unstable angina. Am Heart J 129:1028–1030, 1995.

37. Holzmann M, Zurukzoglu W: Die klinische Bedeutung der negativen und diphasischen U-Wellen in menschlichen EKG. Cardiologia 27:202–214, 1955.

38. Surawicz B, Kemp RL, Bellet S: Polarity and amplitude of the U wave of the electrocardiogram in relation to the T wave. Circulation 15:90–97, 1957.

39. Georgopoulos J, Proudfit WL, Page IH: Relationship between arterial pressure and negative U wave in electrocardiograms. Circulation 23:675–680, 1961.

40. Kemp RL, Surawicz B, Bettinger JC, et al: Prognostic significance of negative U waves in the electrocardiogram in hypertension. Circulation 15:98–101, 1957.

41. Kishida H, Saitoh T, Oikawa K, et al: Negative U-wave as a predictor of antihypertensive treatment effecting regression of echocardiographic hypertrophy in hypertensive patients. Jpn Heart J 40:31–44, 1999.

42. Fu LT, Takahashi N, Yamamoto M, et al: Handgrip induced negative U-wave in the electrocardiogram of hypertensive subjects. Jpn Heart J 22:59–73, 1981.

43. Choo MH, Gibson DG: U waves in ventricular hypertrophy. Possible demonstration of mechano-ventricular coupling. Br Heart J 55:428–433, 1986.

44. Hegglin R: Die Klinik der energetisch-dynamischen Herzinsuffizienz. Basel, Switzerland, S Karger, 1947.

45. Viskin S, Heller K, Barron HV, et al: Postextrasystolic U wave augmentation. A new marker of increased arrhythmic risk in patients without the long QT syndrome. J Am Coll Cardiol 28:1746–1752, 1996.

CHAPTER 21

Load Dependence of Ventricular Repolarization

• • • •

Peter Taggart and Peter Sutton

EFFECT OF VOLUME LOADING

There is now substantial evidence that mechanical stress/strain within the heart alters the electrophysiology and influences the behavior of electrical wave fronts during the cardiac cycle. Alterations of volume within the atria and ventricles alter the stretch on cardiomyocytes. This mechano-electric feedback (MEF) has been shown to affect the timing of electrical recovery (i.e., repolarization) in a wide variety of laboratory models and humans. The time of repolarization at a given location within the heart depends on the time for the activation wave front to reach that site, plus the action potential duration (APD). Mechanical loading has little or no effect on the speed of conduction in the heart,[1-4] but it does alter APD. Thus, altered load effects on repolarization are caused by effects on APD, from a variety of possible causes.

LABORATORY MODELS

After an activation, cardiac muscle cells can not be re-excited until time has elapsed for the recovery of membrane currents and voltage changes to approach resting conditions. This period of inexcitability is termed the *refractory period*. Under normal circumstances, the effective refractory period (ERP) approximates the APD. The overall result of increased ventricular volume loading is a shortening of APD and ERP (Fig. 21–1). For example, it has been shown in isolated canine ventricles contracting isovolumically that increased preload shortened the ERP[5,6] (Fig. 21–2). In isolated rabbit heart, an increase in left ventricular volume resulted in shortening of the ERP of the left ventricular epicardium.[1,7] Other studies in isolated rabbit hearts

showed a shortening of both the APD at 90% repolarization (APD_{90}) and ERP during left ventricular volume increase.[2] Similar results have been obtained in whole animals.[6,8,9] The general conclusion of these studies is that increased loading results in shortening of the APD and ERP. These effects do not depend on circulating catecholamines, autonomic reflexes, or acute ischemia.[1]

HUMANS

Several studies have recorded monophasic action potentials (MAP) as a measure of APD in humans during changes in ventricular pressure and volume. In one study, MAP recordings were obtained from the right ventricle in patients undergoing balloon valvuloplasty for congenital pulmonary stenosis. In these patients, the narrowed pulmonary valve orifice creates an obstruction to right ventricular outflow, resulting in a chronic increase in intracavity pressure and volume. Relieving the obstruction resulted in lengthening of the right ventricular MAP duration at 90% repolarization, coincident with a decrease in intracavity pressure and volume.[10] The QT interval of the electrocardiogram, which reflects APD, is prolonged, as expected from the MAP prolongation. A subsequent transient occlusion of the right ventricular outflow tract with the balloon catheter resulted in an increase in intracavity pressure and shortening of MAP duration and the QT interval.[10] Thus, decreasing intracavity pressure and volume (i.e., decreasing stretch) lengthens the APD and vice versa.

A standard technique used during coronary artery surgery is cardiopulmonary bypass. Venous blood flow returning to the heart is interrupted and siphoned

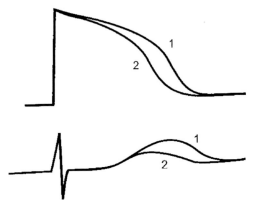

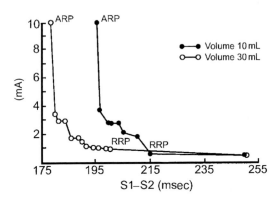

■ Figure 21–1 Diagrammatic illustration of the generally accepted effect of volume loading on action potential duration (APD) and the QT interval of the electrocardiogram. Increased loading shortens APD and the QT interval from control *(1)* to loaded state *(2)*.

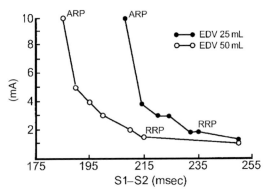

■ Figure 21–2 Effect of volume loading on the effective refractory period (ERP) in the canine left ventricle. In the isovolumic beating heart, increased volume loading from 10 to 30 mL shortened ERP, shifting the strength interval relation to the left *(top)*. A similar effect was obtained in the ejecting heart in response to increasing volume load from 25 to 50 mL *(bottom)*. Coupling intervals of the extrastimulus (S1–S2) are plotted versus the maximum stimulus current (mA) failing to capture the ventricle at that interval. ARP, absolute refractory period; EDV, end-diastolic volume; RRP, relative refractory period. *(From Lerman BB, Burkhoff D, Yue DT, Sagawa K: Mechanoelectrical feedback: Independent role of preload and contractility in modulation of canine ventricular excitability. J Clin Invest 76:1843–1850, 1985, with permission.)*

from a canula placed in the right atrium to a pump/oxygenator. Oxygenated blood is then returned to the circulation through a canula in the ascending aorta, thereby bypassing the heart and lungs. Under these conditions, the ventricles are unloaded, partly empty, and not supporting the circulation. When the coronary artery grafts are completed, the circulation is restored to normal, and bypass is discontinued progressively over a period of 30 to 40 sec. During this phase, the ventricles fill, ventricular pressures increase, and the heart is converted from a nonworking to a working state. MAP recordings from the left ventricular epicardium during this phase of reloading showed shortening of APD_{90} as the left ventricular pressure and volume increased (Fig. 21–3).[11]

It is not uncommon for patients undergoing cardiopulmonary bypass surgery to receive infusions of between 100 and 200 mL, administered as a bolus over 10 to 15 sec, to rectify the hemodynamic appearance of the heart. The increase in circulating volume as a result of the bolus infusion is accompanied by an increase in ventricular loading. A bolus infusion was given during the last 16 to 21 sec of the slow play-out in Figure 21–3, during which there was a progressive increase in radial artery pressure. The increased volume load was accompanied by shortening of APD_{90} from 302 to 284 msec.[11]

Beat-to-beat changes in response to altered loading have been studied in animal models by recording MAP and ERP from the left ventricular epicardium and transiently occluding the ascending aorta, thereby preventing outflow from the left ventricle.[6,8,9,12,13] This technique was adapted for patients undergoing cardiac surgery such that the ascending aorta was occluded abruptly during diastole for one to three beats.[14] The first occluded beat (i.e., nonejecting) was therefore purely afterloaded. The subsequent occluded beats were both preloaded and afterloaded because of the

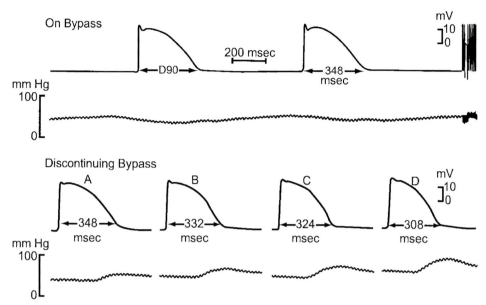

■ **Figure 21–3** Effect of change from an underfilled to a normally filled left ventricle in patients undergoing coronary artery surgery during discontinuing cardiopulmonary bypass. *Top,* Left ventricular epicardial monophasic action potential (MAP) with radial artery pressure during bypass, showing stable MAP as evident from the slow playout and the slow sine wave of the pump pressure. *Bottom,* Progressive increase in radial artery pressure as bypass is discontinued and ventricular pressure and volume are restored, accompanied by a progressive shortening of MAP duration *(A–D). (From Taggart P, Sutton PMI, Treasure T, et al: Monophasic action potentials at discontinuation of cardiopulmonary bypass: Evidence for contraction-excitation feedback in man. Circulation 77:1266–1275, 1988, with permission.)*

combination of not ejecting with the addition of diastolic filling.

Aortic occlusion resulted in an increase in left ventricular pressure and APD_{90} shortening (Fig. 21–4). The majority of the effect was observed on the first occluded beat, that is, in response to afterload. The effect was fully reversible on release of the aortic occlusion and reproducible when the occlusion was repeated.

OVERALL EFFECT: ADDED COMPLEXITY

Although the overall effect of the studies reported previously is for stretch to shorten the APD and refractory period, stretch may also lengthen the APD. *In silico* (modeling) studies have shown that stretch occurring early during repolarization can shorten the APD, whereas stretch occurring late in the repolarization phase prolongs APD.[15] Thus, stretch may shorten or lengthen APD depending on the timing. Several in vivo studies in animal and human hearts have demonstrated depolarizations in late repolarization that resemble early afterdepolarizations (EAD; see the following). This results in late APD lengthening. It is possible that the rate of stretch, as well as the timing, may influence the development of afterdepolarizations.

Regional Heterogeneity

Most of the foregoing studies have measured APD or refractoriness at a single site. Measurements of refractory period at several sites on left ventricular epicardium in an isolated rabbit heart model showed that an increase in left ventricular volume decreased refractoriness in a markedly heterogeneous manner.[1] In the in situ pig heart, a 33% increase in systolic pressure was achieved by aortic cross clamping. This was

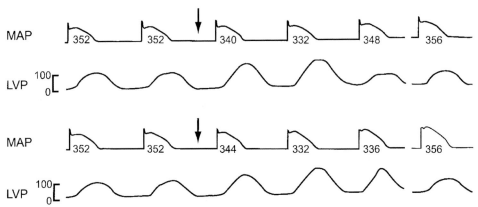

■ **Figure 21–4** Effect of an abrupt increase in left ventricular loading in patients undergoing coronary artery surgery. Left ventricular epicardial monophasic action potentials (MAP) and direct left ventricular pressures (LVP) were recorded during transient occlusion of the ascending aorta for between one and three beats. Two consecutive occlusions are shown. *Arrows* mark the onset of occlusion, which was accompanied by an increase in LVP and shortening of MAP duration. The effect was similar for both occlusions. *(From Taggart P, Sutton P, Lab M, et al: Effect of abrupt changes in ventricular loading on repolarisation induced by transient aortic occlusion in man. Am J Physiol 636:H816–H823, 1992, with permission.)*

accompanied by a reduction in refractory period with a greater change at the apex compared with the base.[12] In another isolated rabbit heart model, up to six MAP were recorded from the left ventricular epicardium during a sustained increase in left ventricular volume. The APD_{90} and refractory periods shortened inhomogeneously.[2]

Interaction with Cycle Length

The effect of load on APD depends on cycle length. In a study in pigs that measured epicardial MAP, the APD of a premature beat was dependent on the length of time since the preceding action potential. During steady state, pacing test pulses with progressively shorter interbeat intervals were introduced. Under control conditions, APD_{70} of the test beats decreased monotonically as the interbeat interval was shortened. When each test beat was loaded by transient aortic occlusion, the APD at the long interbeat intervals was shortened, and the APD at the short interbeat intervals was lengthened. In addition, the maximum slope of the curve relating APD to preceding interval, referred to as the restitution curve, was steepened by 32 msec/100 msec.[16]

In an isolated rabbit heart model, balloon dilation of the left ventricle increased the normal cycle

length–dependent shortening of refractoriness at rapid rates.[3] For example, with steady state pacing at 1000 msec, an increase in left ventricular volume of 1.0 mL shortened the refractory period by 1%; whereas at a cycle length of 250 msec, the same volume increase shortened the refractory period by 21% (Fig. 21–5).

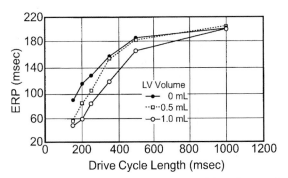

■ **Figure 21–5** Cycle length dependence of the influence of ventricular loading on refractoriness. In an isolated rabbit heart, preparation increasing left ventricular (LV) volume shortened ERP. This effect was more pronounced at shorter basic cycle lengths. *(From Reiter MJ, Landers M, Zetelaki Z, et al: Electrophysiologic effects of acute dilatation in the isolated rabbit heart: Cycle length-dependent effects on epicardial refractoriness and conduction velocity. Circulation 96:4050–4056, 1997, with permission.)*

THE ATRIUM

MEF has been demonstrated in the atrium of both animals and humans. An increase in atrial pressure in an isolated rabbit heart decreased atrial refractory periods and MAP duration.[17] However, a study in canines found that an increase in atrial pressure was associated with an increase in atrial refractory period.[18] In isolated guinea-pig hearts, atrial stretch shortened the APD_{50} and lengthened the APD_{90}; this appeared to be caused by EAD.[19]

In humans, it has been shown that very short or very long A-V intervals were associated with an increase in atrial pressure, atrial size, and the atrial refractory period.[20]

PROARRHYTHMIC EFFECT OF ALTERED LOADING

There is little doubt that increased loading is proarrhythmic. In isolated hearts, a transient stretch produced by volume loading pulses during diastole may induce a depolarization. If that attains sufficient amplitude, it may initiate an action potential. (Because these diastolic depolarizations do not impinge on repolarization, they are discussed elsewhere in this textbook, see chapters 12–14.) Transient stretch during the action potential may result in depolarization during repolarization resembling an EAD (Fig. 21–6). Again, these after-depolarizations may initiate an action potential. The majority of such observations has been made using MAP recordings; as a result, EAD-like deflections have been treated with reservation because of susceptibility of MAP recordings to movement artefact. However, their reproducibility and association with premature ventricular beats makes it highly likely that, at least in the majority of cases, they do represent EAD. Several studies have provided convincing evidence for stretch-induced EAD generating single or repetitive action potentials. Such interventions include transient occlusion of the ascending aorta to produce abrupt stretch in in situ canine hearts,[6] in situ pig hearts,[21] and humans,[14] and occlusion of the right ventricular outflow tract in humans during pulmonary valvuloplasty.[10]

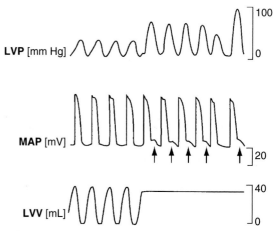

Figure 21–6 Transient dilation or stretch may induce depolarizations during repolarization of the action potential resembling "early afterdepolarizations." An example is shown in an in situ canine heart preparation during transient aortic occlusion. During occlusion, peak left ventricular pressure (LVP) increases abruptly *(top trace)*. The monophasic action potential (MAP) trace *(middle)* shows the development of depolarizations occurring late in the repolarization phase *(arrows)*. LVV, left ventricular volume. *(From Franz MR, Burkhoff D, Yue DT, Sagawa K: Mechanically induced action potential changes and arrhythmia in isolated and in situ canine hearts. Cardiovasc Res 23:213–223, 1989, with permission.)*

Sustained stretch increased the inducibility of ventricular tachycardia and ventricular fibrillation in isolated rabbit hearts[1,22] and in isolated blood-perfused canine ventricles.[23] Left ventricular dilation in isolated rabbit hearts decreased the fibrillation threshold.[24]

PATHOLOGIC HEARTS

There is evidence to suggest that the arrhythmogenic potential of MEF may be enhanced in pathologic hearts. In isolated perfused canine hearts with infarction, an increase in ventricular volume resulted in more pronounced shortening of the ERP in the region of infarction, compared with control areas, and an increase of inducibility of arrhythmias. It was suggested that differential stretch between the normal and infarcted regions resulted in increased dispersion of refractoriness and, hence, an enhanced susceptibility to arrhythmia.[25]

During the ventricular pressure and volume changes associated with the Valsalva maneuver, patients with regional wall motion abnormality frequently demonstrate changes in MAP duration that are different, or even opposite in direction, from subjects with normal wall motion.[26] This could be explained by regional differences in local strain between normally and abnormally contracting segments. This is expected to result in increased heterogeneity of repolarization, which is a well-known substrate for arrhythmia.[27]

Ventricular tachycardia is generally unstable in patients with heart failure, and it more readily degenerates to ventricular fibrillation.[28] Although several mechanisms may be involved, one possibility is MEF.

SUMMARY: CLINICAL IMPLICATIONS

Experiment and theory suggest that MEF may play a significant role in arrhythmogenesis in humans. As indicated previously, there are deflections during repolarization that resemble EAD. That these depolarizations could cause premature action potentials in response to increased loading has been demonstrated in several animal models and in humans. Stretch appears to cause focal tachycardias by inducing afterdepolarizations. Increased loading and stretch also have been shown to shorten the APD and refractory period, both of which are known to facilitate re-entrant arrhythmias. Nevertheless, proof that mechanical factors are a direct cause of either focal tachycardias or re-entrant rhythms in patients currently has not been offered. Several therapeutic interventions such as pharmacologic unloading and ventricular unloading using a balloon-assisted device may be associated with a lessening or termination of arrhythmia. However, several other factors may be influenced by these maneuvers, which makes it difficult to attribute an antiarrhythmic effect directly to a mechanical action. A major difficulty in this respect has been the lack of a stretch-activated channel blocker suitable for clinical use. The (highly nonspecific) stretch-activated channel blocker gadolinium has been shown to block stretch-induced premature ventricular beats in the isolated dog heart,[29] and the recent introduction of the highly specific peptide blocker GsMTx-4

appears to hold some promise (see Chapter 42). This should help to define the role of MEF in arrhythmogenesis in humans and to provide a therapeutic option.

References

1. Reiter MJ, Synhorst DP, Mann DE: Electrophysiologic effects of acute ventricular dilatation in the isolated rabbit heart. Circ Res 62:554–562, 1988.
2. Zabel M, Portnoy S, Franz MR: Effect of sustained load on dispersion of ventricular repolarisation and conduction time in the isolated rabbit heart. J Cardiovasc Electrophysiol 7:9–16, 1996.
3. Reiter MJ, Landers M, Zetelaki Z, et al: Electrophysiologic effects of acute dilatation in the isolated rabbit heart: Cycle length-dependent effects on epicardial refractoriness and conduction velocity. Circulation 96:4050–4056, 1997.
4. Reiter MJ, Zetelaki Z, Kirchhof CJH, et al: Interaction of acute ventricular dilatation and d-sotalol during sustained ventricular tachycardia around a fixed obstacle. Circulation 89:423–431, 1994.
5. Lerman BB, Burkhoff D, Yue DT, Sagawa K: Mechanoelectrical feedback: Independent role of preload and contractility in modulation of canine ventricular excitability. J Clin Invest 76:1843–1850, 1985.
6. Franz MR, Burkhoff D, Yue DT, Sagawa K: Mechanically induced action potential changes and arrhythmia in isolated and in situ canine hearts. Cardiovasc Res 23:213–223, 1989.
7. Hansen DE: Mechanoelectrical feedback effects of altering preload, afterload, and ventricular shortening. Am J Physiol 264:H423–H432, 1993.
8. Dean JW, Dilly SG, Lab MJ: Increased afterload shortens the absolute refractory period in situ ventricle of anaesthetised pig. J Physiol (Lond) 387:7P, 1987.
9. Benditt DG, Kriett JM, Tobler HG, et al: Electrophysiological effects of transient aortic occlusion in intact canine hearts. Am J Physiology 249:H1017–H1023, 1985.
10. Levine JH, Guarnieri T, Kadish AH, et al: Changes in myocardial repolarisation in patients undergoing balloon valvuloplasty for congenital pulmonary stenosis: Evidence for contraction excitation feedback in humans. Circulation 77:70–77, 1988.
11. Taggart P, Sutton PMI, Treasure T, et al: Monophasic action potentials at discontinuation of cardiopulmonary bypass: Evidence for contraction-excitation feedback in man. Circulation 77:1266–1275, 1988.
12. Dean JW, Lab MJ: Regional changes in ventricular excitability during load manipulation of the in situ pig heart. J Physiol (Lond) 429:387–400, 1990.
13. Tobler HG, Gornick CC, Anderson RW, Benditt DG: Electrophysiology properties of the myocardial infarction border zone: Effects of transient aortic occlusion. Surgery 100:150–156, 1986.
14. Taggart P, Sutton P, Lab M, et al: Effect of abrupt changes in ventricular loading on repolarisation induced by transient aortic occlusion in man. Am J Physiol 636:H816–H823, 1992.
15. Kohl P, Day K, Noble D: Cellular mechanisms for cardiac mechano-electric feedback in a mathematical model. Can J Cardiol 14:111–119, 1978.
16. Horner SM, Dick DJ, Murphy CF, Lab MJ: Cycle length dependence of the electrophysiological effects of increased load on the myocardium. Circulation 94:1131–1136, 1996.

17. Ravelli F, Allessie MA: Effects of atrial dilatation on refractory period and vulnerability to atrial fibrillation in isolated Langendorff-perfused rabbit heart. Circulation 96:1686–1695, 1997.
18. Kaseda S, Zipes DP: Contraction-excitation feedback in the atria: A cause of changes in refractoriness. J Am Coll Cardiol 11:1327–1336, 1988.
19. Nazir SA, Lab MJ: Mechanoelectric feedback in the atrium of the isolated guinea-pig heart. Cardiovasc Res 32:112–119, 1996.
20. Klein LS, Miles WM, Zipes DP: Effect of atrioventricular interval during pacing or reciprocating tachycardia on atrial size, pressure and refractory period: Contraction-excitation feedback in human atrium. Circulation 82:60–68, 1990.
21. Lab MJ: Contribution of mechano-electric coupling to ventricular arrhythmias during reduced perfusion. Int J Microcirc Clin Exp 8:433–442, 1989.
22. Reiter MJ, Mann DE, Williams GR: Interaction of hypokalaemia and ventricular dilatation in isolated rabbit hearts. Am J Physiol 265:H1544–H1550, 1993.
23. Hansen DE, Craig CS, Hondeghem LM: Stretch-induced arrhythmias in the isolated canine ventricle: Evidence for the importance of mechanoelectrical feedback. Circulation 81:1094–1105, 1990.
24. Jalal S, Williams GR, Mann DE, Reiter MJ: Effect of ventricular dilatation on fibrillation thresholds in the isolated rabbit heart. Am J Physiol 263:H1306–H1310, 1992.
25. Calkins H, Maughan WL, Weisman HF, et al: Effect of acute volume load on refractoriness and arrhythmia development in isolated chronically infarcted canine hearts. Circulation 79:687–697, 1989.
26. Taggart P, Sutton P, John R, et al: Monophasic action potential recordings during acute changes in ventricular loading induced by the Valsalva manoeuvre. Br Heart J 67:221–229, 1992.
27. Kuo CS, Munkata K, Reddy P, Surawicz B: Characteristics and possible mechanism of ventricular arrhythmia dependent on the dispersion of action potential durations. Circulation 67:1356–1367, 1983.
28. Pratt CM, Eaton T, Francis M, et al: The inverse relationship between left ventricular ejection fraction and outcome of antiarrhythmic therapy: A dangerous imbalance in the risk-benefit ratio. Am Heart J 118:433–440, 1989.
29. Hansen DE, Borganelli M, Stacey GP, Taylor LK: Dose-dependent inhibition of stretch-induced arrhythmias by gadolinium in isolated canine ventricles: Evidence for a unique mode of antiarrhythmic action. Circ Res 69:820–831, 1991.

CHAPTER 22

Mechano-Electric Heterogeneity in Physiologic Function of the Heart

• • • •

Vladimir S. Markhasin and Olga Solovyova

Cardiac cellular heterogeneity has been the focus of increasing attention over the past decade, but research in the area can be traced back to more than 75 years ago. In 1927, Carl Wiggers[1] was the first to propose that the inherent heterogeneity of ventricular activation timing allows for temporal summation of contraction in individual parts (*fasciculi*) of cardiac muscle, facilitating overall mechanical performance of the ventricular myocardium. He also suggested that during the isovolumic phase of ventricular contraction, approximately 20 msec before the onset of ejection, myocardial regions that contract early stretch those that contract later. He proposed that this "entrant phase" of contraction increases mechanical efficiency.[1]

Forty years later, Tyberg and colleagues[2] developed an experimental model of elementary myocardial heterogeneity—the duplex—consisting of two serially connected muscles (one "strong" and one "weak"). They experimentally corroborated the importance of the entrant phase and of the orderly sequence of element activation for optimized mechanical activity in heterogeneous duplexes.

Another two decades later, Brutsaert[3] suggested that spatio-temporal nonuniformity of cardiomyocyte properties was a third key factor that—together with loading conditions and activation/inactivation time course—determines myocardial mechanical performance and efficiency of contraction and relaxation.

This gave rise to a new paradigm of cardiac mechanical function, when A.M. Katz and P.B. Katz[4] suggested that cardiac tissue homogeneity arises from cardiomyocyte heterogeneity. Thus, the preexisting heterogeneity of cardiomyocytes that occurs as a result of adaptation to local mechanical conditions ensures global homogeneity and optimizes mechanical performance. According to this theory, myocardial heterogeneity is a preexisting and static phenomenon—that is, it assumes that the properties of cardiomyocytes do not vary in the course of their interaction.

This chapter summarizes the available evidence to illustrate that: (1) heterogeneity is an inherent property of myocardium; (2) the sequence of element activation in inhomogeneous myocardium plays a key role in its overall electromechanical function; and (3) the heterogeneity of cardiac muscle ensures optimization of overall electromechanical function. This chapter also discusses mechanisms of dynamic interaction between cardiomyocytes in inhomogeneous myocardium and demonstrates the importance of mechano-electric feedback (MEF) in cardiac function.

CARDIOMYOCYTE HETEROGENEITY

Electrical Heterogeneity

Ventricular cardiomyocytes from the sub-epicardial (EPI), mid-myocardial (MID), and sub-endocardial (ENDO) layers differ in their electrophysiologic properties, heart rate dependence, and pharmacologic sensitivity.[5-8] The depolarization rate during the early action potential (AP upstroke) is increased in MID cells in comparison with EPI and ENDO cells, making them similar to cardiac Purkinje cells. APs in EPI cardiomyocytes have a prominent initial repolarization phase with a deep notch, called a spike-and-dome configuration. This is less prominent in MID cells and is absent in ENDO cells. Moreover, in isolated cardiomyocytes, the action potential duration (APD) decreases from MID cells to ENDO and EPI myocytes[9] (Fig. 22–1).

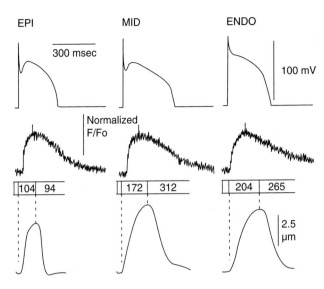

■ Figure 22–1 Transmural differences in action potentials (AP), Ca^{2+} transients, and cell shortening in canine left ventricular cells. Representative AP *(top)*, corresponding normalized Ca^{2+} transients *(below)*, and unloaded cell shortening *(bottom)* recorded from epicardial (EPI), mid-myocardial (MID), and endocardial (ENDO) cardiomyocytes. *(Modified from Cordeiro JM, Greene L, Heilmann C, et al: Transmural heterogeneity of calcium activity and mechanical function in the canine left ventricle. Am J Physiol Heart Circ Physiol 286:H1471–H1479, 2003, with permission.)*

Heterogeneity in AP morphology reflects significant differences in ion current expression, particularly potassium currents.[7,8] A relatively large transient outward current (I_{to}) is seen in EPI and MID cells. This current is responsible for the prominent spike-and-dome morphology. ENDO cells have a much lower I_{to} that eliminates the notch and produces a longer APD at physiologic heart rates. MID cells have a reduced density of the slowly activating delayed rectifier potassium current, I_{Ks},[8] and a strong inward late sodium current, I_{pNa}.[10] In combination, these currents prolong the APD and account for the pronounced heart rate dependence of APD in MID cells.

The sodium-calcium exchange current, I_{NCX}, also differs across the ventricular wall.[11] This current is largest in MID cells, contributing to their long APD and suggesting possible variations in excitation–contraction coupling in different myocardial layers.

The observed differences in AP morphology can be related to the underlying molecular genetics (see Reference 8 for a more detailed discussion of this topic). The normal dispersion of repolarization in cells from various myocardial layers is matched to a differential expression of voltage-gated potassium channels. The role of *KCNH2* (ERG1) and *KCNQ1* (KvLQT1) genes in the generation of the rapidly activating delayed rectifier potassium current, I_{Kr}, and I_{Ks} currents, respectively, was confirmed in myocardial cells. In addition to the variable expression of the Kv α- and β-subunits, there appear to be differences in the expression of Kv channel regulatory molecules. Consistent with this suggestion, the ε isoform of protein kinase C (PKCε) was shown to be differentially distributed in the rat ventricular epicardium and endocardium, and the activation of PKCε has distinct effects on cells from these different layers.

What is the physiologic relevance of the variation in electrophysiologic properties of cardiomyocytes from different layers of the myocardium? Experimental data from human intact heart allowed Franz and colleagues[12] to suggest that *the regional distribution of APD is closely, and inversely, related to the sequence of ventricular depolarization*. Recently, Wan and colleagues[13] confirmed this suggestion by identifying the topographic distribution of APD using cardiomyocytes isolated from different layers of the ventricular wall of the guinea pig. Such a gradient in APD will help to protect the heart from a reverse spread of excitation and re-entry. Thus, the presence of transmural gradients in cellular electrophysiology may contribute to reliable unidirectional propagation of excitation from the endocardium toward the epicardium, and for repolarization in the opposite direction.

Bányász and colleagues[14] and Cordeiro and colleagues[9] showed that AP morphology in different layers of the ventricle correlates with differences in excitation–contraction coupling. This would affect

Ca^{2+} currents through L-type channels, even with no intrinsic differences in the channel structure.

Ca^{2+} Handling Heterogeneity

The gradient of calcium kinetics from different layers has been less thoroughly investigated than the electrophysiologic gradients. An investigation of the base–apex characteristics of Ca^{2+} transients in Langendorff-perfused rabbit heart did not reveal any significant difference.[15] In contrast, in rabbit isolated ventricular cardiomyocytes, there were marked transmural gradients in Ca^{2+} handling.[16] Similar gradients occur in canine ventricular wedge preparations[17] and isolated canine myocytes[9] (see Fig. 22–1).

The time to peak of the Ca^{2+} transient was significantly shorter in canine EPI cells compared with ENDO and MID cells.[9] The peak values of the Ca^{2+} transient did not differ significantly among rabbit cells.[16] In these cells, as well as in canine preparations, the decay of the Ca^{2+} transient was significantly faster in EPI cells compared with the other cell types. There is a close correlation between APD and Ca^{2+} transient duration.[9,16,17] Gradients in Ca^{2+} kinetics were accompanied by differences in Ca^{2+} loading. EPI cells displayed a significantly greater sarcoplasmic reticulum (SR) Ca^{2+} content than ENDO and MID cells.[9] An increase in AP frequency caused an increase in cytosolic free calcium concentration during diastole in canine EPI, and more prominently, ENDO cells.[17] Moreover, the alternations of Ca^{2+} transients at a cycle length of 300 msec were more pronounced in ENDO than EPI cells (85% vs. 15%).[17] Consistent with a faster decline in Ca^{2+} transients in EPI cells, expression of the SR Ca^{2+} adenosine triphosphatase was greater in EPI cells.[17] This may account for their greater SR Ca^{2+} content.

These findings show that there are intrinsic differences in excitation–contraction coupling between cells from different layers of the myocardium, in addition to differences in AP configuration.

Mechanical Heterogeneity

Cazorla and colleagues[18] showed that the sarcomere length–passive tension relation in ferret ventricle is significantly steeper in ENDO compared with EPI cells. Passive tension in ENDO cells at a sarcomere length of 2.0 μm, for example, is more than three times that of EPI cells. These transmural differences in stiffness may be linked to differences in titin isoform expression.[19]

The Frank–Starling relation of sarcomere length versus active tension is steeper in ENDO than in EPI cells from both ferret and rat ventricle.[18] This transmural difference may have a number of explanations. First, the affinity of troponin C (TnC) for calcium may be greater in ENDO than EPI cells. Second, dynamic changes in TnC-calcium affinity during activation of the contractile proteins (increasing Ca^{2+} affinity with increasing number of attached crossbridges; cooperativity) may differ.[20] The number of active crossbridges, in turn, depends on the kinetics of the bridges (the rate of their attachment and detachment). The transmural differences in TnC-calcium affinity may be caused by transmural differences in the distribution of myosin isoforms. In rodents, three isoforms have been described: v_1, v_2, and v_3 (v_1 ensures rapid cycling of crossbridges, v_2 is not active, and v_3 is a slow isoform that is dominant in ENDO cells).[21]

Transmural distinctions in active mechanical properties have been reported in isolated cardiomyocytes from guinea pig[13,22] and dog[9] (see Fig. 22–1). In canine heart, ENDO cells show the following characteristics: (1) the greatest extent of unloaded shortening (freely contracting cells); (2) the smallest rate of shortening (as a percentage of total cell length); (3) the longest time-to-peak shortening; and (4) the slowest relaxation rate.[9] These regional differences correlate well with variations in the Ca^{2+} transient kinetics.

Bogaert and Rademakers[23] used magnetic resonance tagging to study structural, mechanical, and functional heterogeneity in normal human left ventricle. They found that tension is greatest in the subendocardial layers, and that it increases from apex to base during the isovolumic phase of contraction. Also, active myocardial shortening (as a percentage of diastolic length) was largest in the sub-endocardium (as previously reported by Cazorla and colleagues[18]), whereas segment shortening was smaller in basal compared with apical myocardium.

The previous in situ data from humans are in good agreement with data obtained from isolated cells. ENDO cells are stiffer than EPI cells, a property that may protect them from overstretching during the higher end-diastolic tensions in that layer. The length–active tension relation is steeper in ENDO cells, and the tension they develop is greater than that of EPI cells, at matching sarcomere lengths. This steepness helps to reduce the relative load on cross-bridges before the ejection phase and enables ENDO cells to shorten more than EPI cells. The ability to shorten effectively against a load is further facilitated by an intrinsically greater capacity for shortening and a greater duration of contractile activity. As suggested previously, the increased duration is a consequence of differences in a variety of subcellular mechanisms. Finally, the greater capacity of isolated apical cardiomyocytes to shorten under load[13] corresponds well with the greater segment shortening of the apical left ventricle.[23]

Extending the empirical generalization of the inverse relation of APD, to activation sequence, we may summarize that not only the APD but also the duration of the contraction–relaxation cycle and the duration of the Ca[2+] transient are inversely related to the sequence of transmural activation. ENDO cardiomyocytes, which are activated first, have a longer APD, a longer Ca[2+] transient with both a longer time to peak and a slower rate of decay, and a longer contractile cycle (at lower rates of contraction and relaxation; see Fig. 22–1). These data on cardiomyocyte heterogeneity are the basis of the physiologic relevance of mechanical heterogeneity.

MECHANO-ELECTRIC EFFECTS IN HETEROGENEOUS MYOCARDIUM

Identification of the effects of electromechanical heterogeneity on cardiac function is difficult in the intact heart, because cardiomyocytes are continuously subjected to dynamic redistribution of lengths and loads in a complex stress–strain field. Despite ample evidence for the presence of spatio-temporal heterogeneity, little is known about the mechano-electric effects of the interactions between heterogeneous segments of myocardium during the normal cardiac cycle.

Muscle Duplex Approach

Basic effects of the interaction between heterogeneous myocardial elements on the electromechanical activity of each element and the whole system can be mimicked, and experimentally assessed, using a condensed model of cardiac heterogeneity: the duplex. A duplex consists of a pair of dynamically interacting multicellular cardiac muscle preparations that are mechanically interconnected, either in series or in parallel. When connected in parallel, elements interact during isotonic–auxotonic contractions (corresponding to the ejection phase), where mutual shortening–lengthening of elements occurs through the redistribution of internal loads (c.f., Fig. 22–2A). Series elements interact during isometric duplex contractions (simulating the isovolumic phases of cardiac mechanical activity; Fig. 22–3).

The idea of muscle duplexes was first implemented by Tyberg and colleagues,[2] and then applied by Wiegner and colleagues[24] and Shimizu and colleagues.[25] Our group extended the approach, as discussed elsewhere.[26,27] Briefly, we implemented *six* principal duplex configurations, based on *in parallel* and *in series* combinations of biological and virtual (mathematical model) muscle segments. The combinations include (1) in parallel and (2) in series *biological duplex* (two mechanically connected biological samples, such as thin papillary muscles or trabeculae); (3) in parallel and (4) in series *virtual duplex* (two interconnected computational models of cardiac electromechanical activity); and (5) in parallel and (6) in series *hybrid duplex* (a biological sample that mechanically interacts, in real time, with a virtual muscle).[26–30] For all duplex configurations, one can study the element and the system functions in isolation and during mechanical interaction (including isometric, isotonic, and auxotonic modes of contraction). This enables a detailed assessment of the electromechanical characteristics of heterogeneous cardiac muscle preparations.

Electromechanical heterogeneity of the duplex can be controlled through selecting elements from a library of mechano-electric characteristics. In the biological setting, one can increase and decrease heterogeneity between elements with unilateral interventions such as variations in temperature or the application of drugs. In hybrid and virtual duplexes, the virtual elements are

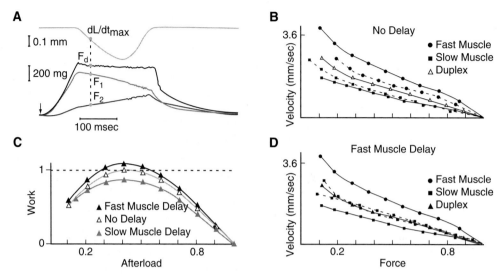

■ **Figure 22–2** Mechanical effects in a parallel biological heterogeneous duplex. *A,* (from *top* to *bottom*) Duplex shortening and total force (F_d) and individual forces (F_1, F_2) recorded of in parallel connected "slow" (25°C) and "fast" (30°C) papillary muscles from rabbit right ventricle under constant afterload imposed on the pair. *Dots* on the traces indicate the time of maximal velocity of shortening. Forces developed at this time (normalized by corresponding isometric peak force [PF]) are plotted versus the maximal velocity to obtain force–velocity relations for each element and the duplex *(B and D).* The relations change because of muscle coupling and the activation sequence. Work performed by the duplex (normalized) against various afterloads (normalized to the duplex PF) is optimized when the fast muscle stimulation is delayed *(C).* *(B and D: Solovyova O, Katsnelson L, Guriev S, et al: Mechanical inhomogeneity of myocardium studied in parallel and serial cardiac muscle duplexes: Experiments and models. Chaos Solitons Fractals 13:1685–1711, 2002, with permission.)*

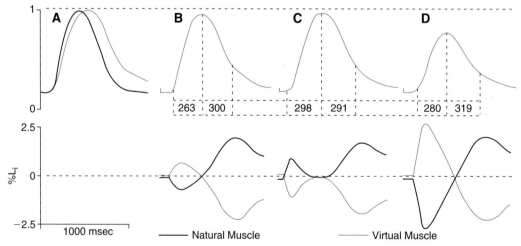

■ **Figure 22–3** Effect of stimulation delays on isometric contractions of an in series hybrid duplex. *A,* Isometric force developed in isolation by a fast natural muscle (papillary muscle from rat right ventricle, 0.3 Hz, 30°C, *dark line*) and a slow virtual muscle *(light line)* used to form the hybrid duplex. *B–D,* (from *top* to *bottom*) Force in the duplex *(top)* and element shortening/lengthening expressed in percentage of the initial length, L_i. Contractions with simultaneous stimulation *(B)* and with 60 msec delay of either the fast muscle *(C)* or the slow muscle *(D).* The time (in msec) to peak force and to 30% relaxation are indicated in the *middle row.*

open to wide variation to simulate physiologic or pathologic electromechanical properties.

For the biological duplexes presented in this chapter, we selected individual muscles that developed nearly equal peak isometric forces, but which displayed a prominent asynchrony in the time courses of force generation or shortening (see Fig. 22–3A).[27,28,30] These fast and slow muscles showed significant differences in mechanical characteristics, such as their length–force and force–velocity relations (see Fig. 22–2B and D).[28] In hybrid and virtual duplexes, we used virtual samples of fast and slow muscles, which displayed mechanical asynchrony corresponding to biological samples. These fast and slow virtual muscles also differed in their Ca^{2+} transients. The mechanically faster virtual muscles generated shorter APD than their slower counterparts (Fig. 22–4A and E), even when the electrical parameters of the models were the same.[30] These differences in APD are examples of MEF. *Dynamic variations in mechanics and Ca^{2+} handling create differences in the electrical behavior of individual cardiomyocytes within tissues,* even when the cells have identical electrical properties at rest.

Duplexes where the elements are mechanically asynchronous, possess different APD, and simulate interactions between transmural layers, where isolated ENDO myocytes contract more slowly and have longer APD than their EPI counterparts. Increasing asynchrony mimics the effects of normal myocardium interacting with pathologic myocardium (hypertrophied myocardium would show slower mechanics and a longer APD[22,31]).

A useful feature of the duplex model is that the temporal relation of the elements is under experimental control. For example, introducing a variable time delay in electrical activation allows one to simulate activation delays. In situ, these delays could occur between distant myocardial segments as a result of the more than 100-fold difference in speed between electrical and mechanical propagation (0.3 to 0.6 m/sec vs. 300 m/sec).

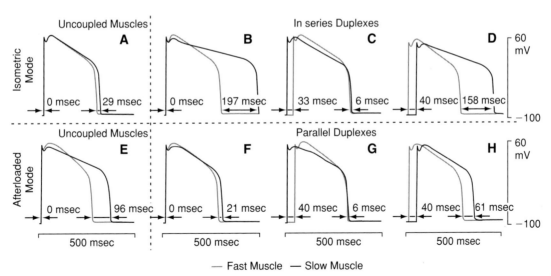

■ **Figure 22–4** Effects of mechanical coupling on action potential duration (APD) and dispersion of repolarization (DR) in elements of heterogeneous virtual duplexes. Shown are AP in a fast *(light lines)* and a slow *(dark lines)* virtual muscle before coupling *(A and E)* and mechanically coupled in series *(B–D)* or in parallel *(F–H)*. *Top line* demonstrates AP in the uncoupled muscles *(A)* and in series duplexes *(B–D)* during isometric contraction. *Bottom line* shows AP in the uncoupled muscles *(E)* and in parallel duplexes *(F–H)* during afterloaded contractions at an afterload of 25% of peak isometric force generated by the preparations. APD difference and DR change caused by (1) mode of contraction; (2) muscle coupling pattern; and (3) excitation sequence (stimulation delay of either the fast muscle *[C and G]* or the slow muscle *[D and H]* during duplex contractions).

Biomechanical Effects of Heterogeneity

In all duplex configurations, the contractile activity of an individual element (quantitatively assessed in length–force and force–velocity relations) is a function of the dynamic interaction with the other element, depending on their individual mechanical properties, electrical activation sequence, and connection patterns.[26,28]

The length–force and force–velocity relations of elements of in parallel duplexes were significantly different from those obtained before mechanical coupling (see Fig. 22–2B). Delayed electrical activation of the faster element of in parallel duplexes (which contracts/relaxes faster in isolation and represents "EPI" contraction patterns) causes the force–velocity and length–force relations of the elements to approach each other, up to a perfect overlap at favorable activation delays (see Fig. 22–2D). Delayed stimulation of the slower element, in contrast, causes these relations to diverge (see Reference 28 for a more detailed discussion of this topic). Furthermore, the physical work performed by duplexes also depends on the activation sequence and increases with fast element stimulation delay (and vice versa; see Fig. 22–2C). These results illustrate that the inherent myocardial heterogeneity, in conjunction with the intrinsic activation sequence, may confer functional homogeneity to the system, together with energetic advantages from work optimization. In contrast, an increase in functional heterogeneity of myocardium or a disturbed activation sequence may lead to a decrease in the capacity of the heart to perform work.

With in series duplexes, isometric peak force is maintained at a maximum level over a wide range (from 0 to 100 msec) of delays in fast element activation (see Fig. 22–3B and C). In contrast, delayed stimulation of the slow element has pronounced negative effects on peak force and speed of contraction–relaxation of the duplex (see Fig. 22–3D).[27] Tyberg and colleagues[2] also showed significantly different effects of stimulation delay on the duplex peak force, depending on the activation sequence in duplexes of strong and weak elements.

Why would the mechanical function of a heterogeneous myocardial system benefit from later activation of faster elements? If the faster element was activated before the slow one (see Fig. 22–3D), it would shorten against slack neighboring tissue (and vice versa), causing dys-synchrony of contraction and reduced system performance. In contrast, delayed activation of the fast element (see Fig. 22–3C) "preloads" it during early contraction (mechanical tuning during entrant phase) and allows elements to synchronize their activity, increasing the efficiency of the system.

Extending the duplex approach, one-dimensional (1D) cardiac tissue models consisting of several mechanically connected (in series) virtual muscle elements were studied.[32] A gradient of mechanical properties of individual elements (e.g., a gradual increase in the velocity of contraction and relaxation), in conjunction with excitation spreading from slow to fast coupled elements, provides the chain with stable contractile responses and tolerance to variations in activation delay of the fastest element. In contrast, force development in 1D models with either inverted excitation sequence or random (including uniform) spatial distribution of mechanical properties is significantly decreased. Interestingly, both homogeneous duplexes and 1D tissue stands, consisting of identical elements (either fast or slow ones), responded to stimulation delays with a decrease in force production.[27,32]

These results allow us to speculate that the pattern of regional mechanical heterogeneity is related to the excitation sequence, with the effect of optimizing the contractile function of normal myocardium.

Effects of Mechanical Interaction on the Electrical Activity of Duplex Elements

Using virtual duplexes,[30] we found significant changes in the APD of fast and slow virtual muscle elements after duplex formation (in parallel and in series; see Fig. 22–4).[27,30] The relative changes in APD were converse: An increase in APD of one muscle coincides with a decrease in the other. These changes correlated with similar changes in the duration of Ca^{2+} transients. Interestingly, the APD differences of in parallel elements decreased because of load redistribution during afterloaded contractions (see Fig. 22–4F), whereas in series contractions of the same element pairs increased the APD differences as a result of length redistribution (see Fig. 22–4B).

Delayed activation of the faster element of an in series duplex during isometric contractions (causing precontraction stretch by the earlier activated slow element) was accompanied by an increase in the APD of the fast muscle and a reduction of APD in the slow muscle. These changes in APD caused a *reduction* in the dispersion of repolarization (DR) by a value that significantly exceeded the initial stimulation delay (see Fig. 22–4C). Thus, and in contrast to the stability of duplex force generation with various delays in fast muscle stimulation (see Fig. 22–3B and C), DR was sensitive to the delay, with values abruptly decreasing after a delayed increase of 0 to 40 msec (see Fig. 22–4B and C). Inverting the electrical activation sequence increased the difference in APD and DR beyond the levels observed in isolation (see Fig. 22–4D). With in parallel duplexes, delayed stimulation of the fast element during afterloaded contractions smoothed the DR, whereas an inverted activation sequence kept it high (see Fig. 22–4G and H). In homogeneous duplexes, delays between element activations always caused a reduction in peak mechanical performance and an increased DR. This suggests that a myocardium with inherent activation delays would benefit from mechanical heterogeneity.[30]

Underlying Mechanisms

Using virtual duplexes, one may examine potential subcellular mechanisms of MEF.[26,28,30] Functional adjustments of the mechanical activity of a duplex element correlate with (and are seemingly controlled by) significant changes in the Ca^{2+} activation of thin filaments (assessed by kinetics of Ca^{2+} binding to TnC). These changes are accompanied by either a convergence or a divergence of cytosolic Ca^{2+} transients of the interacting elements. The mechanically induced modulation of Ca^{2+} transients affects Ca^{2+}-dependent currents, predominantly I_{NCX}. Our models predict that the latter current may be sufficient to trigger the observed changes in AP modulation. Changes in AP repolarization also are influenced by secondary effects of changes in the AP shape on the voltage-sensitive K^+ and Na^+ currents. In both in series and in parallel virtual duplexes, *changes in the APD caused by mechanical interactions are correlated with changes in the Ca^{2+} transient duration.*

In this complex interplay of cellular processes, *mechano-dependent Ca^{2+} kinetics play a key role in the fine adjustment of mechanical and electrical activity.* This allows the myocardium to match local function to global demand.

An open question is whether SR Ca^{2+} loading is affected by the previously discussed interactions (which would be expected from the significant modulation of cytosolic Ca^{2+} kinetics and APD in our models). Preliminary results, obtained in hybrid and virtual duplexes, showed a heterogeneous distribution of SR Ca^{2+} loading in mechanically interacting fast and slow elements. With mechanical coupling, an increase in SR Ca^{2+} loading of the slow element was accompanied by a significant increase in the amplitude and duration of Ca^{2+} transient and an increase in APD. Opposite changes were observed in the fast element.[33] This cross talk could provide a suitable mechanism to maintain adequate Ca^{2+} loading of individual cells, because "weak" cells would be stretched during systole, increasing SR Ca^{2+} and yielding a more forceful contraction. This boost would assist in meeting the external demands, even in the absence of calcium influx through stretch-activated ion channels.

Dynamic deformation of interacting elements, especially a precontractile distension of in series elements during isometric contractions, could activate mechanosensitive channel currents. These could contribute to changes in the AP and to SR loading (a problem that has not yet been addressed in our duplex models).

Summary
Physiologic Relevance of Heterogeneity

The preceding data show that cardiac muscle is structurally and functionally heterogeneous, and that this heterogeneity manifests itself at all stages of functional integration, from the molecular to the whole-organ level. The coordinated electromechanical activity of the heart involves, and in fact requires, a range of physical gradients. These include transmural and apex–base gradients of passive and active mechanical properties, with tension increasing from sub-epicardium to sub-endocardium and from apex to base. Deformation increases from sub-epicardium to sub-endocardium and from base to apex. In addition, there is a sequence of activation of ventricular regions that creates specific temporal gradients from the sub-endocardium to the sub-epicardium and from the apex to the base. Finally, there is a prominent transmural gradient of cardiomyocyte properties, including electrical and mechanical characteristics, and specific features of excitation–contraction coupling (see Fig. 22–1). *A major achievement of the recent decade is the identification and detailed description of the distribution of cell properties along these physical and temporal gradients.*

The dynamic relation, however, between these gradients and their effects on heart function is less well understood. The duplex models of a heterogeneous myocardium allow us to elucidate fundamental aspects of this interaction. The dynamic mechanical interaction (the continuous length and load redistribution) between heterogeneous myocardial elements affects their activity in a way that depends crucially on the pattern of heterogeneity (spatial distribution of electromechanical properties, temporal activation sequence). Under normal physiologic conditions, element heterogeneity confers system homogeneity, optimizing function. Conversely, pathologic disturbances that increase or decrease heterogeneity may reduce cardiac efficiency.

Acknowledgments

This work is the subject of a research collaboration of the Ekaterinburg group with the team of Drs. Noble and Kohl at Oxford University. Mathematical model development and duplex studies were financially supported by two Wellcome Trust Collaborative Research Initiative Grants and by the Russian Foundation for Basic Research.

References

1. Wiggers CJ: Interpretation of the intraventricular pressure curve on the basis of rapidly summated fractionate contractions. Am J Physiol 80:12, 1927.
2. Tyberg JV, Parmley WW, Sonnenblick EH: In-vitro studies of myocardial asynchrony and regional hypoxia. Circ Res 25:569–579, 1969.
3. Brutsaert DL: Nonuniformity: A physiologic modulator of contraction and relaxation of the normal heart. J Am Coll Cardiol 9:341–348, 1987.
4. Katz AM, Katz PB: Homogeneity out of heterogeneity. Circulation 79:712–717, 1989.
5. Wolk R, Cobbe SM, Hicks MN, Kane KA: Functional, structural, and dynamic basis of electrical heterogeneity in healthy and diseased cardiac muscle: Implications for arrhythmogenesis and anti-arrhythmic drug therapy. Pharmacol Ther 84:207–231, 1999.
6. Carmeliet E: Cardiac Cellular Electrophysiology. Amsterdam, Kluwer Academic Publishers, 2002.
7. Antzelevitch C, Fish J: Electrical heterogeneity within the ventricular wall. Basic Res Cardiol 96:517–527, 2001.
8. Nerbonne JM, Guo W: Heterogeneous expression of voltage-gated potassium channels in the heart: Roles in normal excitation and arrhythmias. J Cardiovasc Electrophysiol 13:406–409, 2002.
9. Cordeiro JM, Greene L, Heilmann C, et al: Transmural heterogeneity of calcium activity and mechanical function in the canine left ventricle. Am J Physiol Heart Circ Physiol 286:H1471–H1479, 2003.
10. Sakmann BF, Spindler AJ, Bryant SM, et al: Distribution of a persistent sodium current across the ventricular wall in guinea pigs. Circ Res 87:910–914, 2000.
11. Zygmunt AC, Goodrow RJ, Antzelevitch C: I_{NaCa} contributes to electrical heterogeneity within the canine ventricle. Am J Physiol Heart Circ Physiol 278:H1671–H1678, 2000.
12. Franz MR, Bargheer K, Rafflenbeul W, et al: Monophasic action potential mapping in human subjects with normal electrocardiograms: Direct evidence for the genesis of the t wave. Circulation 75:379–386, 1987.
13. Wan X, Bryant SM, Hart G: A topographical study of mechanical and electrical properties of single myocytes isolated from normal guinea-pig ventricular muscle. J Anat 202:525–536, 2003.
14. Bányász T, Fülöp L, Magyar J, et al: Endocardial versus epicardial differences in L-type calcium current in canine ventricular myocytes studied by action potential voltage clamp. Cardiovasc Res 58:66–75, 2003.
15. Ng GA, Cobbe SM, Smith GL: Non-uniform prolongation of intracellular Ca^{2+} transients recorded from the epicardial surface of isolated hearts from rabbits with heart failure. Cardiovasc Res 37:489–502, 1998.
16. McIntosh MA, Cobbe SM, Smith GL: Heterogeneous changes in action potential and intracellular Ca^{2+} in left ventricular myocyte sub-types from rabbits with heart failure. Cardiovasc Res 45:397–409, 2000.
17. Laurita KR, Katra R, Wible B, et al: Transmural heterogeneity of calcium handling in canine. Circ Res 92:668–675, 2003.
18. Cazorla O, Le Guennec JY, White E: Length-tension relationships of sub-epicardial and sub-endocardial single ventricular myocytes from rat and ferret hearts. J Mol Cell Cardiol 32:735–744, 2000.

19. Cazorla O, Freiburg A, Helmes M, et al: Differential expression of cardiac titin isoforms and modulation of cellular stiffness. Circ Res 86:59–67, 2000.

20. Gordon AM, Regnier M, Homsher E: Skeletal and cardiac muscle contractile activation: Tropomyosin "rocks and rolls." News Physiol Sci 16:49–55, 2001.

21. Litten RZ, Martin BJ, Buchthal RH, et al: Heterogeneity of myosin isozyme content of rabbit heart. Circ Res 57:406–414, 1985.

22. Bryant SM, Shipsey SJ, Hart G: Regional differences in electrical and mechanical properties of myocytes from guinea-pig hearts with mild left ventricular hypertrophy. Cardiovasc Res 35:315–323, 1997.

23. Bogaert J, Rademakers FE: Regional nonuniformity of normal adult human left ventricle. Am J Physiol Heart Circ Physiol 280:H610–H620, 2001.

24. Wiegner AW, Allen GJ, Bing OH: Weak and strong myocardium in series: Implications for segmental dysfunction. Am J Physiol 235:H776–H783, 1978.

25. Shimizu G, Wiegner AW, Gaasch WH, et al: Force pattern of hypoxic myocardium applied to oxygenated muscle preparations: Comparison with effects of regional ischemia on the contraction of non-ischemic myocardium. Cardiovasc Res 32:1038–1046, 1996.

26. Markhasin VS, Katsnelson LB, Nikitina LV, et al: Biomechanics of the inhomogeneous myocardium. Ekaterinburg, Ural Division of the Russian Academy of Sciences, 1999.

27. Markhasin VS, Solovyova O, Katsnelson LB, et al: Mechano-electric interactions in heterogeneous myocardium: Development of fundamental experimental and theoretical models. Prog Biophys Mol Biol 82(1–3):207–220, 2003.

28. Solovyova O, Katsnelson L, Guriev S, et al: Mechanical inhomogeneity of myocardium studied in parallel and serial cardiac muscle duplexes: Experiments and models. Chaos Solitons Fractals 13:1685–1711, 2002.

29. Markhasin VS, Nikitina LV, Routkevich SM, et al: Effects of mechanical interaction between two rabbit cardiac muscles connected in parallel. Gen Physiol Biophys 21:277–301, 2002.

30. Solovyova O, Vikulova N, Katsnelson LB, et al: Mechanical interaction of heterogeneous cardiac muscle segments in silico: Effects on Ca^{2+} handling and action potential. Int J Bifurcat Chaos 13:3757–3782, 2003.

31. Natali AJ, Wilson LA, Peckham M, et al: Different regional effects of voluntary exercise on the mechanical and electrical properties of rat ventricular myocytes. J Physiol 541(pt 3):863–875, 2002.

32. Gur'ev S, Lookin O: Experimental and computer models of mechanically heterogeneous myocardium. J Physiol 552P:P35, 2003.

33. Konovalov P, Solovyova O, Markhasin VS, Kohl P: Local contractility matching to global demand in heterogeneous myocardium: Role of mechanical interaction. Biophys J 84:240a, 2003.

CHAPTER 23

Mechanical Modulation of Cardiac Function: Role of the Pericardium

• • • •

John V. Tyberg

Perhaps because it contains no muscle and seems to be a passive structure, little attention was paid to the role of the pericardium for many years, except to conclude that it prevented excessive cardiac dilation and somehow maintained equality between the outputs of the right (RV) and left ventricle (LV).[1]

TRANSMURAL PRESSURE

The key to the physiology of the pericardium is to understand the critical importance of transmural pressure. The LV, like any elastic chamber, distends in proportion to its transmural pressure, not in proportion to its intracavity pressure per se. Although physicists and engineers understand the distinction, it is frequently overlooked in medicine. Regardless of whether we are aware of it, pressure is always measured in relation to another pressure. Electrical potential (voltage) is always measured in relation to another voltage and, strictly speaking, voltage is a *potential difference.* Analogously, effective distending pressure[2] is a *pressure difference* across the chamber wall—that is, transmural pressure. Although this principle is only rarely important with respect to systolic pressures,[3] it may be critical with respect to LV diastolic pressure under many important circumstances.[4] If we report that left ventricular end-diastolic pressure (LVEDP) = 12 mm Hg, we mean that LVEDP is 12 mm Hg greater than atmospheric pressure, because we measured LVEDP with a transducer that mechanically compared it with atmospheric pressure. However, if pericardial pressure happens to be 4 mm Hg, transmural LVEDP is only 8 mm Hg (transmural LVEDP = LVEDP − pericardial pressure).

Furthermore, if LVEDP increases to 15 mm Hg, but pericardial pressure also increases to 7 mm Hg, transmural LVEDP remains 8 mm Hg and left ventricular end-diastolic volume (LVEDV) will not have changed.

The truth of these statements is persuasively demonstrated by an observation that is commonplace to a cardiac physiologist or a surgeon. Assuming that normal values of right ventricular end-diastolic pressure (RVEDP) and LVEDP are 4 and 12 mm Hg, respectively, consider what happens when the pericardium is opened widely and held back from the heart and when both of those pressures are maintained constant by an infusion of volume. The LV expands somewhat, but the RV and the right atrium (RA) expand substantially, so that they could never be accommodated within the normal pericardium. The chambers of the heart expand because their transmural pressures increase. Because the intracavity pressures remained constant, pericardial pressures could not have been zero when the pericardium was closed. When the pericardium was closed, RVEDP was 4 mm Hg, and pericardial pressure was approximately 4 mm Hg, giving a transmural RVEDP of ~0 mm Hg. When the pericardium was opened, RVEDP was still 4 mm Hg, but because pericardial pressure was then zero, transmural RVEDP was 4 mm Hg. RV volume increased according to the increase in transmural RVEDP. Such observations underscore the importance of the pericardium in preventing excessive dilation of the RV, with its attendant increased irritability,[5] an example of mechano-electric feedback.[6]

Figure 23–1 illustrates these relations.[7] Pressures are represented semiquantitatively by opposing arrows of different lengths and, if unit surface areas are consid-

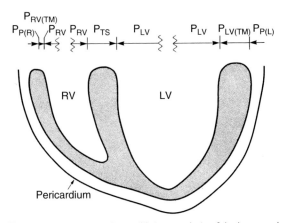

$P_{RV(TM)}$
$P_{P(R)}$ P_{RV} P_{RV} P_{TS} P_{LV} P_{LV} $P_{LV(TM)}$ $P_{P(L)}$

RV   LV

Pericardium

■ **Figure 23–1** A static-equilibrium analysis of the heart and pericardium. *Arrows indicate direction and approximate magnitude of opposing end-diastolic pressures (P), equivalent to opposing forces if the pressures are applied over unit area. At each wall, intracavity pressure is equal to transmural pressure plus the pressure outside the wall. For the left (LV) and right ventricular (RV) free walls, intracavity pressure is equal to transmural (TM) pressure when the pericardium is removed. $P_{P(R)}$ and $P_{P(L)}$, right and left pericardial pressure; P_{TS}, transseptal pressure. (From Tyberg JV: Ventricular interaction and the pericardium. In: Levine HJ, Gaasch WH [eds]: The Ventricle: Basic and Clinical Aspects. Boston, Martinus Nijhoff Publishing, 1985, pp 171–184, with permission.)*

ered, are equivalent to force balances across the LV free wall, the interventricular septum, and the RV free wall. Inertial and viscous effects can be ignored when the heart is approximately stationary at end diastole; therefore, this constitutes a static-equilibrium analysis. At each wall, intracavity pressure is equal to the opposing transmural pressure plus the pressure on the opposite side. As suggested previously, if the pericardium is removed and held back from the heart, pericardial pressure becomes zero (i.e., atmospheric pressure) and intracavity pressure must then be exactly equal to the transmural pressure, which is the rationale for our measurement of pericardial pressure (see later). Except under conditions in which the RV is hypertrophied,[8] RVEDP is approximately equal to pericardial pressure,[9,10] and, except when the RV or the LV are selectively afterloaded by arterial constriction, right and left pericardial pressures are equal.[11] Thus, LV pericardial pressure approximately equals RVEDP, and RVEDP

approximately equals RV pericardial pressure. This implies that transmural RVEDP approaches zero, a contentious conclusion for a time,[12,13] but one that was ultimately verified[14,15] and supported by other investigators.[16]

HOW CAN PERICARDIAL PRESSURE BE MEASURED?

It had long been thought that the relation between LVEDP and LVEDV, so-called diastolic compliance,[17] was practically invariant. Indeed, this assumption was the basis for Sarnoff and Berglund's[18] ventricular function curve analysis in which they used LV filling pressure rather than LVEDV as the measure of LV preload. However, investigators in the 1970s demonstrated that diastolic compliance could change substantially and rapidly—for example, by giving nitroglycerin to a patient with heart failure.[19] My group then suggested that such changes were caused by unappreciated decreases in pericardial pressure,[20] but many thought this hypothesis unlikely because pericardial pressure had been shown to be negative and unchanging, even as RVEDP had been increased to high values by pulmonary artery obstruction.[21]

This prompted a re-examination of what was meant by pericardial pressure and how it should be measured.[22,23] My group compared pericardial pressure measured using a flat, liquid-containing balloon transducer[24] with that measured using an open catheter[21] and compared both pressure measurements with "true" pericardial pressure, which we suggested should be the difference between LVEDP measured with the pericardium closed and that measured with the pericardium open and held back, at the same volume (LVEDV). As explained previously, this rationale was based on our understanding of transmural pressure, such that LVEDP = transmural LVEDP + pericardial pressure. The study demonstrated that the balloon-measured pressure was always correct, but that the open catheter seriously underestimated pericardial pressure unless substantial volumes of liquid (~30 mL) were added to the pericardium. We then measured pericardial pressure in surgical patients who were transiently volume loaded and compared it with mean RA pressure; both pressures increased in parallel and, in

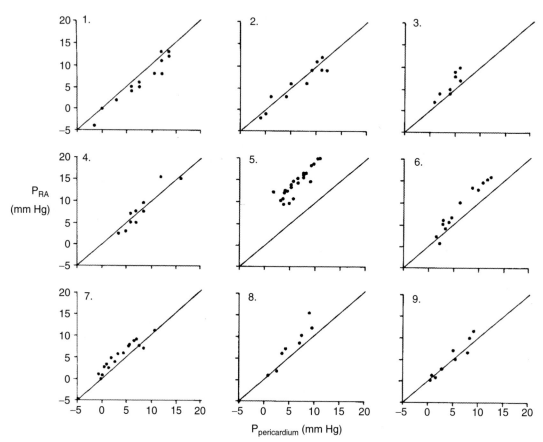

■ **Figure 23–2** Simultaneously measured mean right atrial pressure (P_{RA}; y-axes) and pericardial pressure (x-axes; measured over the left ventricular free wall) in nine patients studied during volume loading before initiation of cardiopulmonary bypass. Note that right atrial pressure increased in proportion to the increase in pericardial pressure in each patient. Note also that, except for one patient (Patient 5), the absolute value of right atrial pressure was equal to pericardial pressure. Thus, pericardial pressure is highly variable and is usually equal to right atrial pressure. *(From Tyberg JV, Taichman GC, Smith ER, et al: The relation between pericardial pressure and right atrial pressure: An intraoperative study. Circulation 73:428–432, 1986, with permission.)*

most cases, were effectively identical[10] (Fig. 23–2). Thus, we concluded that pericardial pressure is changeable acutely, and that it is approximately equal to RV filling pressure under most circumstances.[8] In a normal pericardium without an excess of liquid,[22] pericardial pressure is fundamentally a compressive contact stress[23] and is equal to measured hydrostatic pressure only when special care is taken to eliminate the artifacts caused by the presence of a large catheter.[25] These conclusions have been supported by experimental[16] and clinical[8,26] studies.

IMPLICATIONS FOR THE FRANK–STARLING LAW

When LV filling pressure is used as the parameter of preload in a ventricular function curve analysis,[18] a change in compliance[17] can lead erroneously to the conclusion that LV contractility has changed, as Glantz and Parmley pointed out[27] (Fig. 23–3). If compliance decreases (see Fig. 23–3, middle), LVEDP increases at a given value of LVEDV. That being so, when ventricular systolic performance (i.e., LV stroke work) is eval-

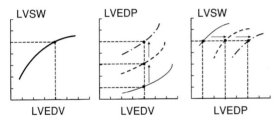

Figure 23–3 Relation of diastolic compliance to contractility. In the presence of constant contractility *(left)*, if diastolic compliance is decreased *(middle)*, it might be mistakenly concluded that contractility is decreased *(right)*. LVSW, left ventricular stroke work; LVEDV, left ventricular end-distolic volume; LVEDP, left ventricular end-diastolic pressure. *(Data from Glantz SA, Parmley WW: Factors which affect the diastolic pressure-volume curve. Circ Res 42:171–180, 1978; reproduced from Tyberg JV, Grant DA, Kingma I, et al: Effects of positive intrathoracic pressure on the evaluation of cardiac performance. In: de Abreu MG, Koch T [eds]: Proceedings of the Second Dresden Postgraduate Course on Mechanical Ventilation, October 26–27, 2001. Lubeck, Drager Medical, 2001, with permission.)*

uated in terms of LVEDP (see Fig. 23–3, right), the ventricular function curve is shifted to the right. This indicates that the same value of LV stroke work is accomplished at increasing values of LVEDP and erroneously suggests that contractility has decreased. LVEDP increases, but LVEDV, the ultimate measure of LV preload, does not, which is consistent with the unchanged value of stroke work.

VENTRICULAR INTERACTION

By ventricular interaction, I mean a reciprocal, complementary change in the volumes of the RV and LV such that when RVEDV increases, LVEDV decreases (and vice versa). Ventricular interaction involves the septum moving toward the LV or the RV and is profoundly diminished when the heart is not constrained by the pericardium[28,29] or other mediastinal structures.[30] The pericardium is relatively stiff compared with the RV or LV myocardium; therefore, as viewed with respect to an "equatorial" cross-sectional plane, the heart is surrounded by an effectively unyielding band or belt. (Small changes in the long axis of the LV may occur, but these are not included in this discus-

sion.) Thus, RVEDV can increase only at the expense of LVEDV. These changes in volume occur because the septum is elastic and moves leftward or rightward with small decreases or increases in the difference between LVEDP and RVEDP (i.e., the *trans*-septal "gradient"; TSG = LVEDP – RVEDP).[31,32] Ventricular interaction is diminished when pericardial pressure is very low and, effectively, it does not occur when the pericardium is open.[29]

Ventricular interaction was illustrated most clearly by a series of studies of the effects of acute pulmonary artery embolization and volume loading, with and without the pericardium.[28,33,34] With the pericardium intact, pulmonary embolization and volume loading appeared to decrease LV diastolic compliance and LV contractility, as evaluated conventionally by plots of LVEDP versus LVEDV and LV stroke work versus LVEDP.[33] However, when diastolic compliance and contractility were evaluated using transmural LVEDP to reflect the effective distending pressure, there was no change in LV compliance or contractility[27] (Fig. 23–4). When the same experiment was repeated after opening the pericardium, ventricular interaction was absent[28] (Fig. 23–5).

Ventricular interaction and its effect on apparent contractility also were illustrated in the newborn lamb.[35] Before the lamb had taken its first breath, pressures and LV performance (stroke work) were measured while blood volume was momentarily increased and decreased by transfusion and withdrawal. These measurements were repeated after ventilation had been initiated, and then again after the pericardium was opened and after it and the lungs had been pulled away from the heart. Ventilation increased LV compliance and apparent contractility (i.e., greater stroke work was performed at the same level of LVEDP), and complete removal of pericardial and pleural constraint to LV filling appeared to further increase compliance and contractility. However, under all these conditions, LV stroke work was predicted by LVEDV or by transmural LVEDP.

As suggested, the constraining effect of the lungs and associated thoracic structures produces measurable effects on LV filling.[36,37] When the chest is closed, pericardial pressure is the sum of pleural pressure and *trans*pericardial pressure (i.e., pericardial pressure – pleural pressure). Pleural pressure (i.e., cardiac fossa pressure) naturally increases with positive end-expiratory

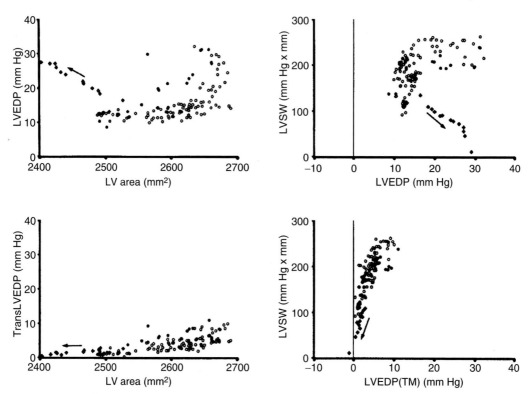

■ **Figure 23–4**   The effect of pericardial pressure on left ventricular (LV) compliance and ventricular function curves in dogs after acute pulmonary embolization and volume loading. In each panel, *arrows* indicate beat-to-beat changes during a preterminal infusion of saline. *Top,* Conventional measures of compliance *(left)* and contractility *(right)* based on LVEDP; *bottom,* transmural LVEDP (LVEDP(TM)). *Top left,* An apparent decrease in LV diastolic compliance, as LVEDP increased while LVEDV (here represented by LV area) decreased. However, the properties of the ventricular wall did not really change as *(bottom left)* the LVEDP(TM)–LV area relation was unchanged, and all the data fell along a single curve. *Top right,* Conventional ventricular function curve indicates that contractility has decreased, as LV stroke work (LVSW) decreased, whereas LVEDP increased. However, *(bottom right)* there was no real change in contractility because there was no shift in the LVSW–LVEDP(TM) relation. Data from Belenkie and colleagues.[33] *(From Tyberg JV, Smith ER: Ventricular diastole and the role of the pericardium. Herz 15:354–361, 1990, with permission.)*

pressure (PEEP), but it is measurable (~5 mm Hg) after volume loading, even in the absence of PEEP.[38] *Trans*pericardial pressure is a measure of the effective distending pressure of the pericardium and thus reflects total cardiac volume.[38,39] Recent work suggests that substantial mediastinal and pleural constraint remains even after surgical pericardiotomy.[30]

Recently, my group demonstrated how the pericardium modulates LV and RV stroke volumes to compensate for sudden changes in atrial volume.[29] In anesthetized dogs, we suddenly infused or removed ~25 mL blood into or from the left atrium (LA) or RA. With infusions, ipsilateral ventricular end-diastolic

transmural pressure, diameter, and stroke volume all increased. With the pericardium closed, there were compensatory decreases in contralateral transmural end-diastolic pressure, diameter, and stroke volume. The sum of the ipsilateral increases and the contralateral decreases in stroke volume approximated the infused volume. Corresponding and opposite changes were seen with blood withdrawals. Changes in LV septum-to-free-wall diameter were inversely related to changes in RV septum-to-free-wall diameter. All these manifestations of direct ventricular interaction were diminished when pericardial pressure was less than 5 mm Hg and were absent when the pericardium was

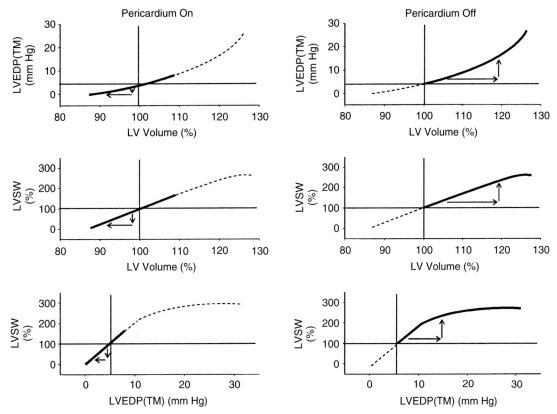

■ **Figure 23–5** Ventricular interaction *(left)*. The effects of volume loading after pulmonary embolism differ qualitatively, depending on whether the pericardium is present. To compare the results of two investigations,[33,34] data were normalized such that LVEDV and LVSW were set equal to 100% when transmural left ventricular end-diastolic pressure (LVEDP(TM); i.e., *left,* LVEDP minus pericardial pressure; *right,* LVEDP) was equal to 5 mm Hg. *Top,* Diastolic compliance (LVEDP(TM) vs. end-diastolic volume); *middle,* LV function (LVSW) in terms of LVEDV; *bottom,* LV function in terms of LVEDP(TM). The left and right paired relations are identical; *thickened lines* indicate the operating regions of the relations, with or without the pericardium. *Paired arrows* tending to describe the sides of a triangle describe the typical effects of volume loading. *Right,* Volume loading increases end-diastolic volume and LVEDP(TM) *(top),* and the increases in LVSW are predicted by both the increases in end-diastolic volume *(middle)* and transmural LVEDP *(bottom).* *Left,* Volume loading **decreases** end-diastolic volume and LVEDP(TM) *(top),* and the magnitudes of the decreases in LVSW are predicted by both the decreases in end-diastolic volume and LVEDP(TM). *(From Tyberg JV, Belenkie I: Mechanical interactions between the respiratory and circulatory systems. In: Bradley TD, Floras JS [eds]: Sleep Disorders and Cardiovascular and Cerebrovascular Disease. New York, Marcel Dekker, 2000, pp 99–112, with permission.)*

opened. Thus, pericardial constraint appears essential for immediate biventricular compensatory responses to acute atrial volume changes. This study not only demonstrated new dynamic aspects of ventricular interaction but also a mechanism whereby pulmonary blood volume is stabilized. Furthermore, it demonstrated that the pericardium acts as a mechanical servo-control system whereby one ventricle can immediately respond to changes in the volume of the other ventri-

cle, adjusting its output to compensate. We suggested that this mechanism might normally be a first line of defense against orthostatic hypotension (i.e., the decrease in arterial blood pressure that results from assuming a standing position). When a person stands up, venous return to the RA is momentarily decreased as blood pools in the lower body. This reduces RVEDV, which, by the mechanism outlined previously, increases LVEDV and LV stroke volume, tending to minimize the hypotension. If pericardial pressure is reduced for any reason, this mechanism might be impaired, and the individual might be more prone to development of orthostatic hypotension (e.g., in both the endurance athlete at rest and the patient with successfully treated heart failure, the pericardium might be "too big for the heart").

Because the complementary changes in RV and LV volumes (i.e., ventricular interaction) occur largely through the displacement of the septum and because the driving force for septal displacement is the TSG, changes in the TSG become a convenient indicator of ventricular interaction. Such considerations led Mirsky and Rankin[40] to observe that the LV is surrounded by the pericardium only over approximately two thirds of its circumference, with the remaining one third being surrounded by the RV. Therefore, because we hold that LVEDV is the most fundamental chamber parameter of preload and the best predictor of systolic performance according to the Frank–Starling Law, it is sometimes useful to modify the definition of transmural pressure accordingly to better account for the contribution of a changing RVEDP and to predict LVEDV.[41]

PHYSIOLOGIC IMPLICATIONS

The paramount importance of transmural pressure has physiologic implications. By recording from single cervical vagal afferent fibers, my group[42] demonstrated that the activity of ventricular mechanoreceptors is dependent on LV transmural pressure and consequent distension, not on intracavity pressure. Similarly, serum atriopeptin (atrial natriuretic peptide) concentrations are dependent on atrial transmural pressure and distension.[43]

These interpretations of pericardial physiology might also have the effect of focusing relatively more attention on changes in LV preload and less on LV contractility, when attempting to understand the basis for changes in systolic performance. As discussed previously,[28,33–35] profound changes in systolic performance can be explained when preload is understood as transmural LVEDP. In healthy dogs, volume loading has negligible effects on stroke volume, although cardiac output increases because of the increased heart rate.[44] However, LVEDV fails to increase when

LVEDP is increased to greater than 10 to 15 mm Hg,[45] which, based on our cumulative experience, could well be caused by pericardial constraint. Similarly, volume loading beyond an LVEDP of 10 to 15 mm Hg fails to increase systolic performance in human subjects,[46] which also could be caused by pericardial constraint.

CLINICAL IMPLICATIONS

Perhaps one of the detrimental effects of an inappropriate PR interval relates to the pericardium. In dogs with atrioventricular block who were paced independently from the RA and RV, we assessed LV diastolic compliance and systolic function when PR intervals were normal and when the atrium and ventricle were stimulated at the same instant (PR interval = 0). In the latter situation, as conventionally assessed, diastolic compliance and systolic performance were decreased because of AV interaction. The unemptied atria compromised the pericardial volume, which increased pericardial pressure and decreased transmural LVEDP and LVEDV for a given value of intracavity LVEDP.[47]

Because pacemaker activity[48] and other heart rate disturbances depend on myocardial stretch,[6] and thus chamber volume, the effects of performing the Valsalva maneuver may be difficult to predict.[49–51] Ventricular volumes decrease during the strain phase of the Valsalva maneuver in healthy subjects (presumably because of a decrease in transmural pressure, despite an increase in intracavity pressure), but not in patients with cardiomyopathy[52] and, perhaps, other cardiac diseases.

Probably the most important clinical implication of these aspects of pericardial physiology is the role of the pericardium in heart failure. In 1946, Howarth, McMichael, and Sharpey-Schafer[53] published a report of the effects of venesection in patients with low-output heart failure. They described a patient with high venous pressure and low cardiac output in whom the removal of 800 mL venous blood almost doubled cardiac output, as venous pressure decreased precipitously. As shown in Figure 23–6, this long-puzzling observation might be explained by the action of the pericardium. As blood was withdrawn from a dog in pacing-induced heart failure,[54] LVEDP decreased as expected. However, because pericardial pressure actu-

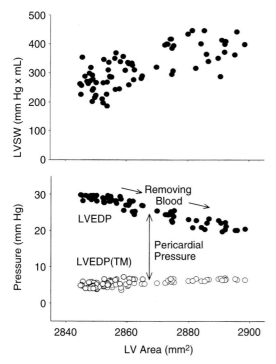

■ **Figure 23–6** Effect of removing blood volume in a dog with pacing-induced heart failure.[54] Removing venous blood decreased LVEDP. However, because pericardial pressure *(vertical arrow)* decreased more than LVEDP, LVEDP(TM) increased, consistent with the increase in LVEDV (i.e., area). In turn, LVSW increased, consistent with the increase in LVEDP(TM) and LVEDV.

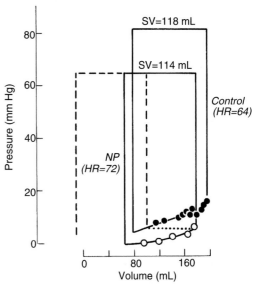

■ **Figure 23–7** The importance of the shift in the LV diastolic pressure–volume relation to the maintenance of stroke volume (SV) after administration of sodium nitroprusside (NP). Because of the shift in the relation, SV was maintained despite large reductions in LVEDP. Had the control pressure–volume relation been followed, this reduction in LVEDP would have corresponded to such a small LVEDV that SV would have decreased greatly. HR, heart rate. Data from Alderman and Glantz.[58] *(From Tyberg JV, Misbach GA, Parmley WW, Glantz SA: Effects of the pericardium on ventricular performance. In: Baan J, Yellin EL, Arntzenius AC [eds]: Cardiac Dynamics. Boston, Martinus Nijhoff, 1980, pp 159–168, with permission.)*

ally decreased more than LVEDP, transmural LVEDP increased. The increase in transmural LVEDP was accompanied by an increase in LVEDV and LV systolic performance (i.e., stroke work).

These observations bring to mind the classical therapy of blood letting—whether effected by venesection or the application of leeches—and raise the question of whether the benefits of nitrate therapy in heart failure are at least partly related to the mechanisms described previously (in addition to decreased mitral regurgitation, if present). Nitrates increase venous capacitance and decrease central venous pressure; therefore, they decrease pericardial pressure,[55] which shifts the LV diastolic pressure–volume relation downward.[19,20,56] LVEDV may increase or decrease slightly, but, if so, much less than would have been expected from the profound decrease in LVEDP. Both nitrates and reduction of blood volume reduce central venous pressure, which decreases pericardial pressure pari passu,[10] thus effectively increasing the compliance of the LV.

As shown in Figure 23–7,[57] a reduction in LV afterload and a modest increase in heart rate typically help to maintain cardiac output after the administration of nitrates.[58] However, the role of pericardium-mediated ventricular interaction is critical. There would be no possibility of reducing LVEDP so much (thereby effectively treating pulmonary edema) and reducing

LVEDV so little (thereby tending to maintain LV preload), except for the downward shift in the diastolic pressure–volume relation, a downward shift that all evidence now suggests is caused by a reduction in pericardial pressure.

Summary

This overview of recent developments in pericardial physiology was incisively anticipated by L. N. Katz in 1955:[4]

Even the use of end-diastolic pressure as an index of end-diastolic volume is not justified. . . . Furthermore, if the expansion of the heart is limited, for example by the pericardium, changes in end-diastolic pressure lose much of their meaning in terms of changes in end-diastolic volume.

With the benefit of this past insight and of the results of more recent experimental work, it is hoped that future generations of clinicians *will not assume* that an intervention that increases LVEDP will necessarily increase stroke volume and cardiac output; *the opposite may occur in some circumstances.* Transmural LVEDP predicts LVEDV, and LVEDV predicts systolic performance (i.e., stroke volume and stroke work); thus, the Frank–Starling Law continues to be useful.

References

1. Shabetai R: The Pericardium. New York, Grune and Stratton, 1981, p 34.
2. Henderson Y, Barringer TBJ: The relation of venous pressure to cardiac efficiency. Am J Physiol 13:352–369, 1913.
3. Haykowsky M, Taylor D, Teo K, et al: Left ventricular wall stress during leg-press exercise performed with a brief Valsalva maneuver. Chest 119:150–154, 2001.
4. Katz LN: Analysis of the several factors regulating the performance of the heart. Physiol Rev 35:91–106, 1955.
5. Levine JH, Guarnieri T, Kadish AH, et al: Changes in myocardial repolarization in patients undergoing balloon valvuloplasty for congenital pulmonary stenosis: Evidence for contraction-excitation feedback in humans. Circulation 77:70–77, 1988.
6. Kohl P, Ravens U: Cardiac mechano-electric feedback: Past, present, and prospect. Prog Biophys Mol Biol 82:3–9, 2003.
7. Tyberg JV: Ventricular interaction and the pericardium. In: Levine HJ, Gaasch WH (eds): The Ventricle: Basic and Clinical Aspects. Boston, Martinus Nijhoff Publishing, 1985, pp 171–184.
8. Boltwood CM, Skulsky A, Drinkwater DC, et al: Intraoperative measurement of pericardial constraint: Role in ventricular diastolic mechanics. J Am Coll Cardiol 8:1289–1297, 1986.
9. Smiseth OA, Refsum H, Tyberg JV: Pericardial pressure assessed by right atrial pressure: A basis for calculation of left ventricular transmural pressure. Am Heart J 108:603–605, 1983.
10. Tyberg JV, Taichman GC, Smith ER, et al: The relation between pericardial pressure and right atrial pressure: An intraoperative study. Circulation 73:428–432, 1986.
11. Smiseth OA, Scott-Douglas NW, Thompson CR, et al: Nonuniformity of pericardial surface pressure in dogs. Circulation 75:1229–1236, 1987.
12. Assanelli D, Lew WYW, Shabetai R, LeWinter MM: Influence of the pericardium on right and left ventricular filling in the dog. J Appl Physiol 63:1025–1032, 1987.
13. Slinker BK, Ditchey RV, Bell SP, LeWinter MM: Right heart pressure does not equal pericardial pressure in the potassium chloride arrested in situ dog heart. Circulation 76:357–362, 1987.
14. Traboulsi M, Scott-Douglas NW, Smith ER, Tyberg JV: The right and left ventricular intracavitary and transmural pressure-strain relationships. Am Heart J 123:1279–1287, 1992.
15. Hamilton DR, Dani RS, Semlacher RA, et al: Right atrial and right ventricular transmural pressures in dogs and humans. Effects of the pericardium. Circulation 90:2492–2500, 1994.
16. Applegate RJ, Johnston WE, Vinten-Johansen J, et al: Restraining effect of intact pericardium during acute volume loading. Am J Physiol Heart Circ Physiol 262:H1725–H1733, 1992.
17. Braunwald E, Ross J Jr: Editorial: The ventricular end-diastolic pressure. Am J Med 34:147–150, 1963.
18. Sarnoff SJ, Berglund E: Ventricular function. 1. Starling's law of the heart studied by means of simultaneous right and left ventricular function curves in the dog. Circulation 9:706–718, 1954.
19. Ludbrook PA, Byrne JD, Kurnik PB, McKnight RC: Influence of reduction of preload and afterload by nitroglycerin on left ventricular diastolic pressure-volume relations and relaxation in man. Circulation 56:937–943, 1977.
20. Tyberg JV, Misbach GA, Glantz SA, et al: A mechanism for the shifts in the diastolic, left ventricular, pressure-volume curve: The role of the pericardium. Eur J Cardiol 7(suppl):163–175, 1978.
21. Kenner HM, Wood EH: Intrapericardial, intrapleural, and intracardiac pressures during acute heart failure in dogs studied without thoracotomy. Circ Res 19:1071–1079, 1966.
22. Smiseth OA, Frais MA, Kingma I, et al: Assessment of pericardial constraint in dogs. Circulation 71:158–164, 1985.
23. Hamilton DR, deVries G, Tyberg JV: Static and dynamic operating characteristics of a pericardial balloon. J Appl Physiol 90:1481–1488, 2001.
24. Holt JP, Rhode EA, Kines H: Pericardial and ventricular pressure. Circ Res 8:1171–1180, 1960.
25. deVries G, Hamilton DR, ter Keurs HEDJ, et al: A novel technique for the measurement of pericardial pressure. Am J Physiol Heart Circ Physiol 280:H2815–H2822, 2001.
26. Dauterman K, Pak PH, Maughan WL, et al: Contribution of external forces to left ventricular diastolic pressure. Implications for the clinical use of the Starling law. Ann Intern Med 122:737–742, 1995.
27. Glantz SA, Parmley WW: Factors which affect the diastolic pressure-volume curve. Circ Res 42:171–180, 1978.
28. Belenkie I, Dani R, Smith ER, Tyberg JV: The importance of pericardial constraint in experimental pulmonary embolism and volume loading. Am Heart J 123:733–742, 1992.

29. Gibbons Kroeker CA, Shrive NG, Belenkie I, Tyberg JV: The pericardium modulates LV and RV stroke volumes to compensate for sudden changes in atrial volume. Am J Physiol Heart Circ Physiol 284:H2247-H2254, 2003.

30. Belenkie I, Kieser TM, Sas R, et al: Evidence for left ventricular constraint during open heart surgery. Can J Cardiol 18:951–959, 2002.

31. Kingma I, Tyberg JV, Smith ER: Effects of diastolic transseptal pressure gradient on ventricular septal position and motion. Circulation 68:1304–1314, 1983.

32. Dong S-J, Beyar R, Zhou Z-N, et al: Determinants of midwall circumferential segmental length of the canine ventricular septum at end diastole. Am J Physiol Heart Circ Physiol 265:H2057–H2065, 1993.

33. Belenkie I, Dani R, Smith ER, Tyberg JV: Ventricular interaction during experimental acute pulmonary embolism. Circulation 78:761–768, 1988.

34. Belenkie I, Dani R, Smith ER, Tyberg JV: Effects of volume loading during experimental acute pulmonary embolism. Circulation 80:178–188, 1989.

35. Grant DA, Kondo CS, Maloney JE, et al: Changes in pericardial pressure during the perinatal period. Circulation 86:1615–1621, 1992.

36. Marini JJ, Culver BH, Butler J: Mechanical effect of lung distension with positive pressure on cardiac function. Am Rev Respir Dis 124:382–386, 1980.

37. Butler J: The heart is in good hands. Circulation 67:1163–1168, 1983.

38. Kingma I, Smiseth OA, Frais MA, et al: Left ventricular external constraint: Relationship between pericardial, pleural and esophageal pressures during positive end-expiratory pressure and volume loading in dogs. Ann Biomed Eng 15:331–346, 1987.

39. Grant DA, Kondo CS, Maloney JE, Tyberg JV: Pulmonary and pericardial limitations to diastolic filling of the left ventricle of the lamb. Am J Physiol Heart Circ Physiol 266:H2327–H2333, 1994.

40. Mirsky I, Rankin JS: The effects of geometry, elasticity, and external pressures on the diastolic pressure-volume and stiffness-stress relations. How important is the pericardium? Circ Res 44:601–611, 1979.

41. Baker AE, Belenkie I, Dani R, et al: Quantitative assessment of the independent contributions of the pericardium and septum to direct ventricular interaction. Am J Physiol Heart Circ Physiol 275:H476–H483, 1998.

42. Wang SY, Sheldon RS, Bergman DW, Tyberg JV: Effects of pericardial constraint on left ventricular mechanoreceptor activity in cats. Circulation 92:3331–3336, 1995.

43. Stone JA, Wilkes PRH, Keane PM, et al: Pericardial pressure attenuates release of atriopeptin in volume-expanded dogs. Am J Physiol Heart Circ Physiol 256:H648–H654, 1989.

44. Vatner SF, Boettcher DH: Regulation of cardiac output by stroke volume and heart rate in conscious dogs. Circ Res 42:557–561, 1978.

45. Boettcher DH, Vatner SF, Heyndrickx GR, Braunwald E: Extent of utilization of the Frank-Starling mechanism in conscious dogs. Am J Physiol Heart Circ Physiol 234:H338–H345, 1978.

46. Parker JO, Case RB: Normal left ventricular function. Circulation 60:4–12, 1979.

47. Linderer T, Chatterjee K, Parmley WW, et al: Influence of atrial systole on the Frank-Starling relation and the end-diastolic pressure-diameter relation of the left ventricle. Circulation 67:1045–1053, 1983.

48. Cooper PJ, Lei M, Cheng LX, Kohl P: Selected contribution: Axial stretch increases spontaneous pacemaker activity in rabbit isolated sinoatrial node cells. J Appl Physiol 89:2099–2104, 2000.

49. Waxman MB, Wald RW, Finley JP, et al: Valsalva termination of ventricular tachycardia. Circulation 62:843–851, 1980.

50. Kohl P, Hunter P, Noble D: Stretch-induced changes in heart rate and rhythm: Clinical observations, experiments and mathematical models. Prog Biophys Mol Biol 71:91–138, 1999.

51. Ambrosi P, Habib G, Kreitmann B, et al: Valsalva manoeuvre for supraventricular tachycardia in transplanted heart recipient. Lancet 346:713, 1995.

52. Little WC, Barr WK, Crawford MH: Altered effect of the Valsalva maneuver on left ventricular volume in patients with cardiomyopathy. Circulation 71:227–233, 1985.

53. Howarth S, McMichael J, Sharpey-Schafer EP: Effects of venesection in low output heart failure. Clin Sci 6:41–50, 1946.

54. Moore TD, Frenneaux MP, Sas R, et al: Ventricular interaction and external constraint account for decreased stroke work during volume loading in CHF. Am J Physiol Heart Circ Physiol 281:H2385–H2391, 2001.

55. Smiseth OA, Manyari DE, Lima JA, et al: Modulation of vascular capacitance by angiotensin and nitroprusside: A mechanism of changes in pericardial pressure. Circulation 76:875–883, 1987.

56. Kingma I, Smiseth OA, Belenkie I, et al: A mechanism for the nitroglycerin-induced downward shift of the left ventricular diastolic pressure-diameter relationship of patients. Am J Cardiol 57:673–667, 1986.

57. Tyberg JV, Misbach GA, Parmley WW, Glantz SA: Effects of the pericardium on ventricular performance. In: Baan J, Yellin EL, Arntzenius AC (eds): Cardiac Dynamics. Boston, Martinus Nijhoff, 1980, pp 159–168.

58. Alderman EL, Glantz SA: Acute hemodynamic interventions shift the diastolic pressure-volume curve in man. Circulation 54:662–671, 1976.

CARDIAC MECHANO-ELECTRIC FEEDBACK AS A PATHOGENIC MECHANISM

• • • •

CHAPTER 24

Mechanically Induced Electrical Remodeling in Human Atrium

• • • •

Jonathan M. Kalman, Prashanthan Sanders, and Joseph B. Morton

In humans, both paroxysmal and chronic atrial fibrillation (AF) are frequently associated with structural heart disease. Common to many of the conditions associated with a high incidence of AF has been the presence of atrial stretch or atrial dilation. Such conditions include congestive heart failure, mitral valve disease, and congenital heart diseases such as atrial septal defect (ASD). Despite this well recognized clinical association, until recently little has been known of the type of electrical remodeling associated with chronic atrial stretch in these conditions and the mechanism that leads to the development of AF. This chapter focuses on the nature of the electrophysiologic substrate for AF in these patients.

Wijffels and colleagues[1] initially described the concept that the atria remodel because of AF in a landmark study in conscious chronically instrumented goats. These investigators observed that although induced AF was initially short-lived, the artificial maintenance of AF resulted in progressive increase of its propensity to become sustained with time providing the seminal observation that "atrial fibrillation begets atrial fibrillation." This persistence of AF has been demonstrated to be associated with an abbreviation of the fibrillatory interval and the atrial effective refractory period (ERP), loss of rate adaptation, increased ERP heterogeneity, and regional conduction slowing.[2–5] Remarkably, similar and consistent observations also have been made in humans after the termination of chronic AF and flutter.[6–9]

Although the initial focus of atrial electrical remodeling was on the role of the atrial ERP, emerging data suggest that the development of structural changes of atrial fibrosis accompanied by conduction slowing is more important for the pathogenesis of chronic AF.[10] These chronic remodeling changes may occur either as a result of sustained atrial arrhythmias, or alternately, of underlying processes such as those mediated by stretch.

As our understanding of the mechanisms underlying AF has grown over recent years, so too has our appreciation of its heterogeneity. This is reflected by the diversity of pathophysiologic processes and underlying conditions that create the substrate for the development of AF. Although recent studies of atrial remodeling have emphasized the importance of rapid atrial rates, attention has also been directed toward the role of stretch and mechano-electric feedback. Atrial stretch appears to play a role in the development of AF in a wide spectrum of clinical conditions, ranging from the acute effects of supraventricular tachycardia (SVT) and myocardial infarction to chronic conditions such as heart failure, mitral regurgitation, ASD, and chronic asynchronous ventricular (VVI) pacing.

This review focuses on changes in atrial electrophysiology occurring as a result of atrial stretch, and also the importance of these changes in providing the electrophysiologic substrate for AF (see also chapters 16 and 17).

EFFECTS OF ACUTE ATRIAL STRETCH ON ATRIAL ELECTROPHYSIOLOGY

Studies in humans of the effects of acute atrial stretch have provided differing and sometimes confusing results. These differences may relate to the different methods of achieving atrial stretch in these studies, the confounding effects of the population under study, and the atrial rate. One method of achieving atrial stretch used simultaneous atrial and ventricular pacing.

Calkins and colleagues[11] reported that simultaneous atrioventricular pacing produced no change in atrial ERP at a drive cycle length of 400 msec in patients without structural heart disease, and they observed no increase in the frequency of AF induction. However, the same group found a decrease in atrial ERP in response to acute changes in atrial pressure brought about by pacing just the final two beats of the drive train at an atrioventricular interval of 0 msec.[12] Tse and colleagues[13] studied patients without structural heart disease and observed that simultaneous atrioventricular pacing caused atrial stretch and was associated with a decrease in right atrial ERP accompanied by an increased propensity for development of AF. In contrast, Klein and colleagues[14] demonstrated an increase in atrial ERP during pacing at a cycle length of 400 msec, associated with an increase in atrial pressure, when the atrioventricular interval was decreased from 160 to 0 msec.

Other studies also have observed a nonuniform increase in atrial ERP in patients without structural heart disease caused by an increase in atrial pressure during simultaneous atrioventricular pacing.[15] There was a significant increase in the atrial ERP measured at the distal coronary sinus and the posterior lateral right atrium, but not at the right atrial appendage. As a result, they observed an increase in the dispersion of ERP.

Antoniou and colleagues[16] studied the effects of acute atrial stretch on the inducibility of AF in patients with a history of paroxysmal AF. In these patients, atrial stretch was induced by volume loading with 0.9% saline to double the right atrial pressure. Whereas at low atrial pressure, AF of greater than 3 min was inducible in 3 of 16 patients, an increase of atrial pressure resulted in persistent AF in 10 patients.

Other studies have examined the impact of atrial stretch brought about by rapid SVT with near simultaneous atrioventricular activation. Although these studies may be confounded by the impact of a rapid rate, they mimic a real clinical situation in which there is an increased risk for AF. Klein and colleagues[14] observed an increase in right atrial ERP associated with an increase in right atrial pressure during SVT. Similarly, Chen and colleagues[17] observed an increase in atrial ERP and dispersion of ERP with an increase in atrial pressure during SVT. Interestingly, these investigators observed a greater dispersion of ERP

with acute atrial stretch in patients with a history of AF.

The reasons for the variable results in these studies on acute atrial stretch may relate to the different populations under study, the wide variation in atrial rate, failure to control for secondary autonomic effects, and the heterogeneous effects of stretch on regional atrial ERP. Indeed, an increase in ERP heterogeneity may be one factor in the proarrhythmic effect of atrial stretch.

At the cellular level, the relative effect of acute mechanical stimulation on modulation of calcium handling (action potential duration [APD] reduction) and stretch-activated ion channel activity (APD lengthening) may also partly explain the apparently opposite effects of acute stretch on shortening/lengthening the ERP. (AP repolarization crossover in which early APD is reduced and late APD is prolonged is discussed in more detail in Chapter 13.)

It is certainly striking that, despite the variation in reported effects on ERP, all studies have demonstrated that acute atrial stretch results in an acute increase in AF inducibility.

EFFECTS OF CHRONIC ATRIAL STRETCH ON ATRIAL ELECTROPHYSIOLOGY

To obtain information regarding the impact of chronic atrial stretch on atrial electrophysiology in humans, it is necessary to study the effects of a variety of pathophysiologic conditions or situations that have in common the development of chronic atrial enlargement.

Asynchronous Pacing

An association between VVI pacing and an increased incidence of AF has been well established. To better understand the mechanism underlying this relation, Sparks and colleagues[18,19] studied the impact of long-term VVI pacing on the electrical properties and mechanical function of the atria. This study was a prospective randomized comparison between 18 patients paced in the VVI mode and 12 patients paced in the DDD (synchronous atrioventricular pacing) mode for 3 months. After chronic VVI pacing, atrial ERP increased significantly in a nonuniform fashion at all sites evaluated (lateral right atrium, right atrial appendage, right atrial septum, and distal coronary sinus). This was associated with prolongation of the P-wave duration and sinus node remodeling. In a parallel study,[19] these authors demonstrated significant enlargement of the atria associated with impairment of atrial mechanical function as evidenced by a decrease in emptying velocities and fractional area change in the left atrial appendage. Importantly, these studies also documented that these changes associated with 3 months of VVI pacing could be reversed by 3 months of physiologic (DDD) pacing.

Recently, the electrophysiologic properties of the atria have been studied in a range of clinical conditions associated with atrial enlargement that provide further information on the substrate for AF.

Mitral Stenosis

Mitral stenosis caused by rheumatic heart disease is frequently complicated by the development of AF. Although the incidence of this condition has diminished significantly in Western communities, it remains a significant illness in many countries worldwide. Fan and colleagues[20] studied electrophysiologic parameters in the right atrium of 31 patients with mitral valve stenosis at the time of percutaneous mitral commissurotomy. Of these, 19 were in chronic AF and 12 in sinus rhythm at the time of the procedure. After cardioversion of AF, these patients demonstrated significantly shortened atrial ERP, sinus node remodeling, and no significant difference in atrial conduction delay to extrastimuli compared with patients in sinus rhythm. At repeat study 3 months after mitral commissurotomy, the atrial ERP had increased significantly from baseline, which was comparable with patients who were in sinus rhythm. Although this increase in ERP may be attributed to reversal of AF-induced remodeling, the study also observed an increase in ERP in the sinus rhythm group immediately after balloon valvuloplasty. This latter observation suggested that under circumstances of mitral stenosis, atrial stretch might reversibly shorten the atrial ERP. There was no change in conduction delay in the AF group after valvuloplasty, but, interestingly, a significant decrease in delay was seen immediately after valvuloplasty in the sinus rhythm group, consistent with the hypothesis that atrial stretch may induce conduction delay. Whether additional, and irreversible, changes in conduction persist in the long-term could not be evaluated in this study. In patients with rheumatic heart disease, it would be expected that the disease itself might lead to regional fibrosis and conduction delay, in addition to the effects of chronic stretch. It should also be emphasized that none of the data in this study were collected from the left atrium, where the most significant electrophysiologic impact of chronic mitral stenosis might occur.

Mitral Regurgitation

Chronic mitral regurgitation is one of the most potent risk factors for the development of AF. In recent years, a number of studies have provided an emerging picture of the substrate for AF in chronic AF. In a chronic canine model of AF, Verheule and colleagues[21] observed a homogeneous increase in left and right atrial ERP. Despite this there was an increase in inducibility of sustained AF and pathologic areas of increased interstitial fibrosis and chronic inflammation.

Tieleman and colleagues[22] measured atrial ERP in a heterogenous group of patients undergoing cardiac surgery: 15 patients with chronic AF, 16 with paroxysmal AF, and 15 with no history of AF. Of these patients, 22 had a history of mitral regurgitation. The authors report that mitral regurgitation was associated with prolongation of the atrial ERP regardless of the underlying atrial rhythm compared with the patients without mitral regurgitation.

These data are consistent with preliminary data from our institution. We studied the electrophysiologic characteristics of 10 patients with severe mitral regurgitation caused by mitral valve prolapse without prior AF, and compared these characteristics with 10 age-matched control subjects. Patients with mitral regurgitation had significant increases in both left and right atrial volumes. These patients demonstrated an increase in atrial ERP at the right atrial septum and in the distal coronary sinus (Fig. 24–1). However, there was an increase in the dispersion of ERP. In addition, patients with mitral regurgitation showed both electro-

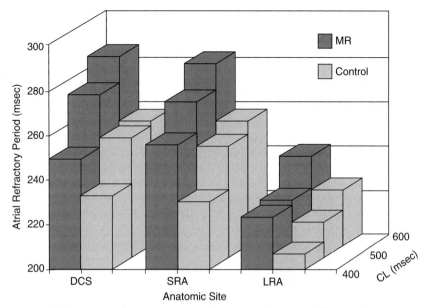

■ **Figure 24–1** Patients with chronic mitral regurgitation (MR) demonstrated increased effective refractory period compared with control patients at the distal coronary sinus (DCS) and the septal right atrium (SRA) at cycle lengths (CL) of 500 and 600 msec (*P* < 0.03). LRA, low right atrium.

physiologic evidence of significant regional conduction delay and prolongation of P-wave duration. Although confirmation of these observations awaits detailed left atrial mapping studies, our findings again suggest that the substrate for AF in patients with chronic mitral regurgitation is likely to be related to atrial enlargement, regional conduction delay, and structural change, rather than to a decrease in the atrial ERP.

Congestive Heart Failure

Congestive heart failure is one of the most common conditions to be complicated by the development of AF, which may occur in up to 30% of patients during the course of the disease. Sanders and colleagues[23] recently described the nature of atrial electrical remodeling in patients with advanced congestive heart failure. Twenty-one patients with congestive heart failure caused by idiopathic or chronic ischemic cardiomyopathy underwent electrophysiologic and electroanatomic evaluation and were compared with 21

age-matched control subjects.[23] Patients with congestive heart failure had extensive electrophysiologic abnormalities. They demonstrated structural and anatomic abnormalities, as well as extensive atrial regions of low-voltage amplitude (Fig. 24–2) and areas of spontaneous electrical silence (scarring).

Together with (and possibly as a result of) these structural changes, there was evidence of significantly impaired atrial conduction. Abnormalities of conduction were observed throughout the right atrium using both conventional and electro-anatomic mapping techniques. There also was anatomically determined regional conduction delay at the crista terminalis (Fig. 24–3). Furthermore, in contrast to the type of atrial remodeling seen in response to rapid atrial rates, patients with congestive heart failure did not demonstrate an abbreviation of the atrial ERP. Indeed, in these patients, there was an increase in ERP at all sites compared with the control group. There was no change in dispersion or the rate adaptation of ERP. These patients also demonstrated impairment of sinus node function. Perhaps as a consequence of the

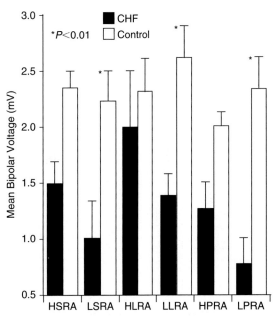

■ **Figure 24–2** Patients with congestive heart failure (CHF) demonstrated lower atrial voltage amplitude in each of the six atrial regions when compared with control patients. HSRA, high septal right atrium; LSRA, low septal right atrium; HLRA, high lateral right atrium; LLRA, low lateral right atrium; HPRA, high posterior right atrium; LPRA, low posterior right atrium.

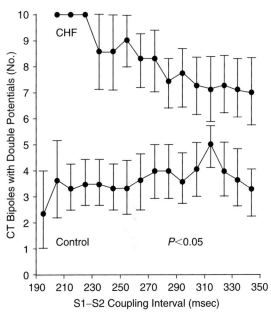

■ **Figure 24–3** A 20-pole mapping catheter (10 bipoles) along the crista terminalis demonstrated that patients with CHF had more bipoles showing double potentials (DP) than control patients, and that the number of bipoles with DP increased in inverse relation to the S1–S2 coupling interval.

demonstrated electrophysiologic abnormalities, these patients had an increased propensity for AF and a significantly increased duration of induced AF.

This study suggests that the substrate for AF in patients with congestive heart failure may be predominantly caused by the development of structural abnormalities and conduction delay, rather than changes in atrial ERP, as occurs in the remodeling because of rapid atrial rates.

Congenital Heart Disease, Atrial Septal Defects, Atrial Stretch, and Atrial Remodeling

The natural history of adults with an ASD and chronic atrial volume overload is characterized by an increased risk for the development of atrial arrhythmias that appears minimally altered by ASD closure. Although

surgical lines of block may form the substrate for "scar-related" atrial macroreentry after surgical ASD repair, the impact of chronic atrial stretch and volume overload on atrial electrophysiology in patients with ASD has been the subject of a recent study. Morton and colleagues[24] studied the right atrial electrophysiologic properties of 13 patients with hemodynamically significant ASD. These patients demonstrated significant prolongation of the atrial ERP at the low lateral right atrium, high lateral right atrium, and high septal right atrium. These changes in ERP were not associated with changes in the heterogeneity of ERP. In addition, these patients demonstrated evidence of anatomically determined functional conduction delay at the crista terminalis (Fig. 24–4). Compared with age-matched control subjects, patients with an ASD had extensive and widely split double potentials recorded along the crista terminalis. Conduction delay at this site increased with increasing prematurity during S2 extrastimulus test-

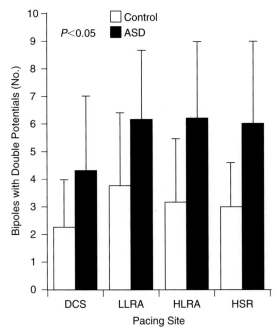

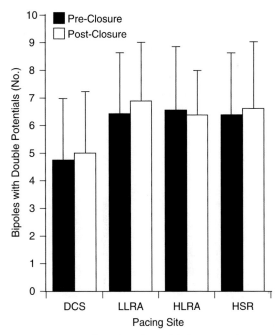

■ **Figure 24–4** Effect of atrial septal defect (ASD) and chronic right atrium stretch on crista terminalis conduction. A 20-pole mapping catheter (10 bipoles) demonstrated that patients with ASD had a greater number of bipoles showing double potentials than control patients when pacing from each of four sites. DCS, distal coronary sinus; LLRA, low lateral right atrium; HLRA, high lateral right atrium; HSR, high septal right.

■ **Figure 24–5** Effect of atrial septal defect (ASD) closure on crista terminalis conduction. Six months after ASD closure (post-closure), the number of bipoles with double potentials had not decreased for pacing at any site when compared with before closure. DCS, distal coronary sinus; LLRA, low lateral right atrium; HLRA, high lateral right atrium; HSR, high septal right.

ing. Importantly, when a proportion of the patients were restudied more than 6 months after ASD closure, these regional abnormalities of conduction persisted (Fig. 24–5). The role of anisotropy and functional conduction delay at the crista terminalis in a range of atrial arrhythmias has been extensively detailed. It has previously been shown that this structure plays an important role in the development of typical atrial flutter,[25] atypical forms of flutter such as lower loop re-entry,[26] and in AF.[27,28]

Patients with an ASD had evidence of sinus node remodeling with significant prolongation of the corrected sinus node recovery time.[24] The authors hypothesized that regional conduction delay formed the substrate for re-entry in patients with an ASD and had an important proarrhythmic effect, despite modest increases in atrial ERP.

Importantly, this study also suggested that these regional conduction abnormalities, presumably a result of chronic atrial stretch and central to the development of arrhythmia substrate, might not reverse when the underlying defect is corrected. Chen and colleagues[29] studied 10 patients with atrial dilation and no history of atrial arrhythmias and found significantly longer atrial ERP compared with 20 control patients with normal atrial size.

Structural Remodeling, Atrial Fibrillation, and the Coexistence of Sinus Node Dysfunction

The studies discussed previously have shed new light on the nature of structural remodeling associated with chronic atrial enlargement, whether it was caused by volume overload or cardiac failure or related to valvular pathology.

The extensive atrial pathology observed in these patients suggests a mechanism that couples AF and sinus node dysfunction (SND). That is, the primary pathologic process leads to diffuse abnormalities. These lead to a loss of functioning atrial myocardium and slowed conduction. This process thus not only creates the substrate for AF, but it also results in destruction of the sinus pacemaker complex.

Sanders and colleagues recently hypothesized that given the widely distributed nature of the functional sinus pacemaker complex[30] and the frequent association of SND with AF, patients with SND would necessarily have widespread atrial abnormalities.[31] They compared electrophysiologic and electro-anatomic properties of the atrium in 16 patients with symptomatic SND with 16 age-matched control subjects. Patients with SND demonstrated similar atrial remodeling to that seen in patients with conditions of chronic atrial stretch. The patients with SND showed a significant increase in atrial ERP without changes in the heterogeneity of ERP, a slowing of atrial conduction, and evidence of anatomically determined conduction delay at the crista terminalis. Electro-anatomic mapping demonstrated the sinus node complex in patients with SND was a localized structure, frequently in the region of the low crista terminalis that corresponds to the site of the largest residual voltage amplitude on voltage mapping. Elsewhere in the atrium, and particularly along the long axis of the original pacemaker complex, there were significant areas of low voltage and electrical silence (or scar). Induced AF persisted for a longer period, or became sustained, in patients with SND. These electrophysiologic abnormalities resembled those seen in conditions of chronic atrial stretch. Why these patients developed such changes in the absence of chronic stretch is unknown, but it is worthwhile to briefly examine the nature of atrial remodeling that occurs with ageing.

Age and Atrial Remodeling

Advancing age is one of the most significant risk factors for the development of AF. It is detected in 3% to 4%

of the population older than 60 years, and it has a prevalence of almost 9% in octogenarians. Recently, Kistler and colleagues[32] described the electrophysiologic and electro-anatomic remodeling that occurs with age. Patients without atrial arrhythmias underwent right atrial mapping, and data were stratified according to age group (30, 30–60, and >60 years). Aging was associated with an increase in atrial refractoriness and both generalized and anatomically determined conduction slowing. Electro-anatomic mapping revealed diffuse areas of low voltage that were associated with regional conduction slowing. There was a significant increase in recorded signals demonstrating fractionation and double potentials with advancing age, particularly in the region of the crista terminalis. These changes also resembled those seen with chronic stretch, although they were less severe and were consistent with the development of atrial fibrosis, which has been found in pathologic studies of aging.

Stretch-Related Triggers

Although this chapter has discussed the role of stretch in development of the atrial substrate required to sustain multiple wavelet re-entry, the triggers that initiate the process may also have a relation to stretch. The most common anatomic locations for these triggers are the pulmonary veins.[33] However, although clinical impression suggests that sudden changes in venous return may stimulate these triggers, by producing pulmonary venous stretch, definitive data are lacking.

There have been a number of recent studies describing the electrophysiologic features of pulmonary vein musculature and why these sleeves of tissue may contribute to the development of AF. Hocini and colleagues,[34] using canine pulmonary veins, found significant conduction delay within the pulmonary veins. This was correlated with myocardial fiber orientation, producing nonuniform anisotropy and fractionated electrograms.[34] Clinically, this is also apparent in patients with paroxysmal AF. They demonstrate decremented conduction to and from the atrium, with documentation of long fractionated electrograms in close juxtaposition to sharp spikes within the pulmonary veins.[35,36] Chen and colleagues[37,38] have demonstrated delayed and early afterdepolarizations after rapid atrial pacing of isolated myocytes from canine pulmonary veins, and they have hypothesized that triggered automaticity may be the mechanism underlying these rapidly firing foci.

However, although these studies have obviously advanced our understanding of pulmonary vein electrophysiology, a link between the observations discussed previously and the role of stretch remains speculative. Clinical studies have suggested that patients with pulmonary vein ectopy initiating AF have significantly dilated pulmonary veins compared with control subjects. This suggests a possible contribution of anatomic remodeling and stretch in predisposing the pulmonary vein to become arrhythmogenic.[39,40] By altering pulmonary vein diameter, chronic atrial stretch may change the wavelength and facilitate the development of re-entry within pulmonary venous muscle bundles. Acute stretch may have similar effects, but it might also result in stretch-induced, calcium-mediated afterdepolarizations.

It is intriguing to hypothesize that atrial stretch contributes to the development of AF, not only by modifying substrate, but also by initiating the triggers.

Summary

Studies in humans of chronic atrial stretch have consistently demonstrated an unchanged or prolonged atrial ERP, which is likely to increase the atrial wavelength, and theoretically protect against the development of AF. As such, these studies have alluded to the important contribution of other factors to formation of the substrate for AF. These factors, in particular, include the development of structural abnormalities, interstitial fibrosis, and, eventually, an apparent loss of functioning atrial myocardium. Associated with these abnormalities is significant generalized conduction slowing, which may also be focused in certain anatomic regions. These changes, which may in part be stretch related and in part reflect primary pathophysiologic processes, do not appear to be reversible once significant structural change has developed.

References

1. Wijffels MC, Kirchhof CJ, Dorland R, et al: Atrial fibrillation begets atrial fibrillation. A study in awake chronically instrumented goats. Circulation 92:1954–1968, 1995.

2. Fareh S, Villemaire C, Nattel S: Importance of refractoriness heterogeneity in the enhanced vulnerability to atrial fibrillation induction caused by tachycardia-induced atrial electrical remodeling. Circulation 98:2202–2209, 1998.

3. Gaspo R, Bosch RF, Talajic M, et al: Functional mechanisms underlying tachycardia-induced sustained atrial fibrillation in a chronic dog model. Circulation 96:4027–4035, 1997.

4. Morillo CA, Klein GJ, Jones DL, et al: Chronic rapid atrial pacing. Structural, functional, and electrophysiological characteristics of a new model of sustained atrial fibrillation. Circulation 91:1588–1595, 1995.

5. Morton JB, Byrne MJ, Power JM, et al: Electrical remodeling of the atrium in an anatomic model of atrial flutter: Relationship between substrate and triggers for conversion to atrial fibrillation. Circulation 105:258–264, 2002.

6. Kamalvand K, Tan K, Lloyd G, et al: Alterations in atrial electrophysiology associated with chronic atrial fibrillation in man. Eur Heart J 20:888–895, 1999.

7. Kumagai K, Akimitsu S, Kawahira K, et al: Electrophysiological properties in chronic lone atrial fibrillation. Circulation 84:1662–1668, 1991.

8. Sparks PB, Jayaprakash S, Vohra JK, et al: Electrical remodeling of the atria associated with paroxysmal and chronic atrial flutter. Circulation 102:1807–1813, 2000.

9. Yu WC, Lee SH, Tai CT, et al: Reversal of atrial electrical remodeling following cardioversion of long-standing atrial fibrillation in man. Cardiovasc Res 42:470–476, 1999.

10. Allessie M, Ausma J, Schotten U: Electrical, contractile and structural remodeling during atrial fibrillation. Cardiovasc Res 54:230–246, 2002.

11. Calkins H, el Atassi R, Leon A, et al: Effect of the atrioventricular relationship on atrial refractoriness in humans. Pacing Clin Electrophysiol 15:771–778, 1992.

12. Calkins H, el Atassi R, Kalbfleisch S, et al: Effects of an acute increase in atrial pressure on atrial refractoriness in humans. Pacing Clin Electrophysiol 15:1674–1680, 1992.

13. Tse HF, Pelosi F, Oral H, et al: Effects of simultaneous atrioventricular pacing on atrial refractoriness and atrial fibrillation inducibility: Role of atrial mechano-electric feedback. J Cardiovasc Electrophysiol 12:43–50, 2001.

14. Klein LS, Miles WM, Zipes DP: Effect of atrioventricular interval during pacing or reciprocating tachycardia on atrial size, pressure, and refractory period. Contraction-excitation feedback in human atrium. Circulation 82:60–68, 1990.

15. Chen YJ, Tai CT, Chiou CW, et al: Inducibility of atrial fibrillation during atrioventricular pacing with varying intervals: Role of atrial electrophysiology and the autonomic nervous system. J Cardiovasc Electrophysiol 10:1578–1585, 1999.

16. Antoniou A, Milonas D, Kanakakis J, et al: Contraction-excitation feedback in human atrial fibrillation. Clin Cardiol 20:473–476, 1997.

17. Chen YJ, Chen SA, Tai CT, et al: Role of atrial electrophysiology and autonomic nervous system in patients with supraventricular tachycardia and paroxysmal atrial fibrillation. J Am Coll Cardiol 32:732–738, 1998.

18. Sparks PB, Mond HG, Vohra JK, et al: Electrical remodeling of the atria following loss of atrioventricular synchrony: A long-term study in humans. Circulation 100:1894–1900, 1999.

19. Sparks PB, Mond HG, Vohra JK, et al: Mechanical remodeling of the left atrium after loss of atrioventricular synchrony. A long-term study in humans. Circulation 100:1714–1721, 1999.

20. Fan K, Lee KL, Chow WH, et al: Internal cardioversion of chronic atrial fibrillation during percutaneous mitral commissurotomy: Insight into reversal of chronic stretch-induced atrial remodeling. Circulation 105:2746–2752, 2002.
21. Verheule S, Wilson EE, Sih H, et al: Alteration in atrial electrophysiology due to chronic atrial dilatation in a canine model of mitral regurgitation. Circulation 104:II-76, 2001.
22. Tieleman RG, Van Gelder IC, Brundel BJJM, et al: Mitral regurgitation is associated with prolongation of the atrial refractory period. Circulation 106:II-370, 2002.
23. Sanders P, Morton JB, Davidson NC, et al: Electrical remodeling of the atria in congestive heart failure: Electrophysiologic and electroanatomic mapping in humans. Circulation 108:1461–1468, 2003.
24. Morton JB, Sanders P, Vohra JK, et al: The effect of chronic atrial stretch on atrial electrical remodeling in patients with an atrial septal defect. Circulation 107:1775–1782, 2003.
25. Olgin JE, Kalman JM, Fitzpatrick AP, et al: Role of right atrial endocardial structures as barriers to conduction during human type I atrial flutter. Activation and entrainment mapping guided by intracardiac echocardiography. Circulation 92:1839–1848, 1995.
26. Cheng J, Cabeen WR Jr, Scheinman MM: Right atrial flutter due to lower loop reentry: Mechanism and anatomic substrates. Circulation 99:1700–1705, 1999.
27. Cox JL, Canavan TE, Schuessler RB, et al: The surgical treatment of atrial fibrillation. II. Intraoperative electrophysiologic mapping and description of the electrophysiologic basis of atrial flutter and atrial fibrillation. J Thorac Cardiovasc Surg 101:406–426, 1991.
28. Liu TY, Tai CT, Chen SA: Treatment of atrial fibrillation by catheter ablation of conduction gaps in the crista terminalis and cavotricuspid isthmus of the right atrium. J Cardiovasc Electrophysiol 13:1044–1046, 2002.
29. Chen YJ, Chen SA, Tai CT, et al: Electrophysiologic characteristics of a dilated atrium in patients with paroxysmal atrial fibrillation and atrial flutter. J Interv Card Electrophysiol 2:181–186, 1998.
30. Boineau JP, Canavan TE, Schuessler RB, et al: Demonstration of a widely distributed atrial pacemaker complex in the human heart. Circulation 77:1221–1237, 1988.
31. Sanders P, Morton JB, Spence SJ, et al: Electrophysiologic and electroanatomic characterization of the atria in sinus node disease: Evidence of diffuse atrial remodeling. Circulation 109:828–832, 2004.
32. Kistler P, Sanders P, Fynn SP, et al: Electrophysiologic and electroanatomic changes in the atrium associated with age. J Am Coll Cardiol 44:109–116, 2004.
33. Haissaguerre M, Jais P, Shah DC, et al: Spontaneous initiation of atrial fibrillation by ectopic beats originating in the pulmonary veins. N Engl J Med 339:659–666, 1998.
34. Hocini M, Ho SY, Kawara T, et al: Electrical conduction in canine pulmonary veins: Electrophysiological and anatomic correlation. Circulation 105:2442–2448, 2002.
35. Tada H, Oral H, Ozaydin M, et al: Response of pulmonary vein potentials to premature stimulation. J Cardiovasc Electrophysiol 13:33–37, 2002.
36. Jais P, Hocini M, Macle L, et al: Distinctive electrophysiological properties of pulmonary veins in patients with atrial fibrillation. Circulation 106:2479–2485, 2002.
37. Chen YJ, Chen SA, Chen YC, et al: Effects of rapid atrial pacing on the arrhythmogenic activity of single cardiomyocytes from pulmonary veins: Implication in initiation of atrial fibrillation. Circulation 104:2849–2854, 2001.
38. Chen YJ, Chen SA, Chang MS, et al: Arrhythmogenic activity of cardiac muscle in pulmonary veins of the dog: Implication for the genesis of atrial fibrillation. Cardiovasc Res 48:265–273, 2000.
39. Lin WS, Prakash VS, Tai CT, et al: Pulmonary vein morphology in patients with paroxysmal atrial fibrillation initiated by ectopic beats originating from the pulmonary veins: Implications for catheter ablation. Circulation 101:1274–1281, 2000.
40. Tsao HM, Yu WC, Cheng HC, et al: Pulmonary vein dilation in patients with atrial fibrillation: Detection by magnetic resonance imaging. J Cardiovasc Electrophysiol 12:809–813, 2001.

CHAPTER 25

Atrial Fibrillation and Dilated Cardiomyopathy

• • • •

A. John Camm and Shamil Yusuf

Dilated cardiomyopathy (DCM) and atrial fibrillation (AF) are two of the most common cardiac ailments encountered in clinical practice. They affect no less than 5 and 2.5 million people, respectively, in the United States alone.[1,2] They both increase with advancing age and have similar predisposing factors, namely hypertension, diabetes, coronary heart disease, and valvular heart disease. However, attributing this high prevalence merely to their common risk factors would belittle a complex inter-relationship that exists between these two disease processes. The prevalence of AF increases sharply with severity of the DCM; however, AF itself is self-perpetuating and progressive, which with time leads to cardiac chamber dilation. Hence, DCM begets AF, which begets AF, which begets DCM. This relation between DCM and AF involves mechanical factors, alterations in electrophysiologic parameters, and neurohormonal activation. The former two of these are explored during the course of this chapter, starting with the mechanisms responsible for AF, moving onto how AF begets DCM, and then to how DCM predisposes to AF. The role of mechano-electric feedback (MEF) between the two is covered in an evidence-based manner, and finally, the mechanisms that might be responsible are discussed (see also Chapters 16 and 17).

MECHANISMS UNDERLYING ATRIAL FIBRILLATION

The mechanisms underlying AF are common to all arrhythmias: abnormal impulse formation, abnormal impulse conduction, or both. In AF, a diverse group of focal mechanisms, such as enhanced normal or abnormal automaticity (e.g., increased or reduced auto-nomic tone), triggered activity (e.g., atrial premature beats, pulmonary vein ectopic foci, accessory atrioventricular [AV] pathways, and acute atrial stretch), or both, can be responsible for abnormal impulse formation. Such focal mechanisms generate early (EAD) or late afterdepolarizations, which when of sufficient magnitude precipitate an extrasystole or repetitive firing. EAD were named as such because they occur during the process of repolarization and delayed afterdepolarizations (DAD) after its completion.

Although abnormalities in impulse generation may trigger AF, it is rarely capable of sustaining it. For this arrhythmia to persist, abnormal impulse conduction by means of re-entry circuits on an appropriate substrate is necessary.

Two types of re-entry circuits are responsible for arrhythmias: macroanatomic re-entry circuits and functionally determined circuits. Functionally determined circuits can occur as a single circuit, producing rapid regular activity, or as multiple wave fronts of irregular activity. It had been postulated by a group of workers as early as 1964 that AF depended on a certain number of wavelets being present in the atria—the *multiple wavelet hypothesis*.[3] If the number of wavelets was high, the statistical probability that they would all extinguish at the same time would be small and AF would persist; with a small number of wavelets present, the chances that they would die out simultaneously are greater and the arrhythmia will self-terminate. Mapping studies in isolated canine heart confirmed this hypothesis and established that the critical number of wavelets required to sustain AF was four to six.[4] In humans, high-density mapping has been applied clinically, and the presence of random re-entry of multiple wandering wavelets during electrically induced AF also has been demonstrated.[5]

The number of wavelets that can coexist simultaneously in the atrium is determined by the following factors:

Atrial tissue mass (or surface area): The number of circuits in the atria increases with the square of the atrial diameter.

Wavelength of the atrial impulse (= atrial refractory period [ARP] × conduction velocity): the shorter the ARP and/or the faster the conduction velocity, the greater the number of circuits in a given tissue mass.

Inhomogeneity in electrophysiologic properties of the atria—that is, either in intra-atrial conduction (enhanced nonuniform anisotropy, locally depressed action potentials) or in recovery of excitability (increased special dispersion in ARP).

FROM ATRIAL FIBRILLATION TO DILATED CARDIOMYOPATHY

Numerous observations over the last 50 years, including reversible cardiac chamber dilation in the presence of AF; a high incidence of left atrial enlargement in patients with rheumatic chronic AF, but not in patients with intermittent AF or sinus rhythm; and normal right and dilated left atrial anatomy in patients with mitral stenosis in sinus rhythm, but biatrial dilation in those with rheumatic and lone AF, have indicated that atrial dilation can be a consequence of, rather than merely possessing a predisposition to, AF.[6] These observations were confirmed by a small study in which 15 patients with AF and normal right and left atrial diameters at baseline were observed prospectively for an average period of 20.6 months.[7] Three orthogonal left atrial dimensions and two right atrial dimensions were measured echocardiographically, and all were found to increase significantly. Also, highly significant increases in calculated left atrial volume (from 45.2 to 64.1 cm^3; $P < 0.001$) and right atrial volume (from 49.2 to 66.2 cm^3; $P < 0.001$) were observed. More recent studies have estimated that the independent contribution of AF to increase in left atrial diameter is about 2.5 mm.[8] This process of arrhythmia-induced atrial dilation, known as atrial remodeling, is not simply confined to the gross anatomy of the atria; it also is a complex multifactorial phenomenon that, in itself, contributes to the self-perpetuating and progressive nature of AF. It can be divided into electrical, contractile, and structural components (Fig. 25–1).[9]

Atrial Fibrillation–Induced Electrical Remodeling of the Atria

Although the term *electrical remodeling of the atria* was not used until 1995,[10] the evidence for this process had been accumulating for almost 15 years. First, the presence of short monophasic action potentials (MAP) had been found to be associated with difficulty in maintaining sinus rhythm after cardioversion. Second, an increased tendency to AF was noted in patients with abnormalities in rate adaptation of their ARP. This observation implied that abnormal rate adaptation of the ARP was a marker of some "cryptic" atrial pathology that caused AF. Third, a loss of rate adaptation of the ARP and a reduction in the atrial action potential

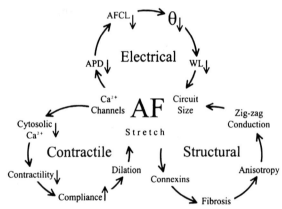

■ **Figure 25–1** The proposed feedback loops for atrial remodeling in atrial fibrillation (AF). Down-regulation of the L-type Ca^{2+} channels results in electrical remodeling and contractile dysfunction. Stretch of the myocardium, resulting from contractile dysfunction and increased atrial compliance, acts as a stimulus for structural remodeling of the atria. The resulting electro-anatomic substrate of AF consists of enlarged atria allowing intra-atrial circuits of small size, caused by a reduction in wavelength (WL; shortening of refractoriness and slowing of conduction, θ) and increased nonisoform tissue anisotropy (zigzag conduction). APD, Action potential duration; AFCL, AF cycle length. *(From Allessie M, Ausma J, Schotten U: Electrical, contractile and structural remodeling during atrial fibrillation. Cardiovasc Res 54:230–246, 2002, with permission.)*

duration (APD) in isolated right atrial tissue of patients with chronic AF was observed.[9] Finally, a reduction in APD in patients with AF was noted to be directly related to the tachycardia.[11]

The concept of electrical remodeling of the atria was given a new impetus by two animal studies in 1995. A rapid atrial–paced (400 per min) dog and pacemaker-induced fibrillation goat model[10,12] both, in addition to confirming the previous observations, showed that long-term rapid atrial pacing or pacemaker maintenance of AF led to a progressive increase in the susceptibility to AF. After 6 weeks of rapid atrial pacing, in 82% of the dogs, episodes of AF lasting longer than 15 min could be induced. In the goat, this effect was even more striking.[12] Whereas during control, only short paroxysms of AF were induced by burst pacing (mean, 6 ± 3 sec), after 2 days of AF, the paroxysms lasted more than 4 hours (mean, 241 ± 459 min); by that time, AF had become sustained in 2 of the 12 animals (>24 hours).

After 2 to 3 weeks, AF was sustained in 90% of the animals (Fig. 25–2). This observation that "atrial fibrillation begets atrial fibrillation" generated unprecedented interest in the underlying molecular mechanisms responsible.

The ionic basis for tachycardia-induced electrical remodeling of the atria has been elucidated from patch clamp experiments and action potential recordings of isolated animal and human atrial cells. The most marked effect is a dramatic reduction in the L-type Ca^{2+} current ($I_{Ca,L}$), which explains the shortening of the APD and the loss of its physiologic rate adaptation.[13] There also is a reduction in the transient outward current (I_{to}),[13,14] but conflicting data on the effect on the sustained component of the ultrarapid delayed rectifier potassium current ($I_{K,ur}$), a reduction demonstrated by some,[13,14] has not been confirmed by others studying a cohort of patients with chronic AF.[15] Pharmacologic probes by which a reduction in $I_{Ca,L}$ and I_{to} can be mimicked showed that in the atrial myocardium, I_{to} is of much less importance for the duration of the action potential than $I_{Ca,L}$.[13]

Atrial Fibrillation–Induced Contractile Remodeling of the Atria

A number of observations from the studies discussed previously and other studies indicated that electrical remodeling alone is not sufficient for AF to be sus-

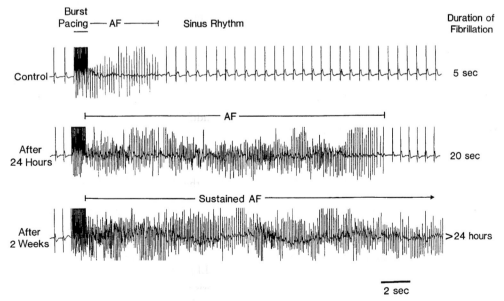

■ **Figure 25–2** Prolongation of the duration of episodes of electrically induced atrial fibrillation (AF) in the goat as a result of electrical remodeling. *(From Wijffels MC, Kirchhof CJ, Dorland R, Allessie MA: Atrial fibrillation begets atrial fibrillation. A study in awake chronically instrumented goats. Circulation 92:1954–1968, 1995, with permission.)*

tained. In the goat model of AF, electrical remodeling was complete and changes in atrial refractoriness were stable within a few days of AF, yet it took an additional 1 to 2 weeks for AF to become persistent. The electrical changes secondary to AF are reversed within a few days of restoration of sinus rhythm regardless of the duration of the AF, yet there is a high recurrence of AF even after allowing a few days for the reverse remodeling. The hypothesis that a "second factor" other than electrical remodeling was required to sustain AF was therefore offered[9] and proved by two studies in the goat model. In the first study, burst pacing was used to induce AF for three consecutive 5-day periods interrupted by 2 days of sinus rhythm.[16] During these 2 days, the electrical remodeling was completely reversed, and the ARP had returned to normal. No significant differences were found in the time required for AF to become sustained during the second or third 5-day episode of AF. In the second study, each episode of induced AF was allowed to continue for a month, after which it was terminated electrically.[17] The ARP was allowed to return to normal before another episode of AF was again induced for another month. Although the time course for electrical remodeling was the same, the time required for development of persistent AF became shorter after each AF episode.

About 40 years ago, investigators had noted a lack of the "a" wave in the atrial pressure curve after cardioversion for AF.[18] This dysfunction in atrial contraction, also known as "atrial stunning," occurs after simultaneous, electrical, or pharmacologic cardioversion and correlates with the duration of the AF. Verapamil is able to prevent this atrial dysfunction after short periods of AF, indicating Ca^{2+} overload to be the transient underlying mechanism. In the goat model of long-standing AF, the contractile ability of the atria is 75% reduced within 2 days and completely abolished within 5 days of the onset of AF. It is accompanied by an increase in atrial size and compliance.[6] All these effects are fully reversed within 2 to 5 days of restoration of sinus rhythm; they follow the same time course as electrical remodeling and are mainly caused by $I_{Ca,L}$ down-regulation. Thus, contractile dysfunction and increase in atrial size during the first few days of AF is a consequence of electrical remodeling of the atria and may perpetuate the arrhythmia, but it is reversible and is not the second factor necessary for maintenance of AF.

Atrial Fibrillation–Induced Structural Remodeling of the Atria

Persistent AF induces more permanent changes in the atria,[9] including the following:

1. Cellular hypertrophy,
2. Perinuclear accumulation of glycogen,
3. Central loss of sarcomeres (myolysis),
4. Alterations in the expression of connexins,
5. Changes in mitochondrial shape,
6. Fragmentation of sarcoplasmic reticulum,
7. Homogeneous distribution of nuclear chromatin,
8. Changes in the quantity and localization of structural cellular proteins,
9. Extracellular fibrosis.

Heterogeneity in cell size and interstitial fibrosis contribute to inhomogeneity in impulse conduction.[9] The role of gap junctions in this process is still unclear, because the data on atrial gap junction structural proteins, the connexins, are inconsistent. In the dog model of AF, an increase in the expression of connexin43 has been reported; in humans, a decrease was found; in the goat model, no change in connexin43 was found, but a decrease in connexin40 was noted. What is clear in the connexin story thus far is that for the speed of propagation of the atrial impulse to be affected, connexin expression needs to be down-regulated by more than 40%. Spatial heterogeneities in connexin expression may create microscopic obstacles for conduction, which do not necessarily disturb the conduction of a broad wave front, but they may serve as turning points or areas of zigzag conduction when the wave front becomes fragmented. In animal models of AF, the previous cellular changes appear to be degenerative, and no signs of programmed cell death are present.[19] In human subjects with AF and atrial dilation, myocytes show a strong terminal deoxynucleotide transferase-mediated dUTP nick-end labeling (TUNEL) reactivity indicative of DNA cleavage and apoptosis.[20] If true, this process would further increase tissue anisotropy, heterogeneity of conduction, and dispersion of the refractoriness. These effects, together with atrial dilation, produce multiple entry and exit points and multiple sites at which unidirectional block occurs, shifting the balance between generation and extinction of wavelets toward the generation of new wave fronts and maintenance of AF. These changes contribute further to atrial dilation and are irreversible and permanent. The only clinical data to date for the prevention of this structural remodeling, and hence of AF, are the use of angiotensin II receptor blockers. In a heterogeneous population with minimal heart disease, angiotensin II receptor blockers have been shown to reduce the recurrence rate of AF.[21]

From Dilated Cardiomyopathy to Atrial Fibrillation

Similar to the evidence of a possible link between AF and cardiac chamber dilation, evidence for the association between DCM and AF has been accumulating over 50 years. As early as 1955, it was noted that the incidence of AF correlated with right and left atrial enlargement in patients with mitral valve disease. Some years later, it was reported that in patients with valve disease or asymmetric septal hypertrophy, AF was rare (3%) when left atrial diameter was less than 40 mm, but common (54%) when it exceeded 40 mm. It was not until the 1990s, however, that large prospective trials established left atrial enlargement to be an independent risk factor for the development of AF; more recently, it also was established as the only predictive factor for the occurrence of AF in mitral regurgitation.[6] The prevalence of AF, however, is not exclusively related to left atrial size, but also to the presence and severity of left ventricular dysfunction with rates less than 5% in patients with New York Heart Association (NYHA) functional Class I symptoms, 50% in those with functional Class IV symptoms, and an intermediate prevalence in patients with NYHA functional Class II and III symptoms.[22]

Dilated Cardiomyopathy–Induced Electrical Remodeling of the Atria

In a canine ventricular pacing–induced heart failure model, atrial ionic remodeling is distinct to that of AF

remodeling.[23] Again, there is a decrease in $I_{Ca,L}$, but this is not as marked as in AF (~30% compared with ~70%); a decrease in I_{to} and a decrease in the slow component of the delayed rectifier potassium current (I_{Ks}) is of a similar magnitude to that of $I_{Ca,L}$, which is not induced by AF. Furthermore, there is an increase in the Na^+-Ca^{2+} exchanger (NCX) current (~45%), which also is not present in tachycardia-induced atrial remodeling. The net electrical effect of these changes is neutral in that $I_{Ca,L}$ reductions are offset by reductions in I_{Ks} and increases in NCX. Hence, the APD in this heart failure model was unaffected at slow rates and increased at faster rates; the APD rate adaptation was reduced, but not as much as much as in AF. Human studies have by and large confirmed the reductions in $I_{Ca,L}$ and I_{to} in the dilated human atria with conflicting data regarding the inwardly rectifying potassium current, I_{K1} (unchanged in dilated atria,[24] but reduced in symptomatic heart failure[25]). All these data are limited, however, by the various disease states, duration of the disease, drug therapy, and the number of patients with AF in each study.

Dilated Cardiomyopathy and Structural Remodeling

DCM is the final end point for a myriad of diseases that affect the heart. It is the consequence of cardiac "remodeling," and its hallmarks include hypertrophy, loss of myocytes, and increased interstitial fibrosis. Three basic mechanisms can account for these phenotypic changes in myocardial structure and function: single gene defects; polymorphic variations in modifier genes (e.g., angiotensin-converting enzyme [ACE] gene); and altered expression of completely normal genes that regulate contractile function, chamber structure, or both. Mechanical stress influences remodeling by the latter of these changes, effecting both intrinsic myocyte contractile function and altered activation of neurohormonal (e.g., adrenergic, renin-angiotensin, endothelin) and cytokine (e.g., tumor necrosis factor-α) signaling pathways. Pressure overload has been shown not only to stimulate myocyte hypertrophy, but also increase physiologic myocyte loss by apoptosis in a rat model, and stretch has been shown to enhance angiotensin II receptor expression in neonatal rat cardiac myocytes. Stretch also activates a number of intracellular and extracellular signaling pathways, including local angiotensin II production, all of which promote cellular hypertrophy, stimulate fibroblast proliferation, and activate matrix protein synthesis leading to tissue fibrosis.[6]

Acute Atrial Stretch and Afterdepolarizations

Mechanical forces acting on atrial tissue or cell membranes convey changes in the electrophysiologic properties of myocytes and are able to generate and maintain AF. In isolated right atrial tissue from both normal and postinfarction rats, stretch-activated depolarizations capable of triggering premature beats and atrial tachyarrhythmias have been clearly demonstrated.[26] These stretch-activated depolarizations, however, rather than being of the classic EAD or DAD types, were not triggered by the preceding action potential and were simply located after the action potential. More conventional EAD and late afterdepolarizations occurring coincidentally with the preceding action potential have been recorded in isolated guinea pig hearts when the atrium was stretched by balloon[27] and in situ pig heart locally stretched by a suction dipole device[28]; DAD also have been recorded in isolated rat atria at increasing diastolic pressure levels.[29] These animal experiments demonstrated that the ability of stretch to trigger premature beats was directly related to the degree of atrial stretch and was greater during swift volume changes, suggesting that the intensity of the stretch and the transient phase are key factors for stretch-induced triggered arrhythmias.

In humans, the pulmonary veins (PV) have been identified as important sources of premature ectopic beats, which in turn trigger AF.[30] This activity emanates from sleeves of left atrial myocardium that extend into the PV. Although, theoretically, this tissue is atrial in origin, its electrophysiologic properties differ from atrial myocardial tissue.[31] In the 79 patients with frequent episodes of paroxysmal AF and 10 control patients studied, distal PV showed the shortest ARP, and right superior PV showed a greater incidence of intra-PV conduction block than left superior PV. Superior and left PV had longer myocardial sleeves than inferior and right PV, respectively. High-

resolution mapping studies in dogs have shown that normal PV have the potential to support re-entry, as well as focal activity, but focal activity appears to originate proximal to the left atrium compared with re-entry tracts, which are more distal.[32] Although, currently, no human studies have looked at the effect of MEF mechanisms in AF of PV origin, a sheep model has been used.[33] Using increased intra-atrial pressure–related AF in nine isolated sheep hearts, the hypothesis that atrial dilation induces arrhythmogenic left atrial sources emanating from the superior PV was tested. In each heart, the intra-atrial pressure was increased from 0 cm H_2O in steps of 5 cm H_2O, with burst pacing being applied to induce AF at each stage after 3 min of stabilization. Once stable AF was induced, the intra-atrial pressure was increased to 30 cm H_2O, and then reduced to 5 cm H_2O. Stable episodes of stretch-related AF (>40 min) were induced in all nine animals. Video movies of the left atrium free wall and left atrium superior PV junction (JPV) were obtained. Electrograms from the right atrium were recorded. At intra-atrial pressures greater than 10 cm H_2O, the maximum dominant frequency (DF_{Max}) was significantly greater in the JPV than in the left atrium free wall (Fig. 25–3).

At less than 10 cm H_2O, DF_{Max} was similar in the JPV and left atrium free wall; DF_{Max} in both JPV and left atrium free wall was significantly greater than in the right atrium. Analysis of excitation direction in JPV showed positive correlation between intra-atrial pressure and the number of waves emanating from the left superior PV, but not from the left atrium free wall (Fig. 25–4). The number of spatio-temporally periodic waves in the JPV correlated with pressure. This study demonstrates that an increase in intra-atrial pressure increases the rate and organization of waves emanating from the superior PV underlying stretch-related AF.

Acute Atrial Stretch and Atrial Fibrillation

The effect of acute dilation on various atrial electrophysiologic parameters has been extensively studied both in animals and humans. The results of the in vitro and in vivo studies are summarized in Chapters 16 and 17. Although isolated atrial preparations under acute

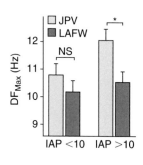

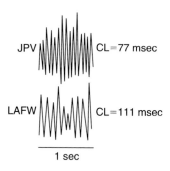

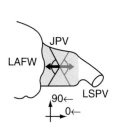

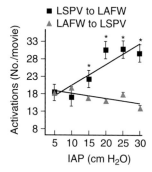

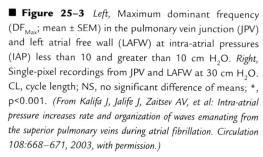

■ **Figure 25-3** *Left,* Maximum dominant frequency (DF_{Max}; mean ± SEM) in the pulmonary vein junction (JPV) and left atrial free wall (LAFW) at intra-atrial pressures (IAP) less than 10 and greater than 10 cm H_2O. *Right,* Single-pixel recordings from JPV and LAFW at 30 cm H_2O. CL, cycle length; NS, no significant difference of means; *, $p < 0.001$. *(From Kalifa J, Jalife J, Zaitsev AV, et al: Intra-atrial pressure increases rate and organization of waves emanating from the superior pulmonary veins during atrial fibrillation. Circulation 108:668–671, 2003, with permission.)*

■ **Figure 25-4** *Left,* Directionality of activity from the pulmonary veins (PV) to left atrial free wall (LAFW; *dark arrow*) and from LAFW to left superior pulmonary vein (LSPV; *light arrow*) assessed at the pulmonary vein junction (JPV). *Right,* Number of activations (mean ± SEM) moving from LSPV to LAFW and from LAFW to LSPV (*$P < 0.01$ compared with LAFW to LSPV as a function of IAP). *(From Kalifa J, Jalife J, Zaitsev AV, et al: Intra-atrial pressure increases rate and organization of waves emanating from the superior pulmonary veins during atrial fibrillation. Circulation 108:668–671, 2003, with permission.)*

stretch conditions consistently show shortening of the MAP duration at early levels of repolarization and complete reversal of these effects after release of the atrial stretch, the in vivo studies provide a more heterogeneous picture from a decrease, increase, or no effect in the ARP. The possible reasons for this may include species differences, varying experimental conditions, different repolarization levels at which APD is determined,[34] and inhomogeneous atrial wall stretch where shortening and lengthening of the atrial refractoriness may occur in the same heart.[35] The in vivo experiments did, however, demonstrate that the effects on the ARP were dependent on the timing (transient increase in pressure shortened the ARP, whereas sustained stretch did not change the refractoriness) and intensity (moderate changes in atrial pressure either increased or had no effect on the ARP, whereas greater changes in atrial pressure invariably decreased the ARP) of atrial stretch.[36,37]

In all these studies, both human and animal, acute atrial stretch increased the inducibility of premature beats and AF. In the Langendorff-perfused volume overload rabbit heart model[38] and in the simultaneous paced human study,[39] the inducibility of AF was directly proportional to the degree of stretch, with

none at 0% stretch and 100% at atrial pressures greater than 10 cm H_2O (Fig. 25–5). Conversely, decreasing the atrial pressure invariably terminated the AF.[38] Furthermore, in addition to these arrhythmogenic effects, atrial dilation may also modulate the rate of the arrhythmia, especially where re-entry is the principal mechanism, such as in atrial flutter.[40]

Chronic Atrial Stretch and Atrial Fibrillation

In a study of dogs with tricuspid regurgitation and pulmonary artery stenosis, although the atrial diameter increased by ~40% after 100 days, APD in vitro was no different from control animals, but the atrial refractoriness was not measured.[41] Atrial arrhythmias did not occur spontaneously, but inducibility and duration increased significantly in this model. Histologic and ultrastructural analysis revealed cardiac hypertrophy and an increase in connective tissue content. In another study of dogs with mitral valve fibrosis and left atrial dilation of as much as six to eight times compared with control dogs, no change in transmembrane potentials was found.[42] Atrial arrhythmias occurred

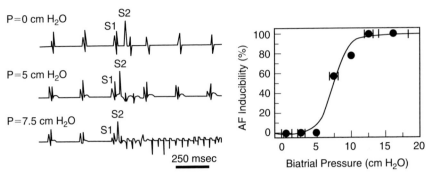

■ **Figure 25–5** Effects of atrial pressure on atrial fibrillation (AF) inducibility in the Langendorff-perfused rabbit heart. *Left,* Earliest possible premature beats at different atrial pressure. *Right,* Inducibility of AF by a single premature stimulus plotted as a function of atrial pressure. *(From Ravelli F, Allessie M: Effects of atrial dilatation on refractory period and vulnerability to atrial fibrillation in the isolated Langendorff-perfused rabbit heart. Circulation 96:1686–1695, 1997, with permission).*

spontaneously in most animals, but the underlying mechanism was not identified. Again, atrial myocyte hypertrophy was present among large amounts of connective tissue. In a goat model of atrial dilation induced by chronic AV block followed by bundle of His ablation, a 12% atrial dilation was accompanied by an increase in the duration of paroxysmal AF from a few seconds during control to several hours. As the ARP and AF intervals in this model of complete AV block were kept constant, this observation could not be attributed to changes in these parameters. In human subjects with complete heart block and ventricular pacing, atrial dilation is accompanied by an increase in the ARP, and these individuals are more prone to AF compared with those with dual-chamber pacing devices.[43] All these studies indicate that the mechanisms underlying *chronic* stretch-induced arrhythmogenesis are different from those induced by *acute* stretch.

Mechanisms Underlying Dilated Cardiomyopathy–Related Arrhythmogenesis

Acute stretch-induced afterdepolarizations are likely to involve stretch-activated ion channels (SAC) as antagonists to these, such as streptomycin and gadolinium are able to suppress mechanically induced afterdepolarizations, whereas calcium channel blockers are

not.[29,44] However, the mechanisms underlying changes in various atrial electrophysiologic parameters during acute stretch are far from clear. Whereas stretch-induced APD shortening was suppressed by streptomycin,[44,45] shortening of the ARP in isolated rabbit heart remained unchanged by gadolinium and by another SAC antagonist, a peptide from a tarantula venom.[46,47] From the observations that calcium channel blockers such as verapamil are able to abolish stretch-induced changes in ARP in both isolated rabbit heart and humans,[48,49] it is conceivable that these changes are a result of modulations in intracellular calcium affected by altered troponin C sensitivity, or by stretch-activated calcium influx, or by both.[50] As for acute stretch-induced AF, this is determined by the shortening of the ARP and atrial dilation, which simultaneously increase the number of wavelets within atria. In humans, the stretch-induced vulnerability to AF was abolished by verapamil independent of autonomic tone, but in the isolated rabbit heart model, this stretch-induced vulnerability and AF maintenance was reduced by SAC blocking agents without preventing stretch-induced shortening of ARP.[34] This indicates that in addition to the shortening of refractoriness, other factors such as autonomic tone; nonuniform distribution of local ARP, probably caused by heterogeneous wall stress; and impairment of atrial wave-front propagation caused by the complex and heterogeneous structure of the atrial wall, may all play a role in the development of AF during stretch.[50]

The mechanism underlying chronic stretch-induced AF is complex, multifactorial, less well established, and less easy to explain. The increase in NCX expression may be quite important in AF promotion; NCX is known to carry transient inward currents that cause DAD and triggered activity.[51,52] In a dog model of ventricular pacing–induced DCM, AF was readily induced by burst atrial pacing but not by single extra stimuli.[53] Therefore, if this is the case, then AF caused by NCX-related triggered activity may be the trigger needed to initiate AF, but this is sustained only in the presence of an appropriate structural substrate. Other factors such as catecholamine excess and metabolic abnormalities may also promote triggered activity.

The key to DCM-related AF is substrate modulation. Cellular hypertrophy sensitizes the myocardium so that smaller mechanical stimuli are able to activate SAC.[54] Tissue fibrosis decreases conduction velocity caused by microscopic zigzagging circuits or depressed propagation in branching muscle bundles, which, in turn, allows multiple small re-entry circuits to stabilize the arrhythmia.[6] The role of DCM-affected atrial connexins in this process again is unknown. Small studies have suggested connexin43 expression is markedly down-regulated in human ventricular DCM tissue, and if so, would further impede impulse conduction and aid zigzagging.[55] These changes produce multiple entry and exit points and multiple sites at which unidirectional block occurs, shifting the balance between generation and extinction of wavelets toward the generation of new wave fronts; fibrosis also increases electrophysiologic dispersion in refractoriness caused by unequal tissue stretch.[35] As a result, a perfect milieu is created for AF propagation. Currently, the only possible therapeutic intervention against the development and progression of this substrate is the use of ACE inhibitors and angiotensin II receptor blockers. Clinically, such agents have proved to be effective against AF in patients with heart failure[56] and left ventricular dysfunction after myocardial infarction.[57]

Conclusion

MEF plays an important role in the genesis of DCM from AF and visa versa, but the precise underlying mechanisms have yet to be elucidated. In the nondilated atria, acute stretch is capable of triggering AF by stimulation of not only the atrial free walls but also the PV. SAC are likely to play a crucial role in this process, and antagonism of these channels offers a novel, exciting, and promising antiarrhythmic approach to the prevention of AF under conditions of increased atrial pressure or volume. Atrial dilation early in AF is caused by electrical remodeling and contractile dysfunction, both of which are reversible. Persistent AF, however, is dependent on atrial dilation and structural changes. These are either initiated and propagated by AF itself or induced by chronic atrial stretch. The role of SAC here is less clear, but in the latter case, there may be a role for NCX in the initiation of AF. In DCM and long-standing AF, a plethora of other intracellular and extracellular mechanisms come into play. These modulate the myocardial substrate so that AF is more easily induced, maintained, and possibly rendered permanent. In such cases, rather than a single class of drugs, multiple agents targeted against the various effectors of myocyte loss, hypertrophy, and interstitial fibrosis, starting with ACE inhibitors/angiotensin II receptor blockers, are crucial for both the prevention and perpetuation of AF and cardiac chamber dilation.

References

1. Nohria A, Lewis E, Stevenson LW: Medical management of advanced heart failure. JAMA 287:628–640, 2002.
2. Benjamin EJ, Wolf PA, D'Agostino RB, et al: Impact of atrial fibrillation on the risk of death: The Framingham Heart Study. Circulation 98:946–952, 1998.
3. Moe GK, Rheinboldt WC, Abildskov JA: A computer model of atrial fibrillation. Am Heart J 67:200–220, 1964.
4. Allessie MA, Lammers WJEP, Bonke FIM, et al: Experimental evaluation of Moe's multiple wavelet hypothesis of atrial fibrillation. In: Zipes DP, Jalife J (eds): Cardiac Electrophysiology and Arrhythmias. New York, Grune & Stratton, 1985, pp 265–275.
5. Cox JL, Canavan TE, Schuessler RB, et al: The surgical treatment of atrial fibrillation. II. Intraoperative electrophysiologic mapping and description of the electrophysiologic basis of atrial flutter and atrial fibrillation. J Thorac Cardiovasc Surg 101:406–426, 1991.
6. Schotten U, Neuberger HR, Allessie MA: The role of atrial dilatation in the domestication of atrial fibrillation. Prog Biophys Mol Biol 82:151–162, 2003.
7. Sanfilippo AJ, Abascal VM, Sheehan M, et al: Atrial enlargement as a consequence of atrial fibrillation. A prospective echocardiographic study. Circulation 82:792–797, 1990.
8. Dittrich HC, Pearce LA, Asinger RW, et al: Left atrial diameter in nonvalvular atrial fibrillation: An echocardiographic study. Stroke Prevention in Atrial Fibrillation Investigators. Am Heart J 137:494–499, 1999.

9. Allessie M, Ausma J, Schotten U: Electrical, contractile and structural remodeling during atrial fibrillation. Cardiovasc Res 54:230–246, 2002.

10. Morillo CA, Klein GJ, Jones DL, Guiraudon CM: Chronic rapid atrial pacing. Structural, functional, and electrophysiological characteristics of a new model of sustained atrial fibrillation. Circulation 91:1588–1595, 1995.

11. Franz MR, Karasik PL, Li C, et al: Electrical remodeling of the human atrium: Similar effects in patients with chronic atrial fibrillation and atrial flutter. J Am Coll Cardiol 30:1785–1792, 1997.

12. Wijffels MC, Kirchhof CJ, Dorland R, Allessie MA: Atrial fibrillation begets atrial fibrillation. A study in awake chronically instrumented goats. Circulation 92:1954–1968, 1995.

13. Yue L, Feng J, Gaspo R, et al: Ionic remodeling underlying action potential changes in a canine model of atrial fibrillation. Circ Res 81:512–525, 1997.

14. Bosch RF, Zeng X, Grammer JB, et al: Ionic mechanisms of electrical remodeling in human atrial fibrillation. Cardiovasc Res 44:121–131, 1999.

15. Grammer JB, Bosch RF, Kuhlkamp V, Seipel L: Molecular remodeling of Kv4.3 potassium channels in human atrial fibrillation. J Cardiovasc Electrophysiol 11:626–633, 2000.

16. Garratt CJ, Duytschaever M, Killian M, et al: Repetitive electrical remodeling by paroxysms of atrial fibrillation in the goat: No cumulative effect on inducibility or stability of atrial fibrillation. J Cardiovasc Electrophysiol 10:1101–1108, 1999.

17. Todd DM, Flynn SP, Walden AP, et al: Repetitive one month periods of atrial electrical remodeling promote stability of atrial fibrillation. Circulation 102:154–155, 2000.

18. Logan WF, Rowlands DJ, Howitt G, Holmes AM: Left atrial activity following cardioversion. Lancet 10:471–473, 1965.

19. Dispersyn GD, Ausma J, Thone F, et al: Cardiomyocyte remodelling during myocardial hibernation and atrial fibrillation: Prelude to apoptosis. Cardiovasc Res 43:947–957, 1999.

20. Aime-Sempe C, Folliguet T, Rucker-Martin C, et al: Myocardial cell death in fibrillating and dilated human right atria. J Am Coll Cardiol 34:1577–1586, 1999.

21. Madrid AH, Bueno MG, Rebollo JM, et al: Use of irbesartan to maintain sinus rhythm in patients with long-lasting persistent atrial fibrillation: A prospective and randomized study. Circulation 106:331–336, 2002.

22. Maisel WH, Stevenson LW: Atrial fibrillation in heart failure: Epidemiology, pathophysiology, and rationale for therapy. Am J Cardiol 91:2D–8D, 2003.

23. Li D, Melnyk P, Feng J, et al: Effects of experimental heart failure on atrial cellular and ionic electrophysiology. Circulation 101:2631–2638, 2000.

24. Le Grand BL, Hatem S, Deroubaix E, et al: Depressed transient outward and calcium currents in dilated human atria. Cardiovasc Res 28:548–556, 1994.

25. Koumi S, Arentzen CE, Backer CL, Wasserstrom JA: Alterations in muscarinic K+ channel response to acetylcholine and to G protein-mediated activation in atrial myocytes isolated from failing human hearts. Circulation 90:2213–2224, 1994.

26. Kamkin A, Kiseleva I, Wagner KD, et al: Mechano-electric feedback in right atrium after left ventricular infarction in rats. J Mol Cell Cardiol 32:465–477, 2000.

27. Nazir SA, Lab MJ: Mechanoelectric feedback in the atrium of the isolated guinea-pig heart. Cardiovasc Res 32:112–119, 1996.

28. Nazir SA, Lab MJ: Mechanoelectric feedback and atrial arrhythmias. Cardiovasc Res 32:52–61, 1996.

29. Tavi P, Laine M, Weckstrom M: Effect of gadolinium on stretch-induced changes in contraction and intracellularly recorded action- and afterpotentials of rat isolated atrium. Br J Pharmacol 118:407–413, 1996.

30. Haissaguerre M, Jais P, Shah DC, et al: Spontaneous initiation of atrial fibrillation by ectopic beats originating in the pulmonary veins. N Engl J Med 339:659–666, 1998.

31. Chen SA, Hsieh MH, Tai CT, et al: Initiation of atrial fibrillation by ectopic beats originating from the pulmonary veins: Electrophysiological characteristics, pharmacological responses, and effects of radiofrequency ablation. Circulation 100:1879–1886, 1999.

32. Arora R, Verheule S, Scott L, et al: Arrhythmogenic substrate of the pulmonary veins assessed by high-resolution optical mapping. Circulation 107:1816–1821, 2003.

33. Kalifa J, Jalife J, Zaitsev AV, et al: Intra-atrial pressure increases rate and organization of waves emanating from the superior pulmonary veins during atrial fibrillation. Circulation 108:668–671, 2003.

34. Franz MR, Bode F: Mechano-electrical feedback underlying arrhythmias: The atrial fibrillation case. Prog Biophys Mol Biol 82:163–174, 2003.

35. Satoh T, Zipes DP: Unequal atrial stretch in dogs increases dispersion of refractoriness conducive to developing atrial fibrillation. J Cardiovasc Electrophysiol 7:833–842, 1996.

36. Calkins H, el-Atassi R, Kalbfleisch S, et al: Effects of an acute increase in atrial pressure on atrial refractoriness in humans. Pacing Clin Electrophysiol 15:1674–1680, 1992.

37. Calkins H, el-Atassi R, Leon A, et al: Effect of the atrioventricular relationship on atrial refractoriness in humans. Pacing Clin Electrophysiol 15:771–778, 1992.

38. Ravelli F, Allessie M: Effects of atrial dilatation on refractory period and vulnerability to atrial fibrillation in the isolated Langendorff-perfused rabbit heart. Circulation 96:1686–1695, 1997.

39. Tse HF, Pelosi F, Oral H, et al: Effects of simultaneous atrioventricular pacing on atrial refractoriness and atrial fibrillation inducibility: Role of atrial mechanoelectrical feedback. J Cardiovasc Electrophysiol 12:43–50, 2001.

40. Ravelli F, Disertori M, Cozzi F, et al: Ventricular beats induce variations in cycle length of rapid (type II) atrial flutter in humans. Evidence of leading circle reentry. Circulation 89:2107–2116, 1994.

41. Boyden PA, Hoffman BF: The effects on atrial electrophysiology and structure of surgically induced right atrial enlargement in dogs. Circ Res 49:1319–1331, 1981.

42. Boyden PA, Tilley LP, Pham TD, et al: Effects of left atrial enlargement on atrial transmembrane potentials and structure in dogs with mitral valve fibrosis. Am J Cardiol 49:1896–1908, 1982.

43. Sparks PB, Mond HG, Vohra JK, et al: Electrical remodeling of the atria following loss of atrioventricular synchrony: A long-term study in humans. Circulation 100:1894–1900, 1999.

44. Nazir SA, Dick DJ, Lab MJ: Mechanoelectric feedback and arrhythmia in the atrium of the isolated Langendorff-perfused guinea pig hearts and its modulation by streptomycin. J Physiol 483P:24–25, 1995.

45. Babuty D, Lab M: Heterogeneous changes of monophasic action potential induced by sustained stretch in atrium. J Cardiovasc Electrophysiol 12:323–329, 2001.

46. Bode F, Katchman A, Woosley RL, Franz MR: Gadolinium decreases stretch-induced vulnerability to atrial fibrillation. Circulation 101:2200–2205, 2000.

47. Bode F, Sachs F, Franz MR: Tarantula peptide inhibits atrial fibrillation. Nature 409:35–36, 2001.
48. Zarse M, Stellbrink C, Athanatou E, et al: Verapamil prevents stretch-induced shortening of atrial effective refractory period in Langendorff-perfused rabbit heart. J Cardiovasc Electrophysiol 12:85–92, 2001.
49. Tse HF, Wang Q, Yu CM, et al: Effect of verapamil on prevention of atrial fibrillation in patients implanted with an implantable atrial defibrillator. Clin Cardiol 24:503–505, 2001.
50. Ravelli F: Mechano-electric feedback and atrial fibrillation. Prog Biophys Mol Biol 82:137–149, 2003.
51. Benardeau A, Hatem SN, Rucker-Martin C, et al: Contribution of Na^+/Ca^{2+} exchange to action potential of human atrial myocytes. Am J Physiol 271:H1151–H1161, 1996.
52. Blaustein MP, Lederer WJ: Sodium/calcium exchange: Its physiological implications. Physiol Rev 79:763–854, 1999.
53. Li D, Fareh S, Leung TK, Nattel S: Promotion of atrial fibrillation by heart failure in dogs: Atrial remodeling of a different sort. Circulation 100:87–95, 1999.
54. Kamkin A, Kiseleva I, Isenberg G: Stretch-activated currents in ventricular myocytes: Amplitude and arrhythmogenic effects increase with hypertrophy. Cardiovasc Res 48:409–420, 2000.
55. Salameh A, Muehlberg K, Mahjour P, et al: Alteration in cardiac connexins in patients with cardiomyopathy. Eur Heart J 24:131, 2003.
56. Gurlek A, Erol C, Basesme E: Antiarrhythmic effect of converting enzyme inhibitors in congestive heart failure. Int J Cardiol 43:315–318, 1994.
57. Pedersen OD, Bagger H, Kober L, Torp-Pedersen C: Trandolapril reduces the incidence of atrial fibrillation after acute myocardial infarction in patients with left ventricular dysfunction. Circulation 100:376–380, 1999.

CHAPTER 26

Natriuretic Peptide and Sudden Cardiac Death in Patients with Congestive Heart Failure

Alan Maisel, Vikas Bhalla, Meenakshi A. Bhalla, and Sanjiv M. Narayan

This chapter discusses the potential diagnostic and prognostic role of natriuretic peptides in patients with congestive heart failure (CHF) at risk for sudden cardiac death (SCD).

SUDDEN CARDIAC DEATH AND ITS RELATION TO CONGESTIVE HEART FAILURE

SCD is defined as unexpected cardiovascular death occurring within an hour of the onset of symptoms, or an unexpected death that was unwitnessed unless a noncardiac cause is confirmed. From a review of death certificates in the United States during 1998 and 1999, SCD accounted for more than 450,000 deaths, or 63% of cardiac deaths among adults 35 years of age.[1]

Of the known predispositions to SCD, structural heart disease remains the most important. As well as being greater in men and older individuals[2] (Fig. 26–1), the incidence of SCD increases 6- to 10-fold in the presence of coronary (see Fig. 26–1) and structural disease (Table 26–1). In an autopsy study of 270 subjects with SCD,[3] 95% showed evidence of a structural abnormality. Indeed, large multicenter studies have confirmed that left ventricular dysfunction of any cause (left ventricular ejection fraction ≤ 40%)[4] is the major identifiable risk factor for SCD.[5,6]

Although SCD is common in patients with significant coronary disease, studies have demonstrated that it primarily follows ventricular tachycardia or fibrillation[7] from scar-related re-entrant arrhythmogenesis,[8] and that acute coronary syndromes are responsible for less than 30% of cases.[5,9]

Other chapters in this textbook suggest mechanisms by which SCD, a primarily electrical entity, could be related strongly to mechanical ventricular dysfunction. This epidemiologic and clinical fact establishes the rationale for using brain (B-type) natriuretic peptide (BNP), a noninvasive serum marker of ventricular wall strain, to indicate potential risk for SCD.

Indeed, the enormous prevalence of CHF and left ventricular dysfunction makes BNP particularly attractive as a potential risk marker for SCD. In the United States alone, CHF affects 4.9 million people, with a current incidence of 550,000 new cases per year. Heart failure accounts for 999,000 hospital discharges annually (a 165% increase since 1979),[10] and its in-hospital mortality and readmission rates are extremely high.[11,12] Although SCD is a major cause of death in patients with CHF, many individuals also die of progressive pump failure (defined as cardiac death with preceding symptomatic or hemodynamic deterioration).[13,14] In a 38-year follow-up of patients in the Framingham Heart Study, the presence of CHF significantly increased overall, and SCD mortality increased by a factor of five (Fig. 26–2).[2]

The relative contribution of SCD to total mortality in CHF varies with an individual's functional status. Although SCD accounts for up to 50% of total mortality in patients with CHF, this proportion is greater in those with milder (New York Heart Association [NYHA] Class I and II) compared with more advanced (NYHA Class III and IV) functional classes. This probably follows from the observation that the

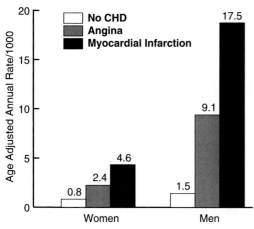

■ **Figure 26–1** Sudden cardiac death (SCD) is related to coronary disease. From a 38-year follow-up in the Framingham Heart Study, SCD was greatest in patients with prior myocardial infarction and in men. CHD, Coronary heart disease. (From Kannel WB, Wilson PW, D'Agostino RB, Cobb J: Sudden coronary death in women. Am Heart J 136:205–212, 1998, with permission.)

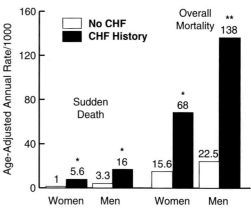

■ **Figure 26–2** Sudden cardiac death is strongly associated with a history of congestive heart failure (CHF), from 38-year follow-up data in the Framingham Heart Study, for men and women. *P < 0.01; **P < 0.001. (From Kannel WB, Wilson PW, D'Agostino RB, Cobb J: Sudden coronary death in women. Am Heart J 136:205–212, 1998, with permission.)

TABLE 26–1 Causes of Sudden Cardiac Death

Ischemic Heart Disease
Coronary heart disease with myocardial infarction or angina
Coronary artery embolism
Nonatherogenic coronary artery disease
Coronary artery spasm

Nonischemic Heart Disease
Coronary heart disease without myocardial infarction or angina
Cardiomyopathy obstructive, nonobstructive, nonischemic
Valvular heart disease
Congenital heart disease
Prolonged QT syndrome
Pre-excitation syndrome
Complete heart block
Myocarditis
Acute pericardial tamponade
Acute myocardial rupture

Noncardiac Disease
Sudden Infant Death syndrome
Drowning
Pickwickian syndrome
Pulmonary embolism
Drug induced
Airway obstruction
No primary heart disease—primary electrical disease, chest wall trauma, Brugada syndrome

absolute contribution of fatal pump failure increases with functional class and disease severity. Nevertheless, absolute SCD incidence also increases with NYHA class, with 1-year SCD mortality ranging from 2% to 4% (NYHA Class I and II) to 5% to 12% (NYHA Class III and IV)[15] (Fig. 26–3).

QUANTIFYING CONGESTIVE HEART FAILURE SEVERITY: THE HISTORY, STRUCTURE, AND PHYSIOLOGY OF NATRIURETIC PEPTIDES

Accurately classifying (or "grading") the severity of CHF is a valuable goal in determining prognosis—and potentially in assigning the relative risk for SCD. Recent studies have caused a great deal of excitement over the use of natriuretic peptides for this purpose.

The history surrounding the development of natriuretic peptides as diagnostic markers for CHF is summarized in Table 26–2. Although the principal peptide is BNP, its primary site of synthesis has since been localized to the ventricular myocardium.

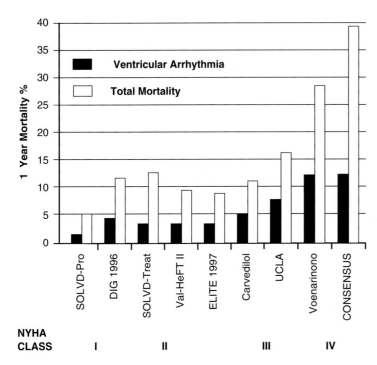

■ **Figure 26–3** Several studies emphasize that mortality increases with the severity of congestive heart failure (New York Heart Association [NYHA] functional class). Although total *(white)* and arrhythmic *(black)* mortality both increase with NYHA functional class, arrhythmias contribute proportionately more to mortality in less ill patients. SOLVD, Studies of Left Ventricular Function; DIG, Digitalis Investigators Group; Val-HeFT, Valsartan Heart Failure Trial; ELITE, Evaluation of Losartan in the Elderly; CONSENSUS, Cooperative North Scandinavian Enalapril Survival Study. *(From Stevenson WG, Stevenson LW: Prevention of sudden death in heart failure. J Cardiovasc Electrophysiol 12:112–114, 2001, with permission.)*

Three major natriuretic peptides—atrial natriuretic peptide (ANP), BNP, and C-type natriuretic peptide (CNP)—have been identified, and all share a 17-amino-acid ring structure (Fig. 26–4). ANP and BNP originate in myocardial cells, whereas CNP is of endothelial origin.[23] Natriuretic peptides are secreted by the heart in response to augmented wall stress, such as from CHF, and result in increased myocardial relax-ation (lusitropy), as well as opposition to the vasocon-strictive, sodium-retaining, and antidiuretic effects of the neurohormonal imbalance initiated by activation of the renin-angiotensin-aldosterone system, the sym-pathetic nervous system, endothelins, and other neu-rohormonal factors.

Specific stimuli vary for the secretion of each natri-uretic peptide. BNP is synthesized, stored, and released

TABLE 26–2   Developmental History of B-Type Natriuretic Peptide as a Marker for Congestive Heart Failure and Wall Strain

Year	Development
1956	Henry and Pearce[16] first observed BNP as a response to balloon stretch of the canine left atrium
1981	de Bold and colleagues[17] injected homogenized atrial tissue into rats and noted a potent natriuretic response
1984	Kangawa and colleagues[18] identified the structure of ANP
1988	Sudoh and colleagues[19] isolated a compound from pig brain that caused natriuretic and diuretic responses similar to ANP
1990	Sudoh and colleagues[20] isolated a structurally distinct member of the natriuretic peptide family, CNP, from pig brain
1991	Minamino and colleagues[21] reported that CNP is expressed to a much greater extent in central nervous system and vascular tissues than in the heart
1991	The primary site of BNP synthesis was localized to the ventricular myocardium[22]

ANP, atrial natriuretic peptide; BNP, B-type natriuretic peptide; CNP, C-type natriuretic peptide.

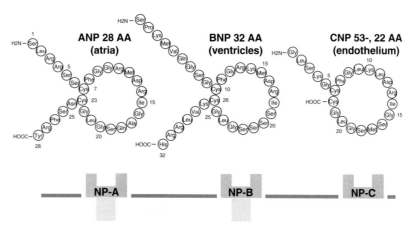

■ **Figure 26–4** Structure of the three major natriuretic peptides. ANP, Atrial natriuretic peptide; BNP, B-type natriuretic peptide; CNP, C-type natriuretic peptide.

primarily by the ventricular myocardium in response to volume expansion and pressure overload,[24–27] whereas ANP is released by atrial and ventricular tissue in response to volume overload.

At the cellular level, volume stretch leads to pulsatile bursts in pre-pro-BNP synthesis, which is then cleaved progressively to pro-BNP and, finally, to BNP and inactive N-terminal pro-BNP.

Because BNP is more stable than ANP and other neurohormones, and because it originates in the ventricles, it is more sensitive to left ventricular dysfunction than ANP and other neurohormones.[28] BNP has been hypothesized to play an important regulatory role in response to acute changes in ventricular volume.[29]

Role of Natriuretic Peptides in Congestive Heart Failure

The correlation of serum BNP concentrations with increased end-diastolic pressure[26,27] closely parallel dyspnea in heart failure, suggesting that this peptide is uniquely suited for use as a neurohormonal index of progressive heart failure.[30] BNP concentrations also parallel NYHA clinical status[31,32] more than does ANP.[29] Thus, BNP has emerged as a strong diagnostic and prognostic indicator of left ventricular dysfunction and heart failure.

Role of B-Type Natriuretic Peptide in the Emergency Care Setting

Several studies have established the role of BNP in the clinical diagnosis of CHF. In 1586 patients presenting to the emergency department with acute dyspnea, admission BNP exceeding 100 pg/mL had a sensitivity of 90% and a specificity of 76% for CHF as opposed to other causes of dyspnea, whereas BNP exceeding 50 pg/mL had a negative predictive value for CHF of 96%.[32] In another study of 321 patients presenting to the emergency department with dyspnea of unknown cause, BNP accurately separated CHF (mean BNP, 759 ± 798 pg/mL) from pulmonary disease (61 ± 10 pg/mL) with a high specificity, sensitivity, and accuracy of 91%. Moreover, comparing patients with heart failure whose dyspnea was caused by chronic obstructive pulmonary disease (COPD; mean BNP 47 ± 23 pg/mL) with patients with COPD whose dyspnea was caused by heart failure (731 ± 764 pg/mL), a BNP value of 94 pg/mL yielded a sensitivity and specificity of 86% and 98%, respectively, and differentiated heart failure from lung disease with an accuracy of 91%.[33]

BNP has been shown in several studies to be an accurate and independent index of heart failure. Moreover, in the studies mentioned previously, BNP predicted CHF in multivariate analyses of history, symptoms, signs, radiologic studies, and laboratory studies.

Combining these results, Maisel[34] and colleagues have proposed an algorithm for using BNP in the diagnosis and management of CHF that is in use at the La Jolla VA Medical Center (La Jolla, CA). In patients with acute dyspnea, a serum BNP value less than 100 pg/mL essentially excludes CHF as the cause of dyspnea, whereas values greater than 400 pg/mL provide a 95% likelihood for CHF. Values between 100 to 400 pg/mL warrant further investigation.[34]

B-Type Natriuretic Peptide and Congestive Heart Failure Prognosis

Studies are increasingly showing that serum BNP levels are highly predictive of subsequent cardiac events. In a study of 325 patients presenting with dyspnea to the emergency department, patients with BNP levels greater than 480 pg/mL had a 51% cumulative probability of death (cardiac and noncardiac), hospital admissions (cardiac), or repeated emergency department visits over the next 6 months. In contrast, only 2.5% of patients with BNP levels less than 230 pg/mL experienced one of these events.[35]

B-TYPE NATRIURETIC PEPTIDE AND THE PREDICTION OF SUDDEN CARDIAC DEATH

Recent studies raise the exciting possibility that BNP may indicate risk for ventricular arrhythmias and SCD, likely by reflecting volume overload and ventricular wall stretch. This association was most impressively demonstrated by Berger and colleagues,[36] who found that BNP levels independently predicted SCD in 452 ambulatory patients with mild to moderate heart failure (NYHA Class I and II) and left ventricular ejection fraction less than 35%. In that study, BNP greater than 130 pg/mL separated patients with high from those with low rates of SCD.

Furthermore, only 1% (1 of 110) of patients with a BNP level less than 130 pg/mL died suddenly, compared with 19% (43 of 227) of patients with BNP levels greater than 130 pg/mL. However, this study requires further confirmation and raises additional questions. First, only 31% of the recruitment population had ischemic left ventricular dysfunction, and these results must be validated in a larger population with coronary disease, who are at greatest risk for SCD (see Fig. 26–1). Second, patients with mild and severe CHF were not well represented in the enrolled population, 12% of whom had NYHA Class I, 34% had NYHA Class II, 33% had NYHA Class III, and 21% had NYHA Class IV. Thus, whether BNP predicts SCD in patients with more (or less) severe CHF also is unclear and worthy of study.

Additional evidence that increased levels of BNP predict ventricular arrhythmias is indirect. Cardiac resynchronization therapy (CRT) is increasingly believed to improve symptoms and reduce mortality[37,38] in patients with moderate to severe CHF and ventricular asynchrony. Many studies have shown that BNP concentrations decrease when CRT therapy is initiated and increase when CRT is subsequently deactivated.[39] Studies also have shown that CRT reduces the incidence of ventricular arrhythmias. Higgins and colleagues[40] studied 32 patients in whom CRT devices with defibrillator capability (CRT-D) were implanted. The study population had a mean age of 65 ± 10 years, 70% of patients had coronary artery disease, and all had CHF: 22% were in NYHA Class II, 65% in Class III, and 13% in Class IV. During a 6-month crossover of CRT-activated to CRT-deactivated therapy, the authors found that patients experienced significantly fewer appropriate device therapies when CRT was activated than when it was not.

However, the link between improvements in CHF and concomitant decreases in BNP level and SCD risk remains somewhat controversial, particularly in the CRT literature. A major negative finding came with the recent Multicenter InSync Randomized Clinical Evaluation Implantable Cardioverter Defibrillator (MIRACLE-ICD) study.[41] This trial examined 369 patients with left ventricular ejection fraction of 35% or less, QRS duration greater than 130 msec, a demonstrated risk for SCD, and NYHA Class III (n = 328) or IV (n = 41). All patients received a CRT-D device, of whom 182 were controls (ICD activated, CRT off) and 187 were active (ICD activated, CRT on). After 6 months of follow-up, patients with active CRT showed improved NYHA functional status and quality of life versus the control group. However, in neither group did the mean BNP concentration change appreciably.

Furthermore, both MIRACLE-ICD and a recent meta-analysis studying 1600 patients from four major CRT trials[37] failed to show a reduction in ventricular arrhythmias or SCD in patients treated with CRT, despite improvements in CHF symptoms and lower mortality rates.

Additional studies are therefore required to clarify the predictive value of BNP for SCD in CHF populations of varying severity. In particular, BNP may better predict SCD when combined with other markers of arrhythmia risk. Promising candidate indices include heart rate variability,[42] the signal-averaged electrocardiogram (ECG),[42-44] and T-wave alternans on the ECG.[44,45]

B-TYPE NATRIURETIC PEPTIDE–GUIDED THERAPY AND PROGNOSIS IN ACUTELY ILL PATIENTS

Mechanistically, because SCD risk is related to the extent of left ventricular dysfunction, therapies resulting in reverse ventricular remodeling may decrease total mortality and morbidity, as well as SCD. Therefore, hypothetically, titration of therapy to BNP levels as an index of pulmonary capillary wedge pressure may reduce the incidence of these end points. Kazanegra and colleagues[46] showed that decreasing levels of BNP correlate with reductions in wedge pressures in patients treated for decompensated CHF (Fig. 26–5). Furthermore, Cheng and colleagues[47] followed the course of 72 patients admitted with decompensated CHF with daily BNP levels and their relation to 30-day readmission rates or death. Patients who were most likely to have a cardiac event had greater BNP levels both at the times of admission and discharge.

Figure 26–6 shows the relation between an increase and decrease in the BNP level with treatment and subsequent end points. Only 16% of patients with a decrease in BNP levels during hospitalization had a subsequent cardiac event, whereas 52% of those with increased BNP levels during treatment had either readmission or cardiac death. Patients whose discharge BNP levels decreased to less than 430 pg/mL had a reasonable likelihood of not being readmitted within the following 30 days. These data were supported by a

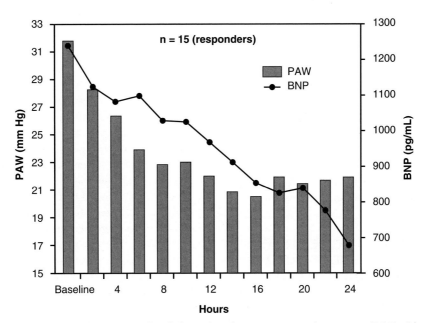

■ **Figure 26–5** The correlation of treatment-induced change in pulmonary artery wedge pressure (PAW) with change in B-type natriuretic peptide (BNP) from baseline. *(From Kazanegra R, Cheng V, Garcia A, et al: A rapid assay for B-type natriuretic peptide correlates with falling wedge pressures in patients treated for decompensated heart failure: A pilot study. J Card Fail 7:21–29, 2001, with permission.)*

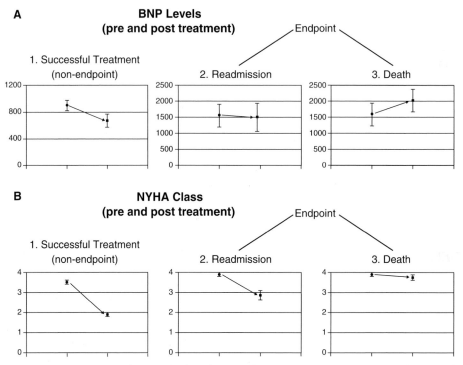

■ **Figure 26–6** B-type natriuretic peptide (BNP) levels and New York Heart Association (NYHA) classification before and after treatment in relation to end points or no end points (successful treatment). Each value represents mean ± SEM and is analyzed by analysis of variance. *(From Cheng V, Kazanagra R, Garcia A, et al: A rapid bedside test for B-type natriuretic peptide predicts treatment outcomes in patients admitted with decompensated heart failure. J Am Coll Cardiol 37:386–391, 2001, with permission.)*

recent study by Bettencourt and colleagues,[48] who found that failure of BNP levels to decrease during hospitalization predicts death and rehospitalization, and that discharge levels less than 250 pg/mL predicted event-free survival.

Measurement of serum BNP levels thus shows promise in monitoring patients with CHF, in tailoring management and titrating their therapy, and in predicting adverse cardiac events and readmissions.

B-TYPE NATRIURETIC PEPTIDE LEVEL–GUIDED THERAPY AND PROGNOSIS IN AMBULATORY PATIENTS

Because BNP levels have been shown to predict SCD in ambulatory patients, it is possible that a BNP-guided treatment strategy may reduce SCD in such

patients. Indeed, in the Acute Infarction Ramipril Efficacy (AIRE) trial, 45% of patients who died suddenly had severe or worsening CHF before death, whereas 39% of sudden deaths were believed to be arrhythmic.[49] Although the monitoring of serum BNP in the outpatient setting has yet to be proven effective in tailoring CHF treatment, several ongoing studies are testing this hypothesis. In a small study, Troughton and colleagues[50] showed that patients who had therapy tailored by BNP levels had fewer hospitalizations and lower mortality than those treated without knowledge of BNP levels. Less directly, that effective CHF treatments correlate with decreasing BNP levels also bodes well for future attempts to tailor therapy in this way.[51,52] Lee and colleagues[53] found that BNP levels in outpatients increased in those showing signs of decompensation, yet BNP levels decreased in those showing improvement in NYHA class. BNP levels may also have value in indicating a number of outpatient states that are indirectly linked with SCD, including volume overload from renal failure or decompensated valvular heart disease, and silent myocardial ischemia in diabetics.[54]

Summary

Epidemiologic and clinical studies have established that SCD, primarily an arrhythmic disorder, is most prevalent in patients with left ventricular dysfunction and CHF. Emerging clinical studies are increasingly demonstrating that increased serum levels of BNP portend an increased risk for SCD, likely by reflecting ventricular wall stretch and volume load. Further clarification of this association, and the possible role of BNP in future indications for implantable defibrillator and CRT, will follow additional clinical and mechanistic studies into the association between mechanical deformation of the ventricles and ventricular arrhythmias.

References

1. Zheng ZJ, Croft JB, Giles WH, Mensah GA: Sudden cardiac death in the United States, 1989 to 1998. Circulation 104:2158–2163, 2001.
2. Kannel WB, Wilson PW, D'Agostino RB, Cobb J: Sudden coronary death in women. Am Heart J 136:205–212, 1998.
3. Chugh SS, Kelly KL, Titus JL: Sudden cardiac death with apparently normal heart. Circulation 102:649–654, 2000.
4. Buxton AE, Lee KL, DiCarlo L, et al: Electrophysiologic testing to identify patients with coronary artery disease who are at risk for sudden death. Multicenter Unsustained Tachycardia Trial Investigators (MUSTT). N Engl J Med 342:1937–1945, 2000.
5. Myerburg RJ: Sudden cardiac death: Exploring the limits of our knowledge. J Cardiovasc Electrophysiol 12:369–381, 2001.
6. Bardy GH: Results from the Sudden Cardiac Death in Heart Failure (SCD-HeFT) trial. ACC Late Breaking Clinical Trials. Presented American College of Cardiology 2004, March 8, 2004, New Orleans, Louisiana.
7. Bayesde Luna A, Coumel P, Leclerq JF: Ambulatory sudden cardiac death: Mechanisms of production of fatal arrhythmia on the basis of data from 157 cases. Am Heart J 117:151–159, 1989.
8. Farb A, Tang AL, Burke AP, et al: Sudden coronary death: Frequency of active coronary lesions, inactive coronary lesions, and myocardial infarction. Circulation 92:1701–1709, 1995.
9. Kuo CS, Munakata K, Reddy CP, Surawicz B: Characteristics and possible mechanism of ventricular arrhythmia dependent on the dispersion of action potential durations. Circulation 67:1356–1367, 1983.
10. American Heart Association: Heart Disease and Stroke Statistics—2003 Update. Dallas, TX, American Heart Association, 2002.
11. Cohn JN, Levine TB, Olivari MT, et al: Plasma norepinephrine as a guide to prognosis in patients with chronic congestive heart failure. N Engl J Med 311:819–823, 1984.
12. Vinson JM, Rich MW, Sperry JC, et al: Early readmission of elderly patients with heart failure. J Am Geriatr Soc 38:1290–1295, 1990.
13. The CONSENSUS Trial Study Group: Effects of enalapril on mortality in severe congestive heart failure. Results of the Cooperative North Scandinavian Enalapril Survival Study (CONSENSUS). N Engl J Med 316:1429, 1987.
14. The SOLVD Investigators: Effect of enalapril on survival in patients with reduced left ventricular ejection fractions and congestive heart failure. N Engl J Med 325:293, 1991.
15. Stevenson WG, Stevenson LW: Prevention of sudden death in heart failure. J Cardiovasc Electrophysiol 12:112–114, 2001.
16. Henry JP, Pearce JW: The possible role of cardiac stretch receptors in the induction of changes in urine flow. J Physiol 131:572–594, 1956.
17. de Bold AJ, Borenstein HB, Veress AT, Sonnenberg H: A rapid and potent natriuretic response to intravenous injection of atrial myocardial extract in rats. Life Sci 28:89–94, 1981.
18. Kangawa K, Fukuda A, Minamino N, Matsuo H: Purification and complete amino acid sequence of beta-rat atrial natriuretic polypeptide (β-rANP) of 5000 daltons. Biochem Biophys Res Commun 119:933–940, 1984.
19. Sudoh T, Kangawa K, Minamino N, Matsuo H: A new natriuretic peptide in porcine brain. Nature 332:78–81, 1988.
20. Sudoh T, Minamino N, Kangawa K, Matsuo H: C-type natriuretic peptide (CNP): A new member of natriuretic peptide family identified in porcine brain. Biochem Biophys Res Commun 168:863–870, 1990.
21. Minamino N, Makino Y, Tateyama H, et al: Characterization of immunoreactive human C-type natriuretic peptide in brain and heart. Biochem Biophys Res Commun 179:535–542, 1991.
22. Hosoda K, Nakao K, Mukoyama M, et al: Expression of brain natriuretic peptide gene in human heart: Production in the ventricle. Hypertension 17:1152–1155, 1991.
23. Stingo AJ, Clavell AL, Heublein DM, et al: Presence of C-type natriuretic peptide in cultured human endothelial cells and plasma. Am J Physiol 263:H1318–H1321, 1992.
24. Klinge R, Hystad M, Kjekshus J, et al: An experimental study of cardiac natriuretic peptides as markers of development of heart failure. Scand J Clin Lab Invest 58:683–691, 1998.
25. Luchner A, Stevens TL, Borgeson DD, et al: Differential atrial and ventricular expression of myocardial BNP during evolution of heart failure. Am J Physiol 274:H1684–H1689, 1998.
26. Maeda K, Tsutamoto T, Wada A, et al: Plasma brain natriuretic peptide as a biochemical marker of high left ventricular end-diastolic pressure in patients with symptomatic left ventricular dysfunction. Am Heart J 135:825–832, 1998.
27. Muders F, Kromer EP, Griese DP, et al: Evaluation of plasma natriuretic peptides as markers for left ventricular dysfunction. Am Heart J 134:442–449, 1997.
28. Yasue H, Yoshimura M, Sumida H, et al: Localization and mechanism of secretion of B-type natriuretic peptide in comparison with those of A-type natriuretic peptide in normal subjects and patients with heart failure. Circulation 90:195–203, 1994.
29. Nakagawa O, Ogawa Y, Itoh H, et al: Rapid transcriptional activation and early mRNA turnover of BNP in cardiocyte hypertrophy. Evidence for BNP as an "emergency" cardiac hormone against ventricular overload. J Clin Invest 96:1280–1287, 1995.

30. Grantham JA, Borgeson DD, Burnett JC: BNP: Pathophysiological and potential therapeutic roles in acute congestive heart failure. Am J Physiol 92:R1077–R1083, 1997.

31. Dao Q, Krishnaswamy P, Kazanegra R, et al: Utility of B-type natriuretic peptide (BNP) in the diagnosis of heart failure in an urgent care setting. J Am Coll Cardiol 37:379–385, 2001.

32. Maisel AS, Krishnaswamy P, Nowak RM, et al, Breathing Not Properly Multinational Study Investigators: Rapid measurement of B-type natriuretic peptide in the emergency diagnosis of heart failure. N Engl J Med 347:161–167, 2002.

33. Morrison LK, Harrison A, Krishnaswamy P, et al: Utility of rapid B-type natriuretic peptide in differentiating congestive heart failure from lung disease. J Am Coll Cardiol 39:202–209, 2002.

34. Maisel A: B-type natriuretic peptide measurements in diagnosing congestive heart failure in the dyspneic emergency department patient. Rev Cardiovasc Med 3(suppl 4):S10–S17, 2002.

35. Harrison A, Morrison LK, Krishnaswamy P, et al: B-type natriuretic peptide predicts future cardiac events in patients presenting to the emergency department with dyspnea. Ann Emerg Med 39:131–138, 2002.

36. Berger R, Huelsman M, Strecker K, et al: B-type natriuretic peptide predicts sudden death in patients with chronic heart failure. Circulation 105:2392–2397, 2002.

37. Bradley DJ, Bradley EA, Baughman KL, et al: Cardiac resynchronization and death from progressive heart failure: A meta-analysis of randomized controlled trials. JAMA 289:730, 2003.

38. Bristow MR, Saxon LA, Boehmer J, et al, Comparison of Medical Therapy, Pacing, and Defibrillation in Heart Failure (COMPANION) Investigators: Cardiac-resynchronization therapy with or without an implantable defibrillator in advanced chronic heart failure. N Engl J Med 350:2140–2150, 2004.

39. Sinha AM, Filzmaier K, Breithardt OA, et al: Usefulness of brain natriuretic peptide release as a surrogate marker of the efficacy of long-term cardiac resynchronization therapy in patients with heart failure. Am J Cardiol 91:755–758, 2003.

40. Higgins SL, Yong P, Sheck D, et al: Biventricular pacing diminishes the need for implantable cardioverter defibrillator therapy. J Am Coll Cardiol 36:824–827, 2000.

41. Young JB, Abraham WT, Smith AL, et al, Multicenter InSync ICD Randomized Clinical Evaluation (MIRACLE ICD) Trial Investigators: Combined cardiac resynchronization and implantable cardioversion defibrillation in advanced chronic heart failure: The MIRACLE ICD Trial. JAMA 289:2685–2694, 2003.

42. Farrell TG, Bashir Y, Cripps T, et al: Risk stratification for arrhythmic events in postinfarction patients based on heart rate variability, ambulatory electrocardiographic variables and the signal-averaged electrocardiogram. J Am Coll Cardiol 18:687–697, 1991.

43. Gomes JA, Cain ME, Buxton AE, et al: Prediction of long-term outcomes by signal-averaged electrocardiography in patients with unsustained ventricular tachycardia, coronary artery disease, and left ventricular dysfunction. Circulation 104: 436–441, 2001.

44. Narayan SM, Cain ME: Non-invasive techniques for assessing arrhythmia risk: T-wave alternans, signal-averaged ECG, and heart rate variability. In: Harrison's Online Textbook of Internal Medicine, 15th ed, New York, McGraw-Hill, 2003.

45. Narayan SM, Lindsay BD, Smith JM: Demonstrating the pro-arrhythmic preconditioning of single premature extrastimuli using the magnitude, phase and temporal distribution of repolarization alternans. Circulation 100:1887–1893, 1999.

46. Kazangera R, Cheng V, Garcia A, et al: A rapid assay for B-type natriuretic peptide correlates with falling wedge pressures in patients treated for decompensated heart failure: A pilot study. J Card Fail 7:21–29, 2001.

47. Cheng V, Kazanagra R, Garcia A, et al: A rapid bedside test for B-type natriuretic peptide predicts treatment outcomes in patients admitted with decompensated heart failure. J Am Coll Cardiol 37:386–391, 2001.

48. Bettencourt P, Ferreira S, Azevedo A, Ferreira A: Preliminary data on the potential usefulness of B-type natriuretic peptide levels in predicting outcomes after hospital discharge in patients with heart failure. Am J Med 113:215–219, 2002.

49. Cleland JG, Erhardt L, Murray G, et al: Effect of ramipril on morbidity and mode of death among survivors of acute myocardial infarction with clinical evidence of heart failure. A report from the AIRE Study Investigators. Eur Heart J 18:41–51, 1997.

50. Troughton RW, Frampton CM, Yandle TG, et al: Treatment of heart failure guided by plasma amino terminal brain natriuretic peptide (N-BNP) concentrations. Lancet 355:1126–1130, 2000.

51. Tsutamoto T, Wada A, Maeda K, et al: Effect of spironolactone on plasma brain natriuretic peptide and left ventricular remodeling in patients with congestive heart failure. J Am Coll Cardiol 37:1228–1233, 2001.

52. Anand IS, Fisher LD, Chiang Y-T, et al, for the Val-HeFT Investigators: Changes in brain natriuretic peptide and norepinephrine over time and mortality and morbidity in the Valsartan Heart Failure Trial (Val-HeFT). Circulation 107:1278–1283, 2003.

53. Lee S-C, Stevens TL, Sandberg SM, et al: The potential of brain natriuretic peptide as a biomarker for New York Heart Association Class during the outpatient treatment of heart failure. J Card Fail 8:149–154, 2002.

54. Bhalla V, Willis S, Maisel AS: B-type natriuretic peptide: The level and the drug—partners in the diagnosis of congestive heart failure. Congest Heart Fail 10:3–27, 2004.

CHAPTER 27

Neurohormonal Antagonists in Relation to Sudden Death in Heart Failure

• • • •

Peter Carson

The relation of mechano-electric stimulation to neurohormonal systems is of great interest with applications from bench to bedside. This chapter discusses work in the settings of postmyocardial infarction (post-MI) and congestive heart failure (CHF).

The inclusion of post-MI studies is an opportunity to study ventricular enlargement under relatively controlled circumstances after an experimental or clinical event. The post-MI data under discussion involve transmural MI, because congestion commonly develops in these patients; this is often considered a "form fruste" of heart failure. These patients are under considerable risk for electrical instability and sudden death.

CONGESTIVE HEART FAILURE

The syndrome of CHF is characterized by increased morbidity and shortened survival.[1] We have come to recognize that patients with heart failure predominantly have impaired systolic *or* impaired diastolic function, although both abnormalities may co-exist. In both circumstances, the heart has undergone extensive remodeling, and the clinical outcomes may differ. Mechano-electric feedback (MEF) factors are expected to differ between systolic and diastolic heart failure.

Focusing on systolic heart failure, multiple factors influence pathologic remodeling. The myocardium's initial response to an event (e.g., MI) that impairs systolic performance is to maintain cardiac output by dilating—a process that enables stroke volume to be maintained with a larger end-diastolic volume by the Frank–Starling mechanism.[2]

The process of remodeling is associated with eccentric hypertrophy in systolic heart failure, whereas concentric hypertrophy is more commonly present in diastolic heart failure.[3] The eccentric hypertrophy involves an increase in myocardial mass without an appreciable increase in wall thickness. This is principally accomplished by an elongation of cardiac myocytes, leading to a marked increase in myocyte volume.[4] Remodeling also involves fibroblasts that produce a collagen network comprising the extracellular matrix, located in the interstitium between myocytes.[5] A stimulus for fibrosis is aldosterone, stimulating specific aldosterone receptors.

As a result of this process of hypertrophy and fibrosis, the heart becomes larger and alters shape, becoming more spherical (Fig. 27–1).[6] Although these changes have been clearly noted after MI, they also occur in noninfarcted myocardium, characteristically in patients with idiopathic-dilated cardiomyopathy, in whom the initiating event is usually unknown.

Trophic factors that stimulate remodeling include hormones, particularly the renin-angiotensin system (RAS) and the sympathetic nervous system.[7] For the former, stretch of myocytes leads to release of angiotensin II,[7] which can induce protein synthesis and produce cardiac cell hypertrophy, eventually leading to overt myocardial hypertrophy.[8] Similarly, adrenergic stimulation of both α and β receptors can result in cardiac myocyte hypertrophy, with adult myocytes particularly influenced by adrenergic pathway.[9] *Norepinephrine* is the principal sympathetic nervous system neurotransmitter and, in excess, is toxic to myocytes.[9] Excess adrenergic stimulation is invariably present in systolic heart failure, and the resulting myocyte loss increases the demand on remaining myocytes to hypertrophy further, with increased dysfunction.[10] Neurohormones are then additionally stimulated, and the cycle repeats. Remodeling is central to the current concepts of the progression of heart failure and the transition from asymptomatic

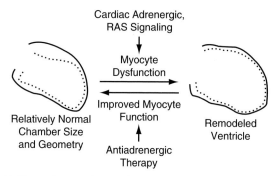

■ **Figure 27–1** Relation of myocyte dysfunction to development and reversal of remodeling and effects of activation of the cardiac adrenergic and renin-angiotensin systems (RAS), as well as antiadrenergic therapy. *(From Eichhorn EJ, Bristow MR: Medical therapy can improve the biologic properties of the chronically failing heart: A new era in the treatment of heart failure. Circulation 94:2285–2296, 1996, with permission.)*

left ventricular dysfunction to symptomatic disease (Fig. 27–2).[1]

NEUROHORMONAL THERAPY AND REMODELING

Part of the proof for the influence of the RAS and the sympathetic nervous system on remodeling involves the effect of specific receptor antagonists.

Renin-Angiotensin System

Positive correlations are present in multiple animal models using RAS inhibitors. In a post-MI rat model, Pfeffer and colleagues[11] demonstrated attenuation of ventricular enlargement in captopril-treated rats. Sabbah and colleagues[10] (microembolization dog model; Fig. 27–3) and McDonald and colleagues[12] (direct current [DC] shock dog model) also demonstrated attenuation of changes in ventricular volume in animals treated with angiotensin-converting enzyme inhibitors (ACEI). Notably, both studies also showed that the β-blocker metoprolol had favorable effects. Because β-blockers inhibit RAS by decreasing renin production, part of their effect on mediating ventricular remodeling may be because of this component of the drug action.

It is unlikely that angiotensin II is solely responsible for the pathologic remodeling of the heart. Spinale and colleagues,[13] in a pig model, noted favorable remodeling effects with an ACEI, but not with an angiotensin receptor blocker (ARB). A favorable effect also was seen with the combination (Table 27–1). These data, together with similar data of McDonald and colleagues,[12] suggest that bradykinin may have a significant role in remodeling, because an ACEI augments bradykinin, whereas an ARB does not.

Clinical data with RAS inhibitors confirm the findings of animal studies. The progressive increase in cardiac size is inhibited. Pfeffer and colleagues[14] and

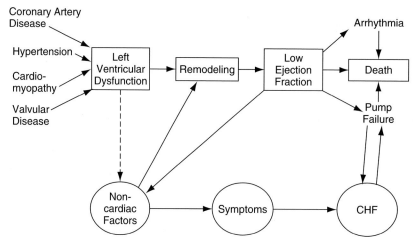

■ **Figure 27–2** The pathogenesis of congestive heart failure (CHF). *(From Cohn JN: Drug therapy: The management of chronic heart failure. N Engl J Med 335:490–498, 1996, with permission.)*

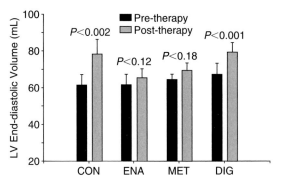

■ **Figure 27–3** Values (mean ± SEM) of left ventricular (LV) end-diastolic volume before and after treatment with either enalapril (ENA), metoprolol (MET), or digoxin (DIG). CON, untreated control dogs. *(From Sabbah HN, Shimoyama H, Kono T, et al: Effects of long-term monotherapy with enalapril, metoprolol, and digoxin on the progression of left ventricular dysfunction and dilation in dogs with reduced ejection fraction. Circulation 89:2852–2859, 1994, with permission.)*

Mitchell and colleagues[15] demonstrated favorable effects on echocardiographic volumes and the shape of the heart in patients after MI. In the established heart failure population of Studies of Left Ventricular Dysfunction (SOLVD), Greenberg and colleagues[16] found that the ACEI enalapril attenuated the progressive increase in ventricular size noted in the placebo group (Fig. 27–4).

More recently, Wong and colleagues[17] noted a modest decrease in ventricular size with the addition of the ARB valsartan to standard therapy, which generally included an ACEI (with a minority on a β-blocker). In a small subgroup without an ACEI, valsartan showed a similar benefit. In the Losartan Heart Failure Survival Study (ELITE II), Konstam and colleagues[18] noted a trend for more favorable effects with captopril than losartan. The available data indicate that renin-angiotensin inhibitors exert modest benefits largely by preventing further remodeling rather than by reversing the process.

Notably, the process of remodeling is also influenced by aldosterone antagonism. Data with spironolactone by Hayashi and colleagues[19] demonstrated favorable post-MI effects that are similar to an ACEI—ventricular size did not increase with treatment—whereas the placebo group did experience enlargement (Fig. 27–5). No heart failure data are currently available.

SYMPATHETIC NERVOUS SYSTEM

In the animal studies discussed previously, Sabbah and colleagues[10] and McDonald and colleagues[12] were among those demonstrating favorable effects of β-blockers on remodeling in animal models. In the microembolization study of Sabbah and colleagues,[10] metoprolol-treated dogs showed improved ejection fraction and ventricular volumes did not increase, unlike the increased volume that occurred in untreated dogs.

TABLE 27–1 Left Ventricular Function and Geometry with Rapid Pacing Heart Failure

	Control	Rapid Pacing	Rapid Pacing and ACEI	Rapid Pacing and AT$_1$ Block	Rapid Pacing and ACEI/AT$_1$ Block
Resting heart rate, bpm	115 ± 4	165 ± 4	141 ± 7	162 ± 5	128 ± 5
Mean arterial pressure, mm Hg	91 ± 3	72 ± 4	77 ± 3	72 ± 3	78 ± 2
LV end-diastolic dimension, cm	3.45 ± 0.07	5.61 ± 0.11	4.95 ± 0.11	5.66 ± 0.10	4.68 ± 0.07
LV fractional shortening, %	39.1 ± 1.0	13.4 ± 1.4	20.9 ± 1.9	16.0 ± 3.4	25.2 ± 0.9

Effects of angiotensin-converting enzyme inhibitor (ACEI), angiotensin II receptor type 1 (AT$_1$) blockade, or combined ACEI and AT$_1$ blockade during the progression of heart failure.
LV, left ventricular.
From Spinale FG, de Gasparo M, Whitebread S, et al: Modulation of the renin-angiotensin pathway through enzyme inhibition and specific receptor blockade in pacing-induced heart failure. I: Effects on left ventricular performance and neurohormonal system. Circulation 96:2385–2396, 1997, with permission.

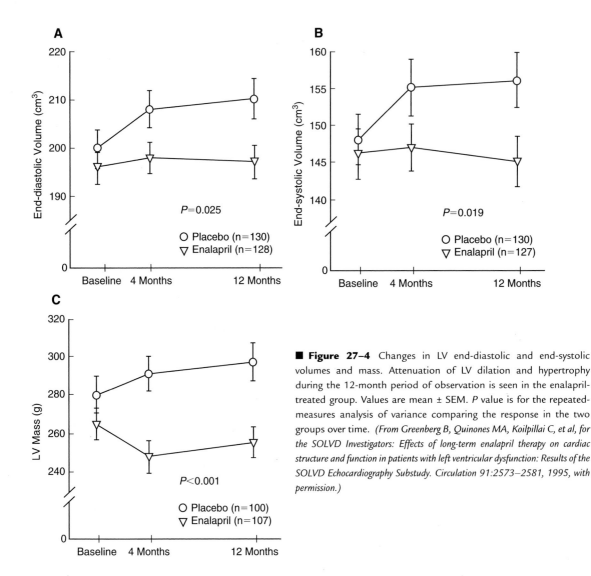

A

B

C

■ **Figure 27–4** Changes in LV end-diastolic and end-systolic volumes and mass. Attenuation of LV dilation and hypertrophy during the 12-month period of observation is seen in the enalapril-treated group. Values are mean ± SEM. *P* value is for the repeated-measures analysis of variance comparing the response in the two groups over time. *(From Greenberg B, Quinones MA, Koilpillai C, et al, for the SOLVD Investigators: Effects of long-term enalapril therapy on cardiac structure and function in patients with left ventricular dysfunction: Results of the SOLVD Echocardiography Substudy. Circulation 91:2573–2581, 1995, with permission.)*

Clinical data with β-blockers have principally focused on improvement in ejection fraction. In fact, in every study of greater than 1 month in duration, a significant improvement in ejection fraction has been noted in heart failure patients treated with β-blockers.[20] Less commonly, ventricular dimensions have been measured.

Hall and colleagues[21] first demonstrated reductions in ventricular volumes with metoprolol tartrate treatment beginning at 3 months. Similarly, Doughty and colleagues[22] showed reduction in ventricular size with carvedilol in the Australian-New Zealand Study. In this latter study, there was a 14 mL/mg difference in left ventricular volume index at 12 months. More recently, Groenning and colleagues[23] published data for metoprolol succinate using magnetic resonance imaging (Fig. 27–6). β-Blockade produced significant reductions in both left ventricular systolic and diastolic volume indices at 6 months.

The magnitude of the antiremodeling effects (25% left ventricular end-diastolic volume and 20% left ventricular end-systolic volume indices) were substantially

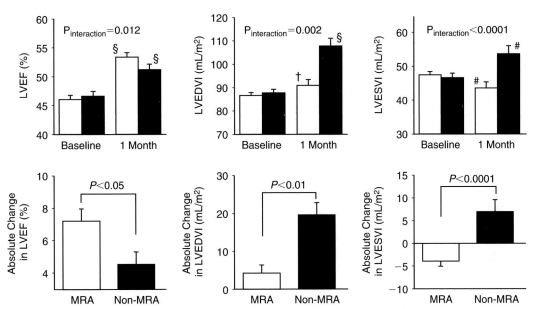

■ **Figure 27–5** LV function and geometry with rapid pacing heart failure. *Top,* Changes in the LV ejection fraction (LVEF), LV end-diastolic volume index (LVEDVI), LV end-systolic volume index (LVESVI) in the two randomized treatment groups from baseline to 1 month later. *Bottom,* Absolute change (value at 1 month minus value at baseline) in LVEF, LVEDVI, and LVESVI. †P < 0.05; #P < 0.01; §P < 0.0001: difference between baseline and 1-month values. Empty columns: treatment with the mineralocorticoid receptor antagonist (MRA) spironolactone; filled columns: non-MRA treated group. *(From Hayashi M, Tsutamoto T, Wada A, et al: Immediate administration of mineralocorticoid receptor antagonist spironolactone prevents post-infarct left ventricular remodeling associated with suppression of a marker of myocardial cologne synthesis in patients with first anterior acute myocardial infarction. Circulation 107:2559–2565, 2003, with permission.)*

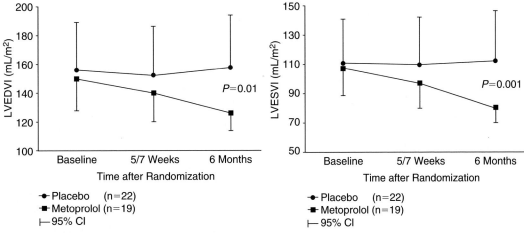

■ **Figure 27–6** Effect of metoprolol treatment on left ventricular function in heart failure. *Left,* LVEDVI over time. *Right,* LVESVI over time. Mean LVEDVI and LVESVI are shown in the metoprolol group and in the placebo group at baseline, 5 or 7 weeks and 6 months after randomization. P values are for the metoprolol group versus the placebo group. CI, confidence interval. *(From Groenning BA, Nilsson JC, Sondergaard L, et al: Antiremodeling effects on the left ventricle during beta-blockade with metoprolol in the treatment of chronic heart failure. J Am Coll Cardiol 36:2072–2080, 2000, with permission.)*

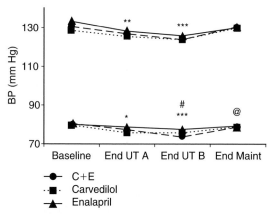

■ **Figure 27–7** Drug effects on mean systolic and diastolic blood pressure (BP) in mild heart failure over time. Significant changes from baseline are denoted by: ***$P < 0.001$, **$P < 0.01$, and *$P < 0.05$ and are valid for all groups; @$P < 0.05$ for the combination group only; # denotes a significant difference between the combination and enalapril groups. C, carvedilol; E, enalapril; UT, up-titration. *(From Remme WJ, Riegger G, Hildebrandt P, et al, on behalf of the CARMEN Investigators and Co-Ordinators: The Benefits of Early Combination Treatment of Carvedilol and An ACE-Inhibitor in Mild Heart Failure and Left Ventricular Systolic Dysfunction. The Carvedilol and ACE-Inhibitor Remodeling Mild Heart Failure Evaluation Trial [CARMEN]. Cardiovasc Drugs Ther 18:57–66, 2004, with permission.)*

greater than previous reports with other agents or other β-blockers (see Fig. 27–6). Together with this effect on ventricular volume, the ejection fraction improved from 29% to 37%. The most recent data involved carvedilol in the Carvedilol and ACE inhibitors remodeling Mild Heart Failure Evaluation (CARMEN).[24] In this study, carvedilol provided greater inhibition of remodeling than enalapril, although the combination provided the greatest effect compared with Enalapril alone (decrease of 5.4 mL/m²; see also Fig. 27–7).

Placed in the context of previous work, the data with clinically used neurohormonal antagonists indicate that β-blockers did more reverse remodeling with a larger reduction in ventricular volumes than ACEI or ARB.

VENTRICULAR ARRHYTHMIAS

St. John Sutton[25] studied the relation of ventricular arrhythmias to heart size in the post-MI substudy of

Survival And Ventricular Enlargement trial (SAVE) (Fig. 27–8). He found a significant increase in ventricular arrhythmias as cardiac dimension or left ventricular mass increased. The substudy was not large enough to reliably assess the impact of ACEI or β-blocker treatment.

Little data exist concerning these effects of neurohormonal antagonists on ventricular arrhythmias in heart failure. The Valsartan Heart Failure Trial (Val-HeFT) II study,[26] involving a comparison of hydralazine isosorbide dinitrate and enalapril, did include ventricular arrhythmia analysis.

The results indicated a reduction of ventricular tachycardia with enalapril. The absence of a placebo group in Val-HeFT II hampered interpretation, and it is worth noting that echocardiographic data did not support a benefit for enalapril over hydralazine isosorbide dinitrate on remodeling, because no change in ventricular dimensions was noted.

CLINICAL OUTCOMES

Mortality in heart failure is substantial. In advanced heart failure, annual mortality rates are similar to aggressive cancer. Even in mild to moderate disease, annual mortality rates are 6% to 10%[27,28] in well treated patients. Currently, the majority of deaths, except in advanced heart failure, are sudden.

The beneficial effects of ACEI and β-blockers on overall mortality in heart failure are well known. Stabilizing electrical activation would involve a reduction in sudden death. Although it is accepted that sudden death may have many possible causes—bradyarrhythmia, myocardial infarction, pulmonary embolus, and aortic dissection—there is little doubt that many of these events are actually lethal arrhythmias.

There are differences in sudden death definitions; therefore, conclusions should be drawn carefully when comparing studies. For ACEI, the data are particularly mixed. The earliest placebo-controlled ACEI trials, Cooperative North Scandinavian Enalapril Survival Study (CONSENSUS)[29] and SOLVD,[30] did not report a benefit for an ACEI in reducing sudden death. In a post-MI population, however, the SAVE data demonstrated a reduction in sudden death.[31] The Val-HeFT data did show a favorable effect on sudden

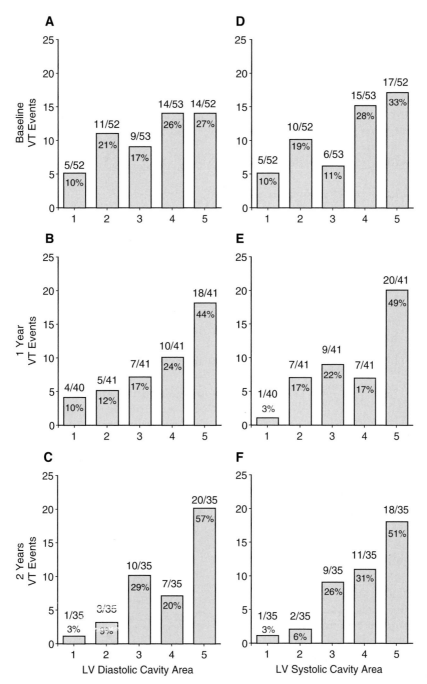

■ **Figure 27–8**   Relation between LV end-diastolic size and ventricular tachycardia (VT) at baseline *(A)*, 1 year *(B)*, and 2 years *(C)*, and relation between LV end-systolic size and VT at baseline *(D)*, 1 year *(E)*, and 2 years *(F)*. Area ranges 1–5 identify quintiles of the studied population. *(From St John Sutton M, Lee D, Rouleau JL, et al: Left ventricular remodeling and ventricular arrhythmias after myocardial infarction. Circulation 107:2577–2582, 2003, with permission.)*

death, although, as noted previously, this study had a positive control comparator of hydralazine and isosorbide dinitrate.

Clinical results with ARB have not shown a favorable effect on sudden death. In ELITE II, losartan did not reduce sudden death compared with captopril.[32] Similarly, as additive therapy in Val-HeFT, valsartan did not reduce sudden deaths.[33] As noted previously, no remodeling effect was seen with losartan in ELITE, and only minor effects were seen with valsartan in Val-HeFT.

Two outcome trials exist with aldosterone antagonists: Eplerenone post-AMI Heart Failure Efficacy and Survival Study (EPHESUS)[34] and Randomized Aldactone (spironolactone) Evaluation Study for Congestive Heart Failure (RALES).[35] In both studies, significant reductions in sudden deaths were noted (21% and 29%, respectively).

The most robust data for neurohormonal antagonists and sudden death involves β-blockers. Earlier trials with these agents—Metoprolol in Dilated Cardiomyopathy (MDC)[36] and Cardiac Insufficiency Bisoprolol Study (CIBIS)[37]—did not show a reduction in sudden death, whereas a later trial with carvedilol did (U.S. Carvedilol program).[38] These data led to speculation that blockade of both β$_1$ and β$_2$ receptors was necessary to reduce sudden death, because metoprolol and bisoprolol were cardioselective and carvedilol was not. However, larger studies established that cardioselectivity did not correlate with sudden death reduction. CIBIS-II (Bisoprolol),[27] Metoprolol Randomized Intervention Trial in Congestive Heart Failure (MERIT-HF),[28] and Carvedilol Prospective Randomized Cumulative Survival Study (COPERNICUS)[39] all demonstrated dramatic 40% to 47% reductions in sudden death. The noncardioselective agent bucindolol was less effective in the Bucindolol Estimation of Survival Trial (BEST), with only a 10% reduction.[40] Although bucindolol has been reported to have intrinsic sympathomimetic properties, it also had less impressive remodeling properties.[40] Therefore, robust reductions in sudden death have been noted, and at least two of the favorable agents, metoprolol succinate and carvedilol, have shown significant antiremodeling effects (Table 27–2).

TABLE 27–2 Sudden Death Reductions in Heart Failure during β-Blocker Mortality Trials

Trial	Active	Placebo	RR
CIBIS-II[27]	71 (5.3%)	132 (10.0%)	−47%
MERIT-HF[28]	79 (4.0%)	132 (6.6%)	−40%
COPERNICUS[39]	48 (4.2%)	88 (7.8%)	−47%

CIBIS, Cardiac Insufficiency Bisoprolol Study; COPERNICUS, Carvedilol Prospective Randomized Cumulative Survival Study; MERIT-HF, Metoprolol Randomized Intervention Trial in Congestive Heart Failure; RR, risk reduction.

Conclusion

Neurohormonal antagonists have shown a range of effects on reversing pathologic remodeling after MI and in heart failure. ACEI produces an attenuation of remodeling and ARB appears to have similar effects. Little data exist for aldosterone antagonists, but expectations are high for these agents because of the relation of aldosterone receptors to fibrosis. β-Blockers exhibit the strongest reverse remodeling effects.

No direct data exist for reduction of ventricular size and reduction of ventricular arrhythmias. However, the significant reduction of sudden death by β-blockers in heart failure suggests a mechano-electric link. MEF is probably of great significance, because pharmacologic reversal of remodeling is the cornerstone of current therapies for heart failure.

References

1. Cohn JN: Drug therapy: The management of chronic heart failure. N Engl J Med 335:490–498, 1996.
2. Ross J, Braunwald E: Studies on Starling's law of the heart: The effects of impeding venous return on performance of the normal and failing human left ventricle. Circulation 30:719–727, 1964.
3. Grossman W, Jones D, McLaurin LP: Wall stress and patterns of hypertrophy in the human left ventricle. J Clin Invest 56:56–64, 1975.
4. Beltrami CA, Finato N, Rocco M, et al: The cellular basis of dilated cardiomyopathy in humans. J Mol Cell Cardiol 27:291–305, 1995.
5. Weber KT, Anversa P, Armstrong PW, et al: Remodeling and reparation of the cardiovascular system. J Am Coll Cardiol 20:3–16, 1992.
6. Katz A: The cardiomyopathy of overload: An unnatural growth response in the hypertrophied heart. Ann Intern Med 121:363–371, 1994.

7. Sadoshima J, Izumo S: Molecular characterization of angiotensin II–induced hypertrophy of cardiac myocytes and hyperplasia of cardiac fibroblasts: Critical role of the AT1 receptor subtype. Circ Res 73:413–423, 1993.

8. Bishopric NH, Sato B, Webster KA: β-Adrenergic regulation of a myocardial actin gene via a cyclic AMP-independent pathway. J Biol Chem 267:20932–20936, 1992.

9. Mann DL, Kent RL, Parsons B, et al: Adrenergic effects on the biology of the adult mammalian cardiocyte. Circulation 85:790–804, 1992.

10. Sabbah HN, Shimoyama H, Kono T, et al: Effects of long-term monotherapy with enalapril, metoprolol, and digoxin on the progression of left ventricular dysfunction and dilation in dogs with reduced ejection fraction. Circulation 89:2852–2859, 1994.

11. Pfeffer JM, Pfeffer MA, Braunwald E: Influence of chronic captopril therapy on the infarcted left ventricle of the rat. Circ Res 57:84–95, 1985.

12. McDonald KM, Rector T, Carlyle PF, et al: Angiotensin-converting enzyme inhibition and beta-adrenoceptor blockade regress established ventricular remodeling in a canine model of discrete myocardial damage. J Am Coll Cardiol 24:1762–1768, 1994.

13. Spinale FG, de Gasparo M, Whitebread S, et al: Modulation of the renin-angiotensin pathway through enzyme inhibition and specific receptor blockade in pacing-induced heart failure: I. Effects on left ventricular performance and neurohormonal system. Circulation 96:2385–2396, 1997.

14. Pfeffer MA, Lamas GA, Vaughan DE, et al: Effect of captopril on progressive ventricular dilatation after anterior myocardial infarction. N Engl J Med 319:80–86, 1988.

15. Mitchell GF, Lamas GA, Vaughan DE, Pfeffer MA: Left ventricular remodeling in the year after first anterior myocardial infarction: A quantitative analysis of contractile segment lengths and ventricular shape. J Am Coll Cardiol 19:1136–1144, 1992.

16. Greenberg B, Quinones MA, Koilpillai C, et al, for the SOLVD Investigators: Effects of long-term enalapril therapy on cardiac structure and function in patients with left ventricular dysfunction: Results of the SOLVD Echocardiography Substudy. Circulation 91:2573–2581, 1995.

17. Wong M, Staszewsky L, Latini R, et al: Valsartan benefits left ventricular structure and function in heart failure: Val-HeFT echocardiographic study. J Am Coll Cardiol 40:970–975, 2002.

18. Konstam MA, Patten RD, Thomas I, et al: Effects of losartan and captopril on left ventricular volumes in elderly patients with heart failure: Results of the ELITE ventricular function substudy. Am Heart J 139:1081–1087, 2000.

19. Hayashi M, Tsutamoto T, Wada A, et al: Immediate administration of mineralocorticoid receptor antagonist spironolactone prevents post-infarct left ventricular remodeling associated with suppression of a marker of myocardial cologne synthesis in patients with first anterior acute myocardial infarction. Circulation 107:2559–2565, 2003.

20. Eichhorn EJ, Bristow MR: Medical therapy can improve the biologic properties of the chronically failing heart: A new era in the treatment of heart failure. Circulation 94:2285–2296, 1996.

21. Hall SA, Cigarroa CG, Marcoux L, et al: Time course of improvement in left ventricular function, mass, and geometry in patients with congestive heart failure treated with β-adrenergic blockade. J Am Coll Cardiol 25:1154–1161, 1995.

22. Doughty RN, MacMahon S, Sharpe N: Beta-blockers in heart failure: Promising or proved? J Am Coll Cardiol 23:814–821, 1994.

23. Groenning BA, Nilsson JC, Sondergaard L, et al: Antiremodeling effects on the left ventricle during beta-blockade with metoprolol in the treatment of chronic heart failure. J Am Coll Cardiol 36:2072–2080, 2000.

24. Remme WJ, Riegger G, Hildebrandt P, et al, on behalf of the CARMEN Investigators and Co-Ordinators: The Benefits of Early Combination Treatment of Carvedilol and An ACE-Inhibitor in Mild Heart Failure and Left Ventricular Systolic Dysfunction. The Carvedilol and ACE-Inhibitor Remodeling Mild Heart Failure Evaluation Trial (CARMEN). Cardiovasc Drugs Ther 18:57–66, 2004.

25. St John Sutton M, Lee D, Rouleau JL, et al: Left ventricular remodeling and ventricular arrhythmias after myocardial infarction. Circulation 107:2577–2582, 2003.

26. Cohn JN, Johnson G, Ziesche S, et al: A comparison of enalapril with hydralazine-isosorbide dinitrate in the treatment of chronic congestive heart failure. N Engl J Med 325:303–310, 1991.

27. CIBIS-II Investigators and Committees: The Cardiac Insufficiency Bisoprolol Study II (CIBIS-II): A randomised trial. Lancet 353:9–13, 1999.

28. MERIT-HF Study Group: Effect of metoprolol CR/XL in chronic heart failure: Metoprolol CR/XL Randomized Intervention Trial in Congestive Heart Failure (MERIT-HF). Lancet 353:2001–2006, 1999.

29. The CONSENSUS Trial Study Group: Effects of enalapril on mortality in severe congestive heart failure: Results of the Cooperative North Scandinavian Enalapril Survival Study (CONSENSUS). N Engl J Med 316:1429–1435, 1987.

30. The SOLVD Investigators: Effect of enalapril on survival in patients with reduced left ventricular ejection fractions and congestive heart failure. N Engl J Med 325:293–302, 1991.

31. Pfeffer MA, Braunwald E, Moye LA, et al, on behalf of the SAVE Investigators: Effect of captopril on mortality and morbidity in patients with left ventricular dysfunction after myocardial infarction: Results of the survival and ventricular enlargement trial. N Engl J Med 327:669–677, 1992.

32. Pitt B, Poole-Wilson PA, Segal R, et al: Effects of losartan compared with captopril on mortality in patients with symptomatic heart failure: Randomised trial—the Losartan Heart Failure Survival Study ELITE II. Lancet 355:1582–1587, 2000.

33. Cohn JN, Tognoni G: A randomized trial of the angiotensin-receptor blocker valsartan in chronic heart failure. N Engl J Med 345:1667–1675, 2001.

34. Pitt B, Remme W, Zannad F, et al: Eplerenone, a selective aldosterone blocker, in patients with left ventricular dysfunction after myocardial infarction. N Engl J Med 348:1309–1321, 2003.

35. Pitt B, Zannad F, Remme WJ, et al: The effect of spironolactone on morbidity and mortality in patients with severe heart failure. N Engl J Med 341:709–717, 1999.

36. Waagstein F, Bristow MR, Swedberg K, et al, for the Metoprolol in Dilated Cardiomyopathy (MDC) Trial Study Group: Beneficial effects of metoprolol in idiopathic dilated cardiomyopathy. Lancet 342:1441–1446, 1993.

37. CIBIS Investigators and Committees: A randomized trial of beta-blockade in heart failure: The Cardiac Insufficiency Bisoprolol Study (CIBIS). Circulation 90:1765–1773, 1994.

38. Packer M, Bristow MR, Cohn JN, et al: The effect of carvedilol on morbidity and mortality in patients with chronic heart failure. US Carvedilol Heart Failure Study Group. N Engl J Med 334:1349–1355, 1996.

39. Packer M, Coats AJS, Fowler MB, et al, for the Carvedilol Prospective Randomized Cumulative Survival Study Group: Effect of carvedilol on survival in severe chronic heart failure. N Engl J Med 344:1651–1658, 2001.

40. The BEST Investigators: A trial of the beta-adrenergic blocker bucindolol in patients with advanced chronic heart failure. N Engl J Med 344:1659–1667, 2001.

CHAPTER 28

Electro-Mechanical Remodeling in Hypertrophy

• • • •

Dirk W. Donker, Harry J. G. M. Crijns, and Paul G. A. Volders

This chapter describes clinical and experimental aspects of electro-mechanical remodeling during long-term hemodynamic overload leading to hypertrophy. The putative role of mechanical stimuli to induce molecular-electrophysiologic changes is discussed. The chapter focuses primarily on the remodeling of ventricular repolarization and its relation to arrhythmogenesis. First, we provide a brief overview of ventricular arrhythmias and sudden cardiac death (SCD) in the general population emphasizing how electrophysiologic changes in the setting of chronic hemodynamic overload can adversely influence these deleterious events.

CLINICAL IMPACT OF VENTRICULAR ARRHYTHMIAS AND SUDDEN CARDIAC DEATH

SCD is responsible for 300,000 to 400,000 victims per year in the United States.[1] In the Maastricht area in The Netherlands, with 182,000 inhabitants, the yearly incidence of out-of-hospital sudden cardiac arrest (death rate, 93%) at the age of 20 to 75 years is approximately 1 per 1000 people.[2] More than 90% of these fatalities occur in patients with coronary artery disease or cardiomyopathies. In the remaining 5% to 10%, no evidence of structural heart disease can be found.

Ventricular arrhythmias are the most frequent cause of sudden death. Often, they are the first manifestation of cardiovascular disease. In a study of patients with sudden arrhythmic death (documented on an ambulatory electrocardiographic [ECG] recorder), ventricular tachyarrhythmias were the terminal event in 83% of the cases, whereas bradyarrhythmias occurred in 17%.[3] Three forms of tachyarrhythmia were distinguished: (1) primary ventricular fibrillation (10% of the 83%); (2) monomorphic ventricular tachycardia or flutter precipitating ventricular fibrillation (75%); and (3) polymorphic ventricular tachycardia, including torsades de pointes (15%).[3] An example of the latter, from our own registry, is shown in Figure 28–1. Fortunately, most often ventricular arrhythmias have less detrimental consequences.

Patients with chronic pathologic overload of the heart (e.g., caused by hypertension, valvular disease, chronic ischemia, and infarction) are at increased risk for fatal arrhythmias[4,5] and prone to develop overt heart failure.[6,7] There is an increase in the frequency and complexity of ventricular ectopy with the progression of heart failure.[8] Total mortality correlates with left ventricular (LV) function and the presence of complex ventricular ectopy.[9] However, a clear correlation between SCD and LV contractile function or ventricular ectopy has not been found. In fact, data from the Vasodilator Heart Failure Trial (Val-HeFT) Study[10] and the Metoprolol Randomised Intervention Trial in Congestive Heart Failure (MERIT-HF) Trial[11] suggest that death is disproportionately sudden in patients with more modest myocardial dysfunction.

Figure 28–1 shows an example of sudden arrhythmic death in a patient with compensated ventricular hypertrophy. The recordings are from an 81-year-old woman with a long-term history of severe aortic stenosis, moderate aortic incompetence, and hypertension leading to concentric LV hypertrophy. Aortic valve replacement was strongly recommended but was refused by the patient. Her last medication comprised enalapril, furosemide, carbamazepine, and venlafaxine. She had been in a vital condition with no clinical signs of circulatory decompensation and a normal ejection fraction of 63% just days before the fatal event.

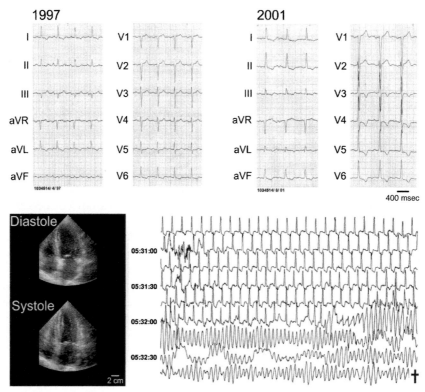

■ **Figure 28–1** Sudden arrhythmic death in a patient with compensated ventricular hypertrophy. *Top,* Twelve-lead electrocardiograms (ECG) in 1997 and 2001 (weeks before death), showing sinus rhythm with normal QT intervals. From 1997 to 2001, the electrical axis changed from horizontal to intermediate, whereas high voltages in the precordial leads and a strain pattern of the ST-T segments developed, compatible with significant hypertrophy. *Bottom left,* Echocardiogram recorded a few days before the fatal event. Cardiac contractile performance was overall good. *Bottom right,* Ambulatory ECG showing the sudden onset of polymorphic ventricular tachycardia degenerating into ventricular fibrillation at 05:32 AM. *(Courtesy of Joep L.R.M. Smeets, MD, PhD, Department of Cardiology, Academic Hospital Maastricht, Netherlands.)*

Pathologic ventricular hypertrophy has long been recognized as an independent risk factor for SCD.[4,6] However, the mechanisms of proarrhythmia in conditions with chronic hemodynamic overload are complex. Even in patients with the same pathology, different mechanisms of tachyarrhythmia prevail. In our patient, the presence of a myocardial substrate with electrical and structural alterations (e.g., fibrosis) must be assumed (based on the recordings shown and literature data). The generation of ventricular ectopic beats, triggering the tachycardia, indicated an arrhythmogenic milieu that was possibly influenced by myocardial ischemia, autonomic dysbalance, local conduction disturbances, and/or the side effects of venlafaxine (with a known proarrhythmic risk; for more

information, see the University of Arizona Health Sciences Center Web site at: www.torsades.org) and furosemide (with a risk for hypokalemia). This case exemplifies the importance of a substrate and triggers for the occurrence of polymorphic ventricular tachycardia in hypertrophy.

ELECTRICAL REMODELING IN CHRONIC CARDIAC OVERLOAD

General Remarks

The poor understanding of arrhythmias in cardiac hypertrophy and failure has instigated numerous studies, both experimental and clinical. A common finding is the presence of structural and electrical reconstitution of the overloaded myocardium. Many of the molecular safeguards of electrical stability undergo functional or expressional alterations, or both, often by genetic reprogramming. Collectively, these alterations are termed *electrical remodeling.*

Electrical remodeling is a key characteristic of normal development, expressing functional adaptation to increasing hemodynamic demands during cardiac growth (e.g., see Reference 12). In congenital and acquired heart disease, when hemodynamic load exceeds physiologic limits, the plasticity of the (mal)adaptive response systems determining electrical stability is challenged. The growing list of molecules affected in such conditions comprises ion channels and transporters, components of the Ca^{2+}-handling machinery, and structural proteins of the myocytes and interstitium.[13] Importantly, their alterations may already be significant in an early stage of overload, when contractility is still adequate to maintain cardiac output at (near-)normal levels. This might explain, at least in part, why a relatively high proportion of patients with compensated or mildly decompensated myocardial function is susceptible to arrhythmias and SCD.

A hallmark of electrical remodeling in hypertrophy and failure, independent of the cause, is prolongation of the ventricular action potential (for excellent reviews, refer to Tomaselli and coworkers[5,13]). For the human heart, action potential prolongation occurs both in compensated hypertrophy[14] and in terminal heart failure.[15,16] In the three-dimensional structure of the heart, regional differences in action potential duration (across the ventricular wall, between the ventricles, and from base to apex) may exaggerate during hypertrophy[17,18] and failure,[19,20] and predispose to ventricular arrhythmias. Conversely, a *reduction* in electrophysiologic gradients may also be proarrhythmic (see Chapter 22). Changes in repolarization may present as perturbations of the normal epicardial to endocardial direction of recovery from electrical activation, which can turn arrhythmogenic.[21] QT-interval labilities in patients with ischemic and nonischemic dilated cardiomyopathy,[22] and other disorders with hypertrophy or failure, are another indication that the substrate for arrhythmias is related, at least in part, to impaired repolarization. Importantly, the presence of

severe repolarization abnormalities can be hidden under a "normal" action potential morphology and duration, or a "normal" QT interval in the surface ECG. In such conditions, a modest challenge of electrical stability can evoke profound proarrhythmic responses.

Repolarization lability in cardiac hypertrophy and failure is commonly based on K^+-channel down-regulation[23,24] and altered Ca^{2+} homeostasis.[25] These changes may have a gene-transcriptional basis,[26,27] although some reports indicate the additional importance of post-transcriptional alterations.[28] Information about the exact time course of electrical changes and underlying molecular mechanisms is scarce. Also, the identity of mechanical or biochemical stimuli that trigger electrical remodeling is largely unknown.

Proarrhythmia in Compensated Ventricular Hypertrophy: The Dog Model with Chronic Complete Atrioventricular Block

A dog model of volume overload caused by complete atrioventricular block (AVB) has been extensively studied. Important electrical, contractile, and structural alterations of the myocardium are found in this model.[18,29] Myocardial adaptation is associated with an enhanced susceptibility to torsades de pointes[18,29] and SCD. Most dogs exhibit compensated contractile function in the chronic stage of AVB (CAVB). Figure 28–2 illustrates the key features of this model as currently known. In vivo electrophysiologic recordings reveal significant QT prolongation with broad-based T waves in CAVB. Monophasic action potential recordings from the endocardium indicate that repolarization prolongation is more prominent in the LV than the right ventricle (RV), leading to exaggerated interventricular dispersion of repolarization. Torsades de pointes occur often spontaneously or can be readily induced by programmed electrical stimulation, repolarization-prolonging drugs, or both, which makes this animal model suitable for chronic studies of proarrhythmia.

At the cellular level, significant down-regulation of the K^+ currents I_{Ks} and I_{Kr},[24] in combination with enhanced Na^+-Ca^{2+} exchange,[31] contribute to the alteration of spatial and temporal action potential hetero-

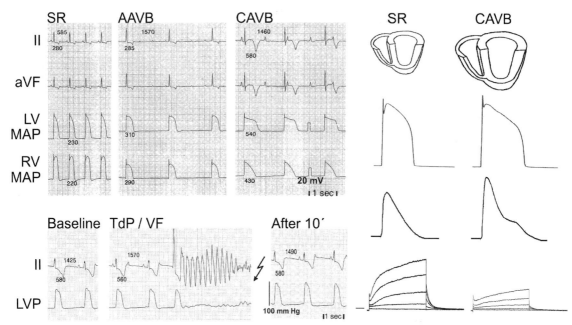

■ **Figure 28–2** Dog model with chronic atrioventricular block (CAVB). *Top left,* Acquired QT prolongation. ECG leads II and aVF and simultaneous monophasic action potential recordings from the endocardium of the left (LV MAP) and right ventricle (RV MAP). *Bottom left,* Spontaneous torsades de pointes (TdP) deteriorating into ventricular fibrillation (VF) with hemodynamic collapse. ECG lead II and LV pressure (LVP) recordings during anesthesia. After successful defibrillation, electrical and hemodynamic stability was regained within minutes. *Right,* Cellular basis of proarrhythmia in dilative ventricular hypertrophy after CAVB. Transmembrane action potential prolongation and enhanced Ca^{2+} release from the sarcoplasmic reticulum (*second* and *third row* from the top, respectively) are typical features. Enhanced Na^+-Ca^{2+}-exchange activity and down-regulation of the delayed-rectifier K^+ current I_{Ks} *(bottom traces)* contribute to action potential prolongation. SR, sinus rhythm; AAVB, Acute atrioventricular block. *(Top left, Reproduced from Volders PGA, Sipido KR, Vos MA, et al: Downregulation of delayed rectifier K^+ currents in dogs with chronic complete atrioventricular block and acquired torsades de pointes. Circulation 100:2455–2461, 1999, by permission of the American Heart Association; bottom left, acknowledgment to Jet D. M. Beekman, Department of Medical Physiology, University Medical Center Utrecht, Netherlands.)*

geneities. In addition, enhanced sarcoplasmic reticulum Ca^{2+} release[31] and an increased Na^+ concentration,[32] together with enhanced Na^+-Ca^{2+} exchange, can cause Ca^{2+}-dependent abnormal impulse formation.[33]

Regarding the K^+ channel down-regulation, important information comes from a recent study of *KCNQ1* and *KCNE1,* the genes encoding for the α and β subunit of the I_{Ks} channel.[27] Results are shown in Figure 28–3. In CAVB, KCNQ1 complementary DNA (cDNA; reverse-transcribed from messenger RNA) decreases by 80% and 90% in the LV and RV, respectively. KCNE1 cDNA diminishes by 70% and 75%. KCNQ1 protein expression in CAVB is decreased by 60% and 45% in the LV and RV, whereas the expression of KCNE1 decreases by 60% and 70%, respectively. The earlier finding of a 50% (LV) and

55% (RV) reduction in I_{Ks} density[24] is in good agreement with this molecular data. Taken together, these findings (and additional results not described here[27]) indicate that the decrease of I_{Ks} involves the regulation of *KCNQ1* and *KCNE1* gene expression at the transcriptional and translational levels.

MISSING LINKS BETWEEN CHRONIC MECHANICAL OVERLOAD AND ELECTRICAL REMODELING

In the previous section, we described the molecular down-regulation of KCNQ1 and KCNE1 proteins that coassemble to form the I_{Ks} channel. For all

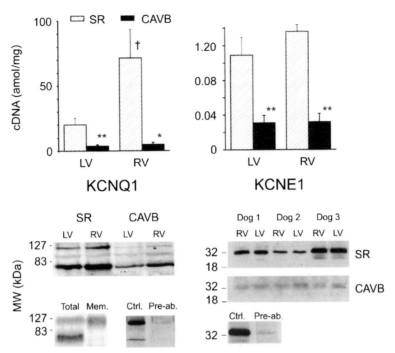

■ **Figure 28–3** Reduction of I_{Ks} in chronic atrioventricular block (CAVB) is caused by down-regulation of KCNQ1 and KCNE1 mRNA and protein expression. *Top,* Competitive multiplex reverse transcription polymerase chain reaction (PCR) showed CAVB-induced reduction of KCNQ1 and KCNE1 complementary DNA (messenger RNA). *Middle left,* Western blot of myocardial proteins from left ventricle (LV) and right ventricle (RV) of a sinus rhythm (SR) and CAVB dog. Probing with KCNQ1 polyclonal antibody identified two bands with molecular weights (MW) of ~72 and ~120 kDa at SR. *Bottom left,* Experiments repeated on total proteins (Total) and membrane proteins (Mem.) isolated from LV cardiac myocytes at SR. Both 72- and 120-kDa bands were recognized in the total protein preparation, but only the 120-kDa band was predominant in proteins isolated from the membrane fraction. At the right, to verify that both bands were linked to KCNQ1, immunoblots were performed using preabsorbed (Pre-ab.) KCNQ1 antibodies. *Middle right,* Western blot of proteins extracted from the LV and RV of SR and CAVB dogs (Dogs 1 to 3) and probed with KCNE1 polyclonal antibody. The KCNE1 antibody recognized a band ~35 kDa and a faint band ~20 kDa in SR. In both blots (left and right), densitometric analysis revealed significant down-regulation of KCNQ1 and KCNE1 proteins during CAVB in both ventricles. *Bottom right,* Control Western blots using proteins probed with anti-KCNE1 antibodies (Ctrl.) or with antibodies preabsorbed against the KCNE1 antigen (Pre-ab.), showing that the 35-kDa antigen contained the KCNE1-specific epitope. $^*P < 0.05$; $^{**}P < 0.01$ (SR vs. CAVB); $^\dagger P < 0.05$ (RV vs. LV). *(Modified from Ramakers C, Vos MA, Doevendans PA, et al: Coordinated down-regulation of KCNQ1 and KCNE1 expression contributes to reduction of I_{Ks} in canine hypertrophied hearts. Cardiovasc Res 57:486–496, 2003, with permission.)*

acquired channelopathies currently known to us, the primary stimuli for down-regulation are unknown. However, mechanical stimuli are obvious candidates.

Recently, we have quantified mechanical overload in the dog model with AVB and found that diastolic stress, diastolic strain (i.e., stretch), systolic strain, and stroke work are all significantly increased at the myocardial level.[34] The imposition of bradycardia-induced volume overload is followed by the development of ventricular hypertrophy and QT prolongation. Whether and how any (or all) of the mechanical changes could influence

I_{Ks} channel expression through transcriptional or translational regulation, or both (or other molecular mechanisms), is an intriguing question.

In contemporary working models of mechano-sensing and -transduction by the cardiac myocyte, a major role is attributed to a protein complex of integrin β_{1D}/talin/melusin at the sarcolemma/Z-disc, whose importance in pressure overload has been demonstrated.[35] In addition, some cardiac mechanical stretch sensor machinery incorporates a protein complex of titin, muscle LIM protein (MLP), and telethonin

(T-cap) interacting at the Z-disc (Fig. 28–4*A*).[36] Defects in the MLP/T-cap complex lead to dilative cardiomyopathy in MLP$^{-/-}$ transgenic mice and a subset of human dilative cardiomyopathy.[36] Furukawa and colleagues[37] have described that the extreme C-terminal region of T-cap binds to the cytoplasmic domain of KCNE1 (=minK; see Fig. 28–4*B*). It is attractive to speculate that this molecular chain of titin/MLP/T-cap/KCNE1 serves as conduit for mechano-electric remodeling. Whether and how the findings of gene-transcriptional and translational alterations[27] fit into this hypothetical scheme remains to be determined.

Mechanical influences could also alter transcriptional activity through the intermediate filament protein desmin. Bloom and colleagues[38] have shown that changes in the spatial arrangement of both the desmin–lamin intermediate filament network and the nuclear envelope–associated chromatin can be induced by mechanical stretch. We have recently found that desmin expression decreases early after the induction of AVB in dogs,[39] parallel to I_{Ks} down-regulation, which could also indicate a mechano-electric link.

More research is needed to answer these important questions of mechano-electric coupling during chronic overload.

REVERSIBILITY OF ELECTRICAL REMODELING BY MECHANICAL UNLOADING?

New insights in the role of mechanical overload derive from studies of cardiac unloading. Different strategies have been successfully proven to decrease LV hypertrophy and improve cardiac contractility after relief from chronically increased mechanical load.[40] Thus, contractile remodeling is potentially reversible, which could also apply to electrical remodeling. Patients treated for hypertension with enalapril[41] and losartan[42] exhibited decreased rate-corrected QT intervals. Several experimental studies showed related findings.[43,44] It is conceivable that the treatment with drugs affects signaling cascades independent of a reduction of mechanical load. However, pure mechanical unloading can also lead to a normalization of altered electrical properties.[45,46] This underscores the importance of mechano-transduction for the reversal of elec-

trical remodeling during unloading, even after months and years of overload.

In contrast, other studies have reported that reverse electrical remodeling is absent during drug treatment,[47] surgical intervention,[48] or ventricular pacing (in CAVB).[49] These issues clearly are not settled (see Chapters 34 to 37). Further investigations are warranted.

ELECTRO-MECHANICAL REMODELING

It can be concluded from the previous sections that chronic mechanical overload might well instigate and modulate electrical remodeling, and vice versa, that altered electrical properties of hypertrophied cardiac myocytes can also influence contraction, and thereby myocardial mechanics.

In rodents, action potential prolongation may set the stage for increased Ca^{2+} transients,[50] thus enhancing contraction and systolic mechanical load. Sah and colleagues[51] have shown that membrane repolarization by the transient outward current, I_{to}, modulates the recruitment and synchronization of sarcoplasmic reticulum Ca^{2+} release through the L-type Ca^{2+} current. Interestingly, the same group demonstrated in quiescent neonatal rat ventricular myocytes that a reduction of Kv4.2/3 (responsible for I_{to}) is followed by hypertrophy, with a proposed causal role for Ca^{2+}-dependent activation of calcineurin.[52] Although the causality has been questioned,[53] these data suggest that the relation between altered electrical properties and cellular hypertrophy may not always incorporate mechanical stimuli.

Based on studies with the Ca^{2+} indicators aequorin[54] and Indo-1,[55] Ca^{2+}-dependent diastolic dysfunction may also directly influence diastolic mechanics.

In the canine model with CAVB, yet another mechanism of electro-mechanical remodeling applies. Action potential prolongation and altered cellular Ca^{2+} and Na^{+} handling contribute to enhanced contractile performance, but also to proarrhythmia.[31] Systolic strain, representing myofiber deformation during contraction, was significantly increased in AVB, in addition to a greater diastolic mechanical load.[34] This can be interpreted as a direct mechanical consequence of the described electrical alterations.

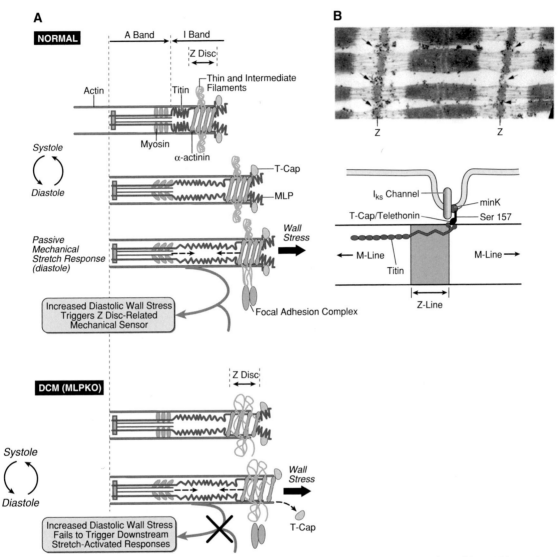

■ **Figure 28–4** *A,* Proposed working model of the cardiac stretch sensor machinery. *Top,* Normal conditions. Titin, anchored between Z-disc and M-line, exhibits elastic "molecular springs" (I band). Titin is able to store force generated by systolic compression (systole), and it largely determines passive myocardial stiffness (diastole). With increasing diastolic wall stress, the titin/MLP/telethonin (T-cap) complex is stretched and mechanical load is sensed. *Bottom,* Loss of the MLP/T-cap complex in knockout mice (MLPKO) causes a defective stretch-sensor function, ultimately leading to dilative cardiomyopathy (DCM), which, in turn, enhances wall stress and mechanical stretch stimuli. *B,* Model for the titin/T-cap/minK complex in cardiac myocytes. *Top,* Detection of T-cap by immunoelectron microscopy in skeletal muscle. T-cap is clustered where membrane structures corresponding to T-tubules and terminal cisternae contact the Z-line periphery *(arrows). Bottom,* Summary of known interactions of titin, T-cap, and minK (=KCNE1). T-cap connects the myofibrillar apparatus to the sarcolemma at the Z-line periphery. Phosphorylation of the C-terminal tail of the T-cap by yet unidentified kinases may regulate the stability of the complex. (See color insert.) *(A, Reproduced from Knöll R, Hoshijima M, Hoffman HM, et al: The cardiac mechanical stretch sensor machinery involves a Z disc complex that is defective in a subset of human dilated cardiomyopathy. Cell 111:943–955, 2002, with permission; B, reproduced from Furukawa T, Ono Y, Tsuchiya H, et al: Specific interaction of the potassium channel β-subunit minK with the sarcomeric protein T-cap suggests a T-tubule-myofibril linking system. J Mol Biol 313:775–784, 2001, with permission.)*

Taken together, the available data suggest that *chronic* mechano-electric feedback forms a closed-loop system with electro-mechanical remodeling, which was presented in detail in the introductory chapters of this book (see Preface).

NEED FOR SERIAL IN VIVO ASSESSMENT OF MYOCARDIAL MECHANICS DURING CHRONIC OVERLOAD

Quantification of the mechanical load imposed on the myocardium during chronic overload could offer mechanistic insights and improve clinical decision making. Recent techniques of tagged magnetic reso-

nance imaging[56] and ultrasound strain-rate imaging[57] may provide this information.

We have developed an alternative method to quantify myocardial mechanics, combining transthoracic echocardiography, invasive LV pressure recordings, and mathematical modeling (Fig. 28–5).[34,58] This method is feasible in anesthetized experimental animals and also in patients. Myofiber stress (σ_f; kPa) is defined as mechanical force per myofiber cross-sectional area and is calculated as:

$$\sigma_f = LVP\left(1 + 3V_{LV}/V_W\right)$$

with V_{LV} and V_W representing LV cavity and wall volume. Natural myofiber strain (e_f; dimensionless), representing deformation, is defined as the natural logarithm of myofiber length (l) relative to its reference

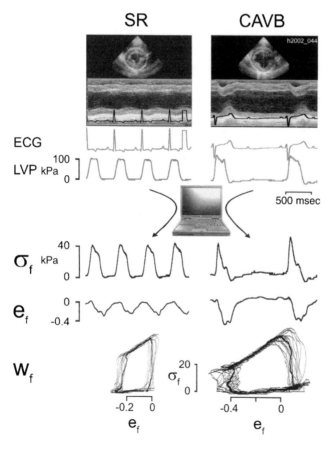

■ **Figure 28–5** Serial quantification of myofiber mechanics throughout the cardiac cycle during chronic ventricular overload. Anesthetized dogs, before (sinus rhythm [SR]) and in chronic atrioventricular block (CAVB; 6 weeks). *Top to bottom,* Echographic M-mode (left ventricular [LV] mid-papillary plane). Endocardial and epicardial borders were delineated to calculate LV cavity and wall volume, incorporating longitudinal axes. LV dimensions during the cardiac cycle were electrocardiogram (ECG)-synchronized with LV pressure (LVP). Note time marker on ECG tracing in SR. A validated mathematical model[58] was used to calculate myofiber stress (σ_f), natural myofiber strain (e_f; dimensionless), and myofiber stroke work (w_f) represented by the area of the σ_f-e_f loop. Note that a negative e_f during systole indicates myofiber shortening. A positive e_f during diastole designates outward deformation; both occur during CAVB.

length (l_{ref}) at beginning of ejection during sinus rhythm:

$$e_f = \ln\left(\frac{1}{l_{ref}}\right) = \frac{1}{3}\ln\left(\frac{\frac{1}{3}V_W + V_{LV}}{\frac{1}{3}V_{W,ref} + V_{LV,ref}}\right)$$

Myofiber stroke work (w_f; kJ/m³/beat) is computed as the area of the σ_f-e_f loop, a local analog of the LV pressure–volume loop:

$$w_f = \oint_{cycle} \sigma_f\, de_f$$

Our approach allows serial mechanical phenotyping during long-term cardiac overload to: (1) characterize the nature and timing of mechanical stimuli throughout the cardiac cycle (see Fig. 28–5); (2) discern the effects of mechanical versus other stimuli of remodeling; (3) define the transition from a functionally compensated to a decompensated state; and (4) evaluate the effects of medical and surgical interventions influencing cardiac overload.

Widespread experimental and clinical application of the aforementioned techniques is awaited and may help to characterize serial mechanical phenotypes in chronic heart disease and their link to electrical and structural remodeling.

CONCLUSIONS

Mechanical load is chronically increased in common cardiac diseases such as hypertension, valvular heart disease, and myocardial infarction. Ventricular hypertrophy often ensues as an adaptational response, but it is associated with significant morbidity and mortality. Electrical remodeling, notably impaired ventricular repolarization, can pose significant problems. It can manifest as prolongation of the ventricular action potential, but it may also be hidden under a "normal" action potential morphology and duration. The underlying alterations of K$^+$ current expression and Ca^{2+} handling often are based on changes of genetic transcription or post-transcriptional modification.

Currently, the role of pathologic mechanical load to the molecular mechanisms initiating and maintaining electrical remodeling is not understood. Recent findings indicate that myofiber stress or strain, or both, are primary mechanical stimuli sensed by the myocytes through protein complexes of integrin β_{1D}/talin/melusin at the sarcolemma/Z-disc and/or titin/MLP/T-cap at the Z-disc. A physical connection between the titin/T-cap complex and the β subunit of the I_{Ks} channel, KCNE1, has been demonstrated and might be involved in the transduction of mechanical overload to K$^+$ channel down-regulation. The translation of these elementary findings to mechano-transduction in the intact heart of humans and animal models requires detailed knowledge of the characteristics of myocardial mechanics during chronic overload. In the dog model with CAVB, increased diastolic stress, diastolic strain, systolic strain, and stroke work are associated with transcriptional changes of the I_{Ks} channel subunits KCNQ1 and KCNE1. A causal role for the mechanical stimuli is speculative and should be investigated at the molecular-genetic level.

The available data on cardiac electrophysiology and mechanics in *chronic* overload convince us that, as in acute studies, electro-mechanical signaling forms a closed-loop system with mechano-electric feedback. Our new approach of calculating mechanics in the intact beating heart may prove useful for understanding how mechano-transduction may lead to remodeling.

Acknowledgments

Dr. Volders is supported by The Netherlands Organization for Health Research and Development (ZonMw 906-02-068). The authors are grateful to Theo Arts, PhD (Departments of Biophysics, Cardiovascular Research Institute Maastricht and Biomedical Engineering, Eindhoven University of Technology, Netherlands) for his excellent scientific contribution. Roel L.H.M.G. Spätjens, BS (Department of Cardiology, Cardiovascular Research Institute Maastricht) prepared the figures.

References

1. Zipes DP, Wellens HJJ: Sudden cardiac death. Circulation 98:2334–2351, 1998.
2. de Vreede-Swagemakers JJM, Gorgels APM, Dubois-Arbouw WI, et al: Out-of-hospital cardiac arrest in the 1990's: A population-based study in the Maastricht area on incidence, characteristics and survival. J Am Coll Cardiol 30:1500–1505, 1997.

3. Bayés de Luna A, Coumel P, Leclercq JF: Ambulatory sudden cardiac death: Mechanisms of production of fatal arrhythmia on the basis of data from 157 cases. Am Heart J 117:151–159, 1989.

4. Haider AW, Larson MG, Benjamin EJ, et al: Increased left ventricular mass and hypertrophy are associated with increased risk for sudden death. J Am Coll Cardiol 32:1454–1459, 1998.

5. Tomaselli GF, Marbán E: Electrophysiological remodeling in hypertrophy and heart failure. Cardiovasc Res 42:270–283, 1999.

6. Kannel WB, Gordon T, Offutt D: Left ventricular hypertrophy by electrocardiogram. Prevalence, incidence, and mortality in the Framingham study. Ann Intern Med 71:89–105, 1969.

7. Rame JE, Ramilo M, Spencer N, et al: Development of a depressed left ventricular ejection fraction in patients with left ventricular hypertrophy and a normal ejection fraction. Am J Cardiol 93:234–237, 2004.

8. Kjekshus J: Arrhythmias and mortality in congestive heart failure. Am J Cardiol 65:42I–48I, 1990.

9. Wilson JR, Schwartz JS, Sutton MS, et al: Prognosis in severe heart failure: Relation to hemodynamic measurements and ventricular ectopic activity. J Am Coll Cardiol 2:403–410, 1983.

10. Cohn JN, Archibald DG, Ziesche S, et al: Effect of vasodilator therapy on mortality in chronic congestive heart failure. Results of a Veterans Administration Cooperative Study. N Engl J Med 314:1547–1552, 1986.

11. Effect of metoprolol CR/XL in chronic heart failure: Metoprolol CR/XL Randomised Intervention Trial in Congestive Heart Failure (MERIT-HF). Lancet 353:2001–2007, 1999.

12. Jeck CD, Boyden PA: Age-related appearance of outward currents may contribute to developmental differences in ventricular repolarization. Circ Res 71:1390–1403, 1992.

13. Armoundas AA, Wu R, Juang G, et al: Electrical and structural remodeling of the failing ventricle. Pharmacol Ther 92:213–230, 2001.

14. Bailly P, Bénitah JP, Mouchonière M, et al: Regional alteration of the transient outward current in human left ventricular septum during compensated hypertrophy. Circulation 96:1266–1274, 1997.

15. Beuckelmann DJ, Näbauer M, Erdmann E: Alterations of K+ currents in isolated human ventricular myocytes from patients with terminal heart failure. Circ Res 73:379–385, 1993.

16. Vermeulen JT, McGuire MA, Opthof T, et al: Triggered activity and automaticity in ventricular trabeculae of failing human and rabbit hearts. Cardiovasc Res 28:1547–1554, 1994.

17. Keung ECH, Aronson RS: Non-uniform electrophysiological properties and electrotonic interaction in hypertrophied rat myocardium. Circ Res 49:150–158, 1981.

18. Volders PGA, Sipido KR, Vos MA, et al: Cellular basis of biventricular hypertrophy and arrhythmogenesis in dogs with chronic complete atrioventricular block and acquired torsades de pointes. Circulation 98:1136–1147, 1998.

19. Näbauer M, Beuckelmann DJ, Überfuhr P, et al. Regional differences in current density and rate-dependent properties of the transient outward current in subepicardial and subendocardial myocytes of human left ventricle. Circulation 93:168–177, 1996.

20. Akar FG, Rosenbaum DS: Transmural electrophysiological heterogeneities underlying arrhythmogenesis in heart failure. Circ Res 93:638–645, 2003.

21. Fish JM, Di Diego JM, Nesterenko V, et al: Epicardial activation of left ventricular wall prolongs QT interval and transmural dispersion of repolarization: Implications for biventricular pacing. Circulation 109:2136–2142, 2004.

22. Berger RD, Kasper EK, Baughman KL, et al: Beat-to-beat QT interval variability: Novel evidence for repolarization lability in ischemic and nonischemic dilated cardiomyopathy. Circulation 96:1557–1565, 1997.

23. Näbauer M, Kääb S: Potassium channel down-regulation in heart failure. Cardiovasc Res 37:324–334, 1998.

24. Volders PGA, Sipido KR, Vos MA, et al: Downregulation of delayed rectifier K+ currents in dogs with chronic complete atrioventricular block and acquired torsades de pointes. Circulation 100:2455–2461, 1999.

25. Sipido KR, Volders PGA, Vos MA, et al: Altered Na/Ca exchange activity in cardiac hypertrophy and heart failure: A new target for therapy? Cardiovasc Res 53:782–805, 2002.

26. Kääb S, Dixon J, Duc J, et al: Molecular basis of transient outward potassium current downregulation in human heart failure: A decrease in Kv4.3 mRNA correlates with a reduction in current density. Circulation 98:1383–1393, 1998.

27. Ramakers C, Vos MA, Doevendans PA, et al: Coordinated down-regulation of KCNQ1 and KCNE1 expression contributes to reduction of I_{Ks} in canine hypertrophied hearts. Cardiovasc Res 57:486–496, 2003.

28. Zicha S, Maltsev VA, Nattel S, et al: Post-transcriptional alterations in the expression of cardiac Na+ channel subunits in chronic heart failure. J Mol Cell Cardiol 37:91–100, 2004.

29. Vos MA, de Groot SHM, Verduyn SC, et al: Enhanced susceptibility for acquired torsade de pointes arrhythmias in the dog with chronic, complete AV block is related to cardiac hypertrophy and electrical remodeling. Circulation 98:1125–1135, 1998.

30. van Opstal JM, Verduyn SC, Leunissen HDM, et al: Electrophysiological parameters indicative of sudden cardiac death in the dog with chronic complete AV-block. Cardiovasc Res 50:354–361, 2001.

31. Sipido KR, Volders PGA, de Groot SHM, et al: Enhanced Ca^{2+} release and Na/Ca exchange activity in hypertrophied canine ventricular myocytes: Potential link between contractile adaptation and arrhythmogenesis. Circulation 102:2137–2144, 2000.

32. Verdonck F, Volders PGA, Vos MA, et al: Increased Na+ concentration and altered Na/K pump activity in hypertrophied canine ventricular cells. Cardiovasc Res 57:1035–1043, 2003.

33. Sipido KR, Volders PGA, Schoenmakers M, et al: Role of the Na/Ca exchanger in arrhythmias in compensated hypertrophy. Ann N Y Acad Sci 976:438–445, 2002.

34. Donker DW, Volders PGA, Borgers M, et al: Increases of systolic fiber strain and end-diastolic fiber stress are the primary local mechanical changes in chronic heart block [abstract]. Eur Heart J 25(suppl): 555, 2004.

35. Brancaccio M, Fratta L, Notte A, et al: Melusin, a muscle-specific integrin β$_1$-interacting protein, is required to prevent cardiac failure in response to chronic pressure overload. Nat Med 9:68–75, 2003.

36. Knöll R, Hoshijima M, Hoffman HM, et al: The cardiac mechanical stretch sensor machinery involves a Z disc complex that is defective in a subset of human dilated cardiomyopathy. Cell 111:943–955, 2002.

37. Furukawa T, Ono Y, Tsuchiya H, et al: Specific interaction of the potassium channel β-subunit minK with the sarcomeric protein T-cap suggests a T-tubule-myofibril linking system. J Mol Biol 313:775–784, 2001.

38. Bloom S, Lockard VG, Bloom M: Intermediate filament-mediated stretch-induced changes in chromatin: A hypothesis for growth initiation in cardiac myocytes. J Mol Cell Cardiol 28:2123–2127, 1996.

39. Donker DW, Volders PGA, Maessen JG, et al: Time frame of myocardial dedifferentiation in canine ventricular hypertrophy [abstract]. J Mol Cell Cardiol 34:A20, 2002.

40. Zafeiridis A, Jeevanandam V, Houser SR, et al: Regression of cellular hypertrophy after left ventricular assist device support. Circulation 98:656–662, 1998.

41. Gonzalez-Juanatey JR, Garcia-Acuna JM, Pose A, et al: Reduction of QT and QTc dispersion during long-term treatment of systemic hypertension with enalapril. Am J Cardiol 81:170–174, 1998.

42. Oikarinen L, Nieminen MS, Toivonen L, et al: Relation of QT interval and QT dispersion to regression of echocardiographic and electrocardiographic left ventricular hypertrophy in hypertensive patients: The Losartan Intervention For Endpoint Reduction (LIFE) study. Am Heart J 145:919–925, 2003.

43. Rials SJ, Wu Y, Xu X, et al: Regression of left ventricular hypertrophy with captopril restores normal ventricular action potential duration, dispersion of refractoriness, and vulnerability to inducible ventricular fibrillation. Circulation 96:1330–1336, 1997.

44. Cerbai E, De Paoli P, Sartiani L, et al: Treatment with irbesartan counteracts the functional remodeling of ventricular myocytes from hypertensive rats. J Cardiovasc Pharmacol 41:804–812, 2003.

45. Rials SJ, Wu Y, Ford N, et al: Effect of left ventricular hypertrophy and its regression on ventricular electrophysiology and vulnerability to inducible arrhythmia in the feline heart. Circulation 91:426–430, 1995.

46. Harding JD, Piacentino V 3rd, Gaughan JP, et al: Electrophysiological alterations after mechanical circulatory support in patients with advanced cardiac failure. Circulation 104:1241–1247, 2001.

47. Kreher P, Ristori MT, Corman B, et al: Effects of chronic angiotensin I-converting enzyme inhibition on the relations between ventricular action potential changes and myocardial hypertrophy in aging rats. J Cardiovasc Pharmacol 25:75–80, 1995.

48. Botchway AN, Turner MA, Sheridan DJ, et al: Electrophysiological effects accompanying regression of left ventricular hypertrophy. Cardiovasc Res 60:510–517, 2003.

49. Peschar M, Vernooy K, Vanagt WY, et al: Absence of reverse electrical remodeling during regression of volume overload hypertrophy in canine ventricles. Cardiovasc Res 58:510–517, 2003.

50. Wickenden AD, Kaprielian R, Kassiri Z, et al: The role of action potential prolongation and altered intracellular calcium handling in the pathogenesis of heart failure. Cardiovasc Res 37:312–323, 1998.

51. Sah R, Ramirez RJ, Backx PH: Modulation of Ca^{2+} release in cardiac myocytes by changes in repolarization rate: Role of phase-1 action potential repolarization in excitation-contraction coupling. Circ Res 90:165–173, 2002.

52. Kassiri Z, Zobel C, Nguyen T-TT, et al: Reduction of I_{to} causes hypertrophy in neonatal rat ventricular myocytes. Circ Res 90:578–585, 2002.

53. Sanguinetti MC: Reduced transient outward K^+ current and cardiac hypertrophy: Causal relationship or epiphenomenon? Circ Res 90:497–499, 2002.

54. Gwathmey JK, Morgan JP: Sarcoplasmic reticulum calcium mobilization in right ventricular pressure-overload hypertrophy in the ferret: Relationships to diastolic dysfunction and a negative treppe. Pflügers Arch 422:599–608, 1993.

55. Maier LS, Brandes R, Pieske B, et al: Effects of left ventricular hypertrophy on force and Ca^{2+} handling in isolated rat myocardium. Am J Physiol 274:H1361–H1370, 1998.

56. Hu Z, Metaxas D, Axel L: In vivo strain and stress estimation of the heart left and right ventricles from MRI images. Med Image Anal 7:435–444, 2003.

57. Herbots L, Maes F, D'Hooge J, et al: Quantifying myocardial deformation throughout the cardiac cycle: a comparison of ultrasound strain rate, grey-scale M-mode and magnetic resonance imaging. Ultrasound Med Biol 30:591–598, 2004.

58. Arts T, Bovendeerd PH, Prinzen FW, et al: Relation between left ventricular cavity pressure and volume and systolic fiber stress and strain in the wall. Biophys J 59:93–102, 1991.

CHAPTER 29

Sudden Death Caused by Chest Wall Trauma (Commotio Cordis)

• • • •

Mark S. Link, N. A. Mark Estes III, and Barry J. Maron

Although sudden deaths of athletes are rare, it has become apparent that a significant percentage of deaths on the athletic field are caused by chest wall blows with a projectile or body part (commotio cordis). This phenomenon has been most frequently observed in young athletes (4 to 18 years old) and may be significantly under-reported. Cardiac workups and autopsies are notable for the lack of any significant cardiac or thoracic abnormalities. Victims are most often found in ventricular fibrillation; resuscitation is possible with early defibrillation.

The incidence of this event has been estimated to be less than 5 deaths per annum in youth baseball,[1-3] but under-reporting and misclassification of deaths surely occur; therefore, the true number of deaths caused by relatively mild chest wall impacts is undoubtedly much greater. Indeed, up to 20% of deaths on the athletic field are caused by chest wall impact.[4] The Commotio Cordis Registry (directed by B.J.M. at the Minneapolis Heart Institute), in its 7-year existence, has documented 156 cases of commotio cordis[3] and is accruing 5 to 15 cases per year (Fig. 29–1). Sudden deaths initially thought to be idiopathic ventricular fibrillation are now more properly classified as commotio cordis.[5,6]

TWO ILLUSTRATIVE CASE REPORTS

A healthy 14-year-old boy was playing touch football with his friends when he was inadvertently struck in the chest by a knee.[7] He immediately described dizziness, and then he collapsed. Cardiopulmonary resuscitation was started; when emergency services arrived 6 min later, he was found in ventricular fibrillation and promptly defibrillated. Ultimately, he recovered completely.

Another case with a less fortunate ending was of a 14-year-old boy competing in a karate match.[4] He was struck in the chest with a hand and collapsed. Resuscitation also was started immediately; he also was found in ventricular fibrillation. Unfortunately, he could not be resuscitated, and he died.

INCIDENCE

In the 19th century, commotio cordis (or cardiac concussion) was defined as cardiac manifestations of chest trauma in individuals, regardless of whether the result was fatal and cardiac morphologic damage was present.[8,9] Early case reports included only adults with severe trauma such as stone throws to the chest or falls from heights.[10] In the 20th century, sudden death caused by low-energy chest wall trauma in sporting activities was reported, and the common understanding of the term *commotio cordis* has been narrowed to those events in which cardiac damage is not present.[1,7,11-20] In baseball, the sport in which the most cases have been documented, the first reported death caused by blunt chest impact was in 1978 and involved a 7-year-old boy struck in the chest by a baseball during a T-ball game.[11] In the 1980s and 1990s, case reports documented several other occurrences of sudden death caused by chest impact, not only in baseball,[14,17] but also in hockey,[18] lacrosse,[16] and softball,[12,13] as well as from fist and knee blows to the chest.[7,14] In addition, an increasing number of syncopal events secondary to chest wall impact (possibly aborted sudden deaths) have been described and are likely caused by nonsustained arrhythmic events.[3,10]

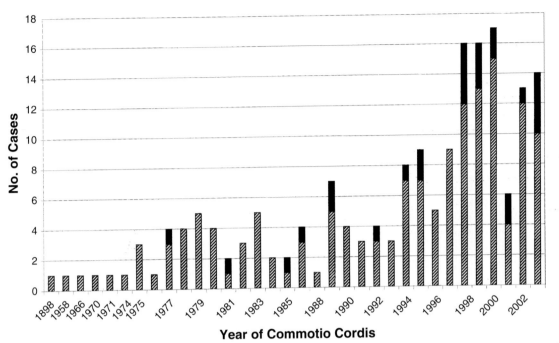

■ Figure 29–1 Number of cases referred to the Commotio Cordis Registry stratified by year of event. Deaths are recorded in *hatched bars*, and survivors are represented by *solid bars*. Note the increasing number of reported cases and increasing likelihood of survivors in more recent years, both of which are likely because of the increased awareness of this phenomenon.

Age and Sex

Commotio cordis, as the current clinical profile suggests, predominantly affects young individuals. In the Commotio Cordis Registry, the mean age is 14 years, with 80% either 18 years or younger (Fig. 29–2).[2,3] It is thought that young athletes are at particular risk because of their more pliable chest wall, which probably facilitates the transmission of chest impact energy to the myocardium. With age, the thoracic cage stiffens, and the chest wall absorbs more of the impact energy. The overwhelming majority of victims are male, and only 4% are female victims.[2,3]

Sporting Activities

Commotio cordis has most commonly been reported in baseball (n = 63), softball (n = 14), ice hockey (n = 14), football (n = 12), and lacrosse (n = 5).[3] In addition, cases occasionally have occurred in a variety of other sports including karate and cricket, as well as nonsports-related contact with a body part, usually a hand, foot, or elbow (Fig. 29–3).

In the Commotio Cordis Registry, competitive sporting activities account for about 60% of cases, whereas about 20% of cases were involved in recreational sports and another 20% in nonsporting activities.[3] Commotio cordis events unrelated to sports are generally caused by chest blows in activities such as playful boxing, as a remedy for hiccups, or child discipline. Fist and hand strikes currently account for 15 (10%) of the reported cases of commotio cordis, including 11 incidents that resulted in criminal prosecution.[21]

Impact Characteristics

In most commotio cordis victims, the impact object is a projectile of the game such as a baseball, hockey puck, or lacrosse ball (Fig. 29–4). However, more

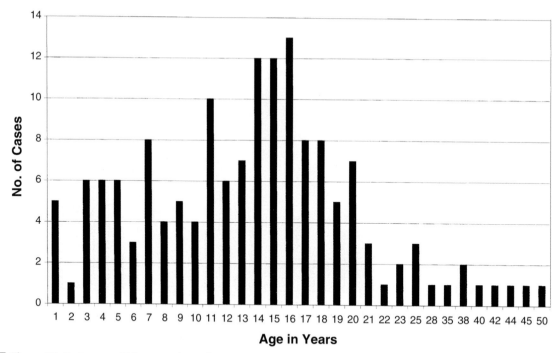

■ **Figure 29-2**   Ages at which commotio cordis events have been documented in the Commotio Cordis Registry. Mean age is 14 years, with 80% of individuals 18 years or younger.

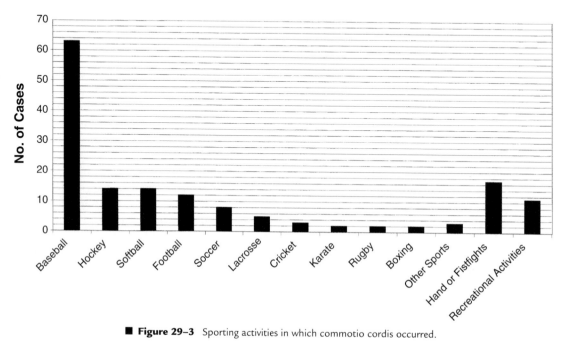

■ **Figure 29-3**   Sporting activities in which commotio cordis occurred.

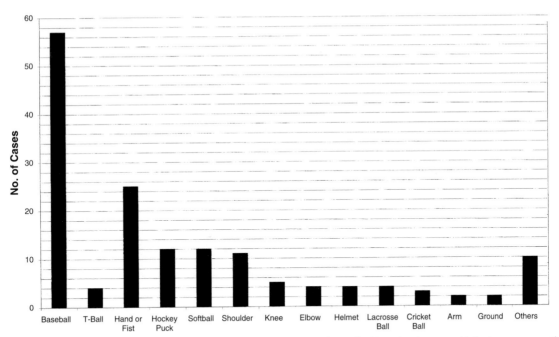

■ **Figure 29–4** Impact objects that have been reported to cause commotio cordis. Note that impacts with body parts currently account for 30% of commotio cordis cases.

recent data from the Commotio Cordis Registry demonstrates that softer projectiles (such as plastic hollow bats or soccer balls) and broader surface blows (by falls to ground, chest wall collision, and football helmets) can cause sudden death. Safety (or softer than standard) baseballs also have been implicated in 4 of the 63 commotio cordis events in baseball, suggesting that absolute protection is not yet possible.

Impact with body parts has accounted for up to 47 of the reported commotio cordis events, including those in sports such as soccer, football, and karate and in nonsporting altercations, disciplining, and play boxing. Varied body parts, including hands (n = 25), shoulders (n = 11), elbows (n = 4), and arms (n = 2) have been implicated. Impacts with air-filled balls including soccer (n = 1), football (n = 1), and tennis balls (n = 1) also have been reported.

Although it is difficult to quantitate the energy or force of chest blows in victims of commotio cordis, it appears that the velocity of the impact object is usually normal for the sport or activity involved. Most victims experienced a commotio cordis event while playing with their peers, not with older and stronger individuals. In youth baseball, the most common sport in which commotio cordis has been reported, a pitched baseball can reach 22 m/sec (50 mph).[22] In baseball, 62 of 63 events have been a result of baseball impact, including 35 fielders, 14 batters, 6 pitchers, and 6 catchers. None of the reported cases had chest wall or cardiac damage to explain death, in contrast to the cases of death reported in motor vehicular accidents in which myocardial contusion or severe cardiac and thoracic damage occur.[23]

In victims of commotio cordis, the chest blows strike the left chest, most directly over the cardiac silhouette. However, the exact location of the chest wall strike cannot always be determined with precision because a precordial bruise is evident at autopsy in only about one third of the cases.[1]

ARRHYTHMIAS AND SURVIVAL

Collapse after impact is immediate in half of the victims, whereas in the other half, it occurs after a brief period of consciousness often marked by extreme lightheadedness.[1] In the 74 cases from the Commotio Cordis Registry in which a postcollapse rhythm was documented, 48 had ventricular fibrillation (Fig. 29–5). After prolonged cardiopulmonary resuscitation, asystole is commonly found.[3] In the few survivors for whom a 12-lead electrocardiogram (ECG) was available, ECG showed marked ST-segment elevation, especially in the anterior leads, which resolved over time, without the development of Q waves or increase of myocardial enzymes.[7,24]

Although commotio cordis initially was reported to be almost invariably fatal, survival currently appears to approach 15%, including some cases with spontaneous resolution that are judged to be aborted events.[3] We believe that the greater likelihood of survival is related to at least two possible factors. The first factor is a reversal of a bias to report only fatal cases; we are becoming aware of many nonfatal cases, with either spontaneous or defibrillated recovery. However, the most important determinant of increased survival is likely the greater recognition of commotio cordis in the community, which probably translates into more timely cardiopulmonary resuscitation and defibrillation. Of 78 Commotio Cordis Registry events in which resuscitation was initiated within 3 minutes, 25% of victims survived, compared with only 8% in whom resuscitation was delayed (>3 minutes).

PREVENTION

Safety or softer than standard baseballs have been recommended by the U.S. Consumer Product Safety Commission to reduce the risk for injury in youth baseball.[26] However, safety baseballs also have been implicated in 4 of the 63 commotio cordis events in baseball. Given the epidemiologic[26,27] and experimental data[28,29] with safety baseballs, we believe that the preponderance of evidence supports their use to reduce risks.

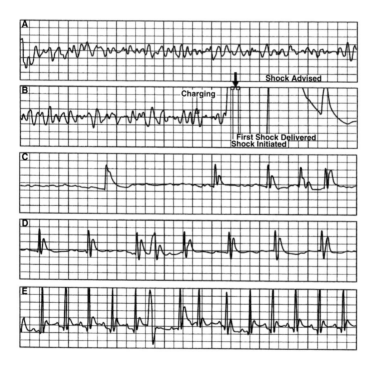

■ **Figure 29–5** Automated external defibrillator tracing documenting ventricular fibrillation and successful defibrillation in a 13-year-old male baseball player struck by a pitched ball. (*Reproduced from Strasburger JF, Maron BJ: Commotio cordis. N Engl J Med 347:1248, 2002, by permission of the Massachusetts Medical Society.*)

Standard, commercially available chest wall protection was worn by about 30% of the commotio cordis victims in organized sports.[1,3] Some chest wall barriers did not adequately cover the left chest wall and precordium; these included at least 8 of 14 hockey players in which chest protection was flawed or inadequate, with respect to the angulation of the shot or displacement of the protector and subsequent direct impact to the precordium when the arms were raised. In addition, five football players were wearing standard shoulder/chest pads that did not cover the precordium, and they experienced a direct hit to the critical area of the chest overlying the heart. However, in others (including three lacrosse goalies, two baseball catchers, and two hockey goalies), the chest wall protector covered the heart; the projectile struck the chest protector, and nonetheless triggered a commotio cordis event.

LEGAL IMPLICATIONS

Commotio cordis may have serious legal implications for the individual responsible for the blow, despite that often the blow occurred in the context of sport or was not intended to cause bodily harm.[21] In fact, one of the first cases of commotio reported in the sporting literature was of a hockey player who was charged with manslaughter when an opponent died after being hit in the chest by a stick.[30] In the Commotio Cordis Registry, there is evidence of seven criminal prosecutions after individuals, typically children, were struck in the chest by a hand or fist.[3,21]

Conclusions

Commotio cordis is an unusual, but devastating, event occurring primarily in young male individuals during sports-related or routine daily activities. Its prevalence is likely underestimated, and self-limited cases caused by nonsustained arrhythmias may be much more common than is believed. Projectiles are generally hard objects including body parts such as shoulder and hands. Sudden death is a result of ventricular fibrillation, and early defibrillation is critical for saving the lives of these young people.

References

1. Maron BJ, Poliac LC, Kaplan JA, Mueller FO: Blunt impact to the chest leading to sudden death from cardiac arrest during sports activities. N Engl J Med 333:337–342, 1995.
2. Maron BJ, Link MS, Wang PJ, Estes III NAM: Clinical profile of commotio cordis: An under-appreciated cause of sudden death in the young during sports and other activities. J Cardiovasc Electrophysiol 10:114–120, 1999.
3. Maron BJ, Gohman TE, Kyle SB, et al: Clinical profile and spectrum of commotio cordis. JAMA 287:1142–1146, 2002.
4. Maron BJ: Sudden death in young athletes. N Engl J Med 349:1064–1075, 2003.
5. Link MS: Commotio cordis, sudden death due to chest wall impact in sports. Heart 81:109–110, 1999.
6. Haq CL: Sudden death due to low-energy chest-wall impact (commotio cordis). N Engl J Med 339:1399, 1998.
7. Link MS, Ginsburg SH, Wang PJ, et al: Commotio cordis: Cardiovascular manifestations of a rare survivor. Chest 114:326–328, 1998.
8. Nélaton A: Elements de Pathologie Chirurgicale, 2nd ed. Paris, Librairie Germer Bateliere, 1876.
9. Meola F: La commozione toracica. Gior Internaz Sci Med 1:923–937, 1879.
10. Nesbitt AD, Cooper PJ, Kohl P: Rediscovering commotio cordis. Lancet 357:1195–1197, 2001.
11. Dickman GL, Hassan A, Luckstead EF: Ventricular fibrillation following baseball injury. Physician and Sports Medicine 6:85–86, 1978.
12. Froede RC, Lindsey D, Steinbronn K: Sudden unexpected death from cardiac concussion (commotio cordis) with unusual legal complications. J Forensic Sci 24:752–756, 1979.
13. Green ED, Simson LR, Kellerman HH, Horowitz RN: Cardiac concussion following softball blow to the chest. Ann Emerg Med 9:155–157, 1980.
14. Frazer M, Mirchandani H: Commotio cordis, revisited. Am J Forensic Med Pathol 5:249–251, 1984.
15. Rutherford GW, Kennedy J, McGhee L: Baseball and softball related injuries to children 5-14 years of age. Washington DC: United States Consumer Product Safety Commission, 1984.
16. Edlich RF, Mayer NE, Fariss BL, et al: Commotio cordis in a lacrosse goalie. J Emerg Med 5:181–184, 1987.
17. Abrunzo TJ: Commotio cordis, the single, most common cause of traumatic death in youth baseball. Am J Dis Child 145:1279–1282, 1991.
18. Kaplan JA, Karofsky PS, Volturo GA: Commotio cordis in two amateur ice hockey players despite the use of commercial chest protectors: Case reports. J Trauma 34:151–153, 1993.
19. Maron BJ, Strasburger JF, Kugler JD, et al: Survival following blunt chest impact induced cardiac arrest during sports activities in young athletes. Am J Cardiol 79:840–841, 1997.
20. Riedinger F, Kummell H: Die Verletzungen und Erkrankungen des Thorax und seines Inhaltes. In von Bergman E, von Bruns P (eds): Handbuch der Praktischen Chirurgie, 2nd ed. Stuttgart: Ferd. Enke, 1903, pp 373–456.
21. Maron BJ, Mitten MJ, Burnett CG: Criminal consequences of commotio cordis. Am J Cardiol 89:210–213, 2002.
22. Seefeldt VD, Brown EW, Wilson DJ, et al: Influence of low-compression versus traditional baseballs on injuries in youth

baseball. East Lansing, MI, Institute for the Study of Youth Sport, July 20, 1993.

23. Tenzer ML: The spectrum of myocardial contusion: A review. J Trauma 25:620–627, 1985.

24. Strasburger JF, Maron BJ: Commotio cordis. N Engl J Med 347:1248, 2002.

25. Deardorff J: Defibrillator crusade saves the day for boy. Chicago Tribune, June 15, 2001.

26. Kyle SB: Youth baseball protective equipment project final report. Washington, DC, United States Consumer Product Safety Commission, 1996.

27. Marshall SW, Mueller FO, Kirby DP, Yang J: Evaluation of safety balls and faceguards for prevention of injuries in youth baseball. JAMA 289:568–574, 2003.

28. Link MS, Wang PJ, Pandian NG, et al: An experimental model of sudden death due to low energy chest wall impact (commotio cordis). N Engl J Med 338:1805–1811, 1998.

29. Link MS, Maron BJ, Wang PJ, et al: Reduced risk of sudden death from chest wall blows (commotio cordis) with safety baseballs. Pediatrics 109:873–877, 2002.

30. Swift EM: A cruel blow; a seemingly harmless slash to the chest resulted in the death of a hockey player in Italy. Now, Jimmy Boni will go on trial for manslaughter. Sports Illustrated, Dec 6, 1993:66–79.

CHAPTER 30

Volume and Pressure Overload and Ventricular Arrhythmogenesis

Michael J. Reiter

• • • •

Ventricular dilation or stretch often is described as a cause of clinical ventricular arrhythmias without much explanation of the nature of the relation. Mechano-electric feedback (MEF), the subject of this textbook, is a potential mechanism for these effects and may be a contributor to ventricular arrhythmias in humans. This chapter considers the role volume and pressure overload might play in facilitating ventricular arrhythmias, elaborates on this hypothesis, and attempts to address three fundamental questions:

1. How do MEF effects observed in animals facilitate ventricular arrhythmias?
2. Do similar phenomena exist in humans?
3. Are these effects arrhythmogenic in humans?

The term MEF is sufficiently broad so as to encompass different phenomena. These vary not only in effect but also mechanistically, temporally, and in terms of their physiologic implications. Extensive discussion of these differences is not required here (see Chapters 1 through 7 for review), except to mention that they are primarily caused by manifestations of mechanosensitive ion channel activity.

The primary mechanical stimulus responsible for MEF remains unclear. Whether pressure or volume overload is the primary determinant of electrophysiologic change has been difficult to determine. Both may have important but different effects. This chapter does not attempt to resolve this distinction and considers pressure and volume overload interrelated.

WHAT MECHANO-ELECTRIC FEEDBACK EFFECTS ARE OBSERVED EXPERIMENTALLY?

The description of stretch effects on the electrophysiologic properties of isolated cells and tissue dates back more than 60 years. In 1943, Bozler[1] postulated a metabolic interaction between contraction and electrical activity based on observations in the turtle ventricle. Ten years later, Dudel and Trautwein[2] described stretch-induced depolarizations. In 1960, Stauch[3] noted a shortening of the QT interval when contraction in the frog ventricle was changed from isotonic to isometric. Subsequent studies in the isolated frog ventricle and isolated muscle preparations demonstrated that stretch could influence resting potential and action potential duration (APD) and was capable of inducing premature ventricular contractions, but these results were thought to be related to cell injury and not physiologically relevant.

The concept that stretch may play a pathophysiologic role is relatively recent and is based primarily on studies of ventricular dilation in isolated hearts and intact animal models. These observations make it clear that the effects of rapid, transient dilation are qualitatively different than those of sustained dilation.

Studies of in situ, cross-circulated,[4] or isolated canine hearts,[4-6] and isolated rabbit hearts[7] demonstrated diastolic depolarizations induced by transient ventricular dilation. Similar depolarizations (detected by optical recordings using voltage-sensitive dyes) can be induced in cultured monolayers of neonatal rat ventricular myocytes by mechanical stimuli using a fluid jet.[8] The magnitude of the stretch-induced depolarization depends on the quantity of the volume pulse, as well as its rapidity and timing.[5-7,9] The provoked depolarization may be of sufficient magnitude to trigger ectopy (Fig. 30–1), nonsustained arrhythmias, or (rarely) sustained arrhythmias and ventricular fibrillation (VF).[9]

Stretch-induced depolarizations are probably mediated by opening of cation nonselective stretch-activated channels (SAC_{CAT}) which can carry an

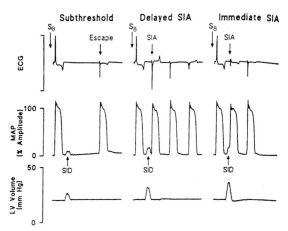

■ Figure 30–1 Stretch-induced depolarizations (SID) in an isolated canine heart preparation. Shown are electrocardiogram (ECG), monophasic action potential recording (MAP), and a left ventricular volume pulse tracing (LV volume). S_8 indicates the timing of the last pacing stimulus in an 8-beat pacing train. After the pacing train, LV volume is transiently increased by a computerized servo-pump. *Left,* A transient 10-mL increase in LV volume produces a SID seen on the MAP recording without triggering an arrhythmia. After 1.5 seconds, there is a ventricular escape beat. Larger volume pulses are seen on the *center* and *right panels,* producing depolarizations of sufficient magnitude to trigger several ectopic beats. *(Reproduced from Stacy GP, Jobe RL, Taylor LK, Hansen DE: Stretch-induced depolarizations as a trigger of arrhythmias in isolated canine left ventricles. Am J Physiol 263:H613, 1992, with permission.)*

inward, depolarizing current when activated at resting membrane potential).

Both depolarization and stretch-induced ventricular ectopy are effectively suppressed by gadolinium.[10] An analogous role for SAC_{CAT} in the atria has been suggested, although most stretch-activated channels in the atria seem to be K^+ selective.[11] Atrial dilation can provoke atrial fibrillation and this dilation-induced atrial fibrillation is prevented by a nontoxic peptide isolated from tarantula spider venom (see Chapters 1 and 4).

The effect of more gradual sustained ventricular dilation of the mammalian ventricle appears to be fundamentally different. In 1985, Lerman and colleagues[12] demonstrated that ventricular dilation, in a cross-circulated isolated canine heart, was associated with a shortening of myocardial refractoriness. About the same time, experiments in the isolated rabbit heart confirmed a decrease in both APD and epicardial

refractoriness secondary to ventricular dilation.[8,13,14] In these experiments, a fluid-filled balloon was anchored within either the left (LV) (typically) or the right ventricle (RV) of Langendorff-perfused isolated hearts. Initially, the balloon volume was adjusted to a nominal end-diastolic pressure (EDP) of 0 mm Hg. Graded volumes then were added or removed from the balloon manually within several seconds. These experiments demonstrated several important characteristics of MEF in isolated hearts:

1. The decrease in refractoriness is rapid (occurring within seconds of balloon dilation) and (within the time constraints of acute experiments) fully reversible.
2. The change in refractoriness is essentially linear with ventricular volume and pressure. Changes in balloon volume associated with increases in left ventricular end-diastolic pressure (LVEDP) from 0 to ~30 mm Hg were associated with 5% to 25% decreases in refractoriness.
3. Changes in epicardial refractoriness were correlated with APD measured with epicardial monophasic action potential (MAP) catheters.
4. The shortening of refractoriness is regionally heterogeneous: When the balloon was anchored within the LV and dilated, there was no change in RV refractoriness. The refractoriness change over the LV epicardium was also heterogeneous.[13,14] When multiple MAP electrodes were used to assess APD during LV dilation in isolated rabbit hearts, most (although not all) sites showed a shortening of APD. The dispersion of APD increased from approximately 27 to 40 msec during constant pacing.[14] Echocardiographic correlation of ventricular dimensions with regional refractoriness suggested that the effective refractory period (ERP) decrease was best correlated with increases in diastolic wall stress.[15]
5. Within the time frame of acute experiments, the effect of dilation on refractoriness did not demonstrate accommodation; that is, the change in refractoriness was maintained without variation for the duration of the dilation.

Subsequent observations in many other models and species have essentially confirmed these observations. An increase in myocardial wall stress leads to a consistent decrease in APD and ventricular refractoriness.

Although the rapidity of the change in APD is consistent with an ion channel effect, the specific channel or channels involved remains uncertain. Zabel and colleagues[14] demonstrated that activation of SAC_{CAT} could account for the decrease in APD, but several observations make this unlikely to be the primary ionic mechanism. First, gadolinium (Gd^{3+}) does not prevent the change in APD at concentrations at which it is a blocker of SAC_{CAT}.[16] Second, the decrease in refractoriness and APD is cycle length–dependent: A greater decrease in refractoriness is observed at shorter cycle lengths.[17,18] Activation of the SAC_{CAT} alone does not explain this cycle length–dependent pattern.

Observations[12] that stretch-induced shortening of APD is associated with, or facilitated by, increases in internal Ca^{2+} may imply that a Ca^{2+}-sensitive channel, a Ca^{2+}-dependent K^+ channel, Na^+-Ca^{2+} exchange, or stretch-modulated voltage-dependent channels (see Chapter 4) may be involved (see Chapters 6 and 22 for further discussion of the effects of stretch on Ca^{2+} kinetics). The influence of stretch on both the L-type Ca^{2+} channel[19] and the slow component of the delayed rectifier potassium current, I_{Ks}[20] (both of which might explain a cycle length–dependent effect) increases the number of potential drivers for the observed changes.

The results of experiments designed to clarify the influence of stretch on myocardial conduction velocity are inconsistent (see Chapter 14). When papillary muscle is subjected to mild stretch, conduction velocity does not change. Conduction slowing is observed with greater degrees of stretch.[21] In intact isolated hearts[13] and in thin epicardial sheets,[17,22] there is no change in conduction velocity. However, Sung and colleagues,[23] using optical mapping in isolated perfused rabbit hearts, found that increased LVEDP (to ~30 mm Hg) decreased apparent conduction velocity by approximately 16%. In these experiments, ventricular loading increased APD (measured at 80% repolarization). The explanation of these divergent findings is not immediately apparent, but it may be related to mechanical arrest and the electromechanical uncoupling agent used.

Animal models suggest that the effects of acute dilation may be greater in the abnormal or chronically dilated myocardium, or under conditions of high sympathetic tone. An increase in LV size decreased ventricular refractoriness more in infarcted than normal myocardium in the dog.[24] Ischemia exaggerated the

decrease in APD seen with dilation in a porcine model.[25] In the isolated dog heart, the likelihood of stretch-induced ventricular ectopy depended on the initial volume (ectopy was more likely when the starting volume was high).[6] In the presence of a pacing-induced cardiomyopathy in dogs, stretch-induced ventricular arrhythmias were more easily provoked.[26] Sympathetic stimulation potentiates the effect of dilation in the in situ porcine heart: Aortic occlusion decreased APD only 2% before, but 5% during, dopamine infusion.[27]

ARRHYTHMOGENIC EFFECTS OF VENTRICULAR DILATION IN ANIMAL MODELS

In the isolated rabbit heart,[13] ventricular ERP was determined by introducing an extrastimulus during continuous ventricular epicardial pacing. Ventricular arrhythmias were frequently induced during the measurement of ERP (Fig. 30–2), when the ventricle was dilated (~35% of captured extrastimuli when the balloon volume was 1.0 mL or more, but less than ~3% when the balloon volume was 0.5 mL or less).

Inducibility of extrasystoles during ventricular dilation, and the absence of spontaneous arrhythmias, suggests the possibility of a re-entrant mechanism. Moe's hypothesis[28] argues that fibrillation requires a minimum number of circulating wavelets, and that inducibility of fibrillation, therefore, will be inversely correlated with the minimum size of the functional re-entry path (proportional to myocardial wavelength = ERP × conduction velocity). Re-entry is favored by conditions that tend to slow conduction, shorten refractoriness, and increase the heterogeneity of repolarization. Inducibility in the isolated rabbit heart that is subjected to either LV dilation (which decreases ventricular refractoriness), hypokalemia (which slows interventricular conduction velocity), or both was correlated with myocardial wavelength. Dilation and hypokalemia were synergistic in facilitating VF.[29] This is analogous to the observation in a canine model that induction of atrial fibrillation was critically dependent on atrial wavelength and the number of mapped circulating wavelets.[30] In a model of re-entrant ventricular tachycardia (VT) around a ring of epicardial tissue in isolated hearts, dilation increased the measured

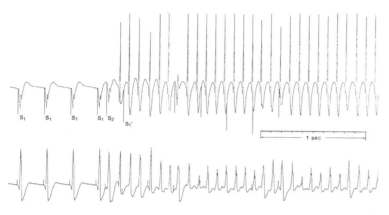

■ **Figure 30–2** Representative recording of ventricular arrhythmia induced during determination of effective refractory period during continuous pacing at high volume. The last 4 stimuli of a 20-beat train (S_1) are seen, followed by an extrastimulus (S_2), which captures and induces a sustained, rapid, ventricular arrhythmia. *(Reproduced from Reiter MJ, Synhorst DP, Mann DE: Electrophysiologic effects of acute ventricular dilatation in the isolated rabbit heart. Circ Res 62:554, 1988, with permission.)*

excitable gap (both spatial and temporal) by decreasing myocardial refractoriness.[22] This increase in the excitable gap appeared to explain arrhythmia acceleration and diminished efficacy of Class III antiarrhythmic agents when the ventricle is dilated.

Myocardial stretch decreases the VF threshold, a measure of the tendency for VF (determined by stimulating the myocardium with a train of pulses of increasing amplitude). This effect has been observed in isolated rabbit[31] and rat hearts.[32] Dilation increases the defibrillation threshold (DFT) in isolated rabbit hearts[33] (Fig. 30–3), the in vivo canine cardiomyopathy model,[34] or the anesthetized pig (see Chapter 35).[35] Dilation decreases the median VF interval, increases the variation in VF cycle lengths (consistent with increased heterogeneity of refractoriness), and increases the complexity of VF.[36]

DO SIMILAR MECHANO-ELECTRIC FEEDBACK PHENOMENA EXIST IN HUMANS?

Effective homeostatic mechanisms and measurement complexities make assessment of MEF more difficult in humans. Nevertheless, numerous observations suggest the existence of MEF in humans (see Chapters 24 through 32) with many similarities to those observed experimentally.

During balloon valvuloplasty in children, Martin and Stanger[37] observed that the corrected QT interval (QTc)

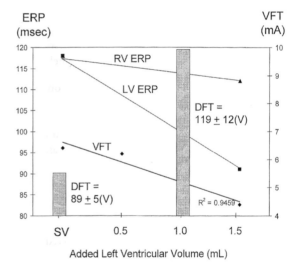

■ **Figure 30–3** Effects of ventricular dilation on epicardial effective refractory period (ERP), ventricular fibrillation threshold (VFT), and defibrillation threshold (DFT) in isolated Langendorff-perfused rabbit hearts. Shown on the abscissa are volumes added to a left ventricular (LV) balloon (SV = starting volume associated with an EDP = 0 mm Hg). Shown are the epicardial ERP of both the dilated left (LV ERP) and nondilated right (RV ERP) ventricles. With an increase in LV volume (associated with an increase in EDP from 0 to 35 mm Hg), the LV ERP decreased from 118 ± 4 to 91 ± 6 msec. RV ERP was unchanged (118 ± 4 to 112 ± 6 msec). VFT and its regression line also are shown. Initial VFT was 6.4 mA decreasing to 4.4 mA with dilation. Bar graphs show the increase in defibrillation threshold from 89 ± 5 peak volts to 119 ± 12 peak volts. These data are not from the same experiments, rather they represent data from Reiter and colleagues,[13] Jalal and colleagues,[31] and Ott and colleagues.[33]

lengthened shortly after dilation. QTc prolongation persisted 16 to 24 hours after valvuloplasty, but was absent 1 to 15 months later. Serial electrocardiograms (ECG) in four patients showed that the QT interval increased over several hours after valvuloplasty. The QT lengthening appeared to peak at ~14 hours and decreased by 36 hours (but it was still longer than before dilation). In 1988, Levine and colleagues[38] studied the effects of balloon valvuloplasty in patients with congenital pulmonic stenosis. In 32 patients studied, the QTc increased from 409 to 441 msec (8%) after successful valvuloplasty. Monophasic action potential duration (MAPD) decreased (~6%) during obstruction of the RV outflow tract by balloon inflation and increased (~6%) after successful dilation. Thus, the total change from obstructed to successfully dilated (although not in the same patient) was about 23 msec, or 11%. Extrasystoles and diastolic depolarizations were observed during balloon inflation.

Taggart and coauthors[39,40] assessed the electrophysiologic effects of increased ventricular stress during coronary artery bypass. During bypass, transient aortic occlusion[39] shortened MAPD from 325 ± 31 to 311 ± 29 msec, and with discontinuance of bypass,[40] LV epicardial MAPD decreased from 288 ± 29 to 261 ± 29 msec (~4%).

In nonanesthetized individuals, Nanthakumar and colleagues[41] used a stimulus T-wave sensing implanted pacemaker to study head-up tilt. When RV volume decreased, a small but significant lengthening of RV repolarization was observed. Although the magnitude of these changes was small (possibly related to the methodology of the measurement and volume manipulation), the effects persisted in the presence of autonomic blockade (0.03 mg/kg i.v atropine, 0.15 mg/kg propranolol).

Pharmacologic unloading with vasodilators also appears to be associated with changes compatible with MEF. In eight patients with coronary artery disease, LV dysfunction, and inducible VT, captopril (48 hours of therapy) increased ERP (from 231 to 249 msec) and the QTc interval.[42]

Ellenbogen and colleagues[43] studied the effects of lower body negative pressure in transplanted (denervated) hearts. In this study, there were modest changes consistent with MEF at a paced cycle length of 400 msec: ERP (baseline 226 ± 12 msec) was increased 4% at a negative pressure of 30 mm Hg (234 ± 21 msec).

Not all studies show consistent effects. Kadish and colleagues[44] compared atrioventricular (AV) sequential pacing at an AV interval of 160 msec to simultaneous atrial and ventricular pacing (AV interval = 0 msec). During AV sequential pacing at an AV interval of 160 msec, LV volume (measured echocardiographically) was greater, but RV ERP *increased* compared with simultaneous pacing. This difference persisted with autonomic blockade. However, simultaneous AV pacing is associated with complex pressure–contraction relations (especially with RV apical pacing) and correlation of RV ERP with LV volumes makes this study difficult to evaluate.

ARE MECHANO-ELECTRIC FEEDBACK EFFECTS ARRHYTHMOGENIC IN HUMANS?

Given the complexity of MEF in humans, it is not surprising that the question of whether MEF may cause arrhythmias is currently unanswered. Are there clinical instances where changes in ventricular volume or pressure are associated with the occurrence of ventricular arrhythmias? Or is MEF a pseudophenomenon without physiologic significance? These questions require consideration of several potentially important and confounding issues.

Is the Magnitude of the Effect in Humans Sufficient to Contribute to Arrhythmias?

Transient mechanical stimulation, although it may provoke isolated ectopy, is less likely to cause sustained arrhythmias. Commotio cordis, in which mechanical impact appears to precipitate ventricular tachyarrhythmia, is an important exception (see Chapters 15 and 29).

Experimentally, MEF can decrease refractoriness 5% to 25% (5 to 30 msec). Quantitatively similar changes are seen in humans under certain conditions. It has been suggested that the effect of MEF on the APD is too small to contribute to ventricular arrhythmias. Support for this concept comes from studies in which an increase in dispersion to nearly 100 msec was required before ventricular arrhythmias could be induced (with a single extrastimulus) in an animal model.[45] However, Gough and colleagues[46] found, in a similar model, that an arc of block could develop between sites having a much smaller difference in refractoriness (e.g., 40 msec), and they pointed out that it is the *distribution* of refractoriness, rather than the absolute degree of inhomogeneity, that is important. Moreover, inhomogeneity is increased with additional extrastimuli or spontaneous ectopy; therefore, quantification of electrophysiologic inhomogeneity required to "permit" ventricular arrhythmias in these situations may be irrelevant.

Are the Effects of Mechano-Electric Feedback Relevant in a Setting of Chronic Dilation, Heart Failure, and Hypertrophy?

The effects of congestive heart failure (CHF) and hypertrophy initially appear to be fundamentally different (exactly opposite) from those expected because of MEF. Ventricular hypertrophy and CHF are associated with APD prolongation, primarily because of down-regulation of various potassium currents. APD lengthening may be arrhythmogenic (because of torsades des pointes, afterdepolarizations) and may contribute to increased heterogeneity of repolarization (favoring re-entry).

Is it appropriate to consider these effects as distinct and unrelated? It seems reasonable that acute dilation on a background of chronic dilation may exaggerate regional differences of repolarization. It is conceivable that the increase in refractoriness seen with CHF is, in part, a compensatory response to an initial shortening of APD seen with acute dilation. The observation that abnormal ion channel expression in CHF is localized in regions of abnormal mechanical activation may be a manifestation of MEF. Considering these two apparently divergent phenomena as separate and unrelated may be overly simplistic (see Chapters 25 to 28).

Are the Clinical Observations Reminiscent of Mechano-Electric Feedback Coincidence or Do They Imply Cause?

There are many situations in which MEF might be the explanation of clinical phenomena (see Reference 16 for a review of this topic). The high incidence of ventricular arrhythmias and sudden death, the propensity for drug-induced arrhythmia acceleration, and the diminished efficacy of antiarrhythmic therapy in patients with CHF all have correlates in the experimental studies of MEF.

LV function is the most important predictor of clinical outcome. LV ejection fraction is the parameter most often examined, but LV dimensions, although less frequently assessed (and more difficult to measure), may be a better predictor. In the Gruppo Italiano per lo Studio della Sopravvivenza nell'Infarto Miocardico (GISSI)-3 study, LV volumes were a *better predictor* of outcome than the LV ejection fraction, or the extent of coronary artery disease.[47] In patients with idiopathic dilated cardiomyopathy and CHF, LV end-diastolic diameter was the *only* variable predictive of survival. It also was predictive of sudden death, independent of ejection fraction and cause, in patients with functional Class III-IV CHF.[48] In humans, DFT appears to be increased by ventricular dilation, again consistent with experimental studies of MEF.[16]

In some studies, hemodynamic decompensation is associated with an increased risk for serious ventricular arrhythmias and degeneration of initially tolerated arrhythmias.[49] Pires and colleagues[49] examined terminal events in 25 patients with implanted defibrillators who experienced out-of-hospital sudden death. Sixteen died of a tachyarrhythmia. Ten of these patients had what was considered an identifiable precipitant, and in 8 of 10, worsening CHF preceded death. MEF may have contributed to the risk for arrhythmia degeneration (Fig. 30–4). In this population, there also was a decrease in first shock defibrillation efficacy, suggesting that CHF influenced DFT.

The effects of pharmacologic vasodilation are consistent with MEF. Vasodilators decrease mortality and sudden death to the degree that they reverse or prevent ventricular dilation. In some studies, these agents prolong refractoriness and decrease ventricular arrhythmias. The effect of β-blocker therapy in reducing overall mortality and sudden death initially appears to be inconsistent with MEF, but it is not. β-Blockade reduces wall stress (by decreasing contractility), chronically increases LV ejection fraction, and reduces LV

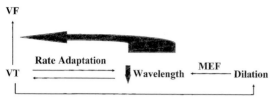

■ **Figure 30–4** Hypothetical relation illustrating a possible role of mechano-electric feedback (MEF) in arrhythmia degeneration. Development of ventricular tachycardia (VT) leads to a shortening of myocardial refractoriness and wavelength caused by the rate-dependent shortening of action potential duration. If VT also leads to an increase in ventricular wall stress recruiting MEF, then there will be a further decrease in myocardial refractoriness (exaggerated because of the underlying tachycardia). A decrease in myocardial wavelength by these multiple mechanisms could lead to arrhythmia acceleration and degeneration of VT into ventricular fibrillation (VF).

end-diastolic volume. Nevertheless, cause and effect is difficult to distinguish, and these relations may be simply circumstantial.

What Are the Results of Studies Assessing Effects of Volume or Pressure Manipulation?

Catheter (mechanically) induced premature ventricular contractions, infrequent commotio cordis, and the observation that sterno-thoracic compression during cardiopulmonary resuscitation can sometimes provoke VF recurrence[50] suggest that rapid mechanical deformation has effects in humans that are similar to those observed in animals.

The influence of sustained stretch is not clear. In both animals and humans, some studies have demonstrated a relation between blood pressure and ventricular arrhythmias. Hypertension (pressure overload) may be arrhythmogenic under certain circumstances. Sideris[51] studied 24 patients; half were given nitroprusside (NP) to reduce blood pressure, and half received metariminol, resulting in a blood pressure increase. When blood pressure decreased, the incidence of ventricular ectopic activity decreased. A correlate of these experiments may be the observation that ventricular unloading can

inhibit ventricular arrhythmias. Ventricular assist devices have been reported to control incessant, and otherwise refractory, ventricular arrhythmias. Mostly anecdotal, case reports often reflect simply a better tolerance of VT. However, some studies have suggested that mechanical unloading can suppress ventricular arrhythmias.[52]

At least three small studies explored the effects of volume manipulation during electrophysiologic evaluation, and no change in VT inducibility with volume loading or unloading was observed. Carlson and colleagues[53] studied 12 patients with coronary artery disease, LV ejection fractions less than 40%, and a history of sustained VT. Electrophysiologic evaluation, including VT induction, was performed at baseline and during NP infusion. During infusion, LV dimensions decreased, but VT inducibility, method of induction, and VT cycle length were not influenced. RV ERP also did not change. Bashir and colleagues[42] studied eight patients, similar to those studied by Carlson. After 48 hours of oral captopril (dose based on target blood pressure reduction of 10%), there was no change in VT inducibility even though RV ERP increased (from 231 ± 26 to 249 ± 23 msec). Kulick and colleagues[54] examined nine patients with a cardiomyopathy (two idiopathic, three alcohol related, and four secondary to hypertension). Mean ejection fraction was approximately 21%. These patients had not experienced a prior spontaneous ventricular arrhythmia. By withholding diuretics and vasodilators for at least 24 hours, acute hemodynamic decompensation was achieved (associated with an increase in right atrial pressure from 8 ± 4 to 16 ± 5 mm Hg and an increase in pulmonary capillary wedge pressure [PCWP] from 20 ± 3 to 33 ± 8 mm Hg). The patients then underwent electrophysiologic evaluation before and during NP administration (right atrial pressure = 11 ± 3 mm Hg; PCWP = 16 ± 3 mm Hg). No difference of inducibility was seen in any patient (all were noninducible under both conditions). RV ERP increased from the "decompensated state" compared with NP infusion (RV apex ERP_{decomp} = 241 ± 20 msec; RV apex ERP_{NP} = 253 ± 14 msec; RV outflow tract ERP_{decomp} = 235 ± 29 msec; RV outflow tract ERP_{NP} = 250 ± 28 msec). All of these studies are limited by the small number of patients, the relatively minor volume manipulation (with variable degrees and rapidity of volume change that was mostly right-sided unloading), and the inability to control other confounding factors (e.g., autonomic tone).

Conclusions

Electrophysiologic changes secondary to changes in ventricular volume and pressure probably do occur in humans. These effects may be arrhythmogenic. Whether the effects are quantitatively sufficient to be clinically important is not yet known. Even if not sufficient to trigger arrhythmias, it seems reasonable to conclude that MEF probably contributes to an electrophysiologic milieu that favors arrhythmias.

Convincing proof of an important arrhythmogenic role for MEF is currently lacking because of the intrinsic complexity of arrhythmogenesis in humans. However, the use of specific blockers for stretch-activated channels may be able to clarify the question in humans. Given the potential importance of MEF, further studies are indicated. These should include large-scale, prospective studies correlating ventricular arrhythmias and sudden death with easily used and accurate methods capable of assessing ventricular refractoriness and wall stress.

References

1. Bozler E: Tonus changes in cardiac muscle and their significance for the initiation of impulses. Am J Physiol 139:477–480, 1943.
2. Dudel J, Trautwein W: Das Aktionpotential und Mechanogramm des Herzmuskels unter dem Einflus der Dehnung. Cardiologie 25:344–362, 1954.
3. Stauch M: The QT interval of the isolated frog heart in isotonic and isometric contraction. Z Kreislaufforsch 49:986–998, 1960.
4. Franz MR, Burkhoff D, Yue DT, Sagawa K: Mechanically induced action potential changes and arrhythmia in isolated and in situ canine hearts. Cardiovasc Res 23:213–223, 1989.
5. Stacy GP, Jobe RL, Taylor LK, Hansen DE: Stretch-induced depolarizations as a trigger of arrhythmias in isolated canine left ventricles. Am J Physiol 263:H613–H621, 1992.
6. Hansen DE, Craig CS, Hondeghem LM: Stretch-induced arrhythmias in the isolated canine ventricle: Evidence for the importance of mechanoelectrical feedback. Circulation 81:1094–1105, 1990.
7. Franz MR, Cima R, Wang D, et al: Electrophysiologic effects of myocardial stretch and mechanical determinants of stretch-activated arrhythmias. Circulation 86:968–978, 1992.
8. Kong C-R, Bursac N, Tung L: Mechanoelectrical excitation in cultured monolayers of cardiac cells [abstract]. Pacing Clin Electrophysiol 26-II:1023, 2003.
9. Bode F, Franz MR, Bonnemeier H, et al: Ventricular fibrillation induced by stretch pulses: Implication for arrhythmogenesis due to commotio cordis [abstract]. Pacing Clin Electrophysiol 26-II:1111, 2003.
10. Hansen DE, Borganelli M, Stacey GP, Taylor LK: Dose-dependent inhibition of stretch-induced arrhythmias by gadolinium in isolated canine ventricles: Evidence for a unique mode of antiarrhythmic action. Circ Res 69:820–831, 1991.
11. Niu W, Sachs F: Dynamic properties of stretch-activated K$^+$ channels in adult rat atrial myocytes. Prog Biophys Mol Biol 82:121–135, 2003.
12. Lerman BB, Burkhoff D, Yue DT, Sagawa K: Mechanoelectrical feedback: Independent role of preload and contractility in modulation of canine ventricular excitability. J Clin Invest 76:1843–1850, 1985.
13. Reiter MJ, Synhorst DP, Mann DE: Electrophysiologic effects of acute ventricular dilatation in the isolated rabbit heart. Circ Res 62:554–562, 1988.
14. Zabel M, Portnoy S, Franz MR: Effect of sustained load on dispersion of ventricular repolarization and conduction time in the isolated rabbit heart. J Cardiovasc Electrophysiol 7:9–16, 1996.
15. Halperin BD, Adler SW, Mann DE, Reiter MJ: Mechanical correlates of contraction-excitation feedback during acute ventricular dilatation. Cardiovasc Res 27:1084–1087, 1993.
16. Reiter MJ: Effects of mechano-electrical feedback: Potential arrhythmogenic influence in patients with congestive heart failure. Cardiovasc Res 32:44–51, 1996.
17. Reiter MJ, Landers M, Zetelaki Z, et al: Electrophysiologic effects of acute dilatation in the isolated rabbit heart: Cycle length dependent effects on epicardial refractoriness and conduction velocity. Circulation 96:4050–4056, 1997.
18. Eckardt L, Kirchhof P, Monnig G, et al: Modification of stretch-induced shortening of repolarization by streptomycin in the isolated heart. J Cardiovasc Pharmacol 36:711–721, 2000.
19. Lyford GL, Strege PR, Shepard A, et al: $_{\alpha1C}$(Ca$_V$1.2) L-type calcium channel mediates mechanosensitive calcium regulation. Am J Physiol Cell Physiol. 283:C1001–C1008, 2002.
20. Wang Z, Mitsuiye T, Noma A: Cell distention-induced increase of the delayed rectifier K$^+$ current in guinea pig ventricular myocytes. Circ Res 78:466–474, 1996.
21. Penefsky ZJ, Hoffman BF: Effects of stretch on mechanical and electrical properties of cardiac muscle. Am J Physiol 204:433–438, 1963.
22. Reiter MJ, Zetelaki Z, Kirchhof CJH, et al: Interaction of acute ventricular dilatation and d-sotalol during sustained reentrant ventricular tachycardia around a fixed obstacle. Circulation 89:423–431, 1994.
23. Sung D, Mills RW, Schettler J, et al: Ventricular filling slows epicardial conduction and increases action potential duration in an optical mapping study of the isolated rabbit heart. J Cardiovasc Electrophysiol 14:739–749, 2003.
24. Calkins H, Maughan WL, Weisman HF, et al: Effect of acute volume load on refractoriness and arrhythmia development in isolated chronically infarcted canine hearts. Circulation 79:687–697, 1989.
25. Horner SM, Lab MJ, Murphy CF, et al: Mechanically induced changes in action potential duration and left ventricular segment length in acute regional ischaemia in the in situ porcine heart. Cardiovasc Res 28:528–534, 1994.
26. Wang Z, Taylor LK, Denney WD, Hansen DE: Initiation of ventricular extrasystoles by myocardial stretch in chronically

dilated and failing canine left ventricle. Circulation 90: 2022–2031, 1994.

27. Horner SM, Murphy CF, Cen B, et al: Sympathomimetic modulation of load-dependent changes in the action potential duration in the in situ porcine heart. Cardiovasc Res 32:148–157, 1996.

28. Moe GK: On the multiple wavelet hypothesis of atrial fibrillation. Arch Int Pharmacodyn Ther 140:183–188, 1962.

29. Reiter MJ, Mann DE, Williams GR: Interaction of hypokalemia and ventricular dilatation in isolated rabbit hearts. Am J Physiol 265:H1544–H1550, 1993.

30. Rensma PL, Allessie MA, Lammers WJ, et al: Length of excitation wave and susceptibility to reentrant atrial arrhythmias in normal conscious dogs. Circ Res 62:395–410, 1988.

31. Jalal S, Williams GR, Mann DE, Reiter MJ: Effect of acute ventricular dilatation on fibrillation thresholds in the isolated rabbit heart. Am J Physiol 263:H1306–H1310, 1992.

32. Rosen S, Lahorra M, Cohen MV, Buttrick P: Ventricular fibrillation threshold is influenced by left ventricular stretch and mass in the absence of ischaemia. Cardiovasc Res 25:458–462, 1991.

33. Ott P, Reiter MJ: Effect of ventricular dilatation on defibrillation threshold in the isolated perfused rabbit heart. J Cardiovasc Electrophysiol 8:1013–1019, 1997.

34. Lucy SD, Jones DL, Klein GJ: Pronounced increase in defibrillation threshold associated with pacing induced cardiomyopathy in the dog. Am Heart J 127:366–376, 1994.

35. Strobel JS, Kay GN, Walcott GP, et al: The effect of ventricular volume on ventricular defibrillation efficacy in pigs [abstract]. J Am Coll Cardiol 1996:327A.

36. Burton FL, Cobbe SM: Effect of sustained stretch on dispersion of ventricular fibrillation intervals in normal rabbit hearts. Cardiovasc Res 39:351–359, 1998.

37. Martin GR, Stanger P: Transient prolongation of the QTc interval after balloon valvuloplasty and angioplasty in children. Am J Cardiol 58:1233–1235, 1986.

38. Levine JH, Guarnieri T, Kadish AH, et al: Changes in myocardial repolarization in patients undergoing balloon valvuloplasty for congenital pulmonary stenosis: Evidence for contraction-excitation feedback in humans. Circulation 77:70–77, 1988.

39. Taggart P, Sutton P, Lab M, et al: Effect of abrupt changes in ventricular loading on repolarization induced by transient aortic occlusion in human. Am J Physiol 263:H816–H823, 1992.

40. Taggart P, Sutton PMI, Treasure T, et al: Monophasic action potentials at discontinuation of cardiopulmonary bypass: Evidence for contraction excitation feedback in man. Circulation 77:1266–1275, 1988.

41. Nanthakumar K, Dorian P, Paquette M, et al: Effect of physiological mechanical perturbation on intact human myocardial repolarization. Cardiovasc Res 45:303–309, 2000.

42. Bashir Y, Sneddon JF, O'Nunain S, et al: Comparative electrophysiological effects of captopril or hydralazine combined with

nitrate in patients with left ventricular dysfunction and inducible ventricular tachycardia. Br Heart J 67:355–360, 1992.

43. Ellenbogen KA, Stambler BS, Wood MA, Mohanty PK: Examination of mechano-electrical feedback in the transplanted human heart. Am J Cardiol 76:51–55, 1995.

44. Kadish AH, Kou WH, Schmaltz S, Morady F: Effect of atrioventricular relationship on ventricular refractoriness in humans. Am J Physiol 259:H1463–H1470, 1990.

45. Kuo CS, Munakata K, Reddy CP, Surawicz B: Characteristics and possible mechanism of ventricular arrhythmia dependent on the dispersion of action potential durations. Circulation 67:1356–1367, 1983.

46. Gough WB, Mehra R, Restivo M, et al: Reentrant ventricular arrhythmias in the late myocardial infarction period in the dog. 13. Correlation of activation and refractory maps. Circ Res 57:432–442, 1985.

47. Nicolosi GL, Latini R, Marino P, et al: The prognostic value of predischarge quantitative two-dimensional echocardiographic measurements and the effects of early lisinopril treatment on left ventricular structure and function after acute myocardial infarction in the GISSI-3 Trial. Gruppo Italiano per lo Studio della Sopravvivenza nell'Infarto Miocardico. Eur Heart J 17:1646–1656, 1996.

48. Lee TH, Hamilton MA, Stevenson LW, et al: Impact of left ventricular cavity size on survival in advanced heart failure. Am J Cardiol 72:672–676, 1993.

49. Pires LA, Lehmann MH, Steinman RT, et al: Sudden death in implantable cardioverter-defibrillator recipients: Clinical context, arrhythmic events and device responses. J Am Coll Cardiol 33:24–32, 1999.

50. Capucci A, Villani GQ, Aschieri D, et al: Sterno-thoracic compression triggers ventricular fibrillation during cardiopulmonary resuscitation. Post-shock ECG analysis in Piacenza Progetto Vita Database [abstract]. Pacing Clin Electrophysiol 26:II-981, 2003.

51. Sideris DA, Kontoyannis DA, Michalis A, et al: Acute changes in blood pressure as a cause of cardiac arrhythmias. Eur Heart J 8:45–52, 1987.

52. Fotopoulous GD, Mason MJ, Walker S, et al: Stabilisation of medically refractory ventricular arrhythmia by intra-aortic balloon counterpulsation. Heart 82:96–100, 1999.

53. Carlson MD, Schoenfeld MH, Garan H, et al: Programmed ventricular stimulation in patients with left ventricular dysfunction and ventricular tachycardia: Effects of acute hemodynamic improvement due to nitroprusside. J Am Coll Cardiol 14:1744–1752, 1989.

54. Kulick DL, Bhandari AK, Hong R, et al: Effect of acute hemodynamic decompensation on electrical inducibility of ventricular arrhythmias in patients with dilated cardiomyopathy and complex nonsustained ventricular arrhythmias. Am Heart J 119:878–883, 1990.

Mortality from Heart Failure: Hemodynamics Versus Electrical Causes

• • • •

Steven N. Singh and Pamela Karasik

Heart failure is characterized by an inability of the heart to pump sufficient amounts of blood to meet the requirements of the body's organs and metabolizing tissues. Systolic heart failure is seen in the presence of decreased ventricular contractility and reduced ejection fraction (EF). In contrast, diastolic heart failure is defined as signs and symptoms of heart failure in the presence of preserved left ventricular contractile function.

In a broad sense, cardiomyopathy has been classified as ischemic or nonischemic. These terms often are loosely defined, and there is some confusion on these definitions. At times there will be some discussion in which the severity of the ischemic disease may not correlate with the severity of the myocardial dysfunction. Nevertheless, these two categories are used for the purposes of this chapter.

Sudden cardiac death often is defined as natural death due to cardiac causes. It is characterized by abrupt loss of consciousness within 1 hour after the onset of symptoms in a person in whom death was unexpected. Although sudden death often is related to an arrhythmia, there are other precipitating causes such as stroke, pulmonary embolism, and acute aortic dissection. In addition, not all sudden death is related to a tachyarrhythmia. Bradycardia and electromechanical dissociation is a common finding, especially in patients with end-stage cardiomyopathy (Fig. 31–1).[1]

Pump failure death is cardiac death that is classified as nonsudden and is characterized by a low-cardiac output state and cardiogenic shock.

EPIDEMIOLOGY

Heart failure affects more than 4 million people in the United States, with 550,000 new cases each year.[2] The prognosis remains poor, but long-term trends show a decline in the incidence of heart failure in women but not men.[3] Between 1950 and 1969, the 1- and 5-year age-adjusted mortality rates among men were 30% and 70%, respectively; from 1990 to 1999, the corresponding rates were 28% and 59%. The corresponding rates in women between 1950 and 1969 were 18% and 57%; from 1990 to 1999, the rates were 24% and 45%, respectively. This translated into an improvement in overall survival rate of about 12% per decade (Fig. 31–2).

The annual mortality rate in heart failure depends on New York Heart Association (NYHA) functional class, EF, and background therapy; it approximates 12%, despite adequate therapy. The modes of death usually are classified as either pump failure or sudden. Recently, the percentage of sudden death exceeds that of pump failure and may be because of the aggressive approaches of new therapies (Table 31–1).[3–10]

MECHANISMS OF ARRHYTHMIA

The mechanisms for arrhythmias implicated in heart failure are complex and include triggered activity (early and late afterdepolarizations), abnormal enhanced automaticity, re-entry, and activation of stretch receptors. The hypertrophied ventricle exhibits an increased propensity for early afterdepolarizations, which may lead to a potentially lethal arrhythmia.[11]

Mechanical stretch from increased ventricular volume can provoke abnormal electrical activity and arrhythmias.[12,13] Abnormal automaticity occurs when spontaneous impulses are generated in partially depolarized fibers because of disease. These impulses may be carried by either sodium or calcium currents depend-

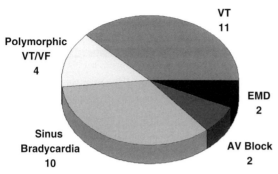

Figure 31–1 Initial rhythm at cardiac arrests in patients with advanced heart failure (n = 29). AV, atrioventricular; EMD, electromechanical dissociation; VF, ventricular fibrillation; VT, ventricular tachycardia. *(Modified from Luu M, Stevenson WG, Stevenson LW, et al: Diverse mechanism of unexpected cardiac arrest in advanced heart failure. Circulation 80:1675–1680, 1989, with permission.)*

ing on the level of maximal diastolic potential. Re-entry is a common mechanism and is responsible for most arrhythmias in patients with heart failure caused by ischemic cardiomyopathy. Such arrhythmias are related to slow conduction in a pathologic substrate.

FACTORS IDENTIFYING INDIVIDUALS AT HIGH RISK

A number of factors have been used to identify individuals at risk for death, including the following: higher NYHA functional class, cardiomegaly on chest radiograph, increased norepinephrine and brain natriuretic peptide levels, presence of atrial fibrillation, bundle branch block, nonsustained ventricular tachycardia (VT) on the electrocardiogram (ECG) or Holter recording, reduced heart rate variability, increased QT dispersion, presence of T-wave alternans, abnormal signal-averaged ECG, and electrophysiologic study–induced sustained VT (Table 31–2).[14–25] Obviously, there are certain limitations on some of these tests. The signal-averaged ECG and electrophysiologic studies are useful in patients with coronary artery disease (CAD), but they are of limited use in patients with nonischemic cardiomyopathy. Also, there is some controversy on the usefulness of each of the previous identifying factors. Nevertheless, a low EF has withstood the test of time and is highly predictive not

only of pump failure death, but also of sudden cardiac death.

OVERVIEW OF THERAPIES AND TRIALS

Several drugs and some devices have been used to treat patients with heart failure (Table 31–3). However, although the data are strong in favor of some, there is still controversy in the use of other drugs and devices.

Drug Therapy

The Digoxin Investigation Group (DIG) trial tested the effects of digoxin against a placebo on survival in patients with heart failure.[26] Although there was no overall difference between the two groups, there was a decrease in deaths caused by heart failure and an increase in deaths caused by sudden arrhythmia. Subsequent analyses showed a decrease in all-cause mortality in patients who had a serum concentration of 0.5 to 0.8 μg/mL digoxin, and a greater mortality rate among women compared with men.[27,28]

Diuretics often are used as maintenance therapy for patients in heart failure. Yet, there is little outcome data. Post-hoc analyses from the Studies of Left Ventricular Dysfunction (SOLVD) database showed that the use of potassium decreasing diuretics was associated with excess mortality from sudden arrhythmic death.[29] This was not the case with potassium-sparing diuretics.

Angiotensin-converting enzyme (ACE) inhibitors have been studied extensively and have shown a clear benefit on survival in patients with heart failure and in those with depressed EF (<40%) after myocardial infarction. In the SOLVD Treatment trial, patients with heart failure treated with enalapril showed a decrease in progression of heart failure mortality but no effect on sudden death mortality.[30]

In contrast, in the Trandolapril Cardiac Evaluation (TRACE)[31] (Fig. 31–3), Acute Infarction and Ramipril Efficacy (AIRE),[32] and Heart Outcome Prevention Evaluation (HOPE)[33] trials, sudden death mortality was reduced with the use of trandolapril and ramipril. These differences may be explained on the

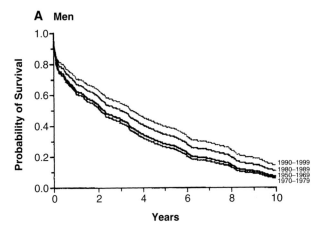

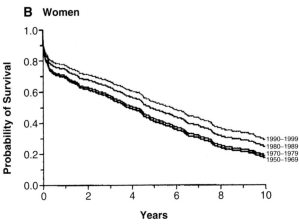

■ **Figure 31–2** Temporal trends in age-adjusted survival of heart failure among men *(A)* and women *(B)*. *(From Levy D, Kenchaiah S, Larson MG, et al: Long-term trends in the incidence of and survival with heart failure. N Engl J Med 347:1397–1402, 2002, with permission.)*

basis of variable tissue penetration among the drugs. Other antiarrhythmic properties include antisympathetic activity, attenuation of mechanical and electrical remodeling, and unloading.

Angiotensin II receptor blockers (ARB) have been compared with ACE inhibitors in patients with heart failure and myocardial infarction. Although there was no difference in total mortality, there was a trend in the reduction of sudden death favoring the ACE inhibitor captopril compared with losartan, a member of ARB.[34] Similarly, in patients with acute myocardial infarction and heart failure, captopril was better than losartan in reducing sudden death.[35]

β-Blockers, once feared, are now mandated therapy in patients with heart failure, even in the most severe cases. It is well known that sympathetic stimulation enhances progression of heart failure and arrhythmogenesis. Therefore, it is not surprising that trials involving β-blockers and heart failure have shown a substantial reduction in deaths from both sudden cardiac death and heart failure (Fig. 31–4).[3-6] With down-regulation of β_1 receptors, there are some data suggesting that the use of a nonselective β-blocker is preferred. In the Carvedilol or Metoprolol European Trial (COMET),[36] there were less total and sudden deaths with the use of carvedilol compared with metoprolol. Notably, in the Cardiac Insufficiency Bisoprolol Study (CIBIS) II trial,[37] whereas patients with sinus rhythm benefited from bisoprolol versus placebo, those in atrial fibrillation did not. The authors speculated that this was not related to a heart rate difference, but perhaps to hypotension caused by the active medication in the atrial fibrillation group.

TABLE 31–1 Total Pump Failure and Sudden Death Mortality Rates in Systolic and Diastolic Heart Failure and in Nonischemic Systolic Heart Failure with Implantable Cardioverter-Defibrillator

Study (Active Treatment Arm)	n	Mean Follow-up (months)	TM (%)	PF (%)	SCD (%)
Systolic Heart Failure					
CIBIS II[4]	1327	15	12	23	31
MERIT-HF[5]	1990	12	7.2	21	54
BEST[6]	1354	24	30	30	44
CARVEDILOL (severe heart failure)[7]	1156	10.4	11.4	NA	NA
EPHESUS[8]	3319	16	14.4	22	34
Val-HeFT[9]	816	23	11.9	16	62
Heart Failure with Preserved LV Function					
Val-HeFT II (ACEI arm)[10]	103	30	17	39	17
CHARM[14]	1514	36.6	11.2*	NA	NA
ICD Trials in Systolic Heart Failure (Nonischemic)					
CAT[45]	50	66	25	NA	0
AMIOVERT[40] (ICD arm)	51	26.4	11.8	50	17
DEFINITE[47] (ICD arm)	229	26	10	30	13

*Cardiovascular death.
ACEI, angiotensin-converting enzyme inhibitor; AMIOVERT, Amiodarone versus Implantable Cardioverter-Defibrillator; BEST, Bucindolol Estimation of Survival Trial; CARVEDILOL, Carvedilol Prospective Randomized Cumulative Survival Study; CAT, Cardiomyopathy Trial; CHARM, Candesartan Cilexetil [Atacand] in Heart Failure Assessment of Reduction Mortality and Morbidity; CIBIS, Cardiac Insufficiency Bisoprolol Study; DEFINITE, Defibrillators in Non-Ischemic Cardiomyopathy Treatment Evaluation; EPHESUS, Eplerenone Post-Acute Myocardial Infarction Heart Failure Efficacy and Survival Study; ICD, Implantable cardioverter-defibrillator; MERIT-HF, Metoprolol Randomized Intervention Trial in Congestive Heart Failure; NA, not available; PF, pump failure; SCD, sudden cardiac death; TM, total mortality; Val-HeFT, Valsartan Heart Failure Trial.

Aldosterone receptor antagonists have been studied in patients with heart failure and have shown benefit in reducing all-cause and sudden death mortality. Such benefits could be related to improvements in electrolyte imbalances, reduction in myocardial fibrosis, and attenuation of the sympathetic nervous system. Although the Randomized Aldactone (spironolactone) Evaluation Study for Congestive Heart Failure (RALES) trial[38] studied only patients with NYHA Class III and IV heart failure, the Eplerenone Post-Acute Myocardial Infarction Heart Failure Efficacy and Survival Study (EPHESUS) trial[39] included patients with myocardial infarction and lesser degrees of heart failure.

Ventricular arrhythmias, documented by ambulatory ECG recordings, often are seen in patients with

TABLE 31–2   Identifying Individuals at High Risk

NYHA functional class	T-wave alternans
Ejection fraction	Baroreflex sensitivity
Electrocardiogram: AF, NSVT, QRS, HR	Signal-averaged electrocardiogram
Chest radiograph: heart size	QT dispersion, QT dynamics
Norepinephrine, brain natriuretic peptide levels	Electrophysiologic study

AF, atrial fibrillation; HR, heart rate; NSVT, nonsustained ventricular tachycardia; NYHA, New York Heart Association.

TABLE 31–3   Pharmacologic and Nonpharmacologic Therapies

Pharmacologic
Digoxin
β-Blockers
Angiotensin-converting enzyme inhibitors
Angiotensin receptor blockers
Aldosterone receptor blockers
Diuretics
Antiarrhythmics

Nonpharmacologic
Biventricular pacing
Implantable cardioverter-defibrillator

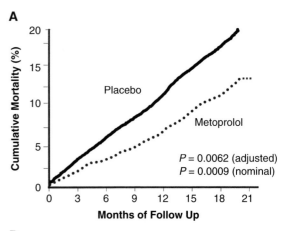

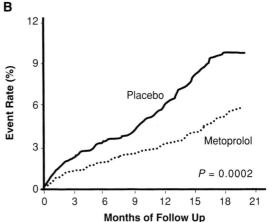

■ **Figure 31–4** Kaplan-Meier plot of total (A) and sudden death (B) mortality.[5]

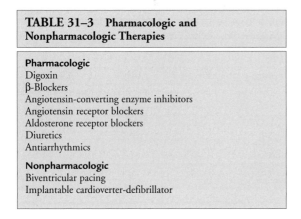

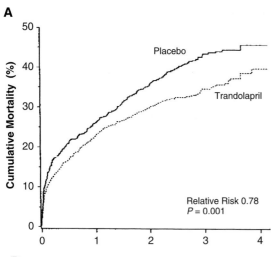

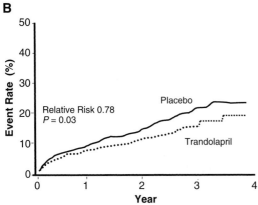

■ **Figure 31–3** Kaplan-Meier plot of total (A) and sudden death (B) mortality. (From Kober L, Torp-Pedersen C, Carlsen JE, et al, for the Trandolapril Cardiac Evaluation [TRACE] Study Group: A clinical trial of the angiotensin-converting enzyme inhibitor trandolapril in patients with left ventricular dysfunction after myocardial infarction. N Engl J Med 333:1670–1676, 1995, with permission.)

heart failure.[15] Almost 50% will have nonsustained VT. The mechanisms responsible for such arrhythmias may include re-entry, triggered activity, abnormal automaticity, and activation of stretch channels. Attempts have been made to suppress these arrhythmias with the use of antiarrhythmic drugs. However, with the exception of the β-blockers, there has been no survival benefit. In fact, the most potent sodium channel blockers—flecainide and propafenone—caused more harm than good.[40,41] Although there was a reduction in all-cause mortality and sudden death in patients with heart failure with amiodarone in the Argentinian Study Group for Prevention of Cardiac Insufficiency (GESICA) trial,[42] there was no such benefit in the Survival Trial of Antiarrhythmic

Therapy in Congestive Heart Failure (CHF-STAT) trial.[15]

In summary, it is clear that ACE inhibitors, β-blockers, and aldosterone receptor blockers are effective not only in reducing sudden arrhythmic death, but reducing all-cause mortality as well. These drugs also have pronounced direct effects on hemodynamics, reducing load, and/or cardiac contractility, but it is not currently clear to what extent these mechanical effects play a role in reduction of "electrophysiologic" mortality. In contrast, the sodium, calcium, and potassium channel blockers (which primarily target electrophysiology, rather than mechanics) have failed to show benefit and, in some instances, show harm.

Device Therapy

The implantable cardioverter-defibrillator (ICD) is effective in improving survival in patients who endured cardiac arrest and in those with hemodynamically intolerable VT, especially with reduced EF.[43] The results of Multicenter Unsustained Tachycardia Trial (MUSTT)[44] showed that patients with CAD, EF less than 40%, and electrophysiologically induced sustained VT had less arrhythmic death when treated with an ICD compared with no therapy or electrophysiologically guided antiarrhythmic therapy. In the Multicenter Automatic Defibrillator Implantation Trial I (MADIT I),[45] patients with CAD, EF of 35% or less, and inducible sustained VT after drug failure were randomized to conventional medical therapy or ICD. The ICD group had a marked reduction in arrhythmic death: 33% in the medical treatment arm versus 5% in the ICD arm. MADIT II[46] randomly assigned patients with CAD with an EF of 30% or less to ICD versus conventional medical therapy. This trial was terminated early because of a 30% relative risk reduction in total mortality. Despite a high-risk population with reduced EF and abnormal signal-averaged ECG, the ICD was not found to be superior to standard therapy in patients undergoing coronary bypass surgery.[47] This was primarily because of a low incidence of sudden cardiac death, the implication being that coronary revascularization is protective.[48]

It is clear from these studies that in individuals at high risk for sudden arrhythmic death, the ICD offers

protection. Of interest, Mitchell and colleagues[49] reviewed the mechanism of death in 320 patients who received the ICD and found that 28% were still classified as sudden. Electromechanical dissociation was common (Fig. 31–5). In patients with nonischemic cardiomyopathy, the role of the ICD is less convincing. In the cardiomyopathy trial (CAT),[50] patients with dilated nonischemic cardiomyopathy were randomized to ICD or a control group. After a mean follow-up of 5.5 years, there was no significant difference in survival.

In the Amiodarone versus Implantable Cardioverter-Defibrillator (AMIOVIRT) trial, the ICD was not found to be superior to amiodarone with respect to all-cause mortality and sudden death.[51] Defibrillators in Nonischemic Cardiomyopathy Treatment Evaluation (DEFINITE), a recently completed trial, showed a reduction in arrhythmic death, as well as a trend toward reduction in total mortality with the use of the ICD in patients with nonischemic dilated cardiomyopathy.[52] In this trial, patients with an EF less than 36% and premature ventricular contraction or nonsustained VT were randomly assigned to either standard medical therapy or an ICD. At 2 years, mortality in the control arm was 13.8% versus 8.1% in the ICD arm ($P = 0.06$). There was a 74% relative reduction in arrhythmic death in the ICD arm ($P < 0.05$). The results of the Sudden Cardiac Death in Heart Failure Trial (SCD-HeFT) were released at the Annual American College of Cardiology Scientific Meeting in

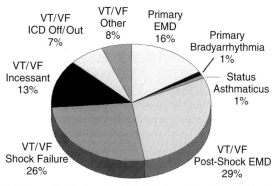

■ **Figure 31–5** Frequency distribution of sudden death in patients with implantable cardioverter-defibrillator (ICD).[49] EMD, electromechanical dissociation; VF, ventricular fibrillation; VT, ventricular tachycardia.

March 2004. In this primary prevention trial, patients with heart failure and EF less than 35% were randomly assigned to ICD, amiodarone, or placebo. Whereas amiodarone provided neither benefit nor harm over placebo, the ICD was associated with a 23% relative risk reduction in total mortality ($P = 0.007$). This was primarily because of a reduction in sudden arrhythmic death. Also presented at this meeting were the results of the Defibrillation in Acute Myocardial Infarction Trial (DINAMIT). Patients (n = 674) with acute myocardial infarction, depressed EF (<35%), and decreased heart rate variability were assigned to ICD or conventional therapy. There was no difference in all-cause mortality, but the ICD significantly reduced sudden arrhythmic death ($P = 0.009$).

Cardiac resynchronization therapy (CRT) is a relatively new therapeutic modality developed to improve myocardial contractility in patients with congestive heart failure and bundle branch block on the ECG. Although early studies suggested hemodynamic improvements, the recently reported Comparison of Medical Therapy, Pacing and Defibrillation in Chronic Heart Failure (COMPANION) trial demonstrated a mortality benefit only when CRT was combined with ICD therapy.[53]

LINK TO MECHANO-ELECTRIC FEEDBACK

It is clear that the ICD reduces sudden cardiac death in patients with heart failure. In SCD-HeFT and DEFI-NITE, it seems that the ICD also provides protection. Thus, the failing overloaded ventricular myocardium must have been the substrate for fatal tachyarrhythmias that were successfully aborted by the ICD in a significant number of patients. Chronic heart failure with its accompanying volume overload is characterized by ventricular remodeling (the "bad" kind) and involves down-regulation of β receptors, increased sympathetic tone, apoptosis and/or fibrotic replacement of myocardial cells, up-regulation of the renin-angiotensin system, electrolyte imbalance, and other "adaptive" mechanisms.

All of these could contribute to the arrhythmogenic substrate or provide arrhythmogenic triggers.

Certainly, a direct electrophysiologic and arrhythmic effect of increased ventricular loading cannot be ruled out in the genesis of fatal arrhythmias in patients with heart failure. It is a common (albeit not systematically studied) observation in the cardiac intensive care unit that acute volume or pressure overload (e.g., during hypertensive crisis) can precipitate VT or ventricular fibrillation (VF).

Ventricular unloading by aggressive diuresis or afterload reduction often promptly acquiesces these arrhythmias. Thus, it can be surmised that stretch-related mechanisms play a role in the load-dependent recurring tachyarrhythmias, which, in patients with ICD, often are successfully aborted.

Summary

Heart failure may be related to either systolic or diastolic dysfunction. The cause is generally classified as ischemic or nonischemic. Death is usually caused by pump failure or sudden fatal arrhythmias. Sudden arrhythmic death is caused by either a tachyarrhythmia or a bradyarrhythmia, the latter being more common in end-stage heart failure. Pharmacologic and non-pharmacologic therapies have made major impacts on how to manage these patients. Future trials should also direct efforts at discerning the specific role of volume or pressure overload in the genesis of fatal arrhythmias in patients with chronic heart failure.

References

1. Luu M, Stevenson WG, Stevenson LW, et al: Diverse mechanism of unexpected cardiac arrest in advanced heart failure. Circulation 80:1675–1680, 1989.
2. Ho K, Pinsky J, Kannel W, Levy D: The epidemiology of heart failure: The Framingham Study. J Am Coll Cardiol 22(suppl A):6A–13A, 1993.
3. Levy D, Kenchaiah S, Larson MG, et al: Long-term trends in the incidence of and survival with heart failure. N Engl J Med 347:1397–1402, 2002.
4. CIBIS II Investigators and Committees: The Cardiac Insufficiency Bisoprolol Study II (CIBIS II): A randomized trial. Lancet 353:9–13, 1999.
5. Hjalmarson A, Goldstein S, Fagerberg B, et al, for the MERIT-HF Study Group: Effects of controlled-release metoprolol on total mortality, hospitalizations, and well-being in patients with heart failure: The Metroprolol CR/XL Randomized Intervention Trial in Congestive Heart Failure. JAMA 283: 1295–1302, 2000.

6. The Beta-Blocker Evaluation of Survival Trial Investigators: A trial of the beta-blocker bucindolol in patients with advanced chronic heart failure. N Engl J Med 344:1659–1667, 2001.

7. Packer M, Coats AJ, Fowler MB, et al, for the Carvedilol Prospective Randomized Cumulative Survival Study Group: Effect of carvedilol on survival in severe chronic heart failure. N Engl J Med 344:1651–1658, 2001.

8. Pitt B, Remme W, Zannad F, et al, for the Eplerenone Post-Acute Myocardial Infarction Heart Failure Efficacy and Survival Study Investigators: Eplerenone, a selective aldosterone blocker, in patients with left ventricular dysfunction after myocardial infarction. N Engl J Med 348:1309–1321, 2003.

9. Cohn JN, O'Connor C, Opasich C, et al: Prognosis and mechanism of death in treated heart failure: Data from the placebo arm of Val-HeFT [abstract]. Circulation 17:2730, 2003.

10. Carson P, Johnson G, Fletcher R, Cohn J: Mild systolic dysfunction in heart failure (left ventricular ejection fraction >35%): Baseline characteristics, prognosis and response to therapy in the vasodilator in heart failure trials (V-HeFT). J Am Coll Cardiol 27:642–649, 1996.

11. Levy D, Garrison RJ, Savage DD, et al: Prognostic implications of echocardiographically determined left ventricular mass in the Framingham Heart Study. N Eng J Med 322:1561–1566, 1990.

12. Tomaselli GF, Beuckelmann DJ, Calkin HG, et al: Sudden death in heart failure: The role of abnormal repolarization. Circulation 90:2534–2539, 1994.

13. Franz M: Stretch activated arrhythmias. In Zipes DP, Jalife J (eds): Cardiac Electrophysiology: From Cell to Bedside. Philadelphia, WB Saunders, 1995, p 592.

14. Yusuf S, Pfeffer MA, Swedberg K, et al: Effects of candesartan in patients with chronic heart failure and preserved left-ventricular ejection fraction: The CHARM-Preserved Trial. Lancet 362:777–781, 2003.

15. Singh SN, Fletcher RD, Fisher SG, et al, for the Survival Trial of Antiarrhythmic Therapy in Congestive Heart Failure: Amiodarone in patients with congestive heart failure and asymptomatic ventricular arrhythmia. N Engl J Med 333: 77–82, 1995.

16. Dries DL, Exner DV, Gersh BJ, et al: Atrial fibrillation is associated with an increased risk for mortality and heart failure progression in patients with asymptomatic and symptomatic left ventricular systolic dysfunction: A retrospective analysis of the SOLVD trials. J Am Coll Cardiol 32:695–703, 1998.

17. Singh SN, Fisher SG, Carson PE, Fletcher RD: Prevalence and significance of nonsustained ventricular tachycardia in patients with premature ventricular contractions and heart failure treated with vasodilator therapy. J Am Coll Cardiol 32: 942–947, 1998.

18. Doval HC, Nul DR, Grancelli HO, et al: Nonsustained ventricular tachycardia in severe heart failure. Independent marker of increased mortality due to sudden death. Circulation 94: 3198–3203, 1996.

19. Iuliano S, Fisher SG, Karasik PE, et al: QRS duration and mortality in patients with congestive heart failure. Am Heart J 143: 1085–1091, 2002.

20. Nul DR, Doval HC, Grancelli HO, et al: Heart rate is a marker of amiodarone mortality reduction in severe heart failure. Circulation 92(suppl I):I-666, 1995.

21. Brendorp B, Elming H, Jun L, et al: QT dispersion has no prognostic information for patients with advanced congestive heart failure and reduced left ventricular systolic function. Circulation 103:831–835, 2001.

22. Barr CS, Naas A, Freeman M, et al: QT dispersion and sudden unexpected death in chronic heart failure. Lancet 343:327–329, 1994.

23. LaRovere MT, Pinna GD, Maestri R, et al: Short-term heart rate variability strongly predicts sudden cardiac death in chronic heart failure patients. Circulation 107:565–570, 2003.

24. Bilchick KC, Fetics B, Djoukeng R, et al: Prognostic value of heart rate variability in chronic congestive heart failure (Veterans Affairs' Survival Trial of Antiarrhythmic Therapy in Congestive Heart Failure). Am J Cardiol 90:24–28, 2002.

25. Stevenson WG, Stevenson LW, Weiss J, Tillisch JH: Inducible ventricular arrhythmias and sudden death during vasodilator therapy of severe heart failure. Am Heart J 116:1447–1454, 1988.

26. The Digitalis Investigation Group: The effect of digoxin on mortality and morbidity in patients with heart failure. N Engl J Med 336:525–533, 1997.

27. Rathore SS, Curtis JP, Wang Y, et al: Association of serum digoxin concentration and outcomes in patients with heart failure. JAMA 289:871–878, 2003.

28. Rathore SS, Wang Y, Krumholz HM: Sex-based differences in the effect of digoxin for the treatment of heart failure. N Engl J Med 347:1403–1411, 2002.

29. Cooper HA, Dries DL, Davis CE, et al: Diuretics and risk of arrhythmic death in patients with left ventricular dysfunction. Circulation 100:1311–1315, 1999.

30. The SOLVD Investigators: Effect of enalapril on survival in patients with reduced left ventricular ejection fractions and congestive heart failure. N Engl J Med 325:293–302, 1991.

31. Kober L, Torp-Pedersen C, Carlsen JE, et al, for the Trandolapril Cardiac Evaluation (TRACE) Study Group: A clinical trial of the angiotensin-converting enzyme inhibitor trandolapril in patients with left ventricular dysfunction after myocardial infarction. N Engl J Med 333:1670–1676, 1995.

32. Cleland JGF, Erhardt L, Murray G, et al, on behalf of the AIRE Study Investigators: Effect of ramipril on morbidity and mode of death among survivors of acute myocardial infarction with clinical evidence of heart failure. A report from the AIRE Study Investigators. Eur Heart J 18:41–51, 1997.

33. The Heart Outcomes Prevention Evaluation Study Investigators: Effects of an angiotensin-converting-enzyme inhibitor, ramipril, on cardiovascular events in high-risk patients. N Engl J Med 342:145–153, 2000.

34. Pitt B, Poole-Wilson PA, Segal R, et al: Randomized trial of losartan versus captopril on mortality in patients with symptomatic heart failure: The losartan heart failure survival study, ELITE II. Lancet 355:1582–1587, 2000.

35. Dickstein K, Kjekshus J, and the OPTIMAAL Steering Committee for the OPTIMAAL Study Group: Effects of losartan and captopril on mortality and morbidity in high-risk patients after acute myocardial infarction: The OPTIMAAL randomized trial. Lancet 360:752–760, 2002.

36. Poole-Wilson PA, Swedberg K, Cleland JG, et al, for the Comet: Comparison of carvedilol and metroprolol on clinical outcomes in patients with chronic heart failure in the carvedilol or metoprolol European trial (COMET): Randomized controlled trial. Lancet 362:7–12, 2003.

37. Lechat P, Hulot JS, Escolano S, et al: Heart rate and cardiac rhythm relationships with bisoprolol benefit in chronic heart failure in CIBIS II Trial. Circulation 103:1428–1433, 2001.

38. Pitt B, Zannad F, Reme WJ, et al, for the Randomized Aldactone Evaluation Study Investigators: The effect of spironolactone on morbidity and mortality in patients with severe heart failure. N Engl J Med 341:709–717, 1999.

39. Pitt B, Remme W, Zannad R, et al, for the Eplerenone Post-Acute Myocardial Infarction Heart Failure Efficacy and Survival Study Investigators: Eplerenone, a selective aldosterone blocker, in patients with left ventricular dysfunction after myocardial infarction. N Engl J Med 348:1309–1319, 2003.

40. The Cardiac Arrhythmia Suppression Trial (CAST) Investigators: Preliminary report. Effect of encainide and flecainide on mortality in a randomized trial of arrhythmia suppression after myocardial infarction. N Engl J Med 321:406–412, 1989.

41. Siebels J, Cappato R, Ruppel R, et al: ICD versus drugs in cardiac arrest survivors: Preliminary results of the cardiac arrest study Hamburg. Pacing Clin Electrophysiol 16:552–558, 1993.

42. Doval HC, Nul DR, Cancelli HO, et al: Randomized trial of low-dose amiodarone in severe congestive heart failure. Lancet 344:493–498, 1994.

43. A comparison of antiarrhythmic therapy with implantable defibrillators in patients resuscitated from near fatal arrhythmias. The antiarrhythmics versus implantable defibrillators (AVID) Investigators. N Eng J Med 337:1576–1583, 1997.

44. Buxton AE, Lee KE, Fisher JD, et al: A randomized study of the prevention of sudden death in patients with coronary disease. Multicenter Unsustained Tachycardia Trial Investigators. N Eng J Med 341:1882–1890, 1999.

45. Moss AJ, Hall WJ, Cannom DS, et al: Improved survival with an implanted defibrillator in patients with coronary disease at high risk for ventricular arrhythmia. Multicenter Automatic Defibrillator Implantation Trial Investigators. N Engl J Med 335:1933–1940, 1996.

46. Moss AJ, Zareba W, Hall WJ, et al, for the Multicenter Automatic Defibrillator Implantation Trial II Investigators: Prophylactic implantation or a defibrillator in patients with myocardial infarction and reduced ejection fraction. N Engl J Med 346:877–882, 2002.

47. Bigger JT, for the Coronary Artery Bypass Graft (CABG) Patch Trial Investigators: Prophylactic use of implanted cardiac defibrillators in patients with high risk for ventricular arrhythmias after coronary artery bypass graft surgery. N Engl J Med 337:1569–1575, 1997.

48. Bigger JT, Whang W, Rottman JN, et al: Mechanisms of death in the CABG Patch trial: A randomized trial of implantable cardiac defibrillator prophylaxis in patients at high risk of death after coronary artery bypass graft surgery. Circulation 99:1416–1421, 2000.

49. Mitchell LB, Pineda EA, Titus JL, et al: Sudden death in patients with implantable cardioverter defibrillators. J Am Coll Cardiol 39:1323–1328, 2002.

50. Bansch D, Antz M, Boczor S, et al, for the CAT Investigators: Primary prevention of sudden cardiac death in idiopathic dilated cardiomyopathy: The Cardiomyopathy Trial (CAT). Circulation 105:1453–1458, 2002.

51. Strickberger SA, Hummel JD, Bartlett TG, et al, for the AMIOVIRT Investigators: Amiodarone versus implantable cardioverter-defibrillator: Randomized trial in patients with nonischemic dilated cardiomyopathy and asymptomatic nonsustained ventricular tachycardia-AMIOVIRT. J Am Coll Cardiol 41:1707–1712, 2003.

52. Kadish A: Defibrillators in non-ischemic cardiomyopathy treatment evaluation (DEFINITE). Presented at the American Heart Association Scientific Meeting, Orlando, 9–12 November 2003.

53. Bristow MR: Cardiac resynchronization therapy (CRT) reduces hospitalization and CRT with ICD reduced mortality in chronic heart failure: The COMPANION Trial. Presented at the American Heart Association Scientific Meeting, Orlando, 9–12 November 2003.

CHAPTER 32

Wall Stress and Arrhythmogenesis in Patients with Left Ventricular Hypertrophy, Dilation, or Both

• • • •

Abdulhalim Salim Serafi and John Vann Jones

Sudden cardiac death (SCD) accounts for 10% to 15% of all deaths in the Western world, with ventricular arrhythmias as the major cause of SCD (World Health Organization Report on SCD, 1985). Despite much attention to this subject, the problem of ventricular arrhythmia remains one of the most fascinating challenges of modern cardiology. The role of wall stress in the pathogenesis of ventricular arrhythmia is under intense investigation. The concept of wall stress is not difficult, although the factors on which it is dependent are complex. Wall stress refers to the amount of tension existing within the myocardial wall at any given moment. Therefore, wall stress refers to the amount of tension exerted on each individual myocardial cell. Wall stress continuously varies throughout the cardiac cycle. Systolic and diastolic components of wall stress are referred to by some researchers as afterload and preload, respectively.

WALL STRESS

The factors that determine ventricular wall stress include ventricular cavity size, myocardial wall thickness, and intraventricular pressure; their relation is governed by the Law of Laplace.[1] This law describes the relation among internal pressure, size, and surface tension in thin-walled hollow vessels and spheres. The Law of Laplace is best exemplified by its characterization of the behavior of soap bubbles and can be described as follows: $T = (P \times R)/2$, where T is surface tension, P is pressure inside the bubble, and R is the internal radius.[2]

Despite that the heart is neither thin-walled nor a perfect sphere, Wood[3] was able to show that the Law

of Laplace could be applied to many hollow viscera, including the heart. In its simplest form, the Laplace equation can be used to calculate the surface tension within the heart, but the thickness of the heart wall means that this calculated "tension," expressed as force per unit length, will be representative only for a specific location within the ventricular wall (e.g., using the ventricular cavity radius for the endocardium). The involvement of radius can be explained by considering the curvature of the wall. As the radius increases, curvature decreases; consequently, a smaller component of the wall tension is angled toward the center of the cavity, generating less pressure. This means that the curvature of the ventricular wall determines how effectively the active wall tension is converted into intraventricular pressure.

There are many causes that lead to increased wall stress, such as hypertension, aortic valve disease, left ventricular aneurysm, and heart failure (Fig. 32–1).

Mean tension is, in fact, dispersed throughout the width of the heart wall, and it has the units of force per unit area (wall stress). The relation between tension and wall stress can be described as follows: mean tension = stress × wall thickness.[4] This leads to a modified Laplace equation: $WS = (P \times R)/2(TH)$, where WS represents wall stress, P represents intraventricular pressure, R represents cavity radius, and TH represents wall thickness.

Because the heart is, in fact, widely accepted as most closely resembling a prolate spheroid, applying the simple spherical formula will result in an 8% error. Although many factors may affect the calculation of wall stress, such as fibrosis, left ventricular dilation, left ventricular hypertrophy (LVH), or cardiomyopathy

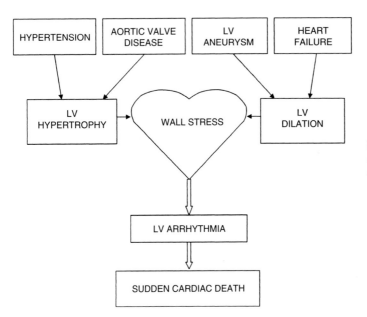

■ **Figure 32–1** Causes of increased wall stress and risk for ventricular arrhythmia. LV, left ventricular.

and hypertension, it is still a useful estimate and can be used as a rough guide to actual wall stress.

There are many difficulties in calculating actual wall stress in the heart. Wall stress is not a fixed number, but rather a continuous function of the spatial position within the wall. However, regardless of actual values, the Laplace equation does show first-order relations among intraventricular pressure, cavity size, wall thickness, and wall stress; therefore, it is possible to make qualitative assessments of the relation between wall stress and ventricular arrhythmias.

Some studies have shown that peak systolic wall stress represents one of the major determinants of myocardial oxygen consumption and ventricular performance, and that it closely relates to the degree of LVH.[5] Other studies have shown that the mortality rates of coronary heart disease are increased among patients with dilated and poorly contracting left ventricles when compared with patients with more normal left ventricular function.[6]

ISCHEMIC HEART DISEASE

There are many factors that contribute to the pathogenesis of ventricular arrhythmia, including ischemic heart disease, which is one of the most common causes of ventricular arrhythmia, especially during the acute stages of myocardial infarction.

For instance, Weaver and colleagues[7] studied survivors of SCD and found that 75% of victims had significant coronary artery disease, although only 20% had more than single-vessel disease and almost half (48%) had an ejection fraction in excess of 50%. Severity of coronary heart disease has not been shown to correlate with occurrence of, or survival from, SCD in the absence of left ventricular dysfunction.[8]

Increased wall stress is an inevitable accompaniment of myocardial dysfunction that plays an important role in the pathogenesis of ventricular arrhythmia.[9] Increased wall stress is known to reduce myocardial performance, and this could be the cause of ventricular arrhythmia due to reduced myocardial function.[10] The Laplace effect and Frank–Starling mechanism act in opposition in myocardial dysfunction. The most important role of the Frank–Starling mechanism is to balance the output of right and left ventricles. Distension of the ventricle increases its contractile force through the Frank–Starling mechanism but reduces the pressure generated by a given force through Laplace's law, thereby reducing mechanical efficiency. In a healthy heart, the gain in contractile energy on the ascending limb of the Starling curve equalizes the Laplace effect. This is not the case, however, in impaired left ventricular function. If right ventricular output starts to exceed left ventricular output, the increase in pulmonary blood volume raises the pressure in pulmonary veins, which increases the filling of the left ventricle, leading to pulmonary congestion and edema.

AORTIC VALVE DISEASE

Patients with symptomatic aortic stenosis have a high prevalence of ventricular arrhythmias before surgery.[11] Arrhythmias in aortic valve disease have been closely linked with left ventricular dysfunction.[12] Arrhythmias are prevalent in both aortic stenosis and aortic incompetence.[13] Aortic stenosis and aortic incompetence are causes of increased wall stress,[14] although by different mechanisms—that is, aortic stenosis by increased intraventricular pressure, and aortic incompetence by left ventricular dilation.

Several studies have shown a decreased incidence of ventricular arrhythmias after aortic valve replacement.[15] Olshausen and colleagues[16] have shown that after aortic valve replacement, improvement in left ventricular function will lead to remarkable reduction in ventricular arrhythmias; this result suggests that when wall stress is relieved, electrophysiology improves.

Rials and colleagues[17] studied the effect of LVH and its regression on ventricular electrophysiology and vulnerability to inducible arrhythmia in the feline heart. They concluded that LVH caused by aortic stenosis in this animal model produces multiple electro-physiologic abnormalities and increased vulnerability to inducible polymorphic ventricular arrhythmia. Cats that show regression of hypertrophy have normal ventricular electrophysiology and have the same low vulnerability to inducible ventricular arrhythmia as sham animals.

Other studies have shown significant regression of LVH after aortic valve replacement in humans.[18] Klein[19] studied the causes of arrhythmias in 102 patients with aortic valve disease. He found that, in the absence of concomitant coronary artery disease, complex arrhythmias were significantly more prevalent in patients with valve disease than in control subjects (40 of 102 vs. 19 of 102). In patients with valve disease without coronary artery disease, complex arrhythmias were significantly more common than in control subjects, even in the presence of coronary artery disease (22 of 65 vs. 4 of 64). In the presence of coronary artery disease, however, no difference in the prevalence of complex arrhythmias was observed between the groups. Klein concluded that among patients with aortic stenosis or aortic regurgitation, arrhythmia occurrence and grade of ventricular ectopic activity were not related to either the degree of aortic stenosis or aortic regurgitation, ventricular hemodynamics, or the presence or absence of concomitant coronary artery disease.

Although it is not surprising that patients with valvular lesions resulting in pressure or volume overload of the myocardium would demonstrate ventricular arrhythmias, the pathophysiologic mechanisms underlying ectopic activity are unclear. In aortic stenosis, coronary artery disease is not associated with a greater incidence of complex arrhythmias, suggesting that myocardial ischemia resulting solely from impaired coronary blood flow is not the primary mechanism involved. The interrelation of increased myocardial mass, degree of ventricular dilation, and ventricular wall stress could be the most important factor.

LEFT VENTRICULAR HYPERTROPHY

To calculate dynamic events in the myocardium throughout the cardiac cycle, the measurement of left ventricular wall thickness has been related to chamber dimensions and pressure. In chronic heart disease, the left ventricular mass has been compared with chamber size, mechanical work, wall forces, and ventricular function in an effort to understand the mechanism of cardiac hypertrophy.

LVH is a compensatory mechanism for ventricular overload and is an independent predictor of cardiovascular morbidity. LVH is either caused by pressure or volume overload.[20] It most often occurs with hypertension, aortic stenosis, and hypertrophic cardiomyopathy. Patients with LVH have a greater rate of cardiac arrhythmias and sudden death, with an incidence of up to 10-fold that of individuals without LVH.[21] Most studies have shown that echocardiographic LVH is associated with ventricular arrhythmia in the presence of other factors such as increased left ventricular mass[22] and electrolyte imbalance (e.g., in potassium and magnesium).[23,24]

Aronow and colleagues[25] observed a hypertensive geriatric population without documented coronary artery disease for an average of 27 months. They showed that patients with LVH were significantly more likely to experience ventricular fibrillation and sudden death than people without LVH (31% vs. 10%).

The mechanisms responsible for the increased risk in patients with LVH are not clearly defined. Previous studies have documented high rates of adverse cardiovascular events in subjects with LVH.[26] Echocardiographic LVH also has been reported to be associated with increased risk for cardiovascular disease and all-cause mortality in hospital and clinical-based studies[27] and in population-based investigations.[28] LVH has been known to be a risk factor for SCD, ventricular arrhythmias, coronary artery disease, and heart failure.[29]

HYPERTENSION

Because increased wall stress is the primary cardiac abnormality in patients with hypertension, it would be expected that there will be an increase in the prevalence of ventricular arrhythmia in patients with hypertension. Treatment with potassium-depleting diuretics is a possible causative factor of ventricular arrhythmia and sudden death in patients with hypertension.[30]

Increased systolic blood pressure, a prime indicator of wall stress, is an adverse prognostic indicator for sudden death after infarction.[31] Other studies in patients with hypertension show that primary myocardial disease has an early latent asymptomatic stage, followed by a symptomatic hypertrophied stage that progresses to an irreversible stage of dilation where the prognosis is poor.[32] Mechanical stretch may have profound electrophysiologic effects in this context.[33]

In patients with hypertension, ventricular wall stress is likely to be a physiologically relevant stimulus, because labile blood pressure causes fluctuations in wall stress. There is evidence in humans that ventricular ectopics can be produced by acute increases in blood pressure.[34,35] Such a proarrhythmic effect is particularly likely in hearts with LVH, which have been

shown to be more susceptible to wall stress–induced arrhythmias than healthy hearts.[23,24]

Loaldi and colleagues[36] have shown that treatment that decreases wall stress in patients with hypertension can produce a parallel reduction in ventricular arrhythmias. They also found that patients with hypertension with compensatory hypertrophy had normal wall stress and, accordingly, no increase in ventricular arrhythmias, whereas those with left ventricular dilation and inadequate hypertrophy had greatly increased arrhythmias.

HEART FAILURE

The Law of Laplace and the effects of ventricular dilation on the mechanics and energetics of myocardial contraction are important factors in heart failure. In a ventricle of normal size during ejection, the average radius decreases significantly. Consequently, the effect of this decrease in diameter on wall tension usually is greater than the opposite effect of the increased pressure. The failing heart often is dilated, and Laplace's law becomes critical. In a dilated ventricle, both the relative and absolute decrease in average radius is much less during the ejection of an equal volume from a healthy heart. Therefore, in a markedly dilated ventricle, the average tension in the myocardial fibers may continue to increase from the beginning of ejection up to the peak systolic pressure.[37] Another finding in dilated ventricles is that the increased tension required to develop a given pressure decreases the rate of myocardial fiber shortening and reduction of ejection volume. Therefore, an important therapeutic goal in the management of heart failure is to reduce cardiac distension by use of diuretics, thereby improving the conversion of the contractile force into pressure.

LEFT VENTRICULAR ANEURYSM

Left ventricular aneurysm (LVA) is a serious complication of acute myocardial infarction that can lead to congestive heart failure, ventricular arrhythmia, and, rarely, thromboembolic events. The usual cause of LVA is acute occlusion of the left anterior descending coronary artery, with LVA formation in the distal part of the anterior wall and septum. LVA act according to the Law of Laplace.

Left ventricular wall tension increases with increasing LV diameter, intracavity pressure, and wall thinning. A large- and thin-walled aneurysm has high wall tension, poor coronary perfusion, and furthers dilation. The ultimate stage of LVA is enlargement, not only of the aneurysm, but of the global LV. Because the impaired LV can not generate high blood pressure, this imposes a limit on the increase in wall tension, protecting against further dilation and rupture that occurs infrequently. Ventricular arrhythmias arise in the border zone between viable and dead myocardium, particularly on the interventricular septum.

Aneurysmectomy and linear repair of LV using cardiopulmonary bypass was introduced by Cooley.[38] This remained the standard procedure until the mid-1980s, when the technique of endoventricular patch plasty (EVPP) gradually took over.[39] The operative goal is to correct the size and geometry of the left ventricle to reduce wall tension and paradoxical movement and to improve systolic function. Intracavitary thrombi are removed, and coronary artery bypass grafting (CABG) is usually performed.

Simple aneurysmectomy, with or without concomitant CABG, often fails to control ventricular arrhythmia, and it is hypothesized that EVPP can have an inherent antiarrhythmic effect.[40] EVPP can reduce wall tension on the interventricular septum and, by sewing the patch there, may act on the arrhythmia substrate like an endocardial excision or cryoablation, converting it to a homogeneous and nonarrhythmogenic scar.

Moreover, because much of the aneurysm sac is retained, EVPP facilities the use of an internal mammary artery graft to the left anterior descending coronary artery, which may be particularly important to improve septal perfusion.

DISCUSSION

The association between increased wall stress and spontaneous or induced ventricular arrhythmias has been documented in well-controlled experimental studies.[41] In clinical studies, increased or variable left ventricular wall stress is a risk factor for ventricular

arrhythmia and SCD.[42] An acute increase of intraventricular pressure or ventricular stretch causes an increase in wall stress that changes the electrophysiologic properties of the heart.[43]

Abnormal wall stress may also cause ventricular arrhythmias in healthy subjects. It has been shown that acute pressure change and wall stress lead to ventricular arrhythmias by affecting one or more of the electrophysiologic properties of the myocardium.[44] Although cardiac mechano-electric feedback has been under intensive study for many years, the precise electrophysiologic mechanisms responsible for ventricular arrhythmias associated with stretch have not been fully elucidated[45] (see Chapters 23, 34, and 36 for discussions on the role of pericardium, hemodynamic unloading, and pericardial constraints, respectively).

Conclusion

All the studies discussed here suggest that ventricular arrhythmias do not appear randomly, but rather depend on the condition of the heart—for example, LVH, LV dilation, LVA, or heart failure.

There is evidence that wall stress may play a role in the pathogenesis of ventricular arrhythmias, whether the underlying cardiac pathology is ischemic heart disease, aortic valve disease, or hypertension.

LV dilation may be responsible for provocation or enhancement of ventricular arrhythmia. The interrelations of increased myocardial mass, degree of ventricular dilation, and ventricular wall stress could be the most important factors in the pathogenesis of ventricular arrhythmias.[46,47]

References

1. Hood WP, Thomson WJ, Rackley CE, Rolett EL: Comparison of calculations of left ventricular wall stress in man from thin-walled and thick-walled ellipsoidal models. Circ Res 24: 575–582, 1969.
2. Horrobin D: The mechanism of breathing. In Horrobin D (ed): Medical Physiology and Biochemistry. London, Edward Arnold, 1968, pp 343–345.
3. Wood RN: A few applications of a physical theorem to membranes in the human body in a state of tension. J Anat Physiol 26:362–370, 1892.
4. Sandler H, Dodge HT: Left ventricular tension and stress in man. Circ Res 13:91–104, 1963.

5. Strauer BE, Beer K, Heitlinger K, Hofling B: Left ventricular systolic wall stress as a primary determinant of myocardial oxygen consumption: Comparative studies in patients with normal left ventricular function, with pressure and volume overload and with coronary heart disease. Basic Res Cardiol 72:301–308, 1977.

6. Bruschke AV, Proudfit WL, Sones FM: Progress study of 590 consecutive non surgical cases of coronary disease followed for 5-9 years. II. Ventriculographic and other correlation's. Circulation 47:1154–1163, 1973.

7. Weaver WD, Lorch GS, Alvarez HA, Cobb LA: Angiographic findings in survivors of sudden death and characteristics of recurrent sudden death [abstract]. Am J Cardiol 37:181, 1976.

8. Grande P, Pedersen A: Myocardial infarct size: Correlation with cardiac arrhythmias and sudden death. Eur Heart J 5:622–627, 1984.

9. James MA, Jones JV: Ventricular arrhythmia in newly presenting untreated hypertensive patients compared with a matched normal population. J Hypertens 7:409–415, 1989.

10. Gunther S, Grossman W: Determinants of ventricular function in pressure overload hypertrophy in man. Circulation 59:679–688, 1979.

11. Serafi AS, Vann Jones J: The relationship between QT dispersion, arrhythmia and left ventricular hypertrophy post aortic valve replacement in patients with aortic stenosis [abstract]. Presented to the British Cardiac Society, Glasgow, April 28, 2003 to May 1, 2003.

12. Schilling G, Finkbeiner T, Elberskirch P, et al: Incidence of ventricular arrhythmias in patients with aortic valve replacement [abstract]. Am J Cardiol 49:894, 1982.

13. Olshausen KV, Amann E, Hofmann M, et al: Ventricular arrhythmias before and late after aortic valve replacement. Am J Cardiol 53:142–146, 1984.

14. Quinones MA, Mokotoff DM, Nouri S, et al: Non-invasive quantification of left ventricular wall stress. Am J Cardiol 45:782–790, 1980.

15. Smith R, Grossman W, Johnson L, et al: Arrhythmias following cardiac valve replacement. Circulation 45:1018–1023, 1972.

16. Olshausen KV, Schwarz F, Apfelbach J, et al: Determinants of the incidence and severity of ventricular arrhythmias in aortic valve disease. Am J Cardiol 51:1103–1109, 1983.

17. Rials SJ, Wu Y, Ford N, et al: Effect of LVH and its regression on ventricular electrophysiology and vulnerability to inducible arrhythmia in the feline heart. Circulation 91:426–430, 1995.

18. Gaasch WH: Left ventricular radius to wall thickness ratio. Am J Cardiol 43:1189–1194, 1979.

19. Klein RC: Ventricular arrhythmias in aortic valve disease: Analysis of 102 patients. Am J Cardiol 53:1079–1083, 1984.

20. Colucci WS, Braunwald E: Pathophysiology of heart failure. In Braunwald F (ed): Heart Disease: A Textbook of Cardiovascular Medicine, 6th ed. Philadelphia, WB Saunders, 2001, pp 503–519.

21. Haider AW, Larson MG, Benjamin EJ, Levy D: Increased left ventricular mass and hypertrophy is associated with increased risk for sudden death. J Am Coll Cardiol 32:1454–1459, 1998.

22. Levy D, Anderson KM, Savage DD, et al: Risk of ventricular arrhythmia's in left ventricular hypertrophy: The Framingham Study. Am J Cardiol 60:560–565, 1987.

23. James MA, Jones JV: An interaction between LVH and potassium in hypertension. J Hypertens 5:1–4, 1991.

24. Evans SJ, Levi AJ, Jones JV: Wall stress induced arrhythmia is enhanced by low potassium and early ventricular hypertrophy in the working rat heart. Cardiovasc Res 29:555–562, 1995.

25. Aronow WS, Epstein S, Schwartz KS, et al: Correlation of complex ventricular arrhythmias detected by ambulatory electrocardiographic monitoring with echocardiographic left ventricular hypertrophy in persons older than 62 years in a long term health care facility. Am J Cardiol 60:85I–93I, 1987.

26. Levy D, Garrison RJ, Savage DD, et al: Prognostic implications of echocardiographically determined left ventricular mass in the Framingham Heart Study. N Engl J Med 322:1561–1566, 1990.

27. Casale PN, Devereux RB, Milner M, et al: Value of echocardiographic left ventricular mass in predicting cardiovascular morbid events in hypertensive men. Ann Intern Med 105:173–178, 1986.

28. Levy D: Left ventricular hypertrophy: Epidemiological insights from the Framingham Heart Study. Drugs 35(suppl 5):1–5, 1988.

29. Kannel WB, Cupples LA, D'Agostino RB: Sudden death risk in overt coronary heart disease: The Framingham Study. Am Heart J 113:799–804, 1987.

30. Moss AJ, Davis HT, DeCamilla J, Bayer LW: Ventricular ectopic beats and their relation to sudden and non-sudden cardiac death after myocardial infarction. Circulation 60:998–1003, 1979.

31. Messerli FH, Ventura HO, Elizardi DJ, et al: Hypertension and sudden death: Increased ventricular ectopic activity in left ventricular hypertrophy. Am J Med 77:18–22, 1984.

32. Hamby R, Catangay P, Apiado O, Khan A: Primary myocardial disease: Clinical haemodynamic and angiocardiographic correlates in 50 patients. Am J Cardiol 25:625–634, 1970.

33. Franz MR: Stretch-activated arrhythmias. In Zipes DP, Jalife J (eds): Cardiac Electrophysiology: From Cell to Bedside, 2nd ed. Philadelphia, WB Saunders, 1994, pp 597–606.

34. Sideris DA, Kontoyannis DA, Michalis L, et al: Acute changes in blood pressure as a cause of cardiac arrhythmias. Eur Heart J 8:45–52, 1987.

35. Taggart P, Sutton P, Lab MJ, et al: Effect of abrupt changes in ventricular loading on repolarization induced by transient aortic occlusion in humans. Am J Physiol 263:H816–H823, 1992.

36. Loaldi A, Pepi M, Agostini P, et al: Cardiac rhythm in hypertension assessed through 24 hour ambulatory electrocardiographic monitoring: Effects of load manipulation with atenolol, verapamil and nifedipine. Br Heart J 50:118–126, 1983.

37. Badeer HS: Current concepts on the pathogenesis of ventricular fibrillation soon after coronary occlusion. Am J Cardiol 11:709–713, 1963.

38. Cooley DA, Collins HA, Morris GC, Chapman DW: Ventricular aneurysm after myocardial infraction: Surgical excision with use of temporary cardiopulmonary bypass. JAMA 167:557–560, 1958.

39. Dor V, Saab M, Coste P, et al: Left ventricular aneurysm: A new surgical approach. Thorac Cardiovasc Surg 37:11–19, 1989.

40. Sinatra R, Macrina F, Braccio M, et al: Left ventricular aneurysmectomy: Comparison between two techniques; early and late results. Eur J Cardiothoracic Surg 12:291–297, 1997.

41. James MA, Jones J: Systolic wall stress and ventricular arrhythmia: The role of acute changes in blood pressure in the isolated working heart. Clin Sci 79:499–504, 1990.

42. Sideris DA, Kontoyannis DA, Michalis L, et al: Acute changes in blood pressure as a cause of cardiac arrhythmias. Eur Heart J 8:45–52, 1987.

43. Calkins H, Levine JH, Kass DA: Electrophysiological effect of varied rate and extent of acute in vivo left ventricular load increase. Cardiovasc Res 25:637–644, 1991.

44. Sideris DA, Toumanidis ST, Kostopulos K, et al: Effect of acute ventricular pressure changes on QRS duration. J Electrocardiol 27:199–202, 1994.

45. Tavi P, Laine M, Weckström M: Effect of gadolinium on stretch-induced changes in contraction and intracellular recorded action and after potentials of rat isolated atrium. Br J Pharmacol 118:407–413, 1996.

46. Jones JV, Serafi AS, James MA: Wall stress and the heart. J Cardiovasc Risk 7:159–161, 2000.

47. Serafi AS, Evans SJ, Jones JV: Arrhythmogenic effect of ventriculography in patients with left ventricular dilatation and/or hypertrophy. Clin Sci (Lond) 95:453–458, 1998.

MECHANO-ELECTRIC FEEDBACK AS A MECHANISM INVOLVED IN THERAPEUTIC INTERVENTIONS

• • • •

CHAPTER 33

Antiarrhythmic Effects of Acute Mechanical Stimulation

• • • •

Peter Kohl, Angie M. King, and Christian Boulin

No procedure in modern medicine has aroused more controversial thought than the attempt to revive the dead.

This statement by Albert Hyman[1] introduced his 1930 article on the mechanical component of "intracardiac therapy"—the injection of drugs into arrested hearts. Hyman noted that, although epinephrine seemed to be the drug of choice, injection of atropine, caffeine, and even dextrose produced similarly favorable results. This apparent drug independence of the intervention led him to propose that the mechanical stimulation, afforded by needle insertion into the myocardium, was sufficient to restart asystolic hearts—a hypothesis that he went on to demonstrate in several patients. In line with the opening statement, through his article, Hyman initiated one of the most controversial debates in medicine of his time.

The use of mechanical interventions to reset disturbed heart rhythms remains a subject of contention. This chapter summarizes the means and antiarrhythmic utility of cardiac mechanical stimulation, recapitulates regulatory aspects, and addresses the mechanisms and potential use of this intervention.

MEANS OF CARDIAC MECHANICAL STIMULATION

Direct Manual Stimulation

Direct mechanical stimulation of cardiac muscle by "finger tap" is a well-established method used by surgeons to prompt rhythmic contractile activity in hearts after induced arrest during open heart surgery. Although this may be one of the most regularly used

mechanical interventions to restore the heartbeat, it is equally one of the least well characterized, in terms of mechanics and mechanisms.

Transthoracic Needle Insertion

Hyman[1] found that the mechanical interaction of a transthoracically inserted needle with the myocardium may resuscitate arrested hearts. He used both straight (for ventricular stimulation) and curved (to reach the right atrial appendage) needles to trigger ectopic beats, followed by temporary or full restoration of sinus rhythm in about 25% of cases. Although his observations are largely of historical interest, transthoracic injection is still used occasionally for emergency cardiac resuscitation, and its mechanical component is worth consideration.

Intracardiac Catheter Tip Prodding

Cardiac catheterization often is associated with induction of premature ventricular beats (PVB). Interestingly, catheter tip interactions with the cardiac wall also can lead to cardioversion from tachyarrhythmia. This was systematically studied by Befeler[2] in 68 patients undergoing diagnostic catheterization. Catheter tip stimulation of atrial and ventricular muscle was found to be effective in reverting atrial tachycardia in 24% of cases, junctional tachycardia in 60%, and ventricular tachycardia (VT) in 14% (another 27% of patients with VT in this study were treated by precordial thump [PT]; see later). Catheter tip–induced conversion of fibrillation was not attempted in this study. Elsewhere, however, there is a case report on successful and maintained cardioversion of chronic atrial fibrillation by catheter prodding.[3]

Intrathoracic Pressure Increase

Several reports have highlighted the link between an abrupt increase in intrathoracic pressure and termination of tachyarrhythmias. This type of mechanical cardioversion can be self-administered[4] by coughing[5] or through the Valsalva maneuver,[6] which has been found to also work in heart transplant recipients.[7]

Extracorporal Impact

The most well-known form of acute cardiac mechanical stimulation is probably PT, a fist thump that is usually applied to the sternum[8] (although cases of successful spinal impact have been reported).[9] First described as a trigger of competent ventricular contraction in asystolic patients,[10] PT has been used to pace hearts[11] or to terminate tachycardia[12] and fibrillation.[13] This procedure also has been proposed for patient self-administration,[14] although not without serious objection.[15]

ANTIARRHYTHMIC EFFECTS

Asystole

In 1920, Schott[10] reported that a single blow to the chest could restore a palpable pulse in a patient with ventricular standstill caused by a Stokes–Adams attack. Building on Schott's observations, it was subsequently shown that rhythmic thumps, applied to the precordium (precordial percussion) of patients in ventricular standstill, can trigger ventricular contractions.[16] These mechanically induced beats have a greater hemodynamic effect than external chest compres-

sion,[17] and they may be used to maintain consciousness in patients during extended periods of ventricular standstill (up to 1.5 hours have been reported).[11] Although of historical and mechanistic interest, asystole caused by Stokes–Adams attacks plays a less prominent role in modern-day Western medicine (because these patients will normally carry an implanted pacemaker).

Tachycardia

Following reports on successful application of PT as a means of restarting asystolic hearts, it was found that PT may also be used to revert VT to normal sinus rhythm (NSR; Fig. 33–1).[8,12] The success rate of optimally performed PT in VT may exceed 40%,[2,18] and the best results are seen if impacts coincide with the electrocardiogram R wave.[19]

Because the timing, relative to the cardiac cycle, of manually applied PT can not be reliably controlled, there is concern about mechanical stimulation during the vulnerable period (T wave), which could have a detrimental effect on heart rhythm (see Chapter 29). The expectation, however, that ill-timed PT would readily convert VT to ventricular fibrillation (VF) has largely not been confirmed,[18] except in patients[20] and experiments[21] involving severe preexisting hypoxia. This highlights that PT is more efficient if applied early in the development of VT, where it appears to pose little risk for rhythm deterioration.[18]

To control impact timing, mechanical stimulators have been developed (Fig. 33–2) that can be triggered through cardiac rhythm monitors.[22,23] In a study by Zoll and colleagues,[22] ventricular excitation was reliably evoked in 8 of 10 patients (9 patients had different cardiac rhythm disturbances including atrial

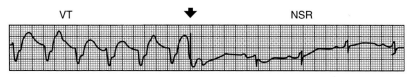

■ **Figure 33–1** Electrocardiogram recording from a patient in ventricular tachycardia (VT). Normal sinus node rhythm (NSR) was reinstated by a single precordial thump *(arrow)* to the lower sternum. *(From Pennington JE, Taylor J, Lown B: Chest thump for reverting ventricular tachycardia. N Engl J Med 283:1192–1195, 1970, with permission.)*

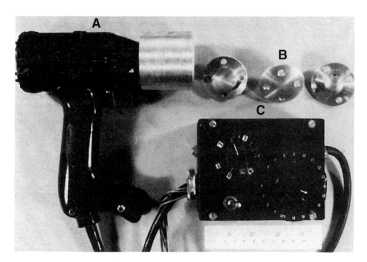

■ **Figure 33–2** Modified industrial stapling gun *(A)* projectiles with varying impact area *(B)* and control box for electrocardiogram synchronization *(C)*, used by Paul Zoll for precordial thump studies. *(From Zoll PM, Belgard AH, Weintraub MJ, Frank HA: External mechanical cardiac stimulation. N Engl J Med 294:1274–1275, 1976, with permission.)*

fibrillation, and 1 patient was in NSR undergoing a hemodynamic study), with not a single observation of repetitive responses, tachycardia, or fibrillation.

Furthermore, it was found that the threshold for external mechanical stimulation of PVB in adults is as low as 0.04 to 1.5 J.[22] This is only a fraction of the energy required for external electrical stimulation (150 J for biphasic and 200 J or more for monophasic defibrillatory stimuli).

Interestingly, this is also several orders of magnitude less than the mechanical energy levels involved in commotio cordis during competitive sports. For example, a standard regulation baseball (weight, 0.142 kg) at a speed of 45 m/sec (value not uncommon for batted balls in major league games) has a kinetic energy of 144 J.

This discrepancy in a key parameter of the mechanical intervention may explain the rarity of negative side effects with PT. In fact, controlled chest impacts, applied at energies 10 times the threshold level for mechanical action potential (AP) stimulation, did

not trigger VT or VF, even if applied during the T wave.[22] Thus, there would appear to be a minimum "permissive" energy level (tens of Joules in the adult), which has to be exceeded before impact timing becomes the decisive factor in determining impact arrhythmogenicity.

Fibrillation

In contrast to the relatively optimistic reports on PT effectiveness in patients with asystole or VT, successful treatment of VF by mechanical interventions has been achieved only occasionally (success rates as low as 2% have been observed).[24] In all reported cases, PT was applied early during the development of VF, either at the verge of deterioration from VT[25] or within the first 10 sec of VF (Fig. 33–3), as verified by electrocardiogram and, occasionally, arterial pressure recordings.[2,26,27]

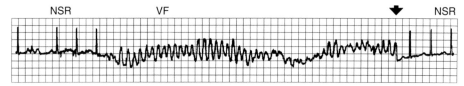

■ **Figure 33–3** Electrocardiogram recording of a patient whose early ventricular fibrillation (VF) was converted to normal sinus rhythm (NSR) by a single precordial thump *(arrow)*. *(From Barrett JS: Chest thumps and the heart beat. N Engl J Med 284:393, 1971, with permission.)*

Overall Utility

The use of mechanical stimulation as a means of cardioversion in the hospital setting shows a large variation among societies, hospitals, and even within single health care organizations. Medical personnel in China, for example, use PT as a matter of course for patients experiencing life-threatening dysrhythmia. In contrast, personnel of specialized cardiac catheter laboratories usually opt for attaching automated defibrillator pads to patients before any intervention is conducted; thus, they do not normally consider application of PT.

Judging by the majority of published reports, PT has the best benefit-to-cost ratio if applied early during the development of serious heart rhythm disturbances. Automated mechanical stimulator technology could overcome concerns about impact timing, location, and energy, as well as ethical issues (e.g., hitting a conscious patient), and, if used as a preventive means (e.g., during patient evacuation or transport), this technology could reduce the time delay between onset of an arrhythmia and the attempted mechanical (or electrical) termination. Interestingly, that is not the prevailing message of current resuscitation advice.

LEGISLATION

History

Formal guidelines for Advanced Life Support (ALS) were first issued by the American Heart Association (AHA) in 1974 (then revised in 1980, 1986, and 1992). The U.K. Resuscitation Council published ALS guidelines in 1984 (updates were published in 1989, 1992, 1995, and 1998). In 2000, the International Liaison Committee on Resuscitation (ILCOR), an association of key international resuscitation organizations, published their first cardiopulmonary resuscitation guidelines, which lay the foundation to ALS worldwide (adopted by, among other organizations, the AHA and the European Resuscitation Council).[28]

Recommendations

In the 1970s and 1980s, ALS guidelines tended to recommend PT for treatment of asystole, VT, and VF. It was believed that, even though success rates of PT differed widely among investigators, the swiftness of delivery, and the overall low incidence of negative side effects, warranted regular PT use. This applied particularly to the clinical setting, where other treatment modalities (such as electrical defibrillators) are available as backups (even though there is some delay). Outside of the hospital, PT was considered appropriate for any pulseless rhythm disturbance.

Since the 1990s, PT has been progressively de-emphasized. In 1992, the AHA removed asystole as an indication. In the 2000 ILCOR guidelines, PT is listed as the first ALS procedure only after witnessed or monitored cardiac arrest (Fig. 33–4), and it is highlighted that PT is unlikely to succeed after more than 30 sec of cardiac arrest. The guidelines have ceased to provide a procedural instruction of how to apply PT. Written descriptions in previous guidelines and explanatory notes described PT as a sharp impact to the lower half of the sternum, delivered from a height of about 20 cm, using the ulnar edge of the tightly clinched fist (see Fig. 33–5 for one of the rare graphic representations).[29] This might be suitably extended by the suggestion to actively retract the fist after full impact, to emphasize the impulse-like nature of the optimal stimulus.

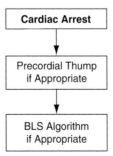

■ **Figure 33–4** Initial sequence of the 2000 International Liaison Committee on Resuscitation (ILCOR) Advanced Life Support flow chart, recommending precordial thump as a first measure after witnessed cardiac arrest, before commencement of Basic Life Support (BLS). *(From de Latorre F, Nolan J, Robertson C, et al: European Resuscitation Council guidelines 2000 for adult advanced life support. Resuscitation 48:211–221, 2001, with permission.)*

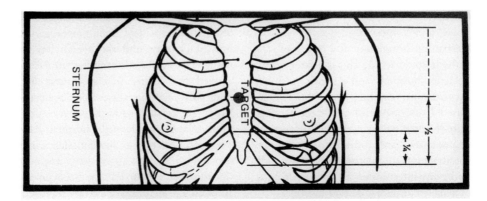

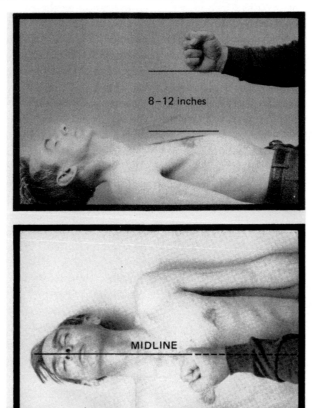

■ **Figure 33–5** "How-to" illustration of precordial thump. *(From Huszar RJ: Emergency Cardiac Care. Bowie, MA, Robert J Brady, 1982, with permission.)*

Thus, PT is currently the first prescribed ALS procedure for witnessed cardiac arrest, but conditions for and style of application are not explained in sufficient detail.

MECHANISMS

General Considerations

The theory underlying PT, which was developed in the 1970s, assumes that the mechanical stimulation causes, through mechano-electric feedback (MEF), a change in myocardial electrical properties.[13,23] This has been proposed particularly to depolarize excitable ventricular tissue and, if the depolarization is large enough, to either trigger ectopic beats in quiescent tissue or obliterate the excitable gap required for re-entrant excitation.[12,27]

Experimental Findings

Experimental studies have overwhelmingly confirmed that stretch of resting myocardium does indeed cause depolarization (see Reference 30 for a review of this topic). If the mechanically induced depolarizations reach the threshold for AP generation (suprathreshold mechanical stimulus), they cause ectopic beats in ventricular tissue preparations.[31] Rhythmic application of suprathreshold mechanical stimuli can be used to mechanically pace quiescent ventricles in isolated perfused hearts,[32] and thus mimic the effects of PT or precordial percussion during asystole in humans.

Mechanically induced depolarizations may be explained by activation of cation nonselective stretch-activated channels (SAC_{CAT}) in ventricular cardiomyocytes.[33] SAC_{CAT} have a reversal potential between 0 and −15 mV, and their activation is capable of triggering AP in isolated cardiomyocytes.[34] Fittingly, pharmacologic inhibition of SAC_{CAT} prevents mechanical induction of PVB in asystolic isolated hearts.[35]

Another group of stretch-activated ion channels is potassium selective (SAC_K), with a reversal potential near −95 mV.[36,37] These channels will have only a moderate effect on resting cells, whose intrinsic transmembrane voltage is near the potassium reversal potential (see Chapters 1 to 4).

In contrast to mechanical effects on the asystolic heart, there is a remarkable paucity of experimental insight into mechanical cardioversion of VT and VF. The few studies reporting successful mechanical termination of VT and VF did not quantify mechanical effects on the heart and could not exclude structural tissue damage, which complicates their interpretation.[38] Nonetheless, the instantaneous conversion from VT and VF to NSR, which was observed in patients and experimental models, suggests that stretch activation of ion channels is likely to play a role in these circumstances. The dynamic interaction of SAC effects with ectopic foci or re-entrant excitation is complex, however, and has not been elucidated in detail.

In VT or VF, some cells will be at resting potential levels, and their response to a mechanical stimulus may be similar to that detailed previously. Other cells will be at various stages of the AP, and the effect of a mechanical stimulus will be affected by the difference between the actual transmembrane potential of a cell and the reversal potential of SAC_{CAT}, SAC_K, or both. This is a highly dynamic setting, and its interpretation benefits from quantitative modeling.

Quantitative Modeling

Impressive improvement in biophysically detailed computer models of the heart has occurred in recent years (see Chapters 22 and 41). It is now possible to address cardiac anatomy, fiber orientation, cell properties, coupling, and regional gradients in mechano-electric factors in simulations of the cardiac electromechanical cycle. These quantitative models have started to possess predictive power, and they can aid data interpretation and hypothesis formation.[39]

We have studied the potential antiarrhythmic effects of a mechanical stimulus in a comparatively simple VT model (figure-of-eight re-entry), using a two-dimensional grid of ventricular cardiomyocytes (Fig. 33–6A). Mechanical impact is simulated through brief (5 msec), impulse-like activation of SAC_{CAT}, SAC_K, or both (stretch-activated conductance 25 nS).

Mechanical activation of SAC_{CAT} (reversal potential −10 mV) reliably terminates re-entry in the ventricular tissue model, exactly through the mechanism proposed

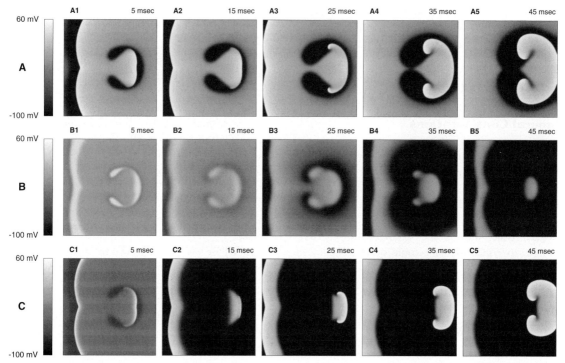

■ **Figure 33–6**   Two-dimensional model (2.5 × 2.5 cm) of ventricular myocardium, consisting of 251 × 251 single-cell models[40] (transmembrane voltage is gray level coded; see Reference 41 for mesh implementation). *A,* Control figure-of-eight re-entry activity. *B,* Mechanical stimulation, modeled by activation for 5 msec of SAC_{CAT} (reversal potential −10 mV; see Chapter 8 for equation), causes depolarization of tissue in the excitable gap and terminates re-entry. *C,* Mechanical stimulation of tissue after simulated ischemic sensitization of SAC_K to stretch shifts net mechanically induced reversal potential to more negative levels (here −35 mV), which prevents depolarization of resting tissue and shortens action potential duration, rendering mechanical stimulation incapable of instantaneously terminating re-entry. (See color insert.) *(Illustration courtesy of Dr. Alan Garny, the Cardiac MEF Lab, University of Oxford.)*

three decades ago: depolarization of the tissue forming the excitable gap (see Fig. 33–6*B*).

Addition of increasing amounts of SAC_K to the population of ion channels activated by the mechanical stimulus moves the reversal potential of the "net stretch-activated current" toward more negative potentials. This reduces the ability to render resting cells inexcitable and shortens AP duration. At a SAC_{CAT} to SAC_K ratio of about 1:0.4 (corresponding to a net stretch-activated reversal potential of −35 mV; see Fig. 33–6*C*), this results in failure to instantaneously terminate VT in the model.

This is of interest in the context of the reported reduction in PT efficacy during preexisting hypoxia.

Hypoxia reduces tissue adenosine triphosphate (ATP), thereby reducing inhibition of ATP-dependent potassium channel, K_{ATP}.

These channels show combined ATP sensitivity and mechanosensitivity in atrial cardiomyocytes.[37] Consequently, ischemia has been shown to potentiate K_{ATP} channel mechanosensitivity.[42]

If ventricular channels have similar properties, preexisting hypoxia may "sensitize" K_{ATP} channels to respond more efficiently to a mechanical stimulus, thereby potentially rendering PT less effective, or even detrimental.

These modeling-derived predictions, although in keeping with clinical insight into PT limitations, require thorough experimental validation. However, they illustrate how clinical consideration, theoretical simulation, and experimental validation may facilitate new directions of study.

NEW INSIGHTS

Clinical Use of Precordial Thump: United States versus United Kingdom

As mentioned previously, there are marked international differences in the approach to mechanical cardioversion. Because it is only since 2000 that the United Kingdom and United States have shared a common set of ALS guidelines, we conducted a questionnaire-based investigation to obtain a glimpse into the current use of PT in the United Kingdom and United States and to relate any differences in clinical utility of PT to the particulars of its application, assessed from verbal descriptions and subsequent biomechanical measurements.

A letter stating the aims of the investigation and a questionnaire relating to "personal experience with PT" was sent to 567 healthcare professionals (United Kingdom: n = 279; United States: n = 288). By March 2004, 95 replies were received (United Kingdom: n = 52; United States: n = 43), with a reported total of 1740 incidents of PT (United Kingdom: n = 813; United States: n = 927).

"Speed of delivery" was ranked by 92.5% of the participants as the most important reason for using PT, whereas "perceived inefficiency" (60.2%), "other established procedures" (45.9%), and "unawareness of technique" (37.8%) were reported to preclude more frequent use of PT. Only 54.3% of professionals were taught PT as part of their curriculum, and no established tools for training or assessment were identified.

There was a pronounced difference in opinions on appropriateness of PT application in VT and VF (Fig. 33–7). U.K. participants ranked onset of VF (89.5%), followed by VF (54.4%), as the prime indications for PT, with VT as a third indication (35.1%). In the United States, the opposite trend was noted, with VT (62.8%) narrowly leading onset of VF (58.1%), and VF as a distant third indication (25.6%).

This correlated with a significantly greater success rate of U.S. healthcare professionals, who reported "at

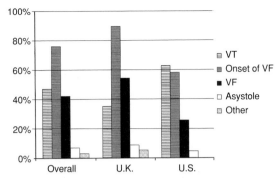

■ Figure 33–7 Prime indications named by U.K. and U.S. healthcare professionals for application of precordial thump. VT, ventricular tachycardia; VF, ventricular fibrillation.

least temporary cardioversion to NSR" in 27.7% of PT applications, compared to only 13.3% in the United Kingdom (Fig. 33–8). Adverse side effects were rare (0.5% of total patients; United Kingdom: 0.8%, United States: 0.2%) and largely of structural nature.

Clearly, this is a limited pilot study, with a comparatively small number of retrospective reports. The data suggest, however, that "earlier application" of PT (during VT and early VF) may have a beneficial effect on the outcome of PT.

Although this may offer a compelling explanation of differences in the clinical utility of PT between the United Kingdom and the United States, it does not rule out a systematic national bias in the actual mechanics of PT application.

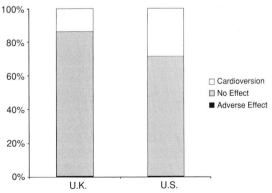

■ Figure 33–8 Differences in U.K. versus U.S. success rates of cardioversion by precordial thump.

Precordial Thump Mechanics

To determine PT mechanics, we developed a "thump-o-meter" to measure preimpact fist speed (Fig. 33–9). Healthcare professionals in both countries (United Kingdom: n = 22; United States: n = 22) performed three PT-like impacts each. Biomechanical recordings were then correlated to reported individual success rates in the application of PT.

Interindividual differences in preimpact fist speed ranged from 0.42 to 8.14 m/sec (Fig. 33–10). Participants with fist speeds of less than 2.25 m/sec reported successful cardioversion in 18% ± 3% of PT cases, compared with 36% ± 2% for those who performed faster impacts ($P < 0.01$).

The national distribution of preimpact fist speeds showed a significantly greater average among U.S. participants (United Kingdom: 1.55 ± 0.68 m/sec; United States: 4.17 ± 1.68 m/sec; $P < 0.01$).

Thus, PT success rates are more than two times greater in the United States than the United Kingdom. This may be related to differences in arrhythmia-targeted by PT, mechanics of PT, or both. A minimum severity of impact appears to be required to achieve optimal mechanical cardioversion rates, which highlights the need for better procedural instructions and training aids, such as a simplified thump-o-meter.

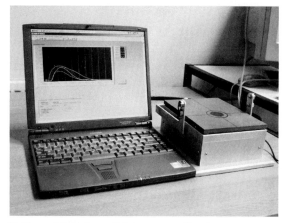

■ **Figure 33–9** Precordial thump recording thump-o-meter.

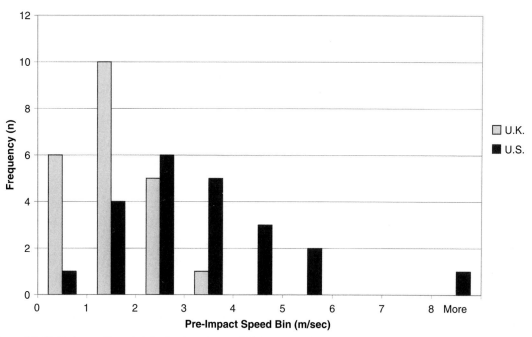

■ **Figure 33–10** Preimpact fist speed distribution of precordial thump recordings, obtained with the thump-o-meter, reveal greater average speeds for U.S. *(black columns)* compared with U.K. participants *(gray columns)*.

Summary

Mechanical stimulation affects cardiac electrophysiology through MEF. Like electrical current discharges, this may either cause or terminate arrhythmias. A potentially important advantage of mechanical energy delivery for cardioversion is that the necessary electrical currents are "generated" onsite—that is, in the heart. The mechanical stimulus is passed on from precordium to cardiac tissue in a direct fashion, without massive "loss" to other regions of the body observed with electrical stimulation (during transthoracic defibrillation in humans, only 4% of the applied current actually traverses the heart).[43] PT therefore allows application of much lower energy levels (reducing trauma) and can be tolerated by the conscious patient.

The insight into mechanisms underlying mechanical cardioversion is still patchy. Given the swift response to mechanical stimulation, it is highly probable that stretch activation of ion channels plays a role in this process. The relative ratio of SAC_{CAT} and SAC_K activation may be involved in determining the success or failure of interventions such as PT, and this ratio may be affected by regional differences in myocardial properties, impact characteristics, or diseases such as myocardial ischaemia.

There would appear to be value in establishing a repository of detailed recordings of patients who underwent targeted mechanical cardioversion (such as acquired by intensive care monitoring systems) and the Oxford Lab is in the process of setting this up. In addition, future progress in our understanding of the use and limitations of mechanical termination of VT and VF requires suitable multicellular experimental (and matching computational) models of these conditions.

Finally, ALS guidelines should be extended by addition of clear procedural instructions regarding the application of PT. Training aids should be introduced to increase the probability of successful mechanical cardioversion (either as stand-alone thump-o-meter type boxes or as part of resuscitation mannequin technology).

Acknowledgments

We thank Patricia Cooper and Alan Garny from the Oxford Cardiac Mechano-Electric Feedback Lab for important contributions to this research. We also thank colleagues at the following hospitals for participation in the fist thump measurements: University of Miami School of Medicine; Florida Hospital Orlando Campus; Royal Brompton Hospital London; Hammersmith Hospital London; and John Radcliffe Hospital Oxford. This study was supported by the British Heart Foundation and the U.K. Medical Research Council.

References

1. Hyman AS: Resuscitation of the stopped heart by intracardiac therapy. Arch Intern Med 46:553–568, 1930.
2. Befeler B: Mechanical stimulation of the heart: Its therapeutic value in tachyarrhythmias. Chest 73:832–838, 1978.
3. Lee HT, Cozine K: Incidental conversion to sinus rhythm from atrial fibrillation during external jugular venous catheterization. J Clin Anesth 9:664–667, 1997.
4. Criley JM, Blaufuss AH, Kissel GL: Cough-induced cardiac compression. Self-administered form of cardiopulmonary resuscitation. JAMA 236:1246–1250, 1976.
5. Wei JY, Greene HL, Weisfeldt ML: Cough-facilitated conversion of ventricular tachycardia. Am J Cardiol 45:174–176, 1980.
6. Waxman MB, Wald RW, Finley JP, et al: Valsalva termination of ventricular tachycardia. Circulation 62:843–851, 1980.
7. Ambrosi P, Habib G, Kreitmann B, et al: Valsalva manoeuvre for supraventricular tachycardia in transplanted heart recipient. Lancet 346:713, 1995.
8. Pennington JE, Taylor J, Lown B: Chest thump for reverting ventricular tachycardia. N Engl J Med 283:1192–1195, 1970.
9. Moore EW, Davies MW: A slap on the back. Anaesthesia 54:308, 1999.
10. Schott E: Über Ventrikelstillstand (Adams-Stokes'sche Anfälle) nebst Bemerkungen über andersartige Arhythmien passagerer Natur. Deutsches Archiv für Klinische Medizin 131:211–229, 1920.
11. Don Michael TAD, Stanford RL: Praecordial percussion in cardiac asystole. Lancet 1:699, 1963.
12. Befeler B, Aranda JM: Termination of ventricular tachycardia by a chest thump over the area of paradoxical pulsation. Am Heart J 94:773–775, 1977.
13. Lown B, Taylor J: Thump-version. N Engl J Med 283:1223–1224, 1970.
14. Conner D, Shander D, Deegan C, et al: Self-administered chest thump for cardioversion of recurrent ventricular tachycardia. Chest 73:877, 1978.
15. Rozanski JJ: Ventricular tachycardia and the chest thump. Chest 74:694–695, 1978.
16. Scherf D, Bornemann C: Thumping of the precordium in ventricular standstill. Am J Cardiol 5:30–40, 1960.
17. Phillips JH, Burch GE: Management of cardiac arrest. Am Heart J 67:265–277, 1964.
18. Goldberg E: Mechanical factors and the electrocardiogram. Am Heart J 93:629–644, 1977.
19. Rajagopalan RS, Appu KSC, Sultan SK, et al: Precordial thump in ventricular tachycardia. J Assoc Physicians India 19:725–729, 1971.

20. Miller J, Tresch D, Horwitz L, et al: The precordial thump. Ann Emerg Med 13:791–794, 1984.
21. Yakaitis RW, Redding JS: Precordial thumping during cardiac resuscitation. Crit Care Med 1:22–26, 1973.
22. Zoll PM, Belgard AH, Weintraub MJ, Frank HA: External mechanical cardiac stimulation. N Engl J Med 294:1274–1275, 1976.
23. Wirtzfeld A, Himmler FC, Forβmann B, et al: External mechanical cardiac stimulation: Methods and possible application. Zeitschrift für Kardiologie 68:583–589, 1979.
24. Barrett JS: Chest thumps and the heart beat. N Engl J Med 284:393, 1971.
25. Caldwell G, Millar G, Quinn E, et al: Simple mechanical methods for cardioversion: Defence of the precordial thump and cough version. Brit Med J 291:627–630, 1985.
26. Baderman H, Roberton NRC: Thumping the precordium. Lancet 2:1293, 1965.
27. Bierfeld JL, Rodriguez-Viera V, Aranda JM, et al: Terminating ventricular fibrillation by chest thump. Angiology 30:703–707, 1979.
28. de Latorre F, Nolan J, Robertson C, et al: European Resuscitation Council guidelines 2000 for adult advanced life support. Resuscitation 48:211–221, 2001.
29. Huszar RJ: Emergency Cardiac Care. Bowie, MA, Robert J Brady, 1982.
30. Kohl P, Hunter P, Noble D: Stretch-induced changes in heart rate and rhythm: Clinical observations, experiments and mathematical models. Prog Biophys Mol Biol 71:91–138, 1999.
31. Kaufmann R, Theophile U: Automatie-fördernde Dehnungseffekte an Purkinje-Fäden, Papillarmuskeln und Vorhoftrabekeln von Rhesus-Affen. Pflugers Arch 297:174–189, 1967.
32. Franz MR, Cima R, Wang D, et al: Electrophysiological effects of myocardial stretch and mechanical determinants of stretch-activated arrhythmias. Circulation 86:968–978, 1992.
33. Craelius W, Chen V, El-Sherif N: Stretch activated ion channels in ventricular myocytes. Biosci Rep 8:407–414, 1988.
34. Craelius W: Stretch-activation of rat cardiac myocytes. Exp Physiol 78:411–423, 1993.
35. Hansen DE, Borganelli M, Stacy GPJ, Taylor LK: Dose-dependent inhibition of stretch-induced arrhythmias by gadolinium in isolated canine ventricles. Evidence for a unique mode of antiarrhythmic action. Circ Res 69:820–831, 1991.
36. Niu W, Sachs F: Dynamic properties of stretch-activated K+ channels in adult rat atrial myocytes. Prog Biophys Mol Biol 82:121–135, 2003.
37. van Wagoner DR: Mechanosensitive gating of atrial ATP-sensitive potassium channels. Circ Res 72:973–983, 1993.
38. Kawakami T, Lowbeer C, Valen G, Vaage J: Mechanical conversion of post-ischaemic ventricular fibrillation: Effects on function and myocyte injury in isolated rat hearts. Scand J Clin Lab Invest 59:9–16, 1999.
39. Kohl P, Sachs F: Mechanoelectric feedback in cardiac cells. Philos Trans R Soc Lond A 359:1173–1185, 2001.
40. Noble D, Varghese A, Kohl P, Noble P: Improved guinea-pig ventricular cell model incorporating a diadic space, I_{Kr} and I_{Ks}, and length- and tension-dependent processes. Can J Cardiol 14:123–134, 1998.
41. Garny A, Kohl P: Mechanical induction of arrhythmias during ventricular repolarisation: Modelling cellular mechanisms and their interaction in 2D. Ann N Y Acad Sci 1015:133–143, 2004.
42. van Wagoner DR, Lamorgese M: Ischemia potentiates the mechanosensitive modulation of atrial ATP-sensitive potassium channels. Ann N Y Acad Sci 723:392–395, 1994.
43. Lerman BB, Deale OC: Relation between transcardiac and transthoracic current during defibrillation in humans. Circ Res 67:1420–1426, 1990.

CHAPTER 34

Termination of Arrhythmias by Hemodynamic Unloading

* * * *

Peter Taggart and Peter Sutton

Theoretical considerations predict that reducing the volume within the heart (i.e., reducing stretch) should be antiarrhythmic. Experimental evidence in animal models supports this contention by the demonstration that increased loading may enhance the inducibility of arrhythmias, and unloading may suppress them. However, clinical evidence currently is incomplete. Although a number of clinical scenarios incorporating unloading are associated with suppression or termination of arrhythmias, the acquisition of hard evidence for a cause-and-effect relation currently has not been possible.

HEMODYNAMIC UNLOADING SHOULD BE ANTIARRHYTHMIC

Two main mechanisms of arrhythmia are re-entry and triggered activity.[1] Re-entry is facilitated by shortening of the refractory period, inhomogeneity of refractoriness, and local conduction slowing. Under normal conditions, the refractory period is mainly voltage dependent and approximates to the action potential duration (APD). Increased volume loading or stretch has been shown to shorten APD and refractoriness in in vitro and in vivo animal studies and in humans.[2–10] In addition, these effects on APD and refractoriness have been shown to be inhomogeneous.[4,11,12] Stretch appears to exert relatively little, if any, effect on conduction velocity.[4,12–14] Increased loading, therefore, would be expected to influence two of the three main requirements for re-entrant arrhythmias in a proarrhythmic manner.

Arrhythmias caused by triggered activity arise from depolarization occurring either during the repolarization phase of the action potential (early afterdepolar-

izations) or after action potential repolarization is complete (delayed afterdepolarizations). If these afterdepolarizations reach sufficient amplitude, they may trigger an action potential and generate a premature beat, or they may trigger a series of action potentials and generate a focal tachycardia. Increased ventricular loading or acute stretch has been shown to induce depolarizations resembling both early and delayed afterdepolarizations.[2,5,8,10,15–17] There also is evidence that stretch alters APD and refractoriness in atrium,[18–23] including in humans.[20,22] However, the effect is less clear than in ventricle, with some studies reporting a lengthening in response to stretch, whereas other studies report a shortening. On the basis of these reports, ventricular or atrial unloading should tend to be protective against focal tachycardias caused by triggered activity. The foregoing theoretical predictions are supported by several studies in different animal models in which arrhythmias were induced by increased stretch or volume loading.

EXPERIMENTAL EVIDENCE THAT HEMODYNAMIC UNLOADING IS ANTIARRHYTHMIC

The majority of experimental work has been directed toward the demonstration of arrhythmia induction by increased hemodynamic loading, rather than arrhythmia termination by decreased loading. Therefore, evidence that hemodynamic unloading is antiarrhythmic is derived, to a large extent, by inference rather than proof.

An abrupt increase in ventricular volume in rabbit and canine ventricles during diastole induces depolarizations resembling delayed afterdepolarizations, premature ventricular beats, and, in some instances, couplets and nonsustained ventricular tachycardia.[5,16,17] The probability of inducing premature beats by an abrupt stretch was greater in the presence of ventricular dilation.[16]

The likelihood of inducing arrhythmia was shown to depend on both the amount of stretch and the rate of increase of the stretch. However, these arrhythmias do not arise from perturbations during action potential repolarization, and therefore are not strictly within the remit of this chapter (see Chapter 21). Several studies have shown that acute stretch or volume loading may cause depolarizations during the terminal phase of the action potential resembling early afterdepolarizations, or may shorten the APD, and hence shorten refractoriness, which, in both cases, may be associated with arrhythmias[5,15,16,24,25] (Figs. 34–1 and 34–2).

In isolated rabbit hearts, the inducibility of arrhythmias was increased substantially when the ventricle was already dilated. The increase in inducibility was accompanied by an increased heterogeneity of refractoriness.[4] In the isolated canine ventricle, the probability of arrhythmia initiation by stretch increases with the volume of diastolic increments[16] (Fig. 34–3). Increased loading decreases the ventricular fibrillation threshold, and unloading increases the threshold.[26] Similarly, increased loading in isolated rabbit hearts

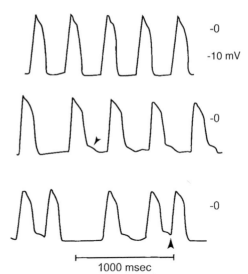

■ **Figure 34–2** Increase in right ventricular pressure and volume, created by the insertion of a balloon catheter into the pulmonary valve orifice before dilating the narrowed valve in patients, induced deflections during repolarization. These deflections resembled early afterdepolarizations *(slanted arrow)* and were associated with spontaneous ectopic beats *(upward arrow)*. *(From Levine JH, Guarnieri T, Kadish AH, et al: Changes in myocardial repolarisation in patients undergoing balloon valvuloplasty for congenital pulmonary stenosis: Evidence for contraction excitation feedback in humans. Circulation 77:70–77, 1988, with permission.)*

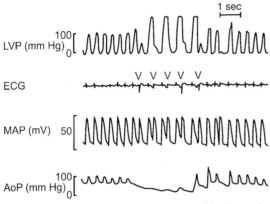

■ **Figure 34–1** Transient aortic occlusion of in situ canine hearts induced afterdepolarizations and arrhythmia. LVP, left ventricular pressure; ECG, electrocardiogram; MAP, monophasic action potential; AoP, aortic pressure; V, ventricular ectopic beat. *(From Franz MR, Burkhoff D, Yue DT, Sagawa K: Mechanically induced action potential changes and arrhythmia in isolated and in situ canine hearts. Cardiovasc Res 23:213–223, 1989, with permission.)*

increases the defibrillation threshold[27] (Fig. 34–4). In rabbit[21] and guinea pig[23] atria, increased loading increases inducibility of atrial fibrillation. In a Langendorff guinea pig heart model, the number of stretch-induced atrial premature beats increased with increased atrial volume loading[23] (Fig. 34–5).

The mechanisms by which changes in loading and stretch influence membrane currents (i.e., mechano-electric transduction) probably involve both stretch-activated cation channels (see Chapter 1) and calcium transients (see Chapter 22). Gadolinium, which blocks many stretch-activated channels, has been shown to block stretch-induced depolarizations and ventricular premature beats[28] (Fig. 34–6).

CLINICAL EVIDENCE

Despite a wealth of experimental evidence for a potential role of mechano-electric feedback (MEF) in the

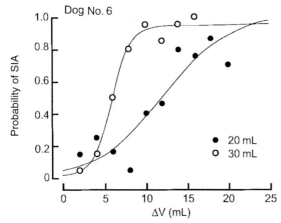

Figure 34–3 In an isolated canine ventricle preparation, the probability of inducing arrhythmia increased as a function of the volume of diastolic increments *(filled circles)*. This effect was enhanced when the baseline volume was increased from 20 to 30 mL *(open circles)*. SIA, Stretch-induced arrhythmia. *(From Hansen DE, Craig CS, Hondeghem LM: Stretch-induced arrhythmias in the isolated canine ventricle: Evidence for the importance of mechanoelectrical feedback. Circulation 81:1094–1105, 1990, with permission.)*

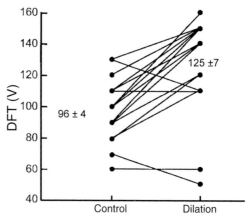

Figure 34–4 Acute ventricular dilation in isolated rabbit hearts increased the defibrillation threshold (DFT) from 96 ± 4 to 125 ± 7 V. *(From Ott P, Reiter MJ: Effect of ventricular dilation on defibrillation threshold in isolated perfused rabbit heart. J Cardiovasc Electrophysiol 8:1013–1019, 1997, with permission.)*

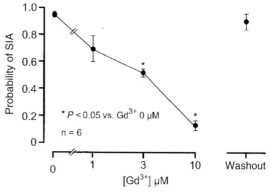

Figure 34–6 Effect of the stretch-activated channel blocker gadolinium (Gd^{3+}) on ventricular arrhythmia inducibility studied in an isolated canine preparation. The probability of the initiation of SIA was reduced by gadolinium in a dose-dependent manner. After washout of the drug, the probability returned to control. *(From Hansen DE, Borganelli M, Stacey GP, Taylor LK: Dose-dependent inhibition of stretch-induced arrhythmias by gadolinium in isolated canine ventricles: Evidence for a unique mode of antiarrhythmic action. Circ Res 69:820–831, 1991, with permission.)*

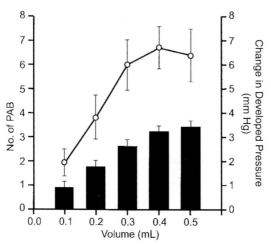

Figure 34–5 Relation between left atrial balloon volume and the incidence of stretch-induced premature atrial beats (PAB) in isolated Langendorff guinea pig hearts. The number of PAB *(black bars)* increased with increased atrial volume loading and increased atrial pressure *(open circles)*. *(From Nazir SA, Lab MJ: Mechanoelectric feedback in the atrium of the isolated guinea-pig heart. Cardiovasc Res 32:112–119, 1996, with permission.)*

Cardiopulmonary Bypass

Many cardiac surgical operations incorporate cardiopulmonary bypass to achieve a bloodless operating field. Deoxygenated blood returning to the heart is diverted through a canula placed in the right atrium to

initiation and termination of arrhythmias, evidence in humans is remarkably limited. However, there are several clinical scenarios in which MEF plays a role.

a pump/oxygenator; then the oxygened blood is returned to the circulation through a canula in the ascending aorta. The circulation thereby bypasses the heart and lungs, whereas maintaining systemic perfusion and coronary flow. During the time the patient is on bypass, the heart is half empty, flaccid, and non-working. At the end of the surgical procedure, the normal circulation is restored, and the heart is refilled and takes over the circulation. Arrhythmias developing at this time may be difficult to manage. It is well known among anesthetists and cardiac surgeons that reverting to the bypass situation (i.e., unloading the heart) may terminate the arrhythmia. A likely explanation for arrhythmias when discontinuing cardiopulmonary bypass (i.e., loading the heart) and the termination of the arrhythmia on reinstating bypass (i.e., unloading the heart) is MEF. In agreement with this suggestion, it has been shown that the process of discontinuing cardiopulmonary bypass (i.e., restoring ventricular loading) shortens APD.[9] The consequent shortening of refractory periods would be expected to facilitate re-entrant arrhythmias such as ventricular tachycardia and ventricular fibrillation. However, proof of a central role of MEF is lacking, and it is clearly not practical to conduct a formal study. Nevertheless, the anecdotal evidence is sufficiently compelling to warrant its inclusion as an example of MEF in humans.

Valsalva Maneuver

The Valsalva maneuver is frequently effective in terminating supraventricular and right ventricular outflow tract arrhythmias. The mechanism of action is traditionally attributed to vagal stimulation. However, the Valsalva maneuver also incorporates large changes in ventricular loading.[29] To perform the Valsalva maneuver, the subject takes in a deep breath, occludes the nostrils by pinching the nose, exhales hard against a closed glottis for 15 sec, and then releases. During the forced expiration phase, the increased intrathoracic pressure impedes venous return and reduces cardiac filling and cardiac output. On release, venous return, cardiac filling, and cardiac output increase rapidly. The heart rate increases during the ventricular unloading and decreases during ventricular reloading caused by

reflexly enhanced sympathetic and parasympathetic nerve activity, respectively.

In a study on patients undergoing cardiac catheterization, monophasic action potentials were recorded from the right ventricular septum during the performance of the Valsalva maneuver.[29] Changes in APD were observed that were probably a function of both autonomic and mechanical effects. Notably, whereas in patients with normal ventricular wall motion, the effect on APD was repeatable and similar among patients, in patients with regional wall motion abnormality, the changes in APD were markedly heterogeneous. These results were attributed to the effects of heterogeneous stretch, and they suggest that regional wall motion abnormality may enhance dispersion of repolarization. In patients with ventricular wall motion abnormality, dispersion of repolarization is sensitive to small changes in volume loading when ventricular load is manipulated by an abrupt alteration in the presence, or absence, of atrial output.[30] Because increased dispersion of repolarization is known to increase arrhythmogenesis, these observations suggest a mechanistic link for the high incidence of arrhythmias in patients with ventricular wall motion abnormality.

Termination of supraventricular tachycardia in orthoptic heart transplant patients by the Valsalva maneuver has been reported, which has been attributed to reduced mechanical stretch of the atria.[31]

Intra-aortic Balloon Assist

Several reports have described the benefit of intra-aortic balloon counterpulsation (IABCP) in the control of ventricular arrhythmias after myocardial infarction and for refractory ventricular arrhythmias.[32–36] One study reported 21 patients with ventricular arrhythmias and severe left ventricular impairment. Ten patients had monomorphic ventricular tachycardia, and 11 had paroxysmal ventricular tachycardia, ventricular fibrillation, or both. The use of IABCP resulted in termination of the arrhythmia in 14 patients and significant reduction in the frequency of episodes of sustained tachycardia in 4 patients. The arrhythmia terminated within 30 to

85 min of commencing IABCP in the 10 patients with incessant monomorphic ventricular tachycardia. Nineteen patients were subsequently discharged from the hospital. The authors suggested that perhaps ventricular unloading (with the increase in mean aortic diastolic pressure) and the decrease in peak systolic pressure would increase coronary blood flow. Ventricular unloading also reduces wall tension and oxygen requirement. This explanation, however, was considered unlikely, because patients with healthy coronary arteries benefited equally with those with significant coronary artery disease, and reversible ischemia was seen in only one patient. Another possibility was a reduction in adrenergic drive because of improved hemodynamic status and general well-being. However, the very nature of the intervention suggests MEF. These various explanations are not mutually exclusive. For example, experiments in canines have shown that ventricular ectopy and tachycardia induced by increasing afterload occur more readily in the presence of induced coronary disease.[16]

Cardiac Assist Devices

In addition to intra-aortic balloon assist, temporary ventricular assist devices are sometimes used—for example, in patients in whom weaning off cardiopulmonary bypass is difficult or impossible. These devices unload the heart by reducing pressure and volume.[37,38] Cardiac constraining devices also are used, whereby pericardium is fashioned as a ventricular support at the time of surgery to reduce postoperative dilation.[39] Both these procedures have been reported to reduce arrhythmia (see Chapters 36 and 37 for discussions on passive ventricular constraints and active cardiac assist devices, respectively).

Pharmacologic Load Reduction

Angiotensin-converting enzyme inhibitors reduce load and reduce mortality in patients with congestive heart failure.[40,41] The reduction in mortality reflects an overall reduction rather than a specific decrease in arrhyth-mic deaths,[40] although there is evidence for a reduction in ventricular tachycardia in these patients.[41]

Summary and Conclusions

There is ample experimental evidence to suggest that ventricular unloading is an effective antiarrhythmic strategy in humans. MEF has been shown to influence several of the key electrophysiologic parameters of arrhythmogenesis, such as APD and refractoriness. Increased hemodynamic loading is proarrhythmic. A cautionary note, however, is necessary when interpreting the experimental findings. The majority of research has focused on the effects of increased loading rather than the effects of unloading. Much of the evidence for the effects of unloading is inferred rather than proven. Evidence that hemodynamic unloading in humans is antiarrhythmic is difficult to acquire because of the following factors: the multiplicity of variables that accompany load manipulation, the lack of feasibility for clinical trials, and the absence of clinically useful blockers for the electrophysiologic effects of load alteration. Hopefully, in the not too distant future, the development of suitable blocking agents will enable the potential of MEF as a therapeutic target.

References

1. Janse MJ, Wit AL: Electrophysiological mechanisms of ventricular arrhythmias resulting from myocardial ischaemia and infarction. Physiol Rev 69:1049–1089, 1989.
2. Lab MJ: Contraction excitation feedback in myocardium: Physiological basis and clinical relevance. Circ Res 50:757–766, 1982.
3. Lerman BB, Burkhoff D, Yue DT, Sagawa K: Mechanoelectrical feedback: Independent role of preload and contractility in modulation of canine ventricular excitability. J Clin Invest 76:1843–1850, 1985.
4. Reiter MJ, Synhorst DP, Mann DE: Electrophysiologic effects of acute ventricular dilatation in the isolated rabbit heart. Circ Res 62:554–562, 1988.
5. Franz MR, Burkhoff D, Yue DT, Sagawa K: Mechanically induced action potential changes and arrhythmia in isolated and in situ canine hearts. Cardiovasc Res 23:213–223, 1989.
6. Franz MR, Cima R, Wang D, et al: Electrophysiologic effects of myocardial stretch and mechanical determinants of stretch-activated arrhythmias. Circulation 86:968–978, 1992.
7. Hansen DE: Mechanoelectrical feedback effects of altering preload, afterload, and ventricular shortening. Am J Physiol 264:H423–H432, 1993.
8. Levine JH, Guarnieri T, Kadish AH, et al: Changes in myocardial repolarisation in patients undergoing balloon valvuloplasty

for congenital pulmonary stenosis: Evidence for contraction excitation feedback in humans. Circulation 77:70–77, 1988.

9. Taggart P, Sutton PMI, Treasure T, et al: Monophasic action potentials at discontinuation of cardiopulmonary bypass: Evidence for contraction-excitation feedback in man. Circulation 77:1266–1275, 1988.

10. Taggart P, Sutton P, Lab M, et al: Effect of abrupt changes in ventricular loading on repolarisation induced by transient aortic occlusion in man. Am J Physiol 636:H816–H823, 1992.

11. Dean JW, Lab MJ: Regional changes in ventricular excitability during load manipulation of the in situ pig heart. J Physiol (Lond) 429:387–400, 1990.

12. Zabel M, Portnoy S, Franz MR: Effect of sustained load on dispersion of ventricular repolarization and conduction time in the isolated rabbit heart. J Cardiovasc Electrophysiol 7:9–16, 1996.

13. Reiter MJ, Zetelakiz, Kirchof CJH, et al: Interaction of acute ventricular dilatation and d-sotalol during sustained ventricular tachycardia around a fixed obstacle. Circulation 89:423–431, 1994.

14. Reiter MJ, Landers M, Zetelaki Z, et al: Electrophysiologic effects of acute dilatation in the isolated rabbit heart: Cycle length-dependent effects on epicardial refractoriness and conduction velocity. Circulation 96:4050–4056, 1997.

15. Lab MJ: Contribution of mechano-electric coupling to ventricular arrhythmias during reduced perfusion. Int J Microcirc Clin Exp 8:433–442, 1989.

16. Hansen DE, Craig CS, Hondeghem LM: Stretch-induced arrhythmias in the isolated canine ventricle: Evidence for the importance of mechanoelectrical feedback. Circulation 81:1094–1105, 1990.

17. Stacy GP, Jobe RL, Taylor LK, Hansen DE: Stretch-induced depolarisations as a trigger of arrhythmias in isolated canine left ventricles. Am J Physiol 263:H613–H621, 1992.

18. Kaseda S, Zipes DP: Contraction-excitation feedback in the atria: A cause of changes in refractoriness. J Am Coll Cardiol 11:1327–1336, 1988.

19. Solti F, Veesey T, Kekesi V, Juhasz-Nagy A: The effect of atrial dilatation on atrial arrhythmias. Cardiovasc Res 23:882–886, 1989.

20. Ravelli F, Disertori M, Cozzi F, et al: Ventricular beats induce variations in cycle length of rapid (type II) atrial flutter in humans: Evidence of leading circle reentry. Circulation 89:2107–2116, 1994.

21. Ravelli F, Allessie MA: Effects of atrial dilation on refractory period and vulnerability to atrial fibrillation in the isolated Langendorff-perfused rabbit heart. Circulation 96:1686–1695, 1997.

22. Klein LS, Miles WM, Zipes DP: Effect of atrioventricular interval during pacing or reciprocating tachycardia on atrial size, pressure and refractory period: Contraction-excitation feedback in human atrium. Circulation 82:60–68, 1990.

23. Nazir SA, Lab MJ: Mechanoelectric feedback in the atrium of the isolated guinea-pig heart. Cardiovasc Res 32:112–119, 1996.

24. Calkins H, Maughan L, Weisman HF, et al: Effects of acute volume load on refractoriness and arrhythmia development in isolated chronically infarcted canine hearts. Circulation 79: 687–697, 1989.

25. Calkins H, Maughan WL, Kass DA, et al: Electrophysiological effect of volume load in isolated canine hearts. Am J Physiol 256:H1697–H1706, 1989.

26. Jalal S, Williams GR, Mann DE, Reiter MJ: Effect of ventricular dilatation on fibrillation thresholds in the isolated rabbit heart. Am J Physiol 263:H1306–H1310, 1992.

27. Ott P, Reiter MJ: Effect of ventricular dilation on defibrillation threshold in isolated perfused rabbit heart. J Cardiovasc Electrophysiol 8:1013–1019, 1997.

28. Hansen DE, Borganelli M, Stacey GP, Taylor LK: Dose-dependent inhibition of stretch-induced arrhythmias by gadolinium in isolated canine ventricles: Evidence for a unique mode of antiarrhythmic action. Circ Res 69:820–831, 1991.

29. Taggart P, Sutton P, John R, et al: Monophasic action potential recordings during acute changes in ventricular loading induced by the Valsalva manoeuvre. Br Heart J 67:221–229, 1992.

30. James PR, Hardman SM, Taggart P: Physiological changes in ventricular filling alter cardiac electrophysiology in patients with abnormal ventricular function. Heart 88:149–152, 2002.

31. Ambrosi P, Habib G, Kreitman B, Metras D: Valsalva manoeuvre for supraventricular tachycardia in transplanted heart recipient. Lancet 346:713, 1995.

32. Willerson JT, Curry GC, Watson JT, et al: Intra-aortic balloon counterpulsation in patients in cardiogenic shock, medically refractory left ventricular failure and/or recurrent ventricular tachycardia. Am J Med 58:183–191, 1975.

33. Hanson EC, Levine FH, Kay HR, et al: Control of post infarction irritability with the intra aortic balloon pump. Circulation 62(2 pt 2):I130–I137, 1980.

34. Culliford AY, Madden MR, Isom OW, et al: Intra-aortic balloon counterpulsation: Refractory ventricular tachycardia. JAMA 239:431–432, 1978.

35. Fotopoulos GD, Mason MJ, Walker S, et al: Stabilisation of medically refractory ventricular arrhythmia by intra-aortic balloon counterpulsation. Heart 82:96–100, 1999.

36. Kurose K, Okamoto K, Sato T, et al: Successful treatment of life threatening tachycardia with high dose propranolol under extracorporeal life support and intraaortic balloon pumping. Jpn Circ J 57:1106–1110, 1993.

37. Pitsis AA, Dardas P, Nikoloudakis N, Burkhoff D: Temporary assist device for post cardiotomy cardiac failure. Ann Thorac Surg 77:1431–1433, 2004.

38. Barbone A, Holmes JW, Heerdt PM, et al: Comparison of right and left ventricular responses to left ventricular assist device support in patients with severe heart failure: A primary role of mechanical unloading underlying reverse remodelling. Circulation 104:670–675, 2001.

39. Oz MC, Artrip JH, Burkhoff D: Direct cardiac compression devices. J Heart Lung Transplant 21:1049–1055, 2002.

40. The CONSENSUS Trial Study Group: Effects of enalapril on mortality in severe congestive heart failure. N Engl J Med 316:1429–1435, 1987.

41. Fletcher RD, Cintron GB, Johnson G, et al, for the V-HeFT 11 VA Cooperative Studies Group: Enalapril decrease prevalence of ventricular tachycardia in patients with chronic congestive heart failure. Circulation 87:V149–V155, 1993.

CHAPTER 35

Mechanical Modulation of Defibrillation Efficacy by Preload Changes

• • • •

Harish Doppalapudi and Raymond E. Ideker

Cardiac size and volume may be altered by cardiac compression or dilation or by changes in preload. Such changes may influence the efficacy of defibrillation by altering the current distribution or by changing the electrophysiologic properties of the myocardium. The former mechanism involves a change in the electric field produced by a shock without a change in the electrophysiologic properties of the myocardium and may be termed *extrinsic* mechano-electric feedback, whereas the latter mechanism involves the traditional concept of mechano-electric feedback and may be termed *intrinsic*. This chapter reviews evidence from animal and human studies, and then discusses the likely mechanisms underlying the influence of cardiac volume changes on defibrillation efficacy. Finally, this chapter discusses some clinical implications of this phenomenon.

EVIDENCE

Animal Studies

A decrease in the size and volume of the ventricles by cardiac compression or by a decrease in cardiac preload has been shown to improve defibrillation efficacy. Idriss and colleagues[1] showed that delivery of a shock during external cardiac compression decreased the 50% effective doses (ED_{50}) required for defibrillation by 37% in voltage, 49% in current, and 63% in energy and shifted the defibrillation dose–response curve to the left in fibrillating pigs (Fig. 35–1). In this study, cardiac compression was achieved by direct mechanical ventricular actuation, and defibrillation was performed using a biphasic waveform shock delivered between a

left ventricular (LV) apex patch and a superior vena cava (SVC) catheter electrode. In another study, Strobel and colleagues[2] inflated a balloon catheter in the inferior vena cava of pigs to decrease the cardiac preload. Although the reduced preload significantly decreased the ED_{50} of voltage (6%), current (12%), and energy (13%) required for defibrillation, this decrease was less than that in the previous study. A biphasic waveform shock was used for defibrillation, but, in contrast to the first study, the shock was delivered between an endocardial right ventricular (RV) lead and an SVC catheter.

Other studies have shown that the defibrillation threshold (DFT) increases with LV dilation and an increase in preload. Using a fluid-filled latex balloon in the LV of isolated Langendorff-perfused rabbit hearts, Ott and Reiter[3] demonstrated a 30% increase in the DFT voltage (which would correspond approximately to a 70% increase in DFT energy) with acute LV dilation. They used a monophasic waveform shock between a patch electrode positioned over the posterior LV and a metallic aortic cannula. Vigh and colleagues[4] investigated the DFT in dogs under three conditions—at baseline, after inducing LV dysfunction with norepinephrine infusion (to achieve an LV ejection fraction < 0.35), and, finally, after volume overload with normal saline (to achieve a pulmonary capillary wedge pressure > 19 mm Hg) in the setting of norepinephrine-induced LV dysfunction. A biphasic waveform was used for defibrillation delivered between a subcutaneous patch and an endovenous RV apex lead. A significant increase of more than 100% in DFT energy compared with baseline was observed only in the last situation—that is, volume overload in the presence of LV dysfunction (Fig. 35–2).

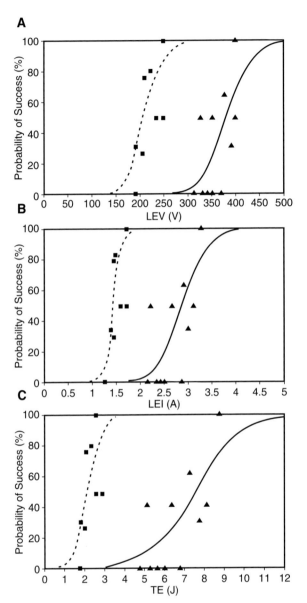

■ **Figure 35–1** Defibrillation shock strength versus probability of success for *(A)* leading edge voltage (LEV), *(B)* leading edge current (LEI), and *(C)* total energy (TE) for a single animal. In each panel, the fitted curves for the normal heart state *(solid line)* and the compressed heart state *(dashed line)* are plotted. For each heart state, the binned raw data points are shown as well *(squares* represent compression; *triangles* represent normal). The data for the normal heart state are positioned to the right of the data for the compressed heart state for each shock parameter. This indicates that shock delivery during cardiac compression improved defibrillation efficacy. *(Modified from Idriss SF, Anstadt MP, Anstadt GL, et al: The effect of cardiac compression on defibrillation efficacy and the upper limit of vulnerability. J Cardiovasc Electrophysiol 6:368–378, 1995, with permission.)*

Human Studies

In 46 patients who underwent implantation of a transvenous defibrillator lead system, Engelstein and colleagues[5] found that patients with DFT greater than 25 J had significantly larger LV volumes (>275 mL; $P < 0.01$) than patients with DFT less than or equal to 25 J. Brooks and colleagues[6] studied 101 consecutive patients requiring an implantable cardioverter-defibrillator (ICD), of

whom 72 underwent successful non-thoracotomy implantation and 29 required thoracotomy for placement of epicardial patches because of high DFT. A smaller cardiac size on chest radiographs and a smaller echocardiographic LV size in diastole were found to be predictors of successful non-thoracotomy implantation. Likewise, in a study of 101 patients who underwent placement of a transvenous defibrillation system, Raitt and colleagues[7] reported that radiographic

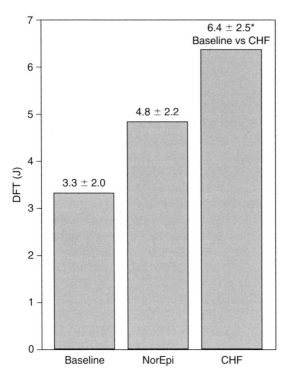

■ **Figure 35–2** Defibrillation threshold measured at baseline, after norepinephrine, and after acute heart failure induction in 10 dogs. A significant difference was noted between baseline and acute congestive heart failure (*P < 0.02). Values are means ± SD. CHF, volume overload simulating congestive heart failure; Norepi, norepinephrine. (*Modified from Vigh AG, Lowder J, Deantonio HJ: Does acute volume overloading in the setting of left ventricular dysfunction and pulmonary hypertension affect the defibrillation threshold? Pacing Clin Electrophysiol 22:759–764, 1999, with permission.*)

cardiac size and echocardiographic LV end-diastolic diameter showed a significant positive correlation with the DFT ($r = 0.36$, $P \leq 0.0003$; and $r = 0.40$, $P \leq 0.0001$, respectively).

Kopp and colleagues[8] studied 95 patients who received ICD. Of these patients, 73 had adequate DFT (≤25 J) and underwent successful nonepicardial lead system implantation. However, in contrast to the studies discussed previously, radiographic heart size and echocardiographic LV size were not found to be predictors of DFT. Klein and colleagues[9] observed no difference in the DFT in 10 patients before or during cardiopulmonary bypass (during which ventricular

volumes are smaller). In a series of eight patients, Haberman and colleagues[10] observed no correlation between the DFT and LV volume.

MECHANISMS

To understand how changes in preload can impact defibrillation, the basic mechanism of defibrillation must be understood.[11] To defibrillate, a shock must not only halt the fibrillation wave fronts, but it also must not create new wave fronts that reinduce fibrillation.[12] A small shock fails to defibrillate because it does not halt all ventricular fibrillation (VF) activation fronts. A stronger shock, still well below the DFT, fails to defibrillate because of re-entry induced by virtual electrodes[13] or shock-induced prolongation of refractoriness and block.[14] A still stronger shock of near DFT strength may fail to defibrillate because of the induction of at least three rapidly activating postshock cycles arising from a focus where the shock field is weak.[15] To defibrillate, a shock must be sufficiently strong that any postshock ectopic cycles of activation are too few or too slow to induce re-entry that degenerates into VF.

Thus, the concept of an initiator and a substrate, as has been previously applied to understanding the initiation of arrhythmias, also applies to defibrillation, with the three or more rapidly activating focal postshock cycles serving as the initiator, and the region of the myocardium where re-entry later develops serving as the substrate.

The ability of a given shock to defibrillate the heart depends on the potential gradient field generated within the myocardium by the shock. There appears to be a minimum potential gradient that must be created throughout the ventricles by the shock to defibrillate consistently.[16] Alteration in current distribution alters the potential gradient field produced by the shock. For a given potential gradient field that is generated, the electrophysiologic properties of the myocardium may determine whether a greater minimum potential gradient is required in the low-gradient areas, and may thus influence the defibrillation efficacy.[17] Changes in preload can influence defibrillation efficacy at both these levels—that is, by alteration of the potential gradient field that is generated by the shock because of alteration in current distribution, and by alteration of the minimum potential gradient field that is required because of alteration in the electrophysiologic properties of the myocardium.

Extrinsic

The first level involves alteration of the potential gradient field generated in the myocardium by an alteration in the current distribution because of a change in ventricular volume or dimensions. Because this mechanism does not involve a direct change in the electrophysiologic properties of the myocardium, it may be termed *extrinsic*.

Compression of the heart decreases the ventricular blood pool by mechanically shunting the blood out of the ventricles. For a given shock strength, decreasing the low-impedance ventricular blood pool results in a greater proportion of the shock current being passed through the high-impedance myocardial tissue.[18] This, in turn, increases the potential gradient in the myocardium. In support of this view, the impedance during defibrillation has been shown to increase with cardiac compression,[1,2] suggesting that less current is shunted through the blood and more current is passed through the myocardium when the volume of blood within the ventricles is decreased by cardiac compression. In the study by Ott and Reiter,[3] however, acute LV dilation has been shown to increase the impedance. Notably, though, in this study, LV dilation was achieved by an inflated, insulated balloon in the LV cavity that offered more resistance to current flow than free blood would.

Compression also decreases the cross-sectional area of the heart. Decreasing chamber dimensions, and hence the distance between shock electrodes, also decreases the distance from the electrodes to the portion of the ventricles most remote from them. Because the potential gradient field in any portion of the myocardium decreases with increasing distance from the shock electrodes, decreasing the distance of the myocardial region that is situated farthest from the shock electrodes would result in a greater minimum potential gradient field throughout the myocardium.

These effects of compression lead to more efficient current distribution, resulting in improvement in defibrillation efficacy.[17] Volume overload of the heart causes the opposite effects, and thus decreases the defibrillation efficacy. Indeed, as shown in Figure 35–3, a computerized simulation of a defibrillation shock delivered to a ventricle with the same volume of myocardium but an increased diameter and cavity size, simulating a dilated ventricle, demonstrates a larger volume of ventricle exposed to a low-potential gradient.[17]

Defibrillation during compression also has been shown to decrease the animal-to-animal variation in the ED_{50} estimate compared with defibrillation without compression.[1] This suggests that geometric differences among animals, either before or after initiation of VF, may account for a proportion of the interanimal variability in defibrillation requirements. Because static cardiac compression creates a more similar cardiac geometry among animals, the potential gradient field for a given defibrillation lead configuration would become more similar across animals.

Intrinsic

For a given potential gradient, mechanical changes can influence the defibrillation efficacy by altering the electrical properties of the myocardium. This may be termed *intrinsic* mechano-electric feedback. The electrophysiologic changes, in turn, can be direct, or they may be mediated through the autonomic nervous system (indirect).

Direct

An increase in preload stretches the ventricle. Various studies in isolated tissue,[19,20] in intact animal heart models,[21–25] and in patients[26] have shown that stretch of the ventricular muscle decreases the action potential duration (APD) and the refractory period, but increases the dispersion of refractoriness, decreases the conduction velocity, and induces depolarizations.

Preload alterations can be considered in terms of static, baseline volume overload and rapid, dynamic volume changes. Likewise, stretch includes acute stretch (caused by rapid, dynamic volume changes) and chronic stretch (gradual, static volume overload). Stretch-induced depolarizations are predominantly caused by acute stretch and are probably mediated through (nonselective) stretch-activated ion channels.[27,28] The changes

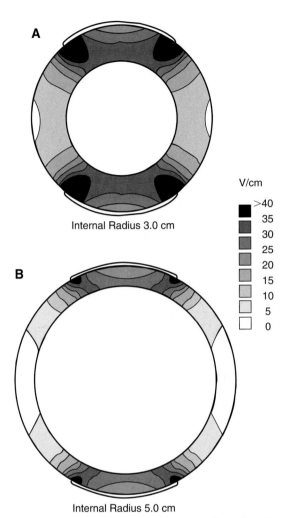

A

Internal Radius 3.0 cm

V/cm

■	>40
■	35
■	30
■	25
■	20
▨	15
▨	10
▨	5
□	0

B

Internal Radius 5.0 cm

■ **Figure 35–3** Computer simulation of effect of cardiac dilation on potential gradient field produced by a 200 V shock. Each circle represents a cross section of the left ventricle. The defibrillation electrodes are curved discs, applied to the top and bottom portions of the heart, and have the same surface area in *A* and *B*. The volume of myocardium is the same in *A* and *B*. *A*, The internal radius of the heart is 3.0 cm; *B*, the internal radius is 5.0 cm. The central portions represent the blood-filled chamber. The conductivity of the myocardium is assumed to be 0.003 S/cm, and the conductivity of the blood is 0.0065 S/cm. The gray level key depicts the resulting potential gradients. The low-gradient area (lighter shades of gray) is considerably larger for the dilated heart *(B)*. (See color insert.) *(Reproduced from Hillsley RE, Wharton JM, Cates AW, et al: Why do some patients have high defibrillation thresholds at defibrillator implantation? Pacing Clin Electrophysiol 17:222–239, 1994, with permission.)* (See color insert.)

in APD and in refractory period can be caused both by acute stretch, through mechanosensitive ion channels, and by chronic stretch, possibly through down-regulation of calcium channels.[27,28] Chronic stretch also causes structural remodeling including connexin expression that can increase anisotropy and cause slowing of conduction.[29,30] All these changes caused by acute or chronic stretch can influence the ability of a shock to defibrillate. They can affect initiation of postshock activation or alter the substrate for re-entry.

Effect on Substrate

A successful defibrillation shock can be classified as type A if the earliest postshock activation appears more than 130 msec after the shock or as type B if it appears less than or equal to 130 msec after the shock.[31] Unsuccessful defibrillation shocks have the same post-shock activation pattern as type B successful shocks of the same shock strength for the first cycle after the shock.[31] However, in the former, the rapid cycles of postshock activation continue until refibrillation occurs through re-entry, whereas in the latter, the ectopic activation cycles terminate, usually in fewer than three cycles in healthy hearts, before re-entry is induced (Fig. 35–4). Thus, altering the substrate may increase the DFT by causing a shock to fail because the one or two rapid postshock cycles induce re-entry in this altered substrate, whereas they would not have induced re-entry in a healthy heart, so that a type B success would have occurred instead. Ventricular dilation (both acute and chronic) decreases the refractory period and increases the dispersion of refractoriness. Chronic volume overload induces structural changes that increase nonuniform anisotropy and cause slowing of conduction, thus facilitating conduction block. Both these effects may facilitate re-entry and cause a shock to fail that would have been a type B success in a heart with a normal substrate.

Effect on Initiation

Acute volume overload (acute stretch) increases the excitability of the myocardium and causes stretch-induced depolarizations.[19,21,24,25] Increased baseline ventricular volume increases the sensitivity to acute stretch-induced depolarizations.[24] Based on our previous discussion that shocks of near-DFT strength fail because of induction of rapidly activating postshock

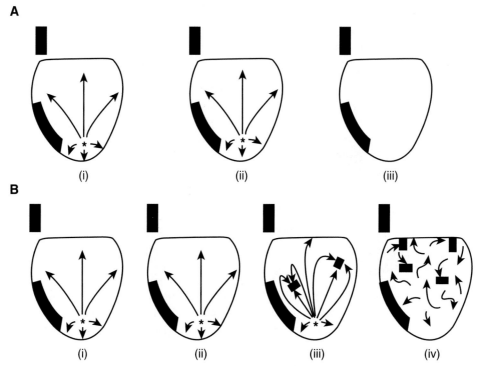

■ **Figure 35–4** Differences in responses after a successful type B shock *(A)* and a failed shock *(B)* delivered from electrodes in the right ventricular apex and the superior vena cava during ventricular fibrillation *(long black bars)*. A, Successful type B shock. After the shock, two cycles of activation arise from a region of the ventricles where the shock field is weak *(asterisk)* and spread over the entire ventricular epicardium *(arrows)*, as shown in (i) and (ii). After the two cycles, spontaneous activations terminate, leaving the ventricles electrically quiescent, as shown in (iii). An organized recovery rhythm is then established. B, Failed shock. Three postshock foci of activation arise from a region where the shock field is weak, as shown in (i), (ii), and (iii). The third activation encounters refractory tissue, so that conduction block occurs *(short black bars)* as shown in (iii), setting up re-entry, which ultimately leads to refibrillation (iv). Thus, the focal activations act as the initiator, and the myocardium where conduction block occurs acts as the substrate in the genesis of refibrillation after a failed shock.

cycles arising from a focus where the shock field is weak, we can conceptualize that volume overload increases the threshold shock field required for noninitiation of focal activations, thus increasing the strength of current required for defibrillation.

Indirect

Changes in preload can cause baroreceptor-mediated alteration of parasympathetic and sympathetic tone. Changes in autonomic tone have been reported to affect ventricular vulnerability and the VF threshold.[32,33] Augmented preload has been shown by

Lerman and colleagues[34] to decrease the ventricular APD and refractoriness through activation of β-adrenergic receptors. This may occur by catecholamine release from intramyocardial nerve endings.[34] These effects are shown to be abolished by β-blockers and by catecholamine depletion. A shortening of APD was reported with dobutamine infusion in another study.[35] As discussed previously, decrease in APD and refractoriness can increase the DFT. Epinephrine has been shown by Sousa and colleagues to increase the DFT.[36] Thus, augmentation of preload can increase the DFT by activating the sympathetic system. However, other studies have shown either a decrease[37,38] or no change[39] in the DFT with adrenergic stimulation.

UPPER LIMIT OF VULNERABILITY/DEFIBRILLATION THRESHOLD CORRELATION

The effect of volume changes on the energy required for defibrillation can help explain why the upper limit of vulnerability (ULV) does not always equal or exceed the DFT. The ULV hypothesis for defibrillation states that, to defibrillate, a shock must not only halt the activation fronts of VF, but it also must not reinitiate VF by the same mechanism that a shock of the same strength during the vulnerable period of paced or sinus rhythm initiates VF.[12,31] A premature electrical stimulus given during the vulnerable period induces re-entry leading to fibrillation when a critical value of potential gradient field, created by the stimulus, intersects a critical degree of refractoriness of the myocardium.

ULV testing is performed by delivering shocks during the T wave when the shock field is most likely to be passing through the critical degree of refractoriness in that part of the ventricle where the shock field is weakest. In contrast, with DFT testing, shocks are delivered during fibrillation with no fixed relation to the repolarization state of the myocardium. A defibrillation shock of slightly less strength than the ULV given during fibrillation may not create a critical point if the tissue, in the region where the shock field is weakest, is not in its vulnerable period; thus, the shock may result in successful defibrillation.[40] Therefore, the ULV should always be greater than or equal to the DFT. However, several investigators have been unable to demonstrate this relation.[1,40]

This discrepancy may result from the fact that cardiac geometry or blood volume, or both, are different during ULV testing than during defibrillation testing. DFT is measured during VF when the cardiac geometry is altered, and the ventricular (especially RV) volume is larger than during ULV determination.[41,42] The latter is performed during the T wave during ventricular systole. These differences in geometry and blood volume may alter the shock-induced myocardial electric field causing the DFT to exceed the ULV.[43]

Maintaining constant cardiac geometry and volume during both ULV testing in paced rhythm and DFT testing in VF keeps the ULV consistently greater than the DFT. This was demonstrated by Malkin and colleagues,[44] who used a rapid-pacing protocol during ULV testing to mimic the electrical or mechanical events, or both, that occur during VF, and by Idriss and colleagues,[1] who used external cardiac compression to maintain similar cardiac geometry and volume with ULV testing during paced rhythm and DFT testing during VF (Fig. 35–5).

CLINICAL IMPLICATIONS

Heart Failure

Heart failure (HF) is a complex pathophysiologic condition in which several different factors, including hemodynamic changes, morphologic alterations, and neurohormonal activation, may influence the DFT. Preload changes can explain the failure of internal defibrillation devices in patients with decompensated HF. As discussed previously, ventricular volume has been shown to be positively correlated with the DFT. Patients with heart failure have a larger baseline LV volume than healthy individuals and tend to have greater DFT. More importantly, acute ventricular dilation (e.g., acute hemodynamic decompensation and acute myocardial ischemia) may result in a significant increase in defibrillation energy requirement. This is because, in addition to the *extrinsic* effects of increased volume, chronic stretch from baseline elevated ventricular volume increases the sensitivity to acute, stretch-induced, electrophysiologic changes.[24] This may result in defibrillation failure in these situations, even if the DFT obtained at the time of implantation was below the programmed or maximum energy delivered by the device.

Volume changes may also have indirect effects on the defibrillation energy requirements in HF. HF usually is associated with cardiac hypertrophy and an increase in LV mass. Chapman and colleagues[45] found a significant positive correlation between LV mass and DFT in humans and dogs. Several studies in animals[2,46,47] and humans[7,8] showed a similar correlation, but other studies did not.[3,5,10,48] Volume overload (chronic stretch) likely does play a role by affecting

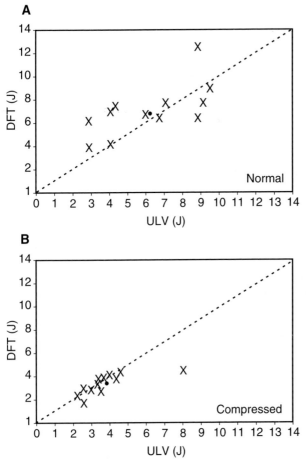

■ **Figure 35–5** Defibrillation threshold (DFT) versus upper limit of vulnerability (ULV) in terms of total energy for the normal *(A)* and compressed *(B)* heart states. *X* represents the mean DFT and mean ULV determined in a single animal. *Solid circles* indicate the mean DFT and mean ULV for all the animals combined. *Dashed lines* represent the unity slope line—the line along which data points are positioned if the ULV and DFT are equal. In *A* (normal heart state), the ULV tends to underestimate the DFT (many points and the *solid circle* positioned above unity slope line), whereas in *B* (compressed heart state), the opposite is true (data points and *solid circle* positioned below unity slope line). *(Modified from Idriss SF, Anstadt MP, Anstadt GL, et al: The effect of cardiac compression on defibrillation efficacy and the upper limit of vulnerability. J Cardiovasc Electrophysiol 6:368–378, 1995, with permission.)*

expression of connexins[29,30] that affect hypertrophy, fibrosis, and other structural changes in HF.

Interestingly, several studies found no correlation between the ejection fraction (EF) and defibrillation efficacy,[5,6,8,47,49] whereas two small studies[7,48] did show a negative correlation. This may be because EF is a poor surrogate of HF (and of volume overload) or because of the different etiologic factors of HF in different patients.

The DFT in HF is affected by LV dilation, hypertrophy, wall thinning, and other chronic alterations. Although most of these changes tend to increase the DFT, some changes (particularly wall thinning) tend to decrease it. Hence, it is difficult to predict the DFT in HF. In a canine model of rapid pacing–induced heart failure, Lucy and colleagues[46] showed a fourfold increase in DFT energy compared with control sub-

jects (Fig. 35–6), and this was significantly correlated with ventricular weight (the ventricular weight being significantly greater in the rapidly paced group). Even when expressed as DFT per gram of ventricular tissue, the authors found a significant increase in DFT in the rapidly paced group compared with control subjects, thus suggesting that both myocardial hypertrophy and LV dysfunction independently affect DFT. They used two sequential monophasic shocks for defibrillation, with the first shock delivered between an anterior RV mesh electrode and a mesh electrode on the left lateral free wall, and the second shock delivered between a posterior RV mesh electrode and the left lateral free wall mesh electrode. Likewise, Huang and colleagues[50] showed that HF, induced by rapid pacing, increased the DFT energy by 180% in dogs when a biphasic

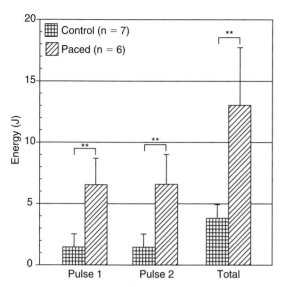

■ **Figure 35–6** Mean defibrillation threshold energy of sequential pulses 1 and 2 and total energy for control and paced animals. Note the minimum energy required to defibrillate hearts of animals with pacing-induced cardiomyopathy was four times greater than that of control animals ($^{**}P < 0.01$). *(Modified from Lucy SD, Jones DL, Klein GJ: Pronounced increase in defibrillation threshold associated with pacing-induced cardiomyopathy in the dog. Am Heart J 127:366–376, 1994, with permission.)*

defibrillation waveform was delivered between an RV apical electrode and an SVC electrode. They also showed that an auxiliary shock to the LV through an electrode in the great cardiac vein decreased the DFT in HF. However, in a similar dog model, Friedman and colleagues[47] found no difference in the ED_{50} or the DFT between failing and nonfailing hearts when a biphasic waveform was delivered between a rectangular cutaneous patch on the left lateral chest wall and an endovenous RV coil. In their study, rapid pacing produced no change in LV mass. However, it induced ventricular cavity dilation and wall thinning, which may have had opposing effects on defibrillation energy requirements, resulting in no net change in the ED_{50} in heart failure.

Prolonged Ventricular Fibrillation

The effects of volume can explain why defibrillation energy requirements may increase with time during VF. Blood is pooled in the venous circulation during VF, so that the right heart becomes progressively distended and the left heart progressively empty over about 3 min of VF.[41,42] Some studies report that defibrillation energy requirements increase with time during VF, whereas other studies report no change in DFT.[1] Interestingly, those studies showing no change in DFT over time used subcutaneous or epicardial patches combined with an endocardial electrode. In the former studies, the increase in DFT may be attributed to increased shunting of current from the endocardial electrode through the increased blood pool of the RV cavity. Therefore, it is important to minimize the duration of VF with endocardial electrodes.

Timing of Shock during Resuscitation

The beneficial effects of compression on defibrillation efficacy suggest that defibrillation efficacy may be improved if shock delivery is timed to peak compression during closed- or open-chest cardiac massage. However, this may not be as important with external defibrillation as it is with internal defibrillation. Internal defibrillation uses small current strengths and is predominantly influenced by the state of the myocardium. External defibrillation, in contrast, involves much greater currents and is influenced by extracardiac and cardiac factors. The relatively small changes in ED_{50} with compression tend to be important when small shock energies are involved (as in internal defibrillation), but they are negligible in the context of high shock energies (with external defibrillation).

Summary

Cardiac volume changes affect the efficacy of defibrillation by altering the current distribution (extrinsic mechano-electric feedback) or by changing the electrophysiologic properties of the myocardium (intrinsic mechano-electric feedback), or both. Cardiac compression and a decrease in preload decrease the DFT, whereas cardiac dilation and an increase in preload increase the DFT. Although patients with heart failure have a larger baseline ventricular volume than the normal level, which tends to increase the DFT, the baseline DFT is difficult to predict because hypertrophy, wall thinning, and other chronic alterations also affect the DFT in HF. Clinical situations causing an increase in ventricular volume, such as acute hemodynamic compensation in patients with heart failure and prolonged VF, tend to increase the DFT.

Acknowledgments

This review is supported in part by National Institutes of Health grant HL-42760.

References

1. Idriss SF, Anstadt MP, Anstadt GL, et al: The effect of cardiac compression on defibrillation efficacy and the upper limit of vulnerability. J Cardiovasc Electrophysiol 6:368–378, 1995.
2. Strobel JS, Kay GN, Walcott GP, et al: Defibrillation efficacy with endocardial electrodes is influenced by reductions in cardiac preload. J Interv Card Electrophysiol 1:95–102, 1997.
3. Ott P, Reiter MJ: Effect of ventricular dilatation on defibrillation threshold in the isolated perfused rabbit heart. J Cardiovasc Electrophysiol 8:1013–1019, 1997.
4. Vigh AG, Lowder J, Deantonio HJ: Does acute volume overloading in the setting of left ventricular dysfunction and pulmonary hypertension affect the defibrillation threshold? Pacing Clin Electrophysiol 22:759–764, 1999.
5. Engelstein ED, Hahn RT, Stein KM, et al: Noninvasive predictors of successful implantation of transvenous defibrillator lead systems. J Am Coll Cardiol, 25 (Spec Issue):110A, 1995.
6. Brooks R, Garan H, Torchiana D, et al: Determinants of successful nonthoracotomy cardioverter-defibrillator implantation: Experience in 101 patients using two different lead systems. J Am Coll Cardiol 22:1835–1842, 1993.
7. Raitt MH, Johnson G, Dolack GL, et al: Clinical predictors of the defibrillator threshold with the unipolar implantable defibrillation system. J Am Coll Cardiol 25:1576–1583, 1995.
8. Kopp DE, Blakeman BP, Kall GJ, et al: Predictors of defibrillation energy requirements with nonepicardial lead systems. Pacing Clin Electrophysiol 18:253–260, 1995.
9. Klein GJ, Jones DL, Sharma AD, et al: Influence of cardiopulmonary bypass on internal cardiac defibrillation. Am J Cardiol 57:1194–1195, 1986.
10. Haberman RJ, Mower MM, Veltri EP, et al: LV mass and defibrillation threshold. Am Heart J 115:1340–1341, 1988.
11. Ideker RE, Chattipakorn N, Gray RA: Defibrillation mechanisms. J Cardiovasc Electrophysiol 11:1008–1013, 2000.
12. Shibata N, Chen PS, Dixon EG, et al: Epicardial activation after unsuccessful defibrillation shocks in dogs. Am J Physiol 255:H902–H909, 1988.
13. Efimov IR, Cheng Y, Van Wagoner DR, et al: Virtual electrode-induced phase singularity—a basic mechanism of defibrillation failure. Circ Res 82:918–925, 1998.
14. Jones JL, Swartz JF, Jones RE, et al: Extracellular field stimulation with symmetrical biphasic defibrillation waveforms

15. Chattipakorn N, Fotuhi PC, Ideker RE: Prediction of defibrillation outcome by epicardial activation patterns following shocks near the defibrillation threshold. J Cardiovasc Electrophysiol 11:1014–1021, 2000.
16. Wharton JM, Wolf PD, Smith WM, et al: Cardiac potential and potential gradient fields generated by single, combined, and sequential shocks during ventricular defibrillation. Circulation 85:1510–1523, 1992.
17. Hillsley RE, Wharton JM, Cates AW, et al: Why do some patients have high defibrillation thresholds at defibrillator implantation? Pacing Clin Electrophysiol 17:222–239, 1994.
18. Sepulveda NG, Wikswo JP Jr, Echt DS: Finite element analysis of cardiac defibrillation current distributions. IEEE Trans Biomed Eng 37:354–365, 1990.
19. Lab MJ: Mechanically dependent changes in action potentials recorded from the intact frog ventricle. Circ Res 42:519–528, 1978.
20. Lab MJ: Transient depolarisation and action potential alterations following mechanical changes in isolated myocardium. Cardiovasc Res 14:624–637, 1980.
21. Franz MR, Cima R, Wang D, et al: Electrophysiological effects of myocardial stretch and mechanical determinants of stretch-activated arrhythmias. Circulation 86:968–978, 1992.
22. Reiter MJ, Synhorst DP, Mann DE: Electrophysiological effects of acute ventricular dilatation in the isolated rabbit heart. Circ Res 62:554–562, 1988.
23. Lerman BB, Burkhoff D, Yue DT, et al: Mechanoelectrical feedback: Independent role of preload and contractility in modulation of canine ventricular excitability. J Clin Invest 76:1843–1850, 1985.
24. Hansen DE, Craig CS, Hondeghem LM: Stretch-induced arrhythmias in the isolated canine ventricle. Circulation 81:1094–1105, 1990.
25. Franz MR, Burkhoff D, Yue DT, et al: Mechanically induced action potential changes and arrhythmia in isolated and in situ canine hearts. Cardiovasc Res 23:213–223, 1989.
26. Taggart P, Sutton PMI, Treasure T, et al: Monophasic action potentials at discontinuation of cardiopulmonary bypass: Evidence for contraction-excitation feedback in man. Circulation 77:1266–1275, 1988.
27. Ravens U: Mechano-electric feedback and arrhythmias. Prog Biophys Mol Biol 82:255–266, 2003.
28. Janse MJ, Coronel R, Wilms-Schopman FJG, et al: Mechanical effects on arrhythmogenesis: From pipette to patient. Prog Biophys Mol Biol 82:187–195, 2003.
29. Kanno S, Saffitz JE: The role of myocardial gap junctions in electrical conduction and arrhythmogenesis. Cardiovasc Pathol 10:169–177, 2001.
30. Severs NJ: Gap junction remodeling in heart failure. J Card Fail 8:S293–S299, 2002.
31. Chen PS, Shibata N, Dixon EG, et al: Activation during ventricular defibrillation in open-chest dogs. Evidence of complete cessation and regeneration of ventricular fibrillation after unsuccessful shocks. J Clin Invest 77:810–823, 1986.
32. Verrier RL, Thompson PL, Lown B: Ventricular vulnerability during sympathetic stimulation: Role of heart rate and blood pressure. Cardiovasc Res 8:602–610, 1974.
33. Han J, Jalon PG, Moe GK: Adrenergic effects on ventricular vulnerability. Circ Res 14:516–524, 1964.

34. Lerman BB, Engelstein ED, Burkhoff D: Mechanoelectrical feedback: Role of β-adrenergic receptor activation in mediating load-dependent shortening of ventricular action potential and refractoriness. Circulation 104:486–490, 2001.

35. Horner SM, Murphy CF, Coen B, et al: Sympathomimetic modulation of load-dependent changes in the action potential duration in the in situ porcine heart. Cardiovasc Res 32:148–157, 1996.

36. Sousa J, Kou W, Calkins H, et al: Effect of epinephrine on the efficacy of the internal cardioverter-defibrillator. Am J Cardiol 69:509–512, 1992.

37. Ruffy R, Schechtman K, Monje E: β-Adrenergic modulation of direct defibrillation energy in anesthetized dog heart. Am J Physiol 248:H674–H677, 1985.

38. Ruffy R, Schechtman K, Monje E, et al: Adrenergically mediated variations in the energy required to defibrillate the heart: Observations in closed-chest, nonanesthetized dogs. Circulation 73:374–380, 1986.

39. Rattes MJ, Sharma AD, Klein GJ, et al: Adrenergic effects on internal cardiac defibrillation threshold. Am J Physiol 253:H500–H506, 1987.

40. Souza JJ, Malkin RA, Ideker RE: Comparison of upper limit of vulnerability and defibrillation probability of success curves using a nonthoracotomy lead system. Circulation 91:1247–1252, 1995.

41. Steen S, Liao Q, Pierre L, et al: The critical importance of minimal delay between chest compressions and subsequent defibrillation: A hemodynamic explanation. Resuscitation 58:249–258, 2003.

42. Mashiro I, Cohn J, Heckel R, et al: Left and right ventricular dimensions during ventricular fibrillation in the dog. Am J Physiol 235:H231–H236, 1978.

43. Idriss SF, Melnick SB, Wolf PD, et al: Predicting the potential gradient field in ventricular fibrillation from shocks delivered in paced rhythm. Am J Physiol 268:H2336–H2344, 1995.

44. Malkin RA, Idriss SF, Walker RG, et al: Effect of rapid pacing and T-wave scanning on the relation between the defibrillation and upper-limit-of-vulnerability dose response curves. Circulation 92:1291–1299, 1995.

45. Chapman PD, Sagar KB, Wetherbee JN, et al: Relationship of left ventricular mass to defibrillation threshold for the implantable defibrillator: A combined clinical and animal study. Am Heart J 114:274–278, 1987.

46. Lucy SD, Jones DL, Klein GJ: Pronounced increase in defibrillation threshold associated with pacing-induced cardiomyopathy in the dog. Am Heart J 127:366–376, 1994.

47. Friedman PA, Foley DA, Christian TF, et al: Stability of the defibrillation probability curve with the development of ventricular dysfunction in the canine rapid paced model. Pacing Clin Electrophysiol 21:339–351, 1998.

48. O'Donoghue S, Platia EV, Mispireta L, et al: Relationships between left ventricular mass and ejection fraction, and defibrillation threshold. J Am Coll Cardiol 15:51A, 1990.

49. Strickberger SA, Brownstein SL, Wilkoff BL, et al: Clinical predictors of defibrillation energy requirements in patients treated with a nonthoracotomy defibrillator system. Am Heart J 131:257–260, 1996.

50. Huang J, Rogers JM, Killingsworth CR, et al: Improvement of defibrillation efficacy and quantification of activation patterns during ventricular fibrillation in a canine heart failure model. Circulation 103:1473–1478, 2001.

CHAPTER 36

Passive Ventricular Containment: A New Treatment Concept for Dilated Cardiomyopathy

• • • •

David A. Kass

Chronic cardiac remodeling is a central feature of the pathophysiology of dilated cardiomyopathy. This process involves structural changes within the extracellular matrix, distortion of the size and shape of cardiomyocytes themselves, and numerous molecular and cellular abnormalities. Under the influence of systemic and locally released neurohormones and abnormal ventricular loading, these abnormalities conspire to limit basal and reserve cardiac function and exacerbate failure. Over the last few decades, the importance of chamber dilation as a feed-forward stimulus to worsened failure has been increasingly recognized.[1,2] Existing treatments with proven efficacy to reduce mortality from both pump failure and sudden cardiac death have had as a common feature the capacity to inhibit and/or reverse chamber dilation/remodeling.[3] Prominent examples are pharmacologic therapies that block the renin-angiotensin-aldosterone system and β-adrenergic system[4–6] and the recently developed pacing-based treatment known as cardiac resynchronization.[7] In the former, remodeling is impeded by blocking detrimental biochemical pathways; in the latter, systolic and energetic improvements caused by more coordinated contraction and redistribution of regional chamber load are involved.

Another approach to limiting chamber dilation is somewhat more direct—that is, to apply a surrounding membrane to the heart that can act as an elastic passive containment.[8–10] In principle, this provides a reminder of a size that the heart should not exceed, perhaps similar to an expensive pair of pants that you still wish to fit into even as years pass. The containment should be elastic, so that the heart can expand intermittently without suffering constrictive physiology, but not

overly so to provide an effective limit to more chronic dilation.

The pericardium does not effectively work as a therapeutic containment for several reasons. It is virtually inflexible once stretched beyond its rest volume, so it provides either no effective restraint to dilation or an extreme constraint.[11] The pericardium also dilates/remodels with chronic failure, but the extent of dilation does not appear to restore the normal reserve space for volume expansion, therefore failing hearts appear to operate closer to the pericardial limit.[12] Other membranes formed first by skeletal muscle tissue and more recently by artificial materials appear to have the requisite properties for an elastic containment. What started out as a surprising observation with skeletal cardiomyoplasty[13] has since led to a new heart failure therapy in which a nonbiologic passive wrap is applied around the heart to keep dilation in check. This strategy appears not only to impede progressive dilation, but actually to reverse dilation and many biochemical and molecular abnormalities that come with it. This chapter reviews the key, albeit initial and still limited, data describing the evolution of this new approach.

DAWN OF A CONCEPT: LESSONS FROM CARDIOMYOPLASTY

In the mid-1980s, pioneering cardiovascular surgeons began to explore the feasibility of creating a muscular booster pump for the heart out of the thin sheet latissimus dorsi muscle. Basic science work had demonstrated the capacity to convert rapid-twitch fatigable skeletal muscle force behavior to a slower nonfatigable cardiac phenotype by cyclic nontetanic stimulation. The excised skeletal muscle was to be wrapped around the heart, and when stimulated using burst electrical impulses, it would contract to assist in systolic ejection. Termed *dynamic cardiomyoplasty* (dCM),[14,15] this treatment began to enter clinical trials by the mid-1990s as part of several multicenter trials in Europe and the United States. However, although conceived as a systolic ventricular assist, subsequent experimental and clinical trial data seemed to point toward a dominant if not primary benefit arising from a passive girdling effect of the wrap.[13,16] Certainly, the notion of a girdle effect had been on the list of potential mechanisms, but few thought it could play such a major role.

Perhaps the first hint that passive action was more important than active assist came in a small but provocative study reported in 1995.[13] Three patients were treated with dCM, and each patient underwent invasive catheterization using pressure–volume analysis to systolic and diastolic function before surgery, and then serially over a 1-year follow-up period. Data with active assist on and off also were compared. As depicted in Figure 36–1*A* and *B,* dCM resulted in a substantial reversal of remodeling, shifting pressure–volume loop data leftward, despite maintenance of stroke volume, and without any compromise in diastolic function. The end-systolic pressure–volume relation shifted to the left, but the diastolic pressure–volume relation remained unaltered. Importantly, this

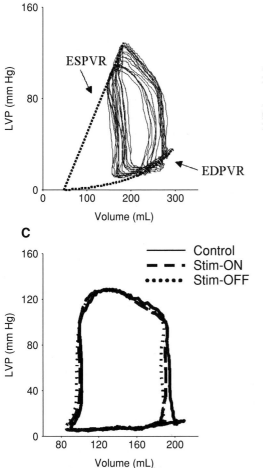

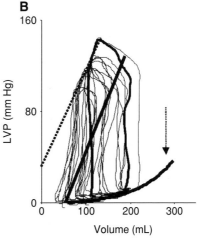

■ **Figure 36–1** *A,B,* Reverse remodeling associated with cardiomyoplasty in human subjects. Pressure–volume relations are obtained in a patient with chronic dilated cardiomyopathy, with cardiac cycles recorded during transient obstruction of the vena cava to vary preload and derive end-systolic and end-diastolic pressure–volume relations (ESPVR and EDPVR, respectively). Baseline data are shown in *A;* the effects of chronic myoplasty are shown in *B* (*vertical arrow,* initial, end-diastolic volume). The baseline ESPVR and EDPVR are superimposed on the latter to show changes. There is a marked left shift of the ESPVR and no significant change in the EDPVR with this chronic myoplasty. Importantly, despite this remodeling effect and improved systolic function, there is no active assist demonstrable in the same patients *(C).* LVP, left ventricular pressure. (*Reproduced from Kass DA, Baughman KL, Pak PH, et al: Reverse remodeling from cardiomyoplasty in human heart failure: External constraint versus active assist. Circulation 91:2314–2318, 1995, with permission.)*

striking chronic effect stood in contrast to the absence of any demonstrable impact on cardiac function when the dCM was acutely turned on (burst stimulation) or off (see Fig. 36–1C). This led to the notion that chronic reverse remodeling was unlikely to be caused by direct systolic assist, but rather might be related to a girdling effect of the muscle. Indeed, the authors speculated that, if correct, an artificial *heart sock* might achieve the same effects, obviating the need for more complex muscle surgery. This prediction was subsequently supported by experimental studies. In a follow-up investigation, cardiac failure was generated in the dog using a rapid-pacing model, and then the animal was treated with a cardiomyoplasty wrap.[16] To assure that systolic assist was not possible, the muscle was stimulated by a standard single-spike pacemaker, which does not induce muscle contraction, although it does convert the muscle to a cardiac phenotype. The results were striking, again showing reversal of chronic remodeling and improvement in contractile function parameters, which were achieved at reduced diastolic pressures and volumes. These results were even more intriguing when contrasted to a parallel study from the same investigators in which the myoplasty wrap was dynamic, with a burst stimulator used to generate a systolic assist.[17] The extent of reverse chamber remodeling and improved cardiac function was similar to if not slightly *less* than that observed with the purely passive wrap, which further emphasizes the value of a girdling mechanism. In fairness, there were several other studies in both animals and humans that found that dCM could provide some systolic assistance.[18] However, that marked reversal of chamber dilation occurred in subjects with no evidence of systolic assistance suggested that an artificial passive wrap might be equally effective.

PASSIVE CONTAINMENT: CHAMBER REMODELING

Stimulated by the cardiomyoplasty experience, scientists began developing a purely passive polymer-based jacket that could surround the heart and provide an elastic containment. Most of the development and experimental and clinical testing to date has used a polyester mesh material (CorCap) developed by Acorn

Cardiovascular (St. Paul, MN).[9,19–21] An alternative device made from Nitinol is under development by Paracor (Sunnyvale, CA), although currently there are no published data to report. Thus, the remaining sections of this chapter focus on results with the Acorn Cardiovascular device.

As depicted in Figure 36–2A and B, the CorCap or cardiac support device (CSD) is applied around the right (RV) and left (LV) ventricles, sutured along a single seam to provide a snug but not constricting envelop surrounding the heart. The material has biaxial inhomogeneous properties and is slightly more distensible in the longitudinal than circumferential axis. Current implantation requires open chest surgery, although a minimally invasive deployment method is under development. Figure 36–2C shows the nonlinear elastic properties of the CorCap. It is more distensible than pericardium, particularly at greater distension ratios.

Initial studies with CSD have largely focused on animals with dilated cardiomyopathy. Using a tachypacing heart failure model in sheep, Power and colleagues[9] reported improved LV fraction shortening, reduced mitral regurgitation, and smaller long-axis dimension in animals treated with the passive containment versus sham. Subsequent studies examined CSD effects on hearts with more severe heart failure induced by this same model and also demonstrated efficacy to impede progressive dilation without inducing constrictive physiology.[22]

However, as the pacing model required sustained rapid heart rates even after placement of the wrap, it was somewhat difficult to clarify the benefits from the containment therapy. This limitation was removed in a diffuse ischemia model in dogs subjected to chronic sequential intracoronary microembolization.[8,21] Once established, heart failure in these animals progresses with chamber dilation and systolic dysfunction. Animals receiving the Acorn Cardiovascular device displayed lower chamber end-diastolic and end-systolic dimensions, increased fractional shortening, and reduced myocyte hypertrophy and interstitial fibrosis.

In a subsequent study, these same investigators asked whether acute volume reduction during placement of the Acorn Cardiovascular support device resulted in even more benefit.[19] Cardiac volumes were reduced during the surgical implant by administration of intravenous dobutamine. The net result was a 25% decline in end-

A

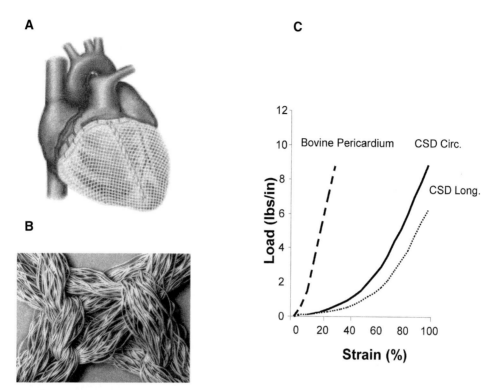

B

C

■ **Figure 36–2** *A,* Cardiac support device (CSD) from Acorn Cardiovascular (St. Paul, MN). The polyester mesh material is applied snugly around the epicardial surface with a suture seam coupling it to the cardiac base and a single longitudinal seam along the anterior intraventricular groove. *B,* High-power image of the mesh material itself. This weave forms a substrate for native fibrous material to form, and the eventual containment is a composite of the polyester mesh and fibrosis. *C,* Stress–strain curves for normal pericardium (bovine example is shown) versus CSD in longitudinal and circumferential orientations. There is slightly more distensibility in the longitudinal direction, which helps to orient the heart toward a more ellipsoidal (i.e., normal) shape. *(A from Saavedra WF, Tunin RS, Paolocci RN, et al: Reverse remodeling and enhanced adrenergic reserve from passive external support in experimental dilated heart failure. J Am Coll Cardiol 39:2069–2076, 2002, with permission.)*

diastolic dimensions 3 months later compared with a 16% increase in dimension in control subjects. Mitral regurgitation and chamber sphericity were reduced. However, whether containment should be applied with the aim of acutely reducing cardiac volumes remains unclear. Uncontrolled clinical studies have suggested that too aggressive a containment can turn into a constraint, and that eliminating the capacity for acute cardiac dilation when it might suddenly be required can be detrimental. Importantly, studies have shown that chronic reverse remodeling occurs with the CSD even when there is little to no acute volume reduction.

A more comprehensive analysis of reverse remodeling based on pressure-volume relations was reported by Saavedra and colleagues.[23] In this study, serial pressure–

volume relations were obtained after development of the failure state, and then 3 to 6 months after placement of the containment device. Figure 36–3A displays example pressure–volume loops and relations before and after chronic CSD implantation. CSD placement resulted in a left shift of the resting pressure–volume loop (see Fig. 36–3A, black lines), as well as the end-systolic pressure–volume relation (ESPVR), consistent with reverse remodeling. This left ESPVR shift was quantified as a decline in ventricular end-systolic volume at a matched pressure within the physiologic range (V_{110}, 110 mm Hg). V_{110} decreased from 44.7 ± 5.2 to 33.9 ± 3.9 mL by chronic CSD treatment ($P < 0.01$). Although individual changes in the diastolic pressure–volume curve varied somewhat,

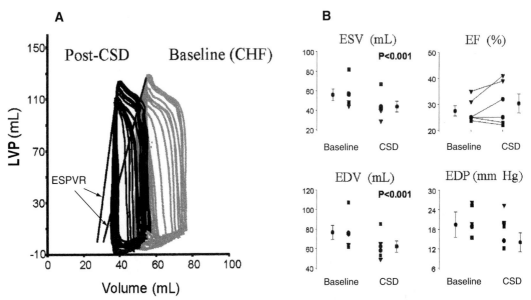

■ **Figure 36–3** *A,* Hemodynamic effects of CSD. Left ventricular pressure–volume relations in an animal with congestive heart failure (CHF) before and after chronic CSD implantation. *Light gray loops* reflect basal conditions; *darker loops* are measured after chronic CSD treatment. There is a left shift of the end-systolic pressure–volume relation and declines in both end-diastolic (EDV) and end-systolic (ESV) chamber volumes. *B,* Right panels show summary data for six animals. Significant declines in ESV and EDV were observed, whereas ejection fraction (EF) tended to increase and end-diastolic pressure (EDP) tended to decline (both individual data and group mean ± SEM). LVP, left ventricular pressure; ESPVR, end-systolic pressure volume relation. *(From Saavedra WF, Tunin RS, Paolocci RN, et al: Reverse remodeling and enhanced adrenergic reserve from passive external support in experimental dilated heart failure. J Am Coll Cardiol 39:2069–2076, 2002, with permission.)*

there was no net difference in chamber compliance based on a monoexponential elastic model (0.09 ± 0.03 before vs. 0.11 ± 0.02 mL^{-1} after CSD; $P > 0.4$). Figure 36–2*B* shows summary data revealing an almost 20% decline in both end-systolic and end-diastolic volumes (both $P < 0.0001$), whereas ejection fraction (EF) and end-diastolic pressure were not significantly altered. Other parameters of systolic function such as the peak rate of pressure increase (2025 ± 130 vs. 1765 ± 67 mm Hg/sec), the linear relation between cardiac work and preload (derived from the same set of pressure–volume loops as in Fig. 36–1*A*; 54.1 ± 11.1 vs. 54.4 ± 9.4 mm Hg), and the isovolumic relaxation (49.9 ± 4.5 vs. 51.7 ± 5.4 msec) were not altered by the CSD. These stabilized results stand in contrast to natural progression data for the failure model itself, where there is progressive systolic depression and chamber dilation.

POSTINFARCTION STUDIES

One of the earliest conceptual targets for a passive containment device was the recently infarcted ventricle. Such hearts commonly experience development of infarct expansion and chamber dilation, contributing to the development of ischemic heart failure. The capacity to ameliorate this remodeling by passive containment was tested by Pilla and colleagues,[24] who used a sheep myocardial infarction model involving open-chest coronary ligation, followed 1 week later by placement of the CSD or sham. Cardiac function was assessed using magnetic resonance imaging. The results pointed to several novel features of this therapy. Although the infarction resulted in LV akinesis of 25 to 30% of the wall, animals receiving the CSD displayed a decline in both absolute and relative akinesis area of more than 50%, whereas this was unaltered in control animals. Although chamber volumes and dimensions were not reported, wall thickness (which included the CSD and related fibrosis in the CSD animals) was significantly greater in the treated animals. Missing from this analysis were also data on ventricular pressures that might identify whether the reduction in infarct size was coupled with changes in diastolic pressure. However, these intriguing results suggest the girdling of infarcted myocardium may be a useful way to decrease the adverse chronic impact it has on chamber geometry and remodeling.

IMPACT ON CARDIAC RESERVE

Most of the reported studies with the CSD device have focused on baseline phenotypes. However, limited data suggest that the benefit maybe more extensive. In particular, Saavedra and colleagues[23] tested the impact of chronic CSD on β-adrenergic reserve in the ischemic failure model. Intravenous dobutamine elicited only a modest systolic response in the baseline failure state, concordant with down-regulation of adrenergic signaling. However, this was considerably enhanced after chronic CSD treatment (Fig. 36–4), as reflected by multiple measures of cardiac performance including cardiac output and external work, EF, and contractility indices. These data are similar to what had been observed with chronic ventricular unloading by means of an assist device. However, in the case of LV assist, where cardiac output is normalized, intrinsic LV workload is reduced profoundly, and systemic and local neurohormonal stimulation are decreased, the CSD method does not itself take over cardiac systolic function. In this case, secondary responses associated with reverse remodeling that lead to improved cardiac function must be invoked. Indeed, in the myocardium from the CSD-treated hearts, isoproterenol-stimulated adenylate cyclase activity was enhanced compared with tissue from non-CSD failure control subjects. However, β-adrenergic receptor density and binding affinity were not altered.[23]

A major concern pertaining to external containment devices is whether they constrict diastolic filling, and thereby Frank–Starling reserve. The pericardium of the failing heart dilates to accommodate myocardial enlargement, but this expansion is generally insuffi-

cient to prevent limitations to preload reserve.[12] The passive properties of the CSD are less abruptly nonlinear compared with pericardium, with a less than 7 mm Hg pressure increase for a 20% volume expansion and a 9 mm Hg increase at 30% expansion. This better enables the material to stretch to accommodate filling volume. Effects of the chronic CSD on preload reserve were studied,[23] and these effects suggested preservation of this mechanism. CSD-treated animals were administered blood volume expanders (dextran) and showed a systolic functional response to preload (see Fig. 36–4). For example, cardiac output increased nearly 100%, and both maximal rate of pressure increase and decline were enhanced. Such responses are not anticipated if there is functional pathophysiologic constriction.

A recent study integrating both mechanisms of cardiac reserve reports improvement in both basal and exercise capacity in sheep with tachypacing-induced cardiac failure that were treated with the Acorn Cardiovascular containment device.[22]

CELLULAR AND MOLECULAR REMODELING

Recent data further support the notion that reverse remodeling induced by a passive containment device includes changes at the cellular and molecular level as well. Sabbah and colleagues[25] found improvement in isolated myocyte shortening, and peak rates of shortening and relengthening that, although still substantially depressed compared with control subjects, were nonetheless almost 100% greater than in cells from untreated failing hearts. Cardiomyocyte area, length, and width were all markedly reduced by the containment therapy, reaching values near healthy control (Fig. 36–5A). Furthermore, these investigators demonstrated substantial reversal of abnormal molecular expression changes typical of heart failure, involving calcium handling and stress response proteins. Proteins such as *p38* mitogen-activated kinase and *p21 ras* are important signaling molecules involved with hypertrophic responses, and their increase is coupled to contractile dysfunction and fibrosis. Both increased markedly with untreated failure but were diminished toward baseline with chronic CSD treatment.

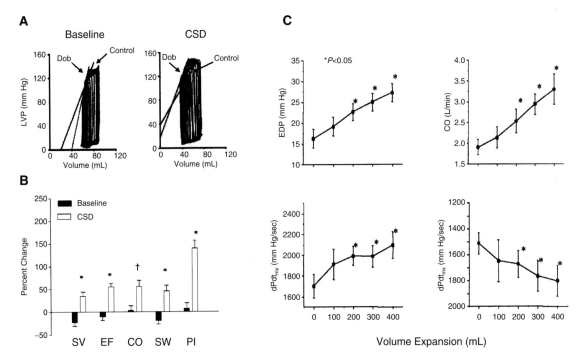

■ **Figure 36–4** Effect of CSD on cardiac contractile (β-adrenergic–stimulated) and preload reserve. *A,* Example pressure–volume loops and relations during acute dobutamine infusion (Dob) stimulation at baseline and after chronic CSD treatment. The predobutamine ESVPR is shown for each case (control). Before CSD placement, the dobutamine response is small, with only a slight left shift of the ESPVR. However, the magnitude of response to this same dose was greatly augmented after chronic CSD treatment. *B,* Summary data for dobutamine-enhanced systolic function before and after CSD treatment. Substantial increases were observed in multiple ejection parameters. Power index (PI): maximal power/EDV^2. *$P < 0.05$, †$P < 0.02$; versus baseline response. *C,* Improved systolic and diastolic function in failing hearts treated with a chronic CSD with acute volume expansion with dextran. For an almost 10 mm Hg increase in EDP, cardiac output increased by nearly 100%, and there were significant changes in both maximal (dPdt$_{mx}$) and minimal (dPdt$_{mn}$) rate of pressure change. Thus, preload-dependent reserve function was not inhibited by CSD placement. CO, cardiac output; EF, ejection fraction; LVP, left ventricular pressure; SV, stroke volume; SW, stroke work. *(Reproduced from Saavedra WF, Tunin RS, Paolocci RN, et al: Reverse remodeling and enhanced adrenergic reserve from passive external support in experimental dilated heart failure. J Am Coll Cardiol 39:2069–2076, 2002, with permission.)*

Abnormalities of calcium-handling proteins such as phospholamban (PLB) and the sarcoplasmic reticular adenosine triphosphatase (SERCA2a) play a central role in systolic depression and relaxation delay in the failing heart. PLB expression declined 40% less than control values in hearts with untreated failure (see Fig. 36–5*B*), but it increased almost twofold in the hearts treated with a device. This was further accompanied by a significant increase in PLB phosphorylation of both serine 16 and threonine 17. Such phosphorylation is important because it is coupled to enhanced SERCA2a calcium

uptake. Although there was a measurable increase in SERCA2a calcium binding affinity, maximal velocity of sarcoplasmic reticulum calcium uptake was not altered by the CSD treatment.

Human Trial Data

Clinical trials of the Acorn Cardiovascular CSD were initiated in 1999. In an early report of the experience in the first 27 patients, Konertz and colleagues[10]

A

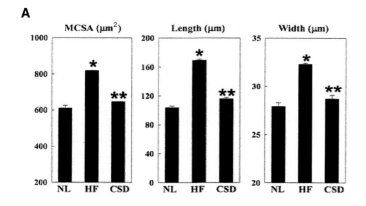

B

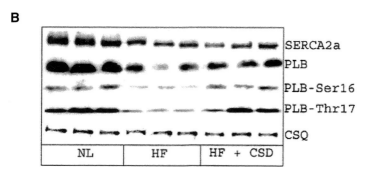

■ **Figure 36–5** Reverse remodeling of myocardial cell morphology and molecular signaling caused by chronic CSD treatment in animal model of ischemic dilated cardiomyopathy. *A*, Myocyte cross-sectional area (MCSA), length, and width are shown for normal hearts (NL), failing hearts (HF), and failing hearts treated with the CSD. The containment device reversed myocyte hypertrophy. *B*, Protein immunoblots for sarcoplasmic reticular adenosine triphosphatase (SERCA2a), phospholamban (PLB), phosphorylated PLB (PLB-Ser16 and PLB-Thr17), and calsequestrin (CSQ, control) in same three groups. Most notable was the decline in PLB and phosphorylated PLB that is improved by chronic treatment with the CSD. *(Reproduced from Sabbah HN, Sharov VG, Gupta RC, et al: Reversal of chronic molecular and cellular abnormalities due to heart failure by passive mechanical ventricular containment. Circ Res 93: 1095–1101, 2003, with permission.)*

reported improvement in heart function class, with 90% of subjects in Class I or II as opposed to 35% before surgery. In the subset of individuals in which echocardiography was obtained, the investigators reported improvement in EF (22% to 28% and 33% at 3 and 6 months, respectively) and a 15% decline in end-diastolic volume.

More detailed analysis recently was presented from this same group in a study by Lembcke and colleagues.[26] Fourteen patients undergoing CSD implantation were examined with contrast-enhanced, electrocardiogram-triggered, electron beam computerized tomography. End-diastolic volumes declined from 383 ± 140 to 311 ± 139 mL, and end-systolic volume decreased from 310 ± 132 to 237 ± 134 mL. There also was a 10% decline in myocardial mass. EF increased similar to previous findings. There was no true control comparison in this analysis, although age- and sex-matched subjects with similar severity of cardiac failure had larger volumes and smaller EF.

Surgical and medical complications associated with the CSD have been generally minimal. In a review of the global surgical experience up to the middle of 2003, Oz and colleagues[27] reported an average implantation time of 27 min, with a mean intraoperative cardiac volume reduction of only 4.6 ± 1%, and no device-related intraoperative complications in this series of 48 safety and feasibility studies. In a subgroup of patients with ischemic heart disease who had undergone concomitant coronary bypass procedures, there was no evidence for constrictive disease, and the containment did not alter coronary flow or flow reserve.[28]

In June 2003, a multicenter, prospective randomized, controlled, clinical trial of the CorCap completed patient enrollment.[29] The study recruited 300 patients from 29 centers across North America. The patient population included two clinical groups: patients with dilated cardiomyopathy (107 patients) and no other primary indication for open heart surgery, and patients with heart failure who were referred for surgical mitral valve repair (193 patients). Half of the patients recruited did not receive the CSD (control group). All patients were receiving optimal medical management, with 97% treated with either an angiotensin-converting enzyme inhibitor or angiotensin receptor blocker, and about 85% treated with a β-blocker. Patients were followed to a common closing date 12 months after the last patient was enrolled (medial follow-up of 22 months). The primary endpoint was a clinical composite with patients classified as improved, same, or worsened based upon the occurrence of death, a major cardiac procedure indicative of heart failure progression, and a change in NYHA class. Preliminary results were presented in November, 2004, at the annual Scientific Sessions of the American Heart Association.[30] In comparison with controls, the odds ratio for improvement based on the composite endpoint was 1.73 (1.07, 2.79; $P = 0.02$) favoring CSD treatment. CSD treated patients displayed a greater decline in left ventricular systolic and diastolic volumes, and improved symptoms as assessed by a quality of life questionnaire. Repeat hospitalizations and adverse events were not different between the groups. These results are encouraging and appear to support both the technical and clinical feasibility of containment device therapy, as well as clinical benefits from the approach.

FUTURE DIRECTIONS AND IMPLICATIONS

Cessation or reversal of progressive chamber remodeling remains an important target for heart failure therapy. The CSD appears to achieve this—and does so remarkably without any primary interaction with the heart's molecular signaling, or by directly assisting systolic or diastolic function. There remain a number of important questions to be answered. For example, how important is the fibrous sheath that intercalates with the CSD material (or alternative materials being tested) in determining the overall effect? It seems likely that net distensibility of the containment material plus fibrosis is less, and that the unstressed volume is smaller, perhaps playing some role in the reverse remodeling. This leaves open the possibility that

material with even less stiffness may also work. Can a containment device serve as a Trojan horse, delivering hormones, proteins to stimulate vascular growth, or even electrical stimulation to resynchronize contraction in hearts that need it? How feasible will it be to implant such devices using minimally invasive surgery, perhaps by a subxiphoid approach? If subsequent surgery is required, or a device must be removed, what are the risks and what approaches are needed? It is possible that the devices can be designed out of biodegradable materials—to provide mechanical containment for a specified period, but then gradually degrade.

Regardless of its ultimate clinical fate, the observations already reported have changed perspectives regarding both the influence of remodeling and the plasticity of the failing heart when such progressive dilation is impeded. Current studies have not determined the impact of containment devices on electrophysiologic remodeling and arrhythmogenicity. However, these features are recognized common causes of heart failure mortality, and their severity often is coupled with cardiac dilation/remodeling. Reverse remodeling by means of containment devices may well prove to be antiarrhythmogenic, and clinical studies hopefully will provide some insights regarding this topic. The notion that a purely passive *support sock* applied to the epicardial surface can up-regulate β-adrenergic responsiveness, reverse myocyte remodeling, and enhance PLB phosphorylation may seem odd at first. Yet, this is clearly the case, and it is heralding a new and exciting treatment for heart failure.

References

1. Udelson JE, Konstam MA: Relation between left ventricular remodeling and clinical outcomes in heart failure patients with left ventricular systolic dysfunction. J Card Fail 8:S465–S471, 2002.
2. Jessup M, Brozena S: Heart failure. N Engl J Med 348: 2007–2018, 2003.
3. Cohn JN, Ferrari R, Sharpe N: Cardiac remodeling—concepts and clinical implications: A consensus paper from an international forum on cardiac remodeling. Behalf of an International Forum on Cardiac Remodeling. J Am Coll Cardiol 35: 569–582, 2000.
4. Konstam MA, Patten RD, Thomas I, et al: Effects of losartan and captopril on left ventricular volumes in elderly patients

with heart failure: Results of the ELITE ventricular function substudy. Am Heart J 139:1081–1087, 2000.

5. Konstam MA, Kronenberg MW, Rousseau MF, et al: Effects of the angiotensin converting enzyme inhibitor enalapril on the long-term progression of left ventricular dilatation in patients with asymptomatic systolic dysfunction. SOLVD (Studies of Left Ventricular Dysfunction) Investigators. Circulation 88:2277–2283, 1993.

6. Doughty RN, Whalley GA, Walsh HA, et al: Effects of carvedilol on left ventricular remodeling after acute myocardial infarction: The CAPRICORN Echo Substudy. Circulation 109:201–206, 2004.

7. St John Sutton MG, Plappert T, Abraham WT, et al: Effect of cardiac resynchronization therapy on left ventricular size and function in chronic heart failure. Circulation 107:1985–1990, 2003.

8. Chaudhry PA, Mishima T, Sharov VG, et al: Passive epicardial containment prevents ventricular remodeling in heart failure. Ann Thorac Surg 70:1275–1280, 2000.

9. Power JM, Raman J, Dornom A, et al: Passive ventricular constraint amends the course of heart failure: A study in an ovine model of dilated cardiomyopathy. Cardiovasc Res 44:549–555, 1999.

10. Konertz WF, Shapland JE, Hotz H, et al: Passive containment and reverse remodeling by a novel textile cardiac support device. Circulation 104:I270–I275, 2001.

11. Chew PH, Yin FCP, Zeger SL: Biaxial stress-strain properties of canine pericardium. J Mol Cell Cardiol 18:567–578, 1986.

12. Dauterman K, Pak PH, Maughan WL, et al: Contribution of external forces to left ventricle diastolic pressure: Implications for the clinical use of the Frank-Starling Law. Ann Intern Med 122:737–742, 1995.

13. Kass DA, Baughman KL, Pak PH, et al: Reverse remodeling from cardiomyopathy in human heart failure: External constraint versus active assist. Circulation 91:2314–2318, 1995.

14. Carpentier A, Chachques JC: Clinical dynamic cardiomyoplasty method and outcome. Semin Thorac Cardiovasc Surg 3:136–139, 1991.

15. Moreira LF, Bocchi EA, Stolf NA, et al: Dynamic cardiomyoplasty in the treatment of dilated cardiomyopathy: Current results and perspectives. J Cardiac Surg 11:207–213, 1996.

16. Patel HJ, Polidori DJ, Pilla JJ, et al: Stabilization of chronic remodeling by asynchronous cardiomyoplasty in dilated cardiomyopathy: Effects of a conditioned muscle wrap. Circulation 96:3665–3671, 1997.

17. Patel HJ, Lankford EB, Polidori DJ, et al: Dynamic cardiomyoplasty: Its chronic and acute effects on the failing heart. J Thorac Cardiovasc Surg 114:169–178, 1997.

18. Schreuder JJ, van der Veen FH, van der Velde ET, et al: Left ventricular pressure-volume relationships before and after cardiomyoplasty in patients with heart failure. Circulation 96:2978–2986, 1997.

19. Chaudhry PA, Anagnostopouls PV, Mishima T, et al: Acute ventricular reduction with the Acorn cardiac support device: Effect on progressive left ventricular dysfunction and dilation in dogs with chronic heart failure. J Card Surg 16:118–126, 2001.

20. Sabbah HN, Kleber FX, Konertz W: Efficacy trends of the acorn cardiac support device in patients with heart failure: A one year follow-up. J Heart Lung Transplant 20:217, 2001.

21. Sabbah HN, Sharov VG, Chaudhry PA, et al: Chronic therapy with the Acorn cardiac support device in dogs with chronic heart failure: Three and six months hemodynamic, histologic and ultrastructural findings. J Heart Lung Transplant 20:189, 2001.

22. Raman JS, Byrne MJ, Power JM, Alferness CA: Ventricular constraint in severe heart failure halts decline in cardiovascular function associated with experimental dilated cardiomyopathy. Ann Thorac Surg 76:141–147, 2003.

23. Saavedra WF, Tunin RS, Paolocci RN, et al: Reverse remodeling and enhanced adrenergic reserve from passive external support in experimental dilated heart failure. J Am Coll Cardiol 39:2069–2076, 2002.

24. Pilla JJ, Blom AS, Brockman DJ, et al: Ventricular constraint using the Acorn cardiac support device reduces myocardial akinetic area in an ovine model of acute infarction. Circulation 106:I207–I211, 2002.

25. Sabbah HN, Sharov VG, Gupta RC, et al: Reversal of chronic molecular and cellular abnormalities due to heart failure by passive mechanical ventricular containment. Circ Res 93:1095–1101, 2003.

26. Lembcke A, Wiese TH, Dushe S, et al: Effects of passive cardiac containment on left ventricular structure and function: Verification by volume and flow measurements. J Heart Lung Transplant 23:11–19, 2004.

27. Oz MC, Konertz WF, Kleber FX, et al: Global surgical experience with the Acorn cardiac support device. J Thorac Cardiovasc Surg 126:983–991, 2003.

28. Raman JS, Power JM, Buxton BF, et al: Ventricular containment as an adjunctive procedure in ischemic cardiomyopathy: Early results. Ann Thorac Surg 70:1124–1126, 2000.

29. Mann DL, Acker MA, Jessup M, et al: Rationale, design, and methods for a pivotal randomized clinical trial for the assessment of a cardiac support device in patients with New York Health Association class III-IV heart failure. J Card Fail. 10:185–92, 2004.

30. Mann, DL for the Acorn Trial Investigators: Results of a multicenter randomized clinical trial for the assessment of a cardiac support device (CSD) in patients with heart failure. Presented at Scientific Sessions 2004 of the American Heart Association, New Orleans, LA, 7–10 November, 2004.

CHAPTER 37

Cardiac Assist Devices: Effects on Reverse Remodeling

Stefan Klotz and Daniel Burkhoff

• • • •

Left ventricular assist devices (LVAD) are commonly used to bridge critically ill patients with heart failure to transplant. All LVAD used for this indication provide volume and pressure unloading of the left ventricle (LV), while simultaneously restoring total systemic blood pressure and blood flow.[1,2]

Although it was generally believed in the past that the massively dilated and dysfunctional hearts of patients with severe end-stage heart failure are irrevocably damaged, in most patients, circulatory support with an LVAD leads to reversal of chamber enlargement, reduction in LV mass, improved global pump function, and normalized ex vivo end-diastolic pressure–volume relations (EDPVR).[2–5] This process has been termed *reverse structural remodeling*. Additional investigation of isolated myocytes and intact isometric LV trabeculae has demonstrated increased contractile function and an enhanced inotropic response to β-adrenergic stimulation after LVAD support, which occurs in conjunction with improved cytosolic Ca^{2+} transients and normalization of some aspects of mitochondrial energetics.[6–8] Taken together, these data indicate that improved LV pump function is not simply the result of changes in chamber size, geometry, and compliance. Recent data indicate that LVAD support also produces other subcellular changes within myocytes that contribute to, or result from, normalized structure, function, or both. This process has been termed *reverse molecular remodeling*. Furthermore, LVAD support may normalize mechano-electric feedback effects by hemodynamic unloading. The concept and implications of this mechanically induced electrical reverse remodeling are discussed in detail in Chapters 16, 17, and 24.

First, this chapter provides an introduction to different types of cardiac assist devices; then evidence supporting the notion of reverse structural and molecular remodeling and implications of this process are reviewed.

CARDIAC ASSIST DEVICES

The concept of mechanical heart support evolved parallel to the development of cardiac transplantation. In 1963, the first use of an implantable LVAD in a human was performed by Hall and colleagues[9] in a patient who had experienced cardiogenic shock after aortic valve replacement. Although circulatory support was adequate, the device was discontinued after 4 days because of severe neurologic injury before device placement. The first successful LVAD implantation in a patient with postcardiotomy failure was performed by DeBakey in 1966.[10] The first LVAD implantation as a bridge to transplantation was performed by Cooley in 1978.[11]

Different Classes of Left Ventricular Assist Devices

The two different classes of LVAD primarily used for long-term support to bridge patients with heart failure to transplant are pusher plate pumps, which propel blood from the LV to the aorta in a pulsatile manner, and axial or centrifugal pumps, which provide nonpulsatile continuous flow. These pumps are implanted either in an intracorporal or extracorporal position.

Intracorporal pusher plate pumps are either pneumatic or electric vented devices, with their pump chambers sitting in their right upper abdominal walls. A sternotomy is needed, but implantation often is possible without the use of cardiopulmonary bypass. An inflow graft is inserted into the LV apex; an outflow graft is frequently connected to the ascending aorta or sometimes to the descending aorta. Explantation of the device is performed through sternotomy during heart transplantation or through a left-sided thoracotomy in cases of cardiac recovery. Examples of implantable pulsatile flow devices are shown in Figure 37–1. The most commonly used devices are the *TCI HeartMate LVAD IP/VE* (Thoratec Corporation, Pleasanton, CA) and the *Novacor LVAD* (World Heart Corporation, Ottawa, Canada). Both LVAD are pneumatic or electric pusher-plate devices, with a maximum stroke volume of ~85 mL and weight of ~1 kg. Porcine valves or bioprosthetic valves are used to achieve unidirectional blood flow.

A new generation of devices with axial flow pumps is currently undergoing clinical testing. Because of the continuous flow properties of axial flow pumps, no valves or compliance chambers are needed in the system. The pump chamber is significantly smaller, and the LVAD therefore can be used in smaller patients (see Fig. 37–1). Relatively simple mechanics and the lack of a compliance chamber may lead to less device failures and lower energy requirements. Impact of continuous flow patterns on end-organ function and cardiac unloading appears comparable with LVAD with pulsatile flow, but further investigations are warranted.[12,13] The *MicroMed DeBakey* (MicroMed Technology, Houston, TX) pump is an electromagnetically actuated, titanium axial flow pump. The axial flow motor contains rotary blades that spin at 7500 to 12,500 rpm and can pump approximately 5 to 6 L/min. The *Jarvik 2000* is a development from the Texas Heart Institute (Houston, TX) and Jarvik Heart Inc. (New York, NY). Similar to the *MicroMed DeBakey* LVAD, it is a valveless axial flow pump with a magnetically driven neodymium-ironboron impeller inside a welded titanium shell. Unique to the device is that it is implanted directly into the LV without the need of an inflow graft. The *HeartMate II LVAD* (Thoratec Corporation) is an implantable rotary blood pump that addresses destination therapy for patients requiring long-term cardiac support. A multicenter European and U.S. clinical trial is scheduled. The *INCOR LVAD* (BerlinHeart AG, Berlin, Germany) is an axial flow pump; it is approved in Europe and Asia, but not in the United States.

All these implantable pulsatile and nonpulsatile devices need a percutaneous driveline, which exits at the right abdominal wall and connects to an external controller and battery packs, which are worn extracorporeally by the patient.

Another group of cardiac assist devices are extracorporal implantable pumps. Their advantage is the use not only as a left heart assist, but also as a biventricular

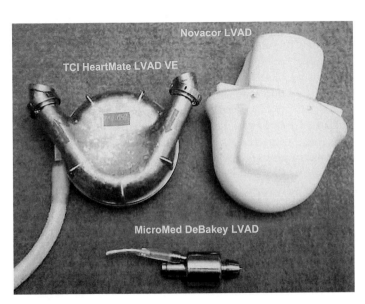

■ **Figure 37–1** The pulsatile TCI HeartMate VE (Thoratec Corporation, Pleasanton, CA) and Novacor LVAD (World Heart Corporation, Ottawa, Canada) and the nonpulsatile MicroMed DeBakey axial flow pump (MicroMed Technology, Houston, TX). A distinctive difference in size is evident between these two different types of cardiac assist devices. LVAD, left ventricular assist device. *(From Klotz S, Deng MC, Stypmann J, et al: Left ventricular pressure and volume unloading during pulsatile versus nonpulsatile left ventricular assist device support. Ann Thorac Surg 77:143–150, 2004, with permission.)*

assist device (BiVAD) or solely as a right heart assist (right ventricular assist device [RVAD]), combined with an easier implantation technique. A disadvantage is the often relatively large drive console with partial or complete immobility of the patient, which limits the quality of life. The pump chamber of the extracorporal devices rests on the upper abdominal wall of the patient. Inflow and outflow cannulae frequently are metal-reinforced and penetrate the skin beneath the costal arch. For right heart assist, the inflow graft is inserted into the right atrium, and the outflow graft is inserted into the pulmonary artery. For left heart assist, connection is the same as for intracorporal LVAD. The *Thoratec device* (Thoratec Corporation) and the *EXCOR VAD* (BerlinHeart AG) are the main extracorporal devices used in the United States and Europe.

LEFT VENTRICULAR ASSIST DEVICE–INDUCED REVERSE STRUCTURAL REMODELING

Pressure and Volume Unloading of the Left Ventricle

In most patients, immediately after LVAD placement, the aortic valve rarely opens, indicating that the LVAD provides most of the hemodynamic support to the body, while also providing volume and pressure unloading for the LV (Fig. 37–2). The echocardiograms in Figure 37–2 show two-dimensional, echocardiographic, long-axis images of the LV cavity during a short venting cycle (when LVAD support is temporarily suspended; see Fig. 37–2A) and within a few minutes after reinitiation of pumping (see Fig. 37–2B).

During device venting, the LV is seen as a dilated structure. When the device is turned on, the ventricle is seen to be collapsed, indicating substantial volume unloading of the LV.

The effect of pressure unloading with LVAD support is presented in Table 37–1. Because of volume unloading of the LV chamber, left atrial pressure declines, which leads to a tremendous decrease in pulmonary pressures. Despite ventricular pressure and volume unloading, cardiac output and systemic blood pressure increase.

Thus, it is clear that the LVAD provides both pressure and volume unloading of the diseased LV, while maintaining adequate systemic perfusion. Furthermore, LVAD-induced hemodynamic unloading may have beneficial effects on terminating ventricular arrhythmia (see Chapter 34 for a detailed discussion of this topic).

Ex Vivo Passive End-Diastolic Pressure–Volume Relation

The chronically increased filling pressures imposed on the failing heart and the heightened neurohormonal bombardment of the myocytes have long been hypothesized to cause the progressive ventricular chamber dilation characteristic of heart failure. As recently as the 1990s it was generally believed that when such remodeling was long-standing and severe (such as observed in patients awaiting heart transplant), these structural abnormalities would be irreversible.

Soon after the introduction of LVAD, however, it was appreciated that these abnormalities were not permanent, but rather could be reversed, at least to some degree. To most specifically study the effect of long-term pressure and volume unloading on heart structure, the technique of the ex vivo passive EDPVR was used. After explantation and preservation with 4°C cardioplegia solution, a compliant, water-filled latex balloon is placed in the LV chamber. While measuring pressure within the balloon, volume is varied from one that achieves an intracavitary pressure of 0 mm Hg to a volume yielding a pressure of at least 30 mm Hg. The pressure–volume point at each volume step is then plotted, resulting in the passive pressure–volume relation for that heart. Such curves have been obtained from normal hearts unsuitable for transplant, hearts explanted from patients undergoing transplant without the need for LVAD support, and hearts that had undergone LVAD support before transplant. Representative ex vivo EDPVR are shown in Figure 37–3. Compared with normal hearts (see open diamonds in Fig. 37–3), the EDPVR of non-LVAD–supported hearts (see open circles in Fig. 37–3) were shifted toward significantly larger volumes, a reflection of the gross dilation and structural remodeling that is typical of end-stage dilated cardiomyopathy. In contrast, LVAD-supported hearts exhibited EDPVR that are

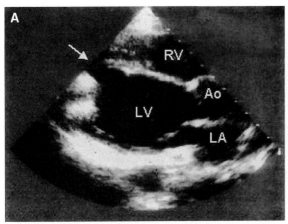 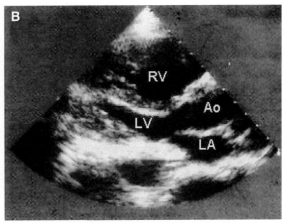

■ **Figure 37–2** Echocardiograms 1 week after LVAD implantation taken at end diastole. *A,* LVAD function is temporarily suspended during a routine venting procedure (the arrow indicates the position of the LAVD flow conduit). End-diastolic dimension is greater than 6 cm, indicating a dilated ventricular cavity. *B,* This image, showing internal dimension of 3 cm, is taken within 1 min after LVAD operation is restored, indicating massive ventricular volume unloading. Ao, aorta ascendens; LA, left atrium; LV, left ventricle; RV, right ventricle. *(From Levin HR, Oz MC, Chen JM, et al: Reversal of chronic ventricular dilation in patients with end-stage cardiomyopathy by prolonged mechanical unloading. Circulation 91:2717–2720, 1995, with permission.)*

shifted significantly toward lower volumes (see filled circles in Fig. 37–3). On consideration that the hemodynamic status of the LVAD recipients at the time of LVAD implantation was worse than that of the non-LVAD–supported patients at the time of heart transplant, it is evident that LVAD support was associated with significant LV reverse functional remodeling. This is caused by a true change in cardiac geometry rather than simply reflecting cardiac decompression.

Accompanying the leftward shift of the EDPVR was a trend for heart mass to decrease (normal: 300 ± 71 g; heart failure: 454 ± 143 g; LVAD support: 346 ± 94 g).

No significant changes in the RV EDPVR are observed. This is expected if the primary mechanism of reverse structural remodeling is caused by the hemodynamic unloading, because the RV does not receive the same profound unloading experienced by the LV. As expected, however, hearts supported by a RVAD have

TABLE 37–1 Hemodynamics with and without Left Ventricular Assist Device Support

Hemodynamics	Non-LVAD Support at Transplant	LVAD Support	
		At Insertion	At Transplant
CVP (mm Hg)	9.5 ± 6.3	13.1 ± 5.3	10.3 ± 5.9
PCWP (mm Hg)	19.8 ± 8.6*	27.1 ± 6.6	12.9 ± 7.2
mPAP (mm Hg)	26.9 ± 9.6*	37.3 ± 9.7	18.2 ± 7.3
mAP (mm Hg)	79.7 ± 11.8†	74.6 ± 8.4	87.9 ± 9.3
CO (L/min)	3.7 ± 1.1‡	4.0 ± 1.2	5.9 ± 1.5
Inotropic support	52%‡	88%	0%

Values are mean ± SD.
*$P < 0.01$; †$P < 0.05$; ‡$P < 0.001$ vs. LVAD support at transplant.
CVP, central venous pressure; PCWP, pulmonary capillary wedge pressure; mPAP, mean pulmonary artery pressure; mAP, mean arterial pressure; CO, cardiac output; LVAD, left ventricular assist device.

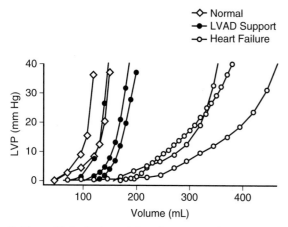

■ Figure 37–3 Ex vivo end-diastolic pressure–volume relations among normal hearts *(open diamonds),* heart failure without LVAD support *(open circles),* and LVAD-supported hearts *(filled circles)* presenting a tremendous leftward shift toward normal hearts. LVP, left ventricular pressure.

shown EDPVR shifts toward lower volumes, similar to what is observed in the LV after LVAD support.

Influence of Left Ventricular Assist Device Support on Myocyte Hypertrophy

Underlying a reverse remodeling of the ventricular chamber must be a reversal of myocyte hypertrophy and elongation. This also is expected because the primary triggers for myocyte hypertrophy in heart failure are hemodynamic overload and neurohormonal activation, both of which are normalized during LVAD support. LVAD support, therefore, should reverse or even normalize myocyte hypertrophy. Zafeiridis and colleagues[14] used isolated myocytes to evaluate changes in myocyte size and shape after LVAD support, and they observed a 60% regression in size. In a similar study from Terracciano and colleagues,[15] LVAD support led to a significant reduction in cell capacitance. In a study from our group, we could show a normalization of the myocyte diameter in LVAD-supported hearts (25.7 ± 4.0 μm; normal hearts: 24.4 ± 3.6 μm) in relation to heart in failure (42.5 ± 8.4 μm). Some histologic samples are shown in Figure 37–4. Furthermore, the extent of hypertrophy regression was a function of the dura-

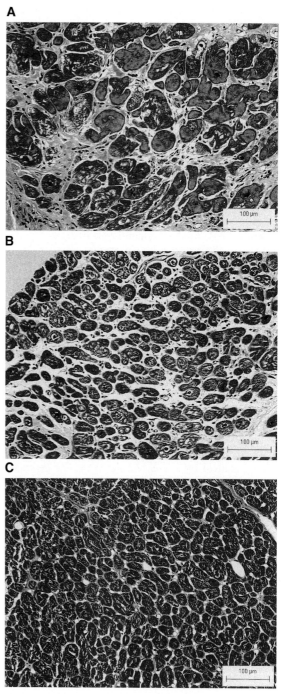

■ Figure 37–4 Normalization of the myocyte diameter in LVAD-supported hearts. Histologic samples representative for end-stage heart failure *(A),* LVAD-supported hearts *(B),* and normal hearts *(C).* (See color insert.)

tion of LVAD support and became evident within as little as 40 days of LVAD support.[16]

Influence of Left Ventricular Assist Device Support on Myocardial Contractile Performance

To measure the contractile strength of the myocardium, isolated endocardial trabeculae were excised from freshly explanted normal hearts, failing hearts, and failing hearts after LVAD support and were mounted in a muscle bath connected to a force transducer. After progressively stretching to the length of maximal force generation, stimulation frequency was increased at 0.5 Hz increments to a maximum of 2.5 Hz, and the response to the β-adrenergic stimulator isoproterenol (4×10^{-6} M) was tested.

At 1 Hz stimulation frequency, developed force generation of normal, LVAD-supported, and non-LVAD–supported hearts (normalized to cross-sectional area) were similar to each other. However, at greater rates of stimulation (force–frequency relation [FFR]), force declined in trabeculae from non-LVAD–supported failing hearts (negative FFR), whereas it increased in the normal and LVAD-supported hearts (positive FFR). Representative force tracings of muscles from these patients are shown in Figure 37–5. Importantly, the FFR of post-LVAD RV trabeculae did not recover significantly.

In the same study, myocardial contraction had improved responsiveness to β-adrenergic stimulation in LVAD-supported trabeculae, whereas the inotropic response to isoproterenol is significantly blunted before LVAD therapy (Fig. 37–6). β-Adrenergic responsiveness is restored not just in the unloaded LV, but in the RV as well. Dipla and colleagues[6] observed similar improvements in isolated myocytes.

Comparable results with regard to FFR and β-adrenergic responsiveness have been obtained from LVAD patients with both ischemic (ICM) and idiopathic dilated cardiomyopathies (DCM). In addition, results of experiments suggest quantitative differences in some of these responses depending on whether the patient was receiving inotropic support before transplantation. This observation suggests that improved β-adrenergic responsiveness after LVAD support may

more closely reflect the withdrawal of inotropic support and improved neurohormonal status than chronic mechanical unloading of the LV.[17]

Nevertheless, these results indicate that, although resting strength may not be significantly influenced, two important mechanisms regulating contractile strength—β-adrenergic responsiveness and frequency of contraction—are restored during LVAD support.

LEFT VENTRICULAR ASSIST DEVICE–INDUCED REVERSE MOLECULAR REMODELING

Evidence for Reverse Molecular Remodeling

The distortion of myocytes that accompanies increased pressure and volume within any heart chamber triggers a sequence of events, many of which are calcium regulated,[18] that eventually leads to remodeling of individual cells. Although physical stretch of the myocardium is believed to be a major regulator of this process, it also involves autonomic neurotransmitters and intracardiac paracrine/autocrine mediators. These individual factors coalesce to produce a cascade of immediate and ultimately prolonged molecular and cellular events mediated, in part, by altered expression of a variety of genes within both myocytes and noncontractile elements of the myocardium.[19]

Increased activity of the sarcoplasmic endoreticular calcium–adenosine triphosphatase subtype 2a (SERCA2a) has been linked with the myocardial FFR, whereas down-regulation of the gene encoding for SERCA2a in heart failure appears to be associated with negative FFR.[5,20] Consistent with these findings, improved force and FFR after LVAD were accompanied by SERCA2a up-regulation. Alterations in the expression and/or function of SERCA2a, the ryanodine-sensitive calcium release channel (RyR), and the sarcolemmal sodium-calcium exchanger (NCX) appears to be associated with various aspects of contractile dysfunction in severe heart failure.[21-25] To limit the impact of variability by having each patient serve as his own control, tissue samples obtained from individual hearts before and after

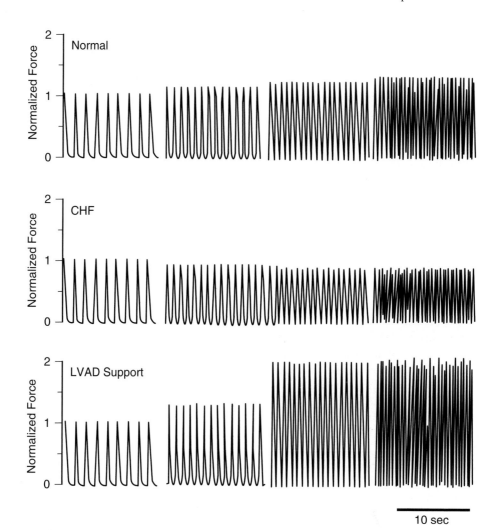

■ **Figure 37–5**   Force tracings from endocardial trabeculae excised from normal, failing (CHF), and LVAD-supported failing hearts. The response to pacing at different frequencies (1, 1.5, 2, and 2.5 Hz) shows progressively decreased systolic performance in heart failure. After LVAD support *(bottom)*, the force-frequency relation is increased. *(From Heerdt PM, Holmes JW, Cai B, et al: Chronic unloading by left ventricular assist device reverses contractile dysfunction and alters gene expression in end-stage heart failure. Circulation 102:2713–2719, 2000, with permission.)*

LVAD support were compared with those harvested from nonfailing hearts and measured by Northern blotting. As shown in Figure 37–7, there was, on average, increased expression of all three genes after LVAD support.[5] Although the RV and LV share a common biochemical milieu, during LVAD support, the LV may be profoundly unloaded, whereas the RV is not.[26]

We took advantage of this difference to test that altered hemodynamic load is the predominant stimulus for increased SERCA2a expression.[7] Using samples taken from both ventricles of the same hearts, LVAD support more than doubled LV SERCA2a protein content. In contrast, there was no significant change in SERCA2a protein within the RV after LVAD support.

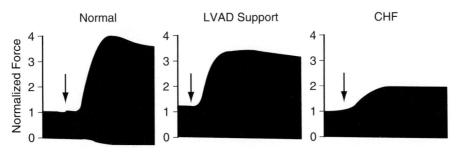

■ Figure 37–6 Force tracings from endocardial trabeculae harvested from normal, failing (CHF), and LVAD-supported hearts during isoproterenol stimulation (arrow). Normal and LVAD-supported trabeculae showed improved responsiveness, whereas the reaction in heart failure is blunted. *(Modified from Marx SO, Reiken S, Hisamatsu Y, et al: Pka phosphorylation dissociates fkbp12.6 from the calcium release channel [ryanodine receptor]: Defective regulation in failing hearts. Cell 101:365–376, 2000, with permission.)*

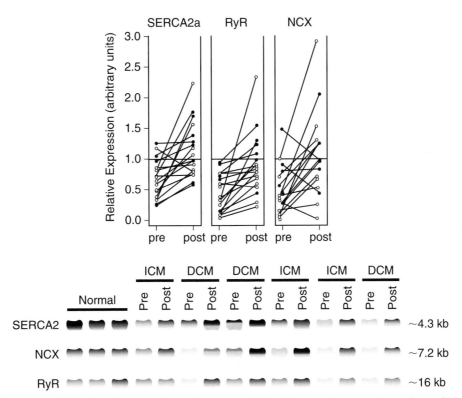

■ Figure 37–7 *Top,* Individual mRNA values (normalized to nonfailing) for sarcoplasmic endoreticulum calcium–adenosine triphosphatase subtype 2a (SERCA2a), the ryanodine receptor (RyR), and the sarcolemmal sodium-calcium exchanger (NCX). *Bottom,* Representative Northern Blots (paired pre- and post-LVAD samples from the same patients) depicting myocardial mRNA for SERCA2a, NCX and RyR. Genes were probed serially, and autoradiographs were developed for differing lengths of time depending on the band intensity. DCM, indiopathic dilated cardiomyopathy; DIM, ischemic dilated cardiomyopathy. *(Modified from Heerdt PM, Holmes JW, Cai B, et al: Chronic unloading by left ventricular assist device reverses contractile dysfunction and alters gene expression in end-stage heart failure. Circulation 102:2713–2719, 2000, with permission.)*

The properties of the RyR, which regulates Ca^{2+} release to the myofilaments, also play a pivotal role in the ability of the sarcoplasmic reticulum (SR) to store and rapidly release Ca^{2+}.[21] The expression of the gene encoding for RyR after LVAD is up-regulated, but with little change in the protein content; this finding is consistent with the fact that blockade of the RyR with an excess of ryanodine had the same effect on Ca^{2+} uptake by SR membranes isolated from both heart failure and LVAD-supported hearts. However, hyperphosphorylation of RyR in failing human myocardium disrupts the normal coupled gating of neighboring receptors, resulting in abnormal ensemble gating patterns, less coordinated SR Ca^{2+} release during excitation, and Ca^{2+} leak during diastole.[27] After LVAD support, these abnormalities are reversed, possibly in response to normalization of the β-adrenergic signaling pathway. Thus, despite subtle changes in gene expression, protein content, or both, it appears that channel or pump function may be more affected by post-translational events. Results of some studies have indicated that with decreased SERCA2a function in heart failure, a compensatory increase in the activity of the NCX occurs as this sarcolemmal protein assumes a greater role in extruding Ca^{2+} during diastole.[20,28,29]

Consistent with this process are data indicating up-regulated myocardial expression of NCX mRNA in human heart failure.[25] However, recent data indicate that levels of NCX protein are not necessarily changed in severe human heart failure,[24] and animal studies have suggested that there can be decreased gene expression and reduced Ca^{2+} flux through the NCX in the setting of cardiac failure.[30-32] Our data showed that LVAD support led to up-regulated gene expression but no change in NCX protein content. Thus, as for RyR, isolated measurement of gene expression may not fully clarify pathophysiologic or LVAD-induced changes of the NCX properties. In a recent study from Terracciano and colleagues,[15] the SR Ca^{2+} content was increased after LVAD support only in patients who showed signs of recovery with explantation of the device. This was combined with increased inactivation in L-type Ca^{2+} currents measured in isolated myocytes.

Furthermore, data have been reported to demonstrate LVAD-induced up-regulation of β-adrenergic and endothelin-A receptors[33,34]; modulation of anti-apoptotic genes[35]; deactivation of nuclear factor-κB[36]; normalization of mitochondrial ultrastructure[37]; and down-regulation of matrix metalloproteinases, tumor necrosis factor-α, and β-tubulin[38-40] (Table 37-2).

TABLE 37-2 Left Ventricular Assist Device–Induced Alterations on the Molecular Level

Molecular Process/Protein	LVAD-Induced Alteration	References
SERCA2a, RyR, NCX	↑	5, 7
PKA phosphorylation of RyR2	Norm (↓)	27
β-Adrenergic receptor	↑	33
Endothelin receptor A	Norm (↑)	34
Antiapoptotic genes	↓	35
NF-κB	↓	36
Mitochondrial ultrastructure	Norm (↑)	37
MMP-1 and MMP-9	↓	38
TIMP-1	↑	46
TNF-α	↓	46
β-tubulin	↓	40
Myocardial ANP and BNP	↓	4
Cardiomyocyte mitochondrial function	↑	8
Metallothionein	↓	48
ERK	↓	47

SERCA2a, sarcoplasmic endoreticular calcium–adenosine triphosphatase subtype 2a; RyR, ryanodine-sensitive calcium release channel; NCX, sarcolemmal sodium-calcium exchanger; PKA, protein kinase A; NF-κB, nuclear factor-kappaB; MMP, matrix metalloproteinase; TIMP, tissue inhibitor of MMP; TNF-α, tumor necrosis factor-α; ANP, atrial natriuretic polypeptide; BNP, brain natriuretic polypeptide; ERK, extracellular signal-related kinases; ↓, down-regulation; ↑, up-regulation; Norm, normalization.

Age, Gender, and Pharmacotherapy

As with underlying disease, the impact of other factors such as age, gender, and pharmacotherapy on reverse remodeling remain largely unexplored. Aging alone has been shown to alter expression of calcium cycling genes (particularly SERCA2a)[41] and to dampen the process of remodeling in response to increased pressure or volume, or both.[42] Similarly, data demonstrating gender-related differences in SR calcium cycling in heart failure[43] indicate the possibility that the fundamental molecular abnormality may be influenced by gender with attendant effects on the nature of any LVAD-induced reversal. Experimental and clinical studies have clearly indicated that drugs such as angiotensin-converting enzyme inhibitors and β-blockers can prevent or reverse structural and perhaps molecular remodeling in the setting of heart failure.[44,45] Angiotensin-converting enzyme inhibitors exert direct effects on ventricular preload and afterload, as well as effects on the neurohormonal system. It has been hypothesized that hemodynamic and neurohormonal factors contribute to the beneficial effects on remodeling. However, whether the use of these drugs during LVAD support alters the nature or time course of reverse remodeling remains unknown.

DISCUSSION

As demonstrated in the data presented previously and in studies in other laboratories, the mechanical unloading of the myocardium provided by LVAD in concert with the associated normalization of cardiac output, systemic blood pressure, and neurohormonal milieu has been shown to induce reverse remodeling of several aspects of ventricular pathophysiology including: (1) reversal of chamber enlargement and normalization of EDPVR[2]; (2) global reduction in LV mass and regression of myocyte hypertrophy[4,14]; (3) increased contractile properties, enhanced inotropic response to β-adrenergic stimulation, increased rates of stimulation, and improved cytosolic Ca^{2+} transients (increased peak, accelerated decay)[6]; and (4) near-normalized expression of genes encoding for proteins involved in calcium metabolism.

Furthermore, LVAD support causes increased receptor density for inotropic activation,[33,34] decreased content or expression in proteins and genes regulating apoptosis,[35,36,46] improved mitochondrial and cellular function and ultrastructure,[8,37,40] reduced activity of stress-inducible proteins and hypertrophy transduction pathways,[47,48] and normalized extracellular matrix proteins and activity.[38]

Despite the multitude of facets of reverse remodeling already identified, it is likely that there are many more currently unexplored aspects of cardiac pathophysiology that are improved by LVAD support as a result of direct mechanical unloading effects. Improved contractile performance, a fundamental indicator that global cellular processes are regaining normal properties, speaks to this fact. Furthermore, the overall reduction in sudden cardiac death during LVAD support, by termination of fatal ventricular arrhythmia (see Chapter 34), is another aspect of electrical remodeling. As studies of this nature grow to include greater numbers of patients, it will also become increasingly important to analyze separately results from patients with different causes of heart failure; myocardial responses to LVAD may differ in the setting of chronic ischemic cardiomyopathy compared with other forms of dilated cardiomyopathy.

The precise mechanisms underlying the various aspects of reverse remodeling remain to be determined. The mechanisms underlying hypertrophy and chamber remodeling in response to pressure and volume loading of the myocardium involve intricately orchestrated up-regulation and down-regulation of a multitude of intracellular signaling cascades; although these mechanisms have been investigated for more than 30 years, they still are not understood. It has been our working hypothesis that reverse remodeling involves the same mechanisms as in remodeling working in the opposite direction. However, additional mechanisms may be in effect. By restoring cardiac output, blood pressure, and renal perfusion, LVAD support leads to normalization of the neurohormonal and cytokine environment, which may have profound effects in normalizing cellular properties.

Some evidence suggests that, in some patients, LVAD support may lead to improvement of global pump function of sufficient magnitude to permit explantation of the device without subsequent transplantation.[26,49] This has led to the concept of using LVAD as a bridge to recovery. The potential of this possibility is strengthened by data demonstrating the global extent to which reverse remodeling occurs. However, a recent study showed that specific changes in excitation coupling, and not regression of cellular hypertrophy, are associated with clinical recovery after LVAD support.[15] Additional data suggest that there is only a low incidence of "full" recovery during LVAD support as assessed by exercise testing with device output turned down.[50] Furthermore, the outcome of a small group of patients that underwent explantation was not uniformly good.[49] Accordingly, weaning from LVAD support is not the current standard of care. Nevertheless, the goal of using LVAD as a bridge to recovery is a worthy pursuit because of the severe imbalance between the number of patients requiring transplant and the number of available donor hearts. Better understanding of the process of reverse remodeling will aid the development of adjunctive therapies and better patient selection criteria and perhaps optimize protocols to improve patient outcome after LVAD explantation.

References

1. McCarthy PM, Savage RM, Fraser CD, et al: Hemodynamic and physiologic changes during support with an implantable left ventricular assist device. J Thorac Cardiovasc Surg 109:409–418, 1995.
2. Levin HR, Oz MC, Chen JM, et al: Reversal of chronic ventricular dilation in patients with end-stage cardiomyopathy by prolonged mechanical unloading. Circulation 91:2717–2720, 1995.
3. McCarthy PM, Nakatani S, Vargo R, et al: Structural and left ventricular histologic changes after implantable LVAD insertion. Ann Thorac Surg 59:609–613, 1995.
4. Altemose GT, Gritsus V, Jeevanandam V, et al: Altered myocardial phenotype after mechanical support in human beings with advanced cardiomyopathy. J Heart Lung Transplant 16:765–773, 1997.
5. Heerdt PM, Holmes JW, Cai B, et al: Chronic unloading by left ventricular assist device reverses contractile dysfunction and alters gene expression in end-stage heart failure. Circulation 102:2713–2719, 2000.
6. Dipla K, Mattiello JA, Jeevanandam V, et al: Myocyte recovery after mechanical circulatory support in humans with end-stage heart failure. Circulation 97:2316–2322, 1998.
7. Barbone A, Holmes JW, Heerdt PM, et al: Comparison of right and left ventricular responses to left ventricular assist device support in patients with severe heart failure: A primary role of mechanical unloading underlying reverse remodeling. Circulation 104:670–675, 2001.
8. Lee SH, Doliba N, Osbakken M, et al: Improvement of myocardial mitochondrial function after hemodynamic support with left ventricular assist devices in patients with heart failure. J Thorac Cardiovasc Surg 116:344–349, 1998.
9. Hall CW, Liotta D, Henly WS, et al: Development of artificial intrathoracic circulatory pumps. Am J Surg 108:685–692, 1964.
10. DeBakey ME: Left ventricular bypass pump for cardiac assistance. Clinical experience. Am J Cardiol 27:3–11, 1971.
11. Cooley DA: Two-staged cardiac replacement. Indian Heart J 34:341–348, 1982.
12. Potapov EV, Loebe M, Nasseri BA, et al: Pulsatile flow in patients with a novel nonpulsatile implantable ventricular assist device. Circulation 102(19 suppl 3):III183–III187, 2000.
13. Klotz S, Deng MC, Stypmann J, et al: Left ventricular pressure and volume unloading during pulsatile versus nonpulsatile left ventricular assist device support. Ann Thorac Surg 77:143–150, 2004.
14. Zafeiridis A, Jeevanandam V, Houser SR, Margulies KB: Regression of cellular hypertrophy after left ventricular assist device support. Circulation 98:656–662, 1998.
15. Terracciano CMN, Hardy J, Birks EJ, et al: Clinical recovery from end-stage heart failure using left-ventricular assist device and pharmacological therapy correlates with increased sarcoplasmatic reticulum calcium content but not with regression of cellular hypertrophy. Circulation 109:2263–2265, 2004.
16. Madigan JD, Barbone A, Choudhri AF, et al: Time course of reverse remodeling of the left ventricle during support with a left ventricular assist device. J Thorac Cardiovasc Surg 121:902–908, 2001.
17. Estrada-Quintero T, Uretsky BF, Murali S, et al: Neurohormonal activation and exercise function in patients with severe heart failure and patients with left ventricular assist system. A comparative study. Chest 107:1499–1503, 1995.
18. Calaghan SC, White E: The role of calcium in the response of cardiac muscle to stretch. Prog Biophys Mol Biol 71:59–90, 1999.
19. Swynghedauw B: Molecular mechanisms of myocardial remodeling. Physiol Rev 79:215–262, 1999.
20. Houser SR, Piacentino V III, Weisser J: Abnormalities of calcium cycling in the hypertrophied and failing heart. J Mol Cell Cardiol 32:1595–1607, 2000.
21. Arai M, Alpert NR, MacLennan DH, et al: Alterations in sarcoplasmic reticulum gene expression in human heart failure. A possible mechanism for alterations in systolic and diastolic properties of the failing myocardium. Circ Res 72:463–469, 1993.
22. Linck B, Boknik P, Eschenhagen T, et al: Messenger RNA expression and immunological quantification of phospholamban and SR-Ca²⁺-ATPase in failing and nonfailing human hearts. Cardiovasc Res 31:625–632, 1996.
23. Go LO, Moschella MC, Watras J, et al: Differential regulation of two types of intracellular calcium release channels during end-stage heart failure. J Clin Invest 95:888–894, 1995.
24. Hasenfuss G, Reinecke H, Studer R, et al: Relation between myocardial function and expression of sarcoplasmic reticulum Ca^{2+}-ATPase in failing and nonfailing human myocardium. Circ Res 75:434–442, 1994.
25. Studer R, Reinecke H, Bilger J, et al: Gene expression of the cardiac Na^+-Ca^{2+} exchanger in end-stage human heart failure. Circ Res 75:443–453, 1994.
26. Muller J, Wallukat G, Weng YG, et al: Weaning from mechanical cardiac support in patients with idiopathic dilated cardiomyopathy. Circulation 96:542–549, 1997.

27. Marx SO, Reiken S, Hisamatsu Y, et al: Pka phosphorylation dissociates fkbp12.6 from the calcium release channel (ryanodine receptor): Defective regulation in failing hearts. Cell 101:365–376, 2000.
28. Flesch M, Schwinger RH, Schiffer F, et al: Evidence for functional relevance of an enhanced expression of the Na$^+$-Ca^{2+} exchanger in failing human myocardium. Circulation 94:992–1002, 1996.
29. Hasenfuss G, Schillinger W, Lehnart SE, et al: Relationship between Na$^+$-Ca^{2+}-exchanger protein levels and diastolic function of failing human myocardium. Circulation 99:641–648, 1999.
30. Yoshiyama M, Takeuchi K, Hanatani A, et al: Differences in expression of sarcoplasmic reticulum Ca^{2+}-ATPase and Na$^+$-Ca^{2+} exchanger genes between adjacent and remote noninfarcted myocardium after myocardial infarction. J Mol Cell Cardiol 29:255–264, 1997.
31. Yao A, Su Z, Nonaka A, et al: Abnormal myocyte Ca^{2+} homeostasis in rabbits with pacing-induced heart failure. Am J Physiol 275(4 pt 2):H1441–H1448, 1998.
32. Dixon IM, Hata T, Dhalla NS: Sarcolemmal calcium transport in congestive heart failure due to myocardial infarction in rats. Am J Physiol 262(5 pt 2):H1387–H1394, 1992.
33. Ogletree-Hughes ML, Stull LB, Sweet WE, et al: Mechanical unloading restores β-adrenergic responsiveness and reverses receptor downregulation in the failing human heart. Circulation 104:881–886, 2001.
34. Morawietz H, Szibor M, Goettsch W, et al: Deloading of the left ventricle by ventricular assist device normalizes increased expression of endothelin ET(a) receptors but not endothelin-converting enzyme-1 in patients with end-stage heart failure. Circulation 102(19 suppl 3):III188–III193, 2000.
35. Bartling B, Milting H, Schumann H, et al: Myocardial gene expression of regulators of myocyte apoptosis and myocyte calcium homeostasis during hemodynamic unloading by ventricular assist devices in patients with end-stage heart failure. Circulation 100(19 suppl):II216–II223, 1999.
36. Grabellus F, Levkau B, Sokoll A, et al: Reversible activation of nuclear factor-κB in human end-stage heart failure after left ventricular mechanical support. Cardiovasc Res 53:124–130, 2002.
37. Heerdt PM, Schlame M, Jehle R, et al: Disease-specific remodeling of cardiac mitochondria after a left ventricular assist device. Ann Thorac Surg 73:1216–1221, 2002.
38. Li YY, Feng Y, McTiernan CF, et al: Downregulation of matrix metalloproteinases and reduction in collagen damage in the failing human heart after support with left ventricular assist devices. Circulation 104:1147–1152, 2001.
39. Razeghi P, Mukhopadhyay M, Myers TJ, et al: Myocardial tumor necrosis factor-α expression does not correlate with clinical indices of heart failure in patients on left ventricular assist device support. Ann Thorac Surg 72:2044–2050, 2001.
40. Aquila-Pastir LA, McCarthy PM, Smedira NG, Moravec CS: Mechanical unloading decreases the expression of β-tubulin in the failing human heart. J Heart Lung Transplant 20:211, 2001.
41. Lakatta EG: Myocardial adaptations in advanced age. Basic Res Cardiol 88(suppl 2):125–133, 1993.
42. Isoyama S, Grossman W, Wei JY: Effect of age on myocardial adaptation to volume overload in the rat. J Clin Invest 81:1850–1857, 1988.
43. Dash R, Frank KF, Carr AN, et al: Gender influences on sarcoplasmic reticulum Ca^{2+}-handling in failing human myocardium. J Mol Cell Cardiol 33:1345–1353, 2001.
44. Weber KT: Cardioreparation in hypertensive heart disease. Hypertension 38(3 pt 2):588–591, 2001.
45. Reiken S, Wehrens XH, Vest JA, et al: β-Blockers restore calcium release channel function and improve cardiac muscle performance in human heart failure. Circulation 107:2459–2466, 2003.
46. Torre-Amione G, Stetson SJ, Youker KA, et al: Decreased expression of tumor necrosis factor-α in failing human myocardium after mechanical circulatory support: A potential mechanism for cardiac recovery. Circulation 100:1189–1193, 1999.
47. Baba HA, Stypmann J, Grabellus F, et al: Dynamic regulation of MEF/Erks and Akt/GSK-3^β in human end-stage heart failure after left ventricular mechanical support: Myocardial mechanotransduction-sensitivity as a possible molecular mechanism. Cardiovasc Res 59:390–399, 2003.
48. Baba HA, Grabellus F, August C, et al: Reversal of metallothionein expression is different throughout the human myocardium after prolonged left-ventricular mechanical support. J Heart Lung Transplant 19:668–674, 2000.
49. Mancini DM, Beniaminovitz A, Levin H, et al: Low incidence of myocardial recovery after left ventricular assist device implantation in patients with chronic heart failure. Circulation 98:2383–2389, 1998.
50. El-Banayosy A, Arusoglu L, Kizner L, et al: Hemodynamic exercise testing reveals a low incidence of myocardial recovery in LVAD patients. J Heart Lung Transplant 20:209–210, 2001.

CHAPTER 38

Cardiac Resynchronization Therapy for Patients with Heart Failure with Ventricular Conduction Delay

• • • •

Angelo Auricchio and Andrew Kramer

The structural, hemodynamic, and neurohumoral changes present in heart failure (HF) are associated with conduction and contraction abnormalities that decrease pump function and increase arrhythmia incidence. About one third of patients with HF and depressed left ventricular (LV) ejection fraction have ventricular conduction delays (VCD), most commonly presenting as a left bundle branch block (LBBB) pattern on surface electrocardiogram (ECG).[1] There is increasing evidence that VCD is an independent risk factor for HF hospitalization, death from pump failure, and death from arrhythmia.[2] Pharmacologic therapy is unable to correct a VCD and its associated negative electromechanical consequences. A relatively new therapy, pre-excitation of the LV free wall with atrial sequential LV or biventricular pacing, can resynchronize the ventricular activation pattern by acting as an electrical bypass, which restores a more coordinated ventricular contraction. This cardiac resynchronization therapy (CRT) can improve cardiac mechanics, facilitate reverse remodeling, and reduce morbidity and mortality of patients with HF with VCD.

ELECTROMECHANICAL ABNORMALITIES INDUCED BY VENTRICULAR CONDUCTION DELAYS

The impressive clinical results with CRT have renewed research interest in the electrical activation patterns associated with VCD. About two thirds of CRT candidates with prolonged QRS present with LBBB morphology, whereas the remaining third exhibit a right bundle branch block (RBBB) morphology (10 to 15%) or diffuse VCD (5 to 10%). VCD also is associated with mechanical dyssynchrony, which depresses ventricular pump function, exacerbating HF symptoms and provoking remodeling. These mechanical consequences constitute a serious component of the HF condition, especially in patients with an LBBB type of conduction pattern.

Abnormal Electrical Activation Sequence

Detailed electrical activation sequence can best be evaluated using catheter-based, three-dimensional, non-fluoroscopic, contact and noncontact mapping techniques.[3,4] These techniques permit in vivo reconstruction of the cardiac anatomy and assessment of the activation sequence with high spatial resolution, enabling detailed characterization of the abnormal electrical activation sequence of each ventricle. Contact mapping produces bipolar recordings that reflect local changes in endocardial electrical events with high sensitivity to rapidly changing signals and a lower sensitivity to slowly changing signals.[5] Noncontact mapping provides unipolar recordings that, from a basket catheter positioned inside the heart chamber, reflect transmural electrical events with equal sensitivity to fast and slow signals.[5]

Ventricular Activation Sequence in Left Bundle Branch Block

Right ventricular (RV) activation sequence in patients with HF and LBBB is quite variable,[6] and usually RV activation pattern is sequential rather than simultaneous (Fig. 38–1). LBBB is associated with a significant delay of the LV trans-septal time (or the time from beginning of the QRS complex to the earliest LV breakthrough), the LV endocardial time, and the LV transmural time (which includes middle and epicardium).[6,7,8]

About one third of patients with HF with LBBB morphology have a normal trans-septal time (i.e., ≤ 20 msec) with an LV breakthrough at an anterior or septo-basal site, probably through one or more septal branches of the His-Purkinje system.[6]

In the remaining patients, the LV breakthrough is a mid-septal or septo-apical site that is associated with an abrupt increase in the trans-septal time, which may result from myocardial rather than fascicular conduction through the septum.[6]

Endocardial and transmural times usually are prolonged in patients with HF, with the latter being most delayed.[7] A "U-shaped" pattern of transmural activation has been observed in almost all patients with LBBB (Fig. 38–2). The functional line of block may emerge from anisotropic conduction through individual myocardial layers that may have developed different electrophysiologic defects in response to HF, and thus have different conduction characteristics. In particular, the line of block may represent a regional transition in layer connectivity or conduction speeds. These conduction transitions can occur at different

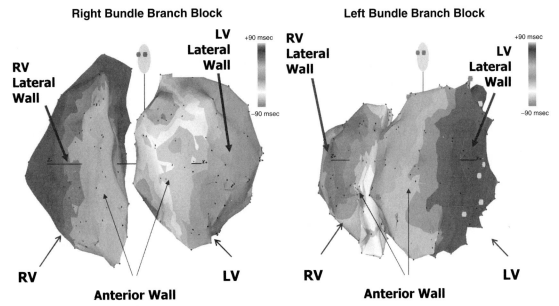

■ **Figure 38–1** Isochronal plot (light gray: −90 msec; dark gray: +90 msec) obtained from patients with right (RBBB; *left*) and left (LBBB; *right*) bundle branch block. In RBBB, the left ventricular (LV) breakthrough site is in the septum, from which activation slowly spreads toward the anterior region, with the right ventricular (RV) lateral wall and the outflow tract being activated last. Total RV activation time in RBBB is always significantly longer than in LBBB. The endocardial spread of activation was similar in both patient populations. Patients with LBBB have a single RV anterolateral breakthrough site. The LV is activated late with respect to the start of QRS, starting from the septum, followed by inferior and finally lateral and posterolateral walls. (See color insert.)

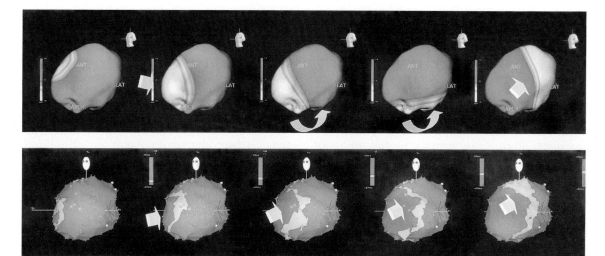

■ **Figure 38–2** Transmural (*top;* gray level coding: white −5 mV; gray +5 mV) and endocardial (*bottom;* gray level coding: light gray indicates spread of activation; the line on the time bar indicates progression from −87 msec to +22 msec) left ventricular (LV) activation in a patient with left bundle branch block QRS morphology. The endocardial activation proceeds uniformly and directly to the lateral and posterolateral wall, ending at the basal region near the mitral valve annulus. In contrast, the transmural activation does not cross from the anterior wall to the lateral wall, but it reaches the lateral or posterolateral regions by propagating inferiorly around the apex and across the inferior wall. This apparent conduction block occurs in the absence of any observable structural defects in the region, such as ischemic scarring, and thus appears to be a functional line of block. (See color insert.)

locations in the same patient depending on where activation is initiated, either spontaneously or with pacing. Thus, each particular propagation pattern may encounter different conduction transitions in these defective ventricles. Analogous to structural conduction blocks, these functional conduction blocks in patients with HF with LBBB could be a frequent source of re-entrant tachycardia, which might account for the high likelihood of sudden death in patients with nonischemic HF.

The specific LV activation sequence cannot be predicted by a LBBB pattern on the ECG. Independent of the QRS duration, patients with LBBB morphology may have an anterior, lateral, or inferior line of block.[6] This electrical heterogeneity is associated with a corresponding heterogeneity of regional mechanical contraction delays in the LV.[9] Because there appears to be a connection between the location of the functional line of block and the region of late contraction, the line of block location may predict where the LV needs to be paced to resynchronize the contraction.

Resynchronization is best achieved by pacing the LV in an area of delayed contraction;[10] by extension,

this may need to be distal to the line of functional block. In patients with HF with QRS less than 150 msec, LV pacing in an anterior location often worsens cardiac function, whereas pacing the same patient at a lateral location may improve cardiac function.[11] Electrical mapping studies have shown that approximately two thirds of patients with QRS duration less than 150 msec exhibit a laterally located line of block, which is consistent with the poor results of LV pacing at an anterior site, which may have been proximal to the line of block. Pacing the LV within the most mechanically delayed site is associated with significantly larger increases in LV ejection fraction and reductions in LV end-systolic volume after several months of CRT.[10]

Left and Right Ventricular Activation in Right Bundle Branch Block

RBBB may be as important a predictor of mortality in patients with HF as LBBB.[12] Currently, there is poor understanding of whether and how CRT will work in patients with HF with RBBB, although retrospective analysis and small studies have indicated that CRT may also benefit these patients.[13,14]

Patients with HF with RBBB QRS morphology have unique LV and RV activation patterns. Indeed, activation of the RV anterior region, lateral region, and outflow tract is delayed, thus mirroring, on the right side of the heart, the pattern of delayed activation observed in the LV of patients with LBBB (see Fig. 38–1). Furthermore, LV activation times and activation sequence frequently are not significantly different between patients with RBBB or LBBB.

Mechanical Dyssynchrony and Hemodynamic Depression

The association between LBBB and abnormal ventricular contraction sequence has been well known for many years.[15] Animal models suggest this is a causal relation.[16,17] In patients with HF, there are three mechanical timing problems arising from LBBB: abnormal left atrioventricular (AV) timing, delayed interventricular timing, and delayed left intraventricular timing.

Left AV timing is altered because the LV contracts much too long after the end of the left atrial (LA) contraction.[18] During this delay, LA systolic pressure decreases before the mitral valve is closed, often resulting in presystolic mitral regurgitation. Also, because the LA pressure is less when the LV finally starts to contract, the LV effective preload is reduced, which reduces the stroke volume by the Frank–Starling mechanism. The delay also causes prolongation of the LV systolic period, which shortens filling time and may cause, or exacerbate, restrictive filling.

Interventricular timing is delayed because the LV contracts later than the RV.[19] Closely associated with this, LV regional contraction patterns are dyssynchronous, most often with a contraction first in the septum, followed by an abnormally delayed lateral wall contraction.[20,21]

Interventricular and intraventricular dyssynchrony reduce LV pump effectiveness, particularly stroke volume, because the early contracting septum is not stiff when the lateral wall contracts, resulting in a loss of work to paradoxical septal motion and fruitless late

contraction of the lateral region after the aortic valve has closed. Thus, the late-contracting lateral wall experiences abnormally increased afterloads and performs nearly twice its normal work. Conversely, the septum is stretched late in systole, which can trigger calcium release to induce aftercontractions and arrhythmia.[22]

Structural Remodeling and Prognosis

Ventricular contraction dyssynchrony creates non-uniformities in regional strain and workload.[23] As a result, there is compensatory hypotrophy in the early-contracting region and hypertrophy in the late-contracting region. These nonuniformities have been shown to be associated with altered expression of regional stress kinase and calcium-handling proteins in the high-stress areas.[24] Thus, mechanical dyssynchrony arising from conduction disorders appears to be a direct cause of ventricular remodeling (Fig. 38–3).

Ventricular remodeling is the hallmark of disease progression in systolic HF. Because it is so strongly associated with mechanical dyssynchrony resulting from VCD, it would be expected that dyssynchrony should predict HF progression. Recently, this was observed using echocardiography to measure LV mechanical dyssynchrony, which was found to be an independent risk factor for hospitalization or mortality in patients with HF.[25,26]

MODULATION OF THE ELECTROMECHANICAL ABNORMALITIES BY CARDIAC RESYNCHRONIZATION

Unlike conventional pacing for bradycardia, CRT requires pacing of both the RV and LV (commonly referred to as biventricular pacing) or pacing of the LV alone to restore a more synchronized ventricular activation and contraction pattern in patients with VCD (typically LV delay). Although this pacing can provide rate support, the unique function of CRT is to improve ventricular pump function, particularly to increase the stroke volume. Thus, CRT usually is delivered by tracking the intrinsic sinus rate and pacing the ventricles

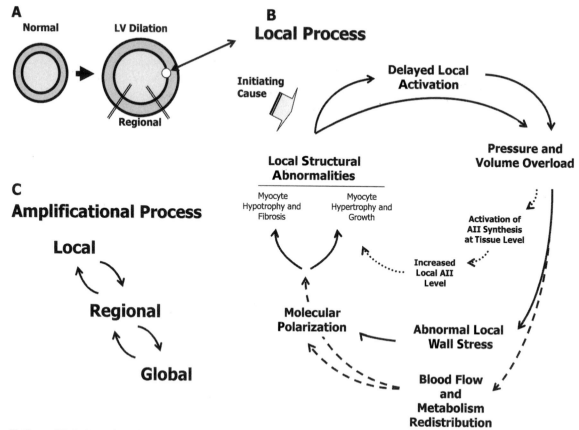

■ **Figure 38–3** Hypothetical vicious cycle through which local conduction disturbances may arise and eventually induce molecular polarization at local and regional levels. LV, left ventricular; AII, Angiotensin II.

after a programmable AV delay. The clinical benefits of CRT are now well established, even though the precise mechanisms of action are still being investigated.

Mechanisms of Cardiac Resynchronization Therapy Action

Generally, it is believed that CRT works by improving the systolic function of the LV without increasing myocardial metabolic demand.[27] By comparison, inotropic drugs increase cellular contractility at the expense of increased metabolic demand, which has been shown to worsen patient condition when administered as a long-term treatment. Biventricular and LV pacing alone can improve most of the timing deficits associated with VCD in patients with HF.[22]

The AV pacing delay with CRT controls the effectiveness of the LV filling pattern and the degree of ventricular pre-excitation or intrinsic fusion. AV timing between the LA and LV can be completely normalized with an AV pacing delay that advances the start of the LV contraction to begin just at the end of LA systole, maximizing the effective preload of the LV.[28] Restoring optimal left AV mechanical timing reduces or eliminates presystolic mitral regurgitation and increases the filling time. Interestingly, RV-only pacing also can restore left AV timing, but it requires shorter AV pacing delays that may create premature closure of the tricuspid valve.

Interventricular and LV intraventricular timing are improved by CRT, but they are not completely normalized. Complete normalization of ventricular contraction would require restoring the intrinsic Purkinje activation sequence. Instead, biventricular and LV pacing spread electrical activation by intramyocardial conduction in a nonintrinsic sequence from the typically lateral LV pacing site. The paced activation sequence improves the ventricular contraction pattern compared with the abnormal intrinsic baseline, which, in turn, improves hemodynamic function compared with baseline. However, the contraction from pacing is not as synchronous as it is when activated by intrafascicular conduction, which proceeds at four times the speed of paced activation and flows from the apex out to and up the ventricular walls to create an optimized squeezing motion.[29,30] In addition, transmural timing may not be normalized by CRT, because activation proceeds by a nonintrinsic sequence through the layers[31] and conduction in each layer may be cellularly altered, which cannot be corrected immediately by pacing.

Conduction–Contraction Relation during Cardiac Resynchronization Therapy

The complex relation between conduction and contraction patterns in patients with HF with ventricular conduction disorder is well illustrated by comparing the effects of biventricular and LV-only pacing. From the beginning, biventricular and LV pacing were found to provide similar degrees of hemodynamic[32,33] and clinical improvement.[34,35] This was unexpected, because it appeared that LV pacing would substitute one conduction delay (RV-to-LV) for another (LV-to-RV), and therefore should not be able to resynchronize ventricular contraction.

In normal canine hearts and nonfailing human hearts, LV pacing at the lateral wall, in fact, creates both conduction delay and mechanical dyssynchrony and worsens hemodynamic function, although not as severely as with RV pacing.[30] In a canine model of HF with LBBB, LV pacing also creates the expected VCD, but, surprisingly, results in a more synchronized LV contraction.[17] Furthermore, these results were observed when pacing at short AV delays to avoid any fusion of paced and intrinsic activations.

However, only epicardial conduction was measured in this study. The paradox that mechanical resynchronization does not require electrical synchrony may be resolved by differences between epicardial and endocardial conduction patterns. In a different study of nonfailing LBBB canine hearts, optimal hemodynamic improvement with LV pacing was, in fact, associated with endocardial electrical synchrony, apparently resulting from fusion of paced and intrinsic activation.[36] Although endocardial and epicardial conduction fuse with intrinsic activation at similar times in normal canines,[37] the failing heart may be different. The paradox could be resolved if, for instance, in the failing heart, endocardial conduction is slow and epicardial conduction is somewhat faster, so that although epicardial conduction is asynchronous with LV, as observed, endocardial electrical and mechanical synchrony could be concordant, which needs to be assessed.

Effect of Cardiac Resynchronization Therapy on Functional Capacity and Ventricular Remodeling

Current clinical evidence supports the value of CRT for patients with moderate or severe chronic heart failure (New York Heart Association [NYHA] functional Class III or IV) caused by ischemic or nonischemic cardiomyopathy and widened QRS duration on surface ECG (generally > 120 msec). Clinical trials consistently have shown that in such patients, functional capacity, quality of life, and exercise tolerance are significantly improved after a few months of CRT.[38] However, about one third of patients with CRT appear not to improve. Whether benefit with CRT can be predicted for individual patients with HF is still a matter of intense investigation.[39] Few data have been collected on CRT in patients with NYHA Class II; currently, this patient group is not routinely recommended for CRT.

Some patients with HF with depressed LV ejection fraction, despite normal duration of the QRS complex, may have echocardiographically assessed mechanical dyssynchrony of similar magnitude as patients with considerably prolonged QRS duration.[40] Although preliminary data suggest that patients with mechanical dyssynchrony, despite normal QRS, may benefit, CRT should not be extended to this group without prospective randomized studies.

Together with hemodynamic improvements, several prospective nonrandomized and randomized trials have shown that reverse remodeling with improvement of functional capacity may occur after the first few months of CRT.[41] The reverse remodeling is time-dependent, being most evident 3 to 6 months after CRT. Unfortunately, data for longer follow-up periods are not available; therefore, it is currently unknown whether the process of remodeling has been indefinitely halted or just delayed by CRT.

Multiple mechanisms may be responsible for the reverse remodeling during CRT, including redistribution of regional ventricular loading and possibly myocardial growth responses to the changed regional workload patterns in the LV, reduction of myocardial

oxygen demand, and reduction or abolition of mitral regurgitation, as well as reduction of sympathetic activity and increase of parasympathetic activity (Fig. 38–4).

Effect of Cardiac Resynchronization Therapy on Mortality and Morbidity

We may speculate that there are three different therapeutic phases with CRT (see Fig. 38–4). The first acute phase starts immediately after implantation and probably lasts 2 to 4 days, during which time most of the changes result from improved hemodynamic and mechanical function. A second phase may follow that

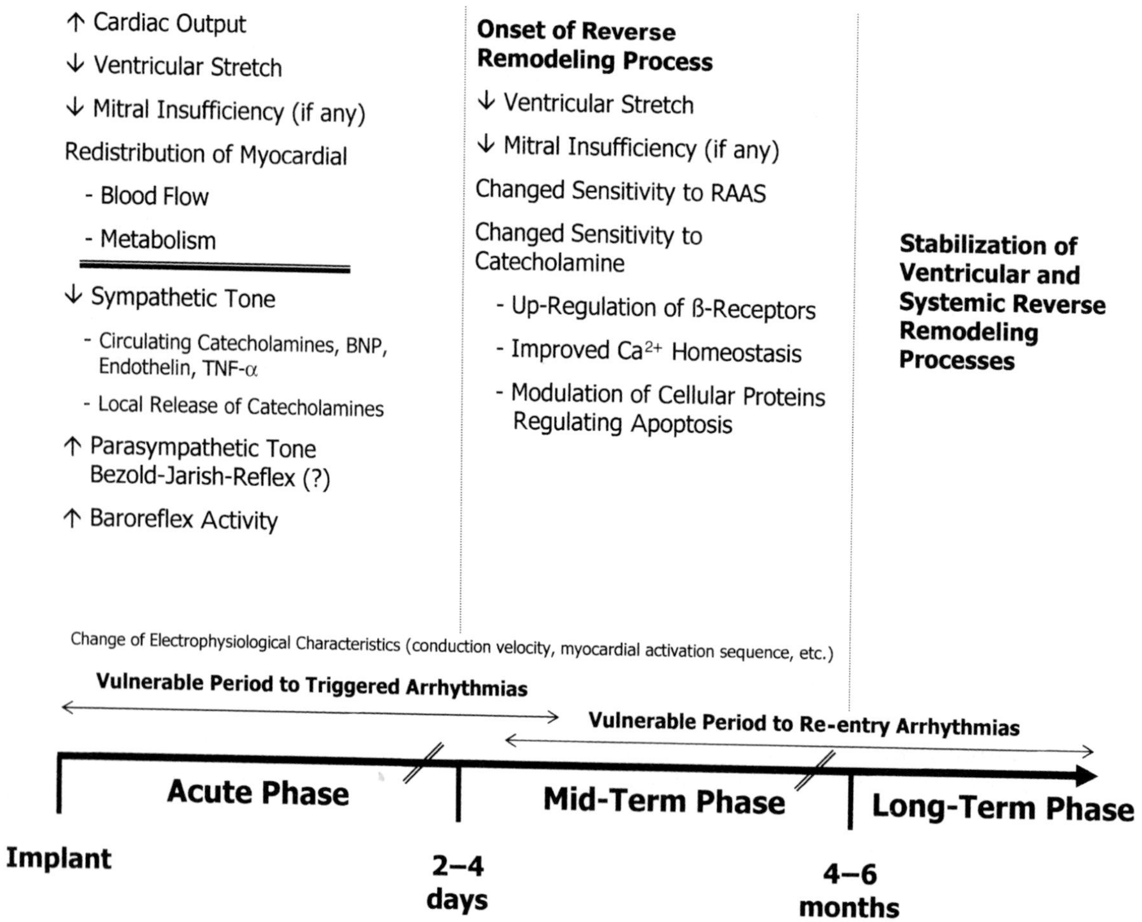

↑ Cardiac Output

↓ Ventricular Stretch

↓ Mitral Insufficiency (if any)

Redistribution of Myocardial

- Blood Flow
- Metabolism

↓ Sympathetic Tone

- Circulating Catecholamines, BNP, Endothelin, TNF-α
- Local Release of Catecholamines

↑ Parasympathetic Tone
Bezold-Jarish-Reflex (?)

↑ Baroreflex Activity

Onset of Reverse Remodeling Process

↓ Ventricular Stretch

↓ Mitral Insufficiency (if any)

Changed Sensitivity to RAAS

Changed Sensitivity to Catecholamine

- Up-Regulation of ß-Receptors
- Improved Ca^{2+} Homeostasis
- Modulation of Cellular Proteins Regulating Apoptosis

Stabilization of Ventricular and Systemic Reverse Remodeling Processes

Change of Electrophysiological Characteristics (conduction velocity, myocardial activation sequence, etc.)

Vulnerable Period to Triggered Arrhythmias

Vulnerable Period to Re-entry Arrhythmias

Acute Phase   **Mid-Term Phase**   **Long-Term Phase**

Implant   **2–4 days**   **4–6 months**

■ **Figure 38–4** Hemodynamic, mechanical, and electrophysiologic changes induced by cardiac resynchronization therapy over time. RAAS, Renin-angiotensin-aldosterone-system; TNFα, tumor necrosis factor α; BNP; B-type natriuretic peptide.

is dominated by morphologic and structural changes related to reverse ventricular mechanical remodeling. According to published data, this phase could last about 6 months. Finally, after 6 to 8 months, there may be a chronic maintenance period, during which the patient's health and condition are relatively stable, prolonging their life and keeping them out of the hospital. It remains to be determined whether and how long CRT can stabilize a HF condition.

The recent Comparison of Medical Therapy, Pacing, and Defibrillation in Heart Failure (COMPANION) trial demonstrated that CRT alone or with defibrillator backup significantly reduced a combined end point of all-cause hospitalization and all-cause mortality compared with best pharmacologic treatment in patients with NYHA Class III-IV HF with an ejection fraction less than 35% and a QRS greater than 120 msec.[42]

All-cause mortality was reduced by a nonsignificant 24% with CRT alone and by a significant 34% with CRT and the defibrillator. However, CRT with or without an implantable cardioverter-defibrillator (ICD) significantly reduced hospital admissions for HF, which could substantially reduce the burden of HF on the healthcare system. These findings are supported by a recent meta-analysis, which calculated a significant (51%) reduction in mortality caused by worsening HF and a significant (29%) decrease in the incidence of hospital admissions for HF decompensation among the represented CRT trials.[38]

Effect of Cardiac Resynchronization Therapy on Ventricular Arrhythmias

Risk for ventricular arrhythmia in patients with HF is increased because of delayed and slowed ventricular activation, alteration of repolarization, excessive sympathetic activity, and structural abnormalities related to fibrosis and ischemia. About one third to one half of deaths in patients with HF is sudden and most likely related to ventricular tachyarrhythmia. Medical antiarrhythmic therapy minimally prevents sudden cardiac death in patients with HF, whereas the ICD has been shown to reduce significantly the incidence of all-cause mortality compared with the best medical therapy in patients with HF of any cause.[43,44]

CRT might be expected to reduce the risk for arrhythmia by improving pump function, reducing sympathetic drive, and stimulating reversal of dilation. Sympathetic nerve activity is reduced abruptly during biventricular pacing in an electrophysiology laboratory setting.[45] On the basis of the heart rate data continuously recorded by implanted CRT devices, heart rate variability (HRV) increases and mean and minimum heart rate decrease after several months of CRT, indicating a likely decrease in sympathetic activity. HRV typically increases quickly in the first 10 to 12 weeks and slowly continues to increase for another 8 to 10 months after the start of CRT. These changes may reflect initial reduction in sympathetic tone caused by immediate increased stroke volume with CRT, followed by continued sympathetic changes as reverse remodeling further improves LV pump function. These reductions in sympathetic activity may be associated with reduced likelihood of tachyarrhythmia.

In contrast, biventricular pacing introduces new electrical activation patterns that may be a new source of arrhythmia; this has been studied recently in patients with nonischemic HF.[31] Normally, the endocardium is activated first by the Purkinje network, followed by the epicardium, yet both layers repolarize at similar times because the epicardium has a shorter action potential duration (APD). With CRT, the transmural activation sequence is reversed by LV epicardial pacing, creating a long transmural repolarization delay, because the endocardium is activated last and has a longer APD. Such changes could be arrhythmogenic in patients at risk for QT prolongation (e.g., in patients receiving APD-prolonging drugs), which can be associated with early afterdepolarizations (EAD). In animals, epicardial LV pacing can facilitate transmural propagation of EAD, resulting in R-on-T-wave extrasystoles. This also has been observed in some patients with HF, in whom LV only or biventricular pacing can trigger recurrent, nonsustained, polymorphic ventricular tachycardia (PVT) or torsades de pointes.[31]

Although of theoretical risk for some individuals, in clinical study populations, CRT has a neutral effect on ventricular arrhythmia. In the CONTAK CD and the InSync ICD studies, arrhythmia incidence was compared for patients with HF receiving an ICD with standard medical care versus those receiving an ICD and

CRT. In a meta-analysis of these studies, there was no significant reduction in ventricular arrhythmias among patients treated with CRT.[38] In the CONTAK CD study, there were no differences between treatment groups in the number of patients receiving appropriate ICD therapy and incidence of ventricular tachycardia (VT) alone, ventricular fibrillation (VF) alone, or both VT and VF.[46] When arrhythmic events were classified into monomorphic VT (MVT) and PVT based on review of electrograms stored by the ICD, there were no differences in MVT events, whereas there were more PVT events in the patients receiving CRT, but the difference was not significant and appeared because of a disproportionate number of PVT episodes in a few patients receiving CRT.[47] Apparently, any positive effects of CRT on MVT are small, whereas some individuals may have increased risk for PVT.

Effect of Cardiac Resynchronization Therapy on Atrial Arrhythmias

Atrial fibrillation is a common supraventricular arrhythmia observed in up to 30% of patients with congestive HF. Paroxysmal and persistent atrial fibrillation are observed with similar frequency in patients with HF. Ischemia and chronic inflammatory processes, or hemodynamic abnormalities such as impaired ventricular filling and AV valve insufficiency, may cause structural abnormalities leading to dilation of the atria, which facilitates the onset and persistence of atrial fibrillation.

HF may also facilitate the onset of atrial fibrillation through neurohumoral mechanisms and changes in the hemodynamic status. There is increasing evidence that the same neurohumoral compensatory mechanisms activated in HF are involved in atrial remodeling, thus creating the anatomic substrate for atrial fibrillation.[48] Another (possibly underappreciated) mechanism in patients with HF is diastolic and systolic mitral regurgitation. The atrial mechanical stimulation created by the regurgitation jet during the atrial vulnerable period may be another significant contributor to the incidence of atrial fibrillation in the HF population.

Definitive data on the effect of CRT on atrial arrhythmias are lacking. It is possible that CRT may influence the onset and duration of atrial arrhythmias, particularly atrial fibrillation. A few cases have been reported in which atrial fibrillation spontaneously converted to sinus rhythm, or previously temporary cardioversions became more permanent after CRT.[49] Atrial size may decrease after several months of CRT because of reduction of diastolic and systolic mitral regurgitation, as well as reduction of sympathetic atrial drive, which may restore and stabilize a normal sinus rhythm.

Conclusions

Treating HF associated with ventricular conduction disorders and mechanical dyssynchrony is a fascinating blend of cardiac mechanics and electrophysiology. It has engendered new electromechanical and pathophysiologic concepts of HF and arrhythmia and a novel device-based treatment: CRT. By correcting the mechanical dyssynchrony caused by VCD, CRT significantly improves functional class, exercise capacity, and quality of life compared with the best pharmacologic HF therapy. CRT also may halt or reverse the cardiac remodeling so closely associated with HF progression and worsening prognosis, and it reduces hospital admissions for HF and possibly all-cause mortality. Although CRT appears to have a neutral effect on arrhythmia, ICD can help prevent the arrhythmic death associated with electromechanical dyssynchrony of the ventricles.

References

1. Xiao H, Roy C, Fujimoto S, Gibson DG: Natural history of abnormal conduction and its relation to prognosis in patients with dilated cardiomyopathy. Int J Cardiol 53:163–170, 1996.
2. Baldasseroni S, De Biase L, Fresco C, et al: Cumulative effect of complete left bundle-branch block and chronic atrial fibrillation on 1-year mortality and hospitalization in patients with congestive heart failure. A report from the Italian network on congestive heart failure (in-CHF database). Eur Heart J 23:1692–1698, 2002.
3. Gepstein L, Hayan G, Ben-Haim SA: A novel method for nonfluoroscopic catheter-based electroanatomical mapping of the heart. In vitro and in vivo accuracy results. Circulation 95:1611–1622, 1997.
4. Schilling RJ, Peters NS, Davies DW: Simultaneous endocardial mapping in the human left ventricle using a noncontact catheter: Comparison of contact and reconstructed electrograms during sinus rhythm. Circulation 98:887–898, 1998.
5. De Bakker JMT, Hauer RNW, Simmens TA: Activation mapping: Unipolar versus bipolar recording. In Zipes DP, Jalife J

(eds): Cardiac Electrophysiology: From Cell to Bedside, 3rd ed. pp 1068–1078, Philadelphia, Saunders, 1999.

6. Auricchio A, Fantoni C, Regoli F, et al: Characterization of left ventricular activation in patients with heart failure and left bundle branch block. Circulation 109:1133–1139, 2004.

7. Vassallo JA, Cassidy DM, Marchlinski FE, et al: Endocardial activation of left bundle branch block. Circulation 69:914–923, 1984.

8. Rodriguez L-M, Timmermans C, Nabar A, et al: Variable patterns of septal activation in patients with left bundle branch block and heart failure. J Cardiovasc Electrophysiol 14:135–141, 2003.

9. Fung JW-H, Yu C-M, Yip G, et al: Variable left ventricular activation pattern in patients with heart failure and left bundle branch block. Heart 90:17–19, 2004.

10. Ansalone G, Giannantoni P, Ricci R, et al: Doppler myocardial imaging to evaluate the effectiveness of pacing sites in patients receiving biventricular pacing. J Am Coll Cardiol 39:489–499, 2002.

11. Butter C, Auricchio A, Stellbrink C, et al: Pacing Therapy for Chronic Heart Failure II Study Group. Effect of resynchronization therapy stimulation site on the systolic function of heart failure patients. Circulation 104:3026–3029, 2001.

12. Hesse B, Diaz LA, Snader CE, et al: Complete bundle branch block as an independent predictor of all-cause mortality: Report of 7073 patients referred for nuclear exercise testing. Am J Med 110:253–259, 2001.

13. Garrigue S, Reuter S, Labeque J-N, et al: Usefulness of biventricular pacing in patients with congestive heart failure and right bundle branch block. Am J Cardiol 88:1436–1441, 2001.

14. Dubin AM, Feinstein JA, Reddy VM, et al: Electrical resynchronization: A novel therapy for the failing right ventricle. Circulation 107:2287–2289, 2003.

15. Grines CL, Bashore TM, Boudoulas H, et al: Functional abnormalities in isolated left bundle branch block. The effect of interventricular asynchrony. Circulation 79:845–853, 1989.

16. Liu L, Tockman B, Girouard S, et al: Left ventricular resynchronization therapy in a canine model of left bundle branch block. Am J Physiol Heart Circ Physiol 282:H2238–H2244, 2002.

17. Leclercq C, Faris O, Tunin R, et al: Systolic improvement and mechanical resynchronization does not require electrical synchrony in the dilated failing heart with left bundle-branch block. Circulation 106:1760–1763, 2002.

18. Auricchio A, Salo RW: Acute hemodynamic improvement by pacing in patients with severe congestive heart failure. Pacing Clin Electrophysiol 20:313–324, 1997.

19. Kerwin WF, Botvinick EH, O'Connell JW, et al: Ventricular contraction abnormalities in dilated cardiomyopathy: Effect of biventricular pacing to correct interventricular dyssynchrony. J Am Coll Cardiol 35:1221–1227, 2000.

20. Curry CW, Nelson GS, Wyman BT, et al: Mechanical dyssynchrony in dilated cardiomyopathy with intraventricular conduction delay as depicted by 3D tagged magnetic resonance imaging. Circulation 101:e2, 2000.

21. Breithardt OA, Stellbrink C, Kramer AP, et al: Echocardiographic quantification of left ventricular asynchrony predicts an acute hemodynamic benefit of cardiac resynchronization therapy. J Am Coll Cardiol 40:536–545, 2002.

22. Leclercq C, Kass DA: Retiming the failing heart: Principles and current clinical status of cardiac resynchronization. J Am Coll Cardiol 39:194–201, 2002.

23. Vernooy K, Verbeek XA, Peschar M, Prinzen FW: Relation between abnormal ventricular impulse conduction and heart failure. J Interv Cardiol 16:557–562, 2003.

24. Spragg DD, Leclercq C, Loghmani M, et al: Regional alterations in protein expression in the dyssynchronous failing heart. Circulation 108:929–932, 2003.

25. Bader H, Garrigue S, Lafitte S, et al: Intra-left ventricular electromechanical asynchrony. A new independent predictor of severe cardiac events in heart failure patients. J Am Coll Cardiol 43:248–256, 2004.

26. Cho G-Y, Park W-J, Han S-W, et al: Doppler tissue imaging assessment of dyssynchronicity is a powerful predictor of mortality in severe congestive heart failure with normal QRS duration [abstract]. J Am Coll Cardiol 43:361A, 2004.

27. Nelson GS, Berger RD, Fetics BJ, et al: Left ventricular or biventricular pacing improves cardiac function at diminished energy cost in patients with dilated cardiomyopathy and left bundle-branch block. Circulation 102:3053–3059, 2000.

28. Auricchio A, Ding J, Spinelli JC, et al: Cardiac resynchronization therapy restores optimal atrioventricular mechanical timing in heart failure patients with ventricular conduction delay. J Am Coll Cardiol 39:1163–1169, 2002.

29. Yu Y, Kramer A, Spinelli J, et al: Biventricular mechanical asynchrony predicts hemodynamic effect of uni- and biventricular pacing. Am J Physiol Heart Circ Physiol 285:H2788–H2796, 2003.

30. Peschar M, de Swart H, Michels KJ, et al: Left ventricular septal and apex pacing for optimal pump function in canine hearts. J Am Coll Cardiol 41:1218–1226, 2003.

31. Medina-Ravell VA, Lankipalli RS, Yan G-X, et al: Effect of epicardial or biventricular pacing to prolong QT interval and increase transmural dispersion of repolarization. Circulation 107:740–746, 2003.

32. Kass DA, Chen CH, Curry C, et al: Improved left ventricular mechanics from acute VDD pacing in patients with dilated cardiomyopathy and ventricular conduction delay. Circulation 99:1567–1573, 1999.

33. Auricchio A, Stellbrink C, Block M, et al: The effect of pacing chamber and atrioventricular delay on acute systolic function of paced patients with congestive heart failure. Circulation 99:2993–3001, 1999.

34. Auricchio A, Stellbrink C, Sack S, et al: Long-term clinical effect of hemodynamically optimized cardiac resynchronization therapy in patients with heart failure and ventricular conduction delay. J Am Coll Cardiol 39:2026–2033, 2002.

35. Touiza A, Etienne Y, Gilard M, et al: Long-term left ventricular pacing: Assessment and comparison with biventricular pacing in patients with severe congestive heart failure. J Am Coll Cardiol 38:1966–1970, 2001.

36. Verbeek XA, Vernooy K, Peschar M, et al: Intra-ventricular resynchronization for optimal left ventricular function during pacing in experimental left bundle branch block. J Am Coll Cardiol 42:558–567, 2003.

37. Faris OP, Evans FJ, Dick AJ, et al: Endocardial versus epicardial electrical synchrony during LV free-wall pacing. Am J Physiol Heart Circ Physiol 285:H1864–H1870, 2003.

38. Bradley DJ, Bradley EA, Baughman KL, et al: Cardiac resynchronization and death from progressive heart failure: A meta-analysis of randomized controlled trials. JAMA 289:730–740, 2003.

39. Auricchio A, Yu CM: Beyond the measurement of QRS complex toward mechanical dyssynchrony: Cardiac resynchronisa-

tion therapy in heart failure patients with a normal QRS duration. Heart 90:479–481, 2004.

40. Yu CM, Lin H, Zhang Q, Sanderson JE: High prevalence of left ventricular systolic and diastolic asynchrony in patients with congestive heart failure and normal QRS duration. Heart 89:54–60, 2003.

41. St John Sutton MG, Plappert T, Abraham WT, et al: Effect of cardiac resynchronization therapy on left ventricular size and function in chronic heart failure. Circulation 107:1985–1990, 2003.

42. Bristow MR, Saxon LA, Boehmer J, et al: Cardiac-resynchronization therapy with or without an implantable defibrillator in advanced chronic heart failure. N Engl J Med 350:2140–2150, 2004.

43. Moss AJ, Zareba W, Hall WJ, et al: Prophylactic implantation of a defibrillator in patients with myocardial infarction and reduced ejection fraction. N Engl J Med 346:877–883, 2002.

44. Grimm W, Alter P, Maisch B: Arrhythmia risk stratification with regard to prophylactic implantable defibrillator therapy in patients with dilated cardiomyopathy: Results of MACAS, DEFINITE, and SCD-HeFT. Herz 29:348–352, 2004.

45. Hamdan MH, Zagrodzky JD, Joglar JA, et al: Biventricular pacing decreases sympathetic activity compared with right ventricular pacing in patients with depressed ejection fraction. Circulation 102:1027–1032, 2000.

46. Higgins SL, Hummel JD, Niazi IK, et al: Cardiac resynchronization therapy for the treatment of heart failure in patients with intraventricular conduction delay and malignant ventricular tachyarrhythmias. J Am Coll Cardiol 42:1454–1459, 2003.

47. McSwain RL, Schwartz RA, deLurgio DB, et al: Cardiac resynchronization therapy does not increase the incidence of polymorphic ventricular tachycardia in patients with CHF [abstract]. Heart Rhythm 1(suppl):S60, 2004.

48. Goette A, Honeycutt C, Langberg JJ: Electrical remodeling in atrial fibrillation: Time course and mechanisms. Circulation 94:2968–2974, 1996.

49. Malinowski K: Spontaneous conversion of permanent atrial fibrillation into stable sinus rhythm after 17 months of biventricular pacing. Pacing Clin Electrophysiol 26:1554–1555, 2003.

Drugs Interacting with Mechano-Electric Feedback: Proarrhythmia, Remodeling, and Apoptosis

• • • •

Paulus Kirchhof and Günter Breithardt

THE TIME SCALE OF MECHANO-ELECTRIC FEEDBACK: A CONTINUUM

Although the term *mechano-electric feedback* (MEF) is most often used to describe the electrophysiologic effect of short stretches (milliseconds or seconds), the electrophysiologic and proarrhythmic alterations in response to chronically increased cardiac stretch are clinically more relevant. Chronic pressure overload (e.g., caused by untreated arterial hypertension or aortic stenosis) not only causes adaptational cardiac hypertrophy, but also several concurrent changes in cardiac electrophysiology: The cardiac action potential is prolonged, probably because of altered ionic currents, reduced intercellular coupling, and redistribution of gap junctional proteins, myocyte hypertrophy, or interstitial fibrosis.[1-4] Furthermore, intracellular calcium (Ca^{2+}) handling adapts in an attempt to maximize the contractile response to an action potential. To achieve these molecular adaptations to chronically increased stretch, the cell can reactivate fetal gene programs. In addition, proapoptotic signals are induced by mechanical stretch.[5] This effect occurs within minutes, indicating that there may be a continuum between acute and chronic forms of MEF, although they are mediated by different mechanisms ranging from activation of ion channels and altered regulation of proteins to contractile remodeling reflected by cellular hypertrophy and increased interstitial fibrosis (Fig. 39–1).

The electrophysiologic effects mediated by stretch-activated channels in response to acute MEF are partially opposed by those in response to chronic pressure overload—that is, shortening of the action potential versus prolongation of the action potential.[6] This chapter discusses the electrophysiologic consequences of cardiac adaptation to chronic stretch. These alterations are part of the adaptation to an increased cardiac workload—a longer action potential results in a longer contraction—but may predispose the heart to dangerous proarrhythmic effects of cardiac and noncardiac drugs. This chapter concludes with perspectives regarding how these electrophysiologic maladaptations may be prevented or treated pharmacologically.

Reduced Repolarizing Currents, Structural Remodeling, and Altered Intracellular Ca^{2+} Handling Facilitate Drug-Induced Arrhythmias

Electrophysiologic adaptations to chronic pressure overload prolong the cardiac action potential by reducing outward, repolarizing currents. An increased cell size, local fibrosis, and altered expression and function of gap junctions (i.e., connections that are responsible for the intercellular flow of current) decrease intercellular contacts. These changes accentuate regional differences in action potential duration and morphology and make the heart more susceptible to a specific form of polymorphic ventricular tachycardia called torsades de pointes.[7-9] Although torsades de pointes often are referred to as arrhythmias in patients with the inherited long QT syndrome, so-called acquired torsades de pointes are a rare but feared side effect of cardiovascular and other drugs that prolong the cardiac action potential, usually by reducing the rapidly activating

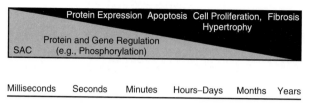

■ **Figure 39–1** Time dependence of different cellular and structural adaptational mechanisms caused by mechano-electric feedback depending on the duration of the mechanical stress. Acute stretch—milliseconds to seconds—activates stretch-activated channels (SAC; this topic is discussed throughout this textbook). When the stretch persists for several seconds, regulatory cellular processes such as protein phosphorylation and gene expression are altered. This affects protein expression and thereby cellular function. When an increased stretch persists for seconds to minutes, proapoptotic signaling pathways are activated, resulting in increased cardiomyocyte apoptosis. Even longer periods of mechanical stimulation cause, among other structural adaptational processes, cellular hypertrophy, increased interstitial fibrosis, and decreased intercellular coupling.

component of the delayed rectifier potassium current, I_{Kr}.[9,10] (Updated lists of drugs that may induce proarrhythmic effects are available at the University of Arizona Health Sciences Center Web site: www.torsades.org.)

Genetic Factors and Chronic Stretch Reduce the Repolarization Reserve

Proarrhythmia caused by action potential–prolonging drugs is a "patient-specific" effect—that is, there is an individual predisposition to drug-induced proarrhythmia.[11] Genetic factors—for example, mutations or polymorphisms in the genes coding for repolarizing currents,[12] alterations in genes coding for proteins involved in drug metabolism, or gender—may predispose an individual patient to proarrhythmia. The majority of patients never experience arrhythmias, despite the presence of reduced repolarization reserve, cardiac hypertrophy, and fibrosis.[9,11] The adaptational process that results from chronically increased mechanical stress provokes similar functional changes—that is, reduced net repolarizing currents.[13] The final outcome of these genetically determined or adaptational changes is a so-called reduced repolarization reserve.[14] Such a reduced repolarization reserve can be clinically assessed as an abnormal prolongation of the QT interval when patients with acquired torsades de pointes are challenged with potassium channel blockers.[15] An episode of drug-induced torsades de pointes may be initiated with transient factors such as bradycardia[16] or hypokalemia.

Structural Alterations in Response to Chronic Stretch

The chronic adaptive response to increased pressure also has structural consequences, including increased cell size, altered expression and function of gap junctions, and reduced intercellular coupling via interstitial fibrosis. These microstructural changes accentuate regional differences in activation and repolarization, which are measurable as increased anisotropy of conduction and regional dispersion of ventricular repolarization.[17] Increased heterogeneity of repolarization increases the susceptibility to ventricular arrhythmias in response to ectopy during the vulnerable period,[18] whereas anisotropic conduction can cause wave break and functional re-entry.[19,20]

Altered Ca²⁺ Handling in Response to Chronic Stretch

Intracellular Ca^{2+} handling also is altered in the hypertrophied heart, probably as a response to the chronically increased workload of each cardiac cell. Models of hypertrophy often show increased Ca^{2+} transients but normal diastolic Ca^{2+}.[3,21,22] This adaptational process leads, among other translational and regulatory mechanisms, to an increased expression and activity of calmodulin-dependent protein kinase II (CaMKII).[3,23,24]

This increased expression facilitates Ca^{2+} influx into the cell and Ca^{2+}-induced Ca^{2+} release from the sarcoplasmic reticulum, subsequently causing triggered activity and afterdepolarizations.[3,23,25] Figure 39–2

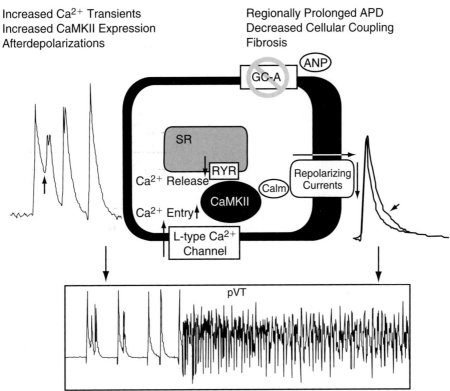

Figure 39–2 Electrophysiologic consequences and molecular mechanisms of chronic volume and pressure overload in a mouse model of deletion of the atrial natriuretic peptide (ANP) receptor guanylyl cyclase A (GC-A).[3] The net repolarizing current of the cardiac action potential is reduced, as reflected by prolonged ventricular action potential duration (APD). Cardiac hypertrophy, increased cell size, increased interstitial fibrosis, and the preponderance of the stretch signal in the left ventricle increase regional inhomogeneity of APD. Focal cardiac fibrosis also forms potential re-entrant circuits. These processes create a substrate for functional re-entry (right side of scheme). In addition, Ca^{2+} transient amplitude is increased, and expression levels of Ca^{2+}-calmodulin-dependent protein kinase II (CaMKII) are increased. These changes are triggers for afterdepolarizations and the occurrence of polymorphic ventricular tachycardias (pVT; left side of scheme and bottom). The combination of this CaMKII-dependent trigger for arrhythmias and a functional substrate for re-entry allows for spontaneous occurrence of pVT with bradycardia. In this model, pharmacologic blockade of CaMKII suppresses ventricular arrhythmias. Similar mechanisms of arrhythmias were identified in models with increased expression of CaMKII and CaMKIV.[23] RYR, ryanodine receptor; SR, sarcoplasmic reticulum; Calm, calmodulin. (See color insert.)

summarizes these changes. When combined in the hypertrophied heart, these adaptive changes form a substrate for functional re-entry and may provide a trigger for ventricular tachycardias. In fact, extreme ventricular hypertrophy in response to chronic arterial hypertension and hypervolemia,[3] or in response to heart-directed expression of CaMKIV,[23] is sufficient to provoke polymorphic ventricular tachycardias when combined with bradycardia, similar to the combination of bradycardia and a mutated *SCN5A* channel

that causes long QT syndrome.[16] Interestingly, either direct blockade of CaMKII or prevention of activation of CaMKII by Ca^{2+}-channel blockade is sufficient to prevent such arrhythmias,[3] similar to the effect of CaMKII blockade in preventing drug-induced torsades de pointes.[26,27] These data can explain the clinical observation that the combination of the action potential–prolonging drug quinidine with the Ca^{2+} channel blocker verapamil leads to a low incidence of drug-induced proarrhythmia.[28]

Stretch-Induced Apoptosis: Mechano-Electric Feedback of a Different Sort?

Apoptosis, or programmed cell death, describes a specific form of histologically "traceless" cell death that was first characterized by lack of inflammation.[29] Apoptosis is part of the normal prenatal and postnatal development of the heart,[30] but it also occurs under abnormal conditions.[31,32] More specifically, apoptosis is increased in response to chronically increased left ventricular pressure (e.g., in hypertensive cardiomyopathy).[33] In addition to chronically increased stretch, short increases in left ventricular pressure and volume reversibly activate proapoptotic signaling pathways (see Fig. 4 in Reference 5), and relief from chronic pressure overload by a left ventricular assist device reverses activation of proapoptotic signaling pathways.[5] In response to long-lasting stretch signals, apoptosis may be induced by mitogen-activated protein kinases/externally regulated kinases,[5] by activation of calcineurin,[34] or by intracellular Ca^{2+} overload (e.g., provoked by a decreased function of the cardiac Na^+-Ca^{2+} exchanger).[35] Hence, activation of apoptotic cell death not only is a consequence of long-term increased tension and pressure, but it also mediates some of the cellular responses that occur within minutes after the onset of increased stretch.

Apoptosis is increased in several arrhythmogenic diseases including atrial fibrillation[36] and arrhythmogenic right ventricular cardiomyopathy.[37] Proarrhythmic effects of increased apoptosis may include reduced intercellular coupling and formation of microreentrant circuits around islets of apoptotic cells. There is indirect evidence that increased apoptosis contributes to the maintenance ("domestication") of atrial fibrillation.[38] If confirmed in dedicated studies examining its electrophysiologic consequences, stretch-induced apoptosis may contribute to the formation of an arrhythmogenic substrate in response to stretch.

Drugs Can Prevent Acute and Chronic Adaptation to Cardiac Stretch

A tarantula-derived peptide that blocks stretch-activated channels can prevent atrial fibrillation induced by acute stretch[39] (see Chapter 42). Chronic treatment with verapamil appears to prevent drug-induced proarrhythmia,[28] probably by preventing Ca^{2+}-mediated activation of CaMKII[3,23] and subsequent suppression of afterdepolarizations, the trigger for drug-induced torsades de pointes.

Long-term pharmacologic inhibition of the angiotensinogen-angiotensin system, conversely, can partially prevent the adaptive cardiac response to chronically increased cardiac load in experimental models of heart failure[40,41] and in clinical studies.[42,43] Interestingly, these antihypertrophic effects may translate into antiarrhythmic effects: angiotensin-converting enzyme (ACE) inhibitors partially prevent structural remodeling in atrial fibrillation,[38] and pharmacologic blockade of ACE reduces the incidence of atrial fibrillation in patients with structural heart disease[44,45] and reduces atrial fibrosis in experimental heart failure.[46]

Preventing the hypertrophic response to increased workload also could be the key to understanding why drugs that block the renin-angiotensin-aldosterone system—for example, angiotensin receptor blockers[47] (see Chapter 7) or aldosterone antagonists[48,49]—prevent sudden death in clinical trials. In addition to interfering with the renin-angiotensin-aldosterone system, aldosterone antagonists may prevent hypokalemia known to trigger torsades-like arrhythmias. These hypotheses require experimental and clinical validation. Table 39–1 summarizes these effects.

Conclusion: Take-Home Messages

Drugs can aggravate stretch-induced proarrhythmic effects and prevent the electrophysiological changes associated with acute or chronic stretch. Altered intracellular Ca^{2+} handling, reduced repolarization reserve, induction of cardiac myocyte apoptosis, and stimulation of hypertrophic cell growth all combine to form a substrate for functional re-entry in a heart challenged with long-lasting stretch stimuli. In addition, altered Ca^{2+} handling, specifically an increased activation of cytoplasmic CaMKII, provokes afterdepolarizations and triggers ventricular arrhythmias in the hypertrophied heart. These adaptations to long-lasting stretch have maladaptational electrophysiologic consequences that appear to contribute to drug-

TABLE 39–1   **Arrhythmogenic Responses to Chronic Stretch and Pharmacological Interventions Aimed at Their Treatment**

Factors		Interventions
Inherited Predisposition		
Genetic predisposition	Gender, *formes frustes* of LQTS (i.e., LQTS-causing mutations without obvious phenotype), altered drug metabolism	—
Substrate Modification		
Reduced repolarization reserve	Reduced ion channel expression and function	Avoidance of action potential–prolonging drugs
Structural remodeling	Increased cardiomyocyte apoptosis, cellular hypertrophy, increased interstitial fibrosis, decreased intercellular coupling, increased heart size	Antihypertensive agents (?); ACE inhibitors/angiotensin receptor blockers; aldosterone blockers
Triggers		
Altered Ca^{2+} handling	Increased L-type Ca^{2+} channel activity, increased CaMKII activity, increased Ca^{2+} release from the SR increased Ca^{2+} load of the SR, increased Ca^{2+} leak from the SR	Verapamil; CaMKII inhibitors (not yet clinically available); prevention of bradycardia (?)

ACE, angiotensin-converting enzyme; CAMKII, calmodulin-dependent protein kinase II; LQTS, long QT syndrome; SR, sarcoplasmic reticulum.

induced proarrhythmia, sudden cardiac death and atrial fibrillation.

Pharmacologic blockade of the renin-angiotensin-aldosterone system reduces remodeling and hypertrophy, thereby reducing arrhythmogenic consequences in response to chronic stretch in the ventricle and the atrium. Pharmacologic blockade of the L-type Ca^{2+} channel (e.g., by verapamil) prevents activation of CaMKII, and thereby may eliminate the trigger for drug-induced proarrhythmia.[28]

Understanding the interactions among genetic predispositions to arrhythmias; the arrhythmogenic substrate that forms in response to chronic stretch stimuli; the triggering events; and, potentially, the dangerous effects of acute stretch stimuli in hearts already exposed to chronic stretch is a task of future studies.

References

1. Cerbai E, Barbieri M, Li Q, Mugelli A: Ionic basis of action potential prolongation of hypertrophied cardiac myocytes isolated from hypertensive rats of different ages. Cardiovasc Res 28:1180–1187, 1994.
2. Spach MS, Heidlage JF, Dolber PC, Barr RC: Electrophysiological effects of remodeling cardiac gap junctions and cell size: Experimental and model studies of normal cardiac growth. Circ Res 86:302–311, 2000.
3. Kirchhof P, Fabritz L, Begrow F, et al: Ventricular arrhythmias, increased cardiac calmodulin kinase II expression, and altered repolarization kinetics in ANP-receptor deficient mice. J Mol Cell Cardiol 36:691–700, 2004.
4. Zhuang J, Yamada KA, Saffitz JE, Kleber AG: Pulsatile stretch remodels cell-to-cell communication in cultured myocytes. Circ Res 87:316–322, 2000.
5. Baba H, Stypmann J, Grabellus F, et al: Dynamic regulation of MEK/Erks and Akt/GSK-3β in human end-stage heart failure after left ventricular mechanical support: Myocardial mechanotransduction-sensitivity as a possible molecular mechanism. Cardiovasc Res 59:390–399, 2003.
6. Guo W, Kamiya K, Yasui K, et al: Paracrine hypertrophic factors from cardiac non-myocyte cells downregulate the transient outward current density and Kv4.2 K+ channel expression in cultured rat cardiomyocytes. Cardiovasc Res 41:157–165, 1999.
7. Dessertenne F: La tachycardie ventriculaire à deux foyers opposés variables [Ventricular tachycardia with 2 variable opposing foci]. Arch Mal Coeur 59:263–272, 1966.
8. Vos MA, Verduyn SC, Gorgels AP, et al: Reproducible induction of early afterdepolarizations and torsade de pointes arrhythmias by d-sotalol and pacing in dogs with chronic atrioventricular block. Circulation 91:864–872, 1995.
9. Haverkamp W, Breithardt G, Camm AJ, et al: The potential for QT prolongation and proarrhythmia by non-antiarrhythmic drugs: Clinical and regulatory implications. Report on a policy conference of the European Society of Cardiology. Eur Heart J 21:1216–1231, 2000.

10. Redfern WS, Carlsson L, Davis AS, et al: Relationships between preclinical cardiac electrophysiology, clinical QT interval prolongation and torsade de pointes for a broad range of drugs: Evidence for a provisional safety margin in drug development. Cardiovasc Res 58:32–45, 2003.

11. Haverkamp W, Mönnig G, Schulze-Bahr E, et al: Physician-induced torsade de pointes—therapeutic implications. Cardiovasc Drugs Ther 16:101–109, 2002.

12. Paulussen AD, Gilissen RA, Armstrong M, et al: Genetic variations of KCNQ1, KCNH2, SCN5A, KCNE1, and KCNE2 in drug-induced long QT syndrome patients. J Mol Med 82:182–188, 2004.

13. Swynghedauw B, Chevalier B, Charlemagne D, et al: Cardiac hypertrophy, arrhythmogenicity and the new myocardial phenotype. II. The cellular adaptational process. Cardiovasc Res 35:6–12, 1997.

14. Roden DM: Mechanisms and management of proarrhythmia. Am J Cardiol 82:49I–57I, 1998.

15. Kääb S, Hinterseer M, Näbauer M, Steinbeck G: Sotalol testing unmasks altered repolarization in patients with suspected acquired long-QT-syndrome: A case-control pilot study using i.v. sotalol. Eur Heart J 24:649–657, 2003.

16. Fabritz L, Kirchhof P, Franz MR, et al: Effect of pacing and mexiletine on dispersion of repolarisation and arrhythmias in hearts of SCN5A ð-KPQ (LQT3) mice. Cardiovasc Res 57:1085–1093, 2003.

17. Spach MS, Josephson ME: Initiating reentry: The role of nonuniform anisotropy in small circuits. J Cardiovasc Electrophysiol 5:182–209, 1994.

18. Kirchhof P, Fabritz L, Zabel M, Franz MR: The vulnerable period for low and high energy T wave shocks: Role of dispersion of repolarisation and effect of d-sotalol. Cardiovasc Res 31:953–962, 1996.

19. van Rijen HV, Eckardt D, Degen J, et al: Slow conduction and enhanced anisotropy increase the propensity for ventricular tachyarrhythmias in adult mice with induced deletion of connexin43. Circulation 109:1048–1055, 2004.

20. Derksen R, van Rijen HV, Wilders R, et al: Tissue discontinuities affect conduction velocity restitution: A mechanism by which structural barriers may promote wave break. Circulation 108:882–888, 2003.

21. Sipido KR, Volders PG, de Groot SH, et al: Enhanced Ca^{2+} release and Na/Ca exchange activity in hypertrophied canine ventricular myocytes: Potential link between contractile adaptation and arrhythmogenesis. Circulation 102:2137–2144, 2000.

22. Shorofsky SR, Aggarwal R, Corretti M, et al: Cellular mechanisms of altered contractility in the hypertrophied heart: Big hearts, big sparks. Circ Res 84:424–434, 1999.

23. Wu Y, Temple J, Zhang R, et al: Calmodulin kinase II and arrhythmias in a mouse model of cardiac hypertrophy. Circulation 106:1288–1293, 2002.

24. Zhang T, Maier LS, Dalton ND, et al: The δC isoform of CaMKII is activated in cardiac hypertrophy and induces dilated cardiomyopathy and heart failure. Circ Res 92:912–919, 2003.

25. Maier LS, Zhang T, Chen L, et al: Transgenic CaMKIIδC overexpression uniquely alters cardiac myocyte Ca^{2+} handling: Reduced SR Ca^{2+} load and activated SR Ca^{2+} release. Circ Res 92:904–911, 2003.

26. Mazur A, Roden DM, Anderson ME: Systemic administration of calmodulin antagonist W-7 or protein kinase A inhibitor H-8 prevents torsade de pointes in rabbits. Circulation 100:2437–2442, 1999.

27. Anderson ME, Braun AP, Wu Y, et al: KN-93, an inhibitor of multifunctional Ca^{++}/calmodulin-dependent protein kinase, decreases early afterdepolarizations in rabbit heart. J Pharmacol Exp Ther 287:996–1006, 1998.

28. Fetsch T, Bauer P, Engberding R, et al: Prevention of atrial fibrillation after cardioversion: Results of the PAFAC trial. Eur Heart J 25:1385–1394, 2004.

29. Kerr J, Wyllie A, Currie A: Apoptosis: A basic biological phenomenon with wide ranging implications in tissue kinetics. Br J Cancer 26:239–257, 1972.

30. James TN: Normal and abnormal consequences of apoptosis in the human heart. Annu Rev Physiol 60:309–325, 1998.

31. Narula J, Haider N, Virmani R, et al: Apoptosis in myocytes in end-stage heart failure. N Engl J Med 335:1182–1189, 1996.

32. Pacifico A, Henry PD: Structural pathways and prevention of heart failure and sudden death. J Cardiovasc Electrophysiol 14:764–775, 2003.

33. Gonzalez A, Fortuno MA, Querejeta R, et al: Cardiomyocyte apoptosis in hypertensive cardiomyopathy. Cardiovasc Res 59:549–562, 2003.

34. Wang Z, Kutschke W, Richardson KE, et al: Electrical remodeling in pressure-overload cardiac hypertrophy: Role of calcineurin. Circulation 104:1657–1663, 2001.

35. Wakimoto K, Kobayashi K, Kuro OM, et al: Targeted disruption of Na^+/Ca^{2+} exchanger gene leads to cardiomyocyte apoptosis and defects in heartbeat. J Biol Chem 275:36991–36998, 2000.

36. Aime-Sempe C, Folliguet T, Rucker-Martin C, et al: Myocardial cell death in fibrillating and dilated human right atria. J Am Coll Cardiol 34:1577–1586, 1999.

37. Mallat Z, Tedgui A, Fontaliran F, et al: Evidence of apoptosis in arrhythmogenic right ventricular dysplasia. N Engl J Med 335:1190–1196, 1996.

38. Cardin S, Li D, Thorin-Trescases N, et al: Evolution of the atrial fibrillation substrate in experimental congestive heart failure: Angiotensin-dependent and -independent pathways. Cardiovasc Res 60:315–325, 2003.

39. Bode F, Sachs F, Franz M: Tarantula peptide inhibits atrial fibrillation. Nature 409:6818–6819, 2001.

40. Rials SJ, Wu Y, Xu X, et al: Regression of left ventricular hypertrophy with captopril restores normal ventricular action potential duration, dispersion of refractoriness, and vulnerability to inducible ventricular fibrillation. Circulation 96:1330–1336, 1997.

41. Cerbai E, Crucitti A, Sartiani L, et al: Long-term treatment of spontaneously hypertensive rats with losartan and electrophysiological remodeling of cardiac myocytes. Cardiovasc Res 45:388–396, 2000.

42. Pfeffer MA, McMurray JJ, Velazquez EJ, et al: Valsartan, captopril, or both in myocardial infarction complicated by heart failure, left ventricular dysfunction, or both. N Engl J Med 349:1893–1906, 2003.

43. McMurray JJ, Ostergren J, Swedberg K, et al: Effects of candesartan in patients with chronic heart failure and reduced left-ventricular systolic function taking angiotensin-converting-enzyme inhibitors: The CHARM-Added trial. Lancet 362:767–771, 2003.

44. Vermes E, Tardif JC, Bourassa MG, et al: Enalapril decreases the incidence of atrial fibrillation in patients with left ventricular dysfunction: Insight from the Studies Of Left Ventricular Dysfunction (SOLVD) trials. Circulation 107:2926–2931, 2003.

45. Pedersen OD, Bagger H, Kober L, Torp-Pedersen C: Trandolapril reduces the incidence of atrial fibrillation after

acute myocardial infarction in patients with left ventricular dysfunction. Circulation 100:376–380, 1999.

46. Li D, Shinagawa K, Pang L, et al: Effects of angiotensin-converting enzyme inhibition on the development of the atrial fibrillation substrate in dogs with ventricular tachypacing-induced congestive heart failure. Circulation 104:2608–2614, 2001.

47. Lindholm LH, Dahlof B, Edelman JM, et al: Effect of losartan on sudden cardiac death in people with diabetes: Data from the LIFE study. Lancet 362:619–620, 2003.

48. Pitt B, Remme W, Zannad F, et al: Eplerenone, a selective aldosterone blocker, in patients with left ventricular dysfunction after myocardial infarction. N Engl J Med 348:1309–1321, 2003.

49. Pitt B, Zannad F, Remme WJ, et al: The effect of spironolactone on morbidity and mortality in patients with severe heart failure. Randomized Aldactone Evaluation Study Investigators. N Engl J Med 341:709–717, 1999.

Evolving Concepts in Measuring Ventricular Strain in the Human Heart

• • • •

Elliot McVeigh

IMPROVEMENTS IN MAGNETIC RESONANCE IMAGING TECHNIQUES AND HARDWARE

Magnetic resonance imaging (MRI) is capable of measuring the motion of myocardium principally because the tissue can be marked and tracked over time. The markers can either be a pattern of saturated magnetization or a pattern of encoded signal phase; both of these patterns can be applied to the entire myocardium in a few milliseconds. Imaging the deformation of the patterns can be performed with a variety of standard methods. The increased imaging gradient switching rates currently available on commercial MRI scanners have led to a dramatic increase in the efficiency of data acquisition, yielding cardiac movies with high temporal resolution and short imaging times.[1] Also, techniques for field-of-view reduction, or zooming into the region around the heart alone, have decreased data acquisition times by factors of two to four; these techniques have been captured under the rubric of image acceleration techniques.[2-4]

These improvements have enabled real-time image acquisitions at up to 30 frames per second for image voxel sizes of $2 \times 2 \times 8$ mm. Also, if approximately 10 repeated heartbeats are identical and can be used to accumulate data, movies derived from these composite data can have more than 200 frames per second. If greater spatial resolution is required, data accumulation over repeated heartbeats can be used to push that limit to a resolution representing the reproducibility of the position of the heart from beat to beat.

Traditional gating strategies for acquiring cardiac data in phase with the electrocardiogram are becoming complemented with wireless gating strategies in which properties of the raw data are measured to infer both the cardiac and respiratory phases at the moment of data acquisition.[5] These techniques are currently viable because the data can be acquired at a rate that is great enough to support partial image reconstruction with sufficient quality to evaluate at what point in the cardiac/respiratory cycle the data were obtained. This is a topic of active research, and important developments likely will be seen during the next 5 years.

MOTION-ENCODING STRATEGIES

This chapter examines two principal types of motion encoding: myocardial tagging and pulsed field gradient methods. Myocardial tagging methods modulate the grayscale value of image pixels in a predetermined pattern (such as a set of parallel sheets), and the deformation of the pattern is imaged through time.[6] In pulsed field gradient methods, the position of the magnetization is instantaneously "marked" by inducing the position-dependent phase with a short gradient pulse. At a later time, a gradient pulse with the opposite polarity is used to refocus the magnetization; however, if tissue has moved in the time between these two gradient pulses, there will be a residual phase on the magnetization that is proportional to the displacement.

MYOCARDIAL TAGGING

Cardiac tagging uses a simple principle. A saturation pattern is placed in the imaging volume, and the volume is imaged after some time delay; *the change in shape of the saturation pattern in the image reflects the change in shape of the underlying body containing the saturation pattern.*[6,7] The principle of "tagging" spins was first proposed by Morse and Singer[8] to measure bulk blood flow. It was demonstrated by Zerhouni and colleagues[9] that the same principle could be used to visually mark tissue with tagged magnetization to measure the more complex deformations of the heart. Axel and Dougherty[10,11] subsequently proposed an efficient scheme for generating parallel planes of saturation throughout the entire imaging volume. Many investigators have proposed refinements and extensions of these methods for generating more complex saturation patterns in both two- (2D) and three-dimensional (3D) images,[12–22] and recently tagging has been coupled with rapid echo-train imaging[23,24] and steady-state free precession imaging.[25,26] High-resolution imaging of tagging grids also has been achieved with projection reconstruction imaging methods.[27–29]

In the last few years, developments have continued in tagging methods. The following section examines the extremes in spatial and temporal resolution that have been achieved.

High Temporal and Spatial Resolution Tagged Magnetic Resonance Imaging

A straightforward method for acquiring high-resolution MR images is to apply the 3D Fourier encoding technique. In this method, slice-selective pulses are not used to isolate a thin imaging slice; phase encoding is used in the slice selection direction. This 3D Fourier acquisition results in thin slices, but it requires an extended imaging time to obtain all the necessary data; hence, a cardiac- and respiratory-gated acquisition must be used. The spacing between tag sheets can be dramatically reduced with the thinner slices obtained with 3D imaging, because the adjacent tag sheets will not blur together during times of high through-slice shear strain. Ennis and colleagues[30] have invoked cardiac/respiratory gating and reduced data acquisition techniques[31] to obtain 3D volumes of tagged myocardium with 8-msec time resolution and 0.5- × 1.4- × 5-mm voxels over the entire heart. The

high-resolution direction is oriented perpendicular to the parallel tag sheets so that the detection of the tag position is most accurate.[6] The tag sheets may be placed close together giving up to five tags across the heart wall (Fig. 40–1). These data sets contain approximately 1500 individual tag intersections in short-axis images for tracking tissue motion throughout the myocardium. The drawback of this imaging mode is the long total acquisition time; therefore, the motions measured must be reproducible from beat to beat over 0.5 to 2 hours. This condition can be achieved in a healthy, ventilated, paced animal. Wireless gating techniques are being developed so that high-resolution imaging techniques can be used in free breathing, nonpaced subjects.

Image Analysis for Tagged Magnetic Resonance Imaging

Direct viewing of movies obtained with tag patterns provides an excellent method for evaluating myocardial function and the relative timing of the onset of local shortening and relaxation. However, if quantitative measurements of myocardial strain over the entire myocardium are required, the myocardium must be segmented and the position of the tag sheets estimated.[32–36] This image analysis task has undergone continuous development over the past decade; however, it remains *the* rate-limiting step in using myocardial tagging for quantitative analysis. In the early development of myocardial tagging, a full study consisted of approximately 200 images to be segmented; currently, with high-resolution in the time and spatial dimension, up to 5000 images need to be segmented. Therefore, depending on the number of images acquired, the tag detection can take many hours or even days of analysis time. For the large studies, this can be politely described as exasperating for the user. Although some early work for directly calculating the motion field from the grayscale tagged images has been reported,[37] the problem of tag detection has been a major motivation for investigators to move to techniques that do not require image segmentation for quantitative analysis (such as the methods described in Pulsed Field Gradient Methods).

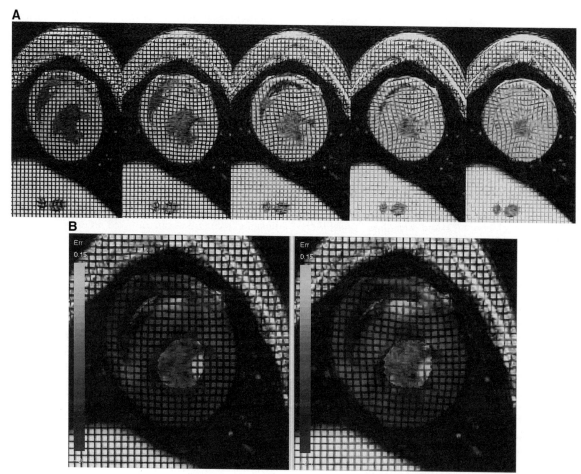

■ **Figure 40–1** *A*, An example of high temporal and spatial resolution tagging achieved with cardiac- and respiratory-gated, three-dimensional, tagged magnetic resonance imaging. This panel shows five time frames selected from a 55-frame movie; each frame is separated by 56 msec. Note the high number of tags across the heart wall. *B*, Two time frames of systolic contraction in a paced canine heart. The calibration bar represents the amount of radial thickening at each location computed from the tag deformation; light gray represents 15% thickening (top of the calibration bar), and dark gray represents 15% thinning (bottom of the calibration bar). The *left panel* is at the first onset of contraction; the *right panel* is 40 msec later. Note the transmural gradient thickening observed in the anterior septum (12 o'clock position in the left ventricle). This early contraction is likely from an activation that escaped from the paced atrium into the septum. (See color insert for B.) *(Data provided by Dan Ennis, National Heart Lung and Blood Institute.)*

Strain Computation from Tagged Magnetic Resonance Imaging

In a tagged MRI movie sequence, a single slice in space is imaged at different time intervals after the application of the tagging pattern. The heart moves in and out of this single slice over the heart cycle; therefore, interpolation must be used to calculate the trajectory of a single position on the myocardium from multiple tagged images that sample that region over the heart cycle. The nature of the interpolation (both through space and time) is the distinction between the different methods used for motion tracking.[38-40] Once the displacement field has been computed in a Lagrangian coordinate system (i.e., a coordinate system attached to the heart), then the strain of the myocardium can be obtained by computing spatial derivatives of the displacement field. A comparison of four techniques undertaken by Declerck and colleagues[41] showed that a 4D B-spline[42,43] model of the myocardial displacement field seemed to be the best overall method for computing the strain field.

PULSED FIELD GRADIENT METHODS

Harmonic Phase Imaging Methods

In the harmonic phase (HARP) imaging method,[44] a simple sinusoidal tagging pattern is applied to the myocardium. These tags are provided by the method called SPAtial Modulation of Magnetization, or SPAMM.[10] If the image is reconstructed with raw data that are centered around the frequency of this sinusoid in Fourier space, the magnitude image will be a low-resolution estimate of the amount of signal in the sinusoidal pattern. The phase of the image will show a banding pattern that deforms with myocardial motion. Relative motion between movie frames of HARP images can be computed from the phase differences between those frames; hence, *motion can be measured without detecting the position of the underlying tags*. The drawback is that the image is a relatively low-resolution representation of the deformation field because a small window of the raw data was used to reconstruct the HARP images. However, that a small region of the raw

data is acquired means that the imaging can be performed rapidly.[45] The same encoding principle can be used to measure longitudinal strain while imaging in the short-axis plane.[46]

Displacement Encoding Using Stimulated Echoes

Displacement Encoding using Stimulated Echoes (DENSE) imaging techniques[47] use the phase of image pixels to encode the net displacement of a piece of tissue over time. Transverse magnetization is position encoded by a short gradient pulse, stored as longitudinal magnetization during the "mixing time" (denoted TM), and then refocused before image data acquisition by an unencoding gradient pulse. The unencoding gradient pulse causes the transverse magnetization to refocus at a phase angle that is linearly proportional to the displacement that occurred during the mixing time. Unfortunately, only half of the original transverse magnetization is recovered. However, *the DENSE image has displacement estimates on the same spatial scale as the image pixel grid, and those displacement estimates do not require image segmentation.* Figure 40–2 shows an example of the high-resolution estimates of myocardial displacement that are achieved with DENSE. These properties make DENSE an attractive method for quantitative estimates of strain

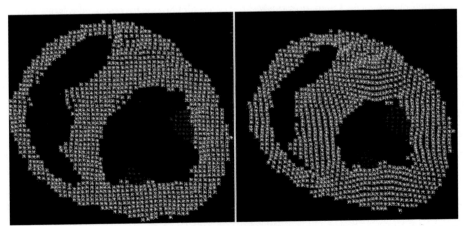

■ **Figure 40–2** Two frames from a displacement encoding using stimulated echoes (DENSE) acquisition of a canine heart from the onset of shortening to mid-systole. Note the number of displacement estimates yielding excellent data for strain in the left and right ventricular walls. Transmural patterns of the myocardial strain can be mapped with this technique. *(Data courtesy Han Wen, National Heart Lung and Blood Institute.)*

and displacement. Direct visualization of the myocardial deformation is not available, but it can be achieved by driving the motion of synthetic tags on the heart with the underlying measured displacement measurements. A number of variants of the DENSE technique have been developed to increase the signal-to-noise ratio of the displacement estimates.[48,49] One drawback of DENSE is that it is a phase-based technique. There are many causes of phase errors in imaging pixels around the heart, such as magnetic field inhomogeneities, chemical shift (frequency shifts in the resonance of different chemical species), motion of the blood, and motion during breathing. Unfortunately, when the value of the phase of a pixel *is* the motion estimate, that estimate is susceptible to error from these many sources.

Clinical Applications of Myocardial Tagging

All of the methods described previously in this chapter are immediately available for clinical use in humans because MRI is widely available and carries virtually no risks. Myocardial tags can be used to create a visual appreciation of local wall motion and strain, making it easier for the physician to detect asynchronous or hypokinetic function in ischemic tissue. These methods currently are not used frequently because MRI scanners are not widely available for cardiologists to obtain data for their patients. As stated previously, a major impediment to the widespread use of these techniques for quantitative estimates of motion and strain in the clinic is the large effort required to segment the heart wall borders and the tagging pattern.

SIMULTANEOUS MEASUREMENT OF STRAIN AND ELECTRICAL ACTIVATION

To evaluate the relation between electrical excitation and the onset of mechanical contraction, MR tagging experiments have been performed during ectopic pacing in anesthetized healthy dogs.[50–52] When systolic contraction was evoked by right atrial pacing, the left ventricle was excited through the normal pathway of the Purkinje system, and the pattern of mechanical activation was found to be uniform as a function of position. However, when the heart was paced from a ventricular site, significant asynchronous and spatially heterogeneous contraction was observed, reflecting the underlying delays in electrical activation. More recently, a 128- or 256-epicardial electrode sock array was used to obtain electrical maps immediately before and after myocardial tagging studies were performed, and the two data sets registered using external markers on the sock array.[53] Surprisingly, the tagged MR images were of good quality when obtained with the epicardial sock in place. This experimental setup now gives us the ability to study the relation of the temporal kinetics of the electrical and mechanical function during myocardial contraction and relaxation in vivo, as shown by the results in Figure 40–3. High-resolution, coregistered, fiber angle maps in the same heart also will allow for the investigation of the underlying architectural substrate of this function.[54]

Experimental preparations can be used to obtain an underlying model for the relation between mechanical state and the electrical behavior of the myocardium. Many outstanding questions about mechano-electric feedback can be addressed. For example, as discussed in Chapter 20, it has been observed that the U wave timing appears to depend on mechanical events. When the relation between the end of T wave and the second heart sound undergoes a change, the U wave follows the second heart sound and not the T wave.[55] The precise temporal relation can be measured between the inscription of the U wave and the onset of stretching during relaxation in the circular layers of the ventricular myocardium and endocardial components of the heart. It is assumed that the endocardial components stretch after the circular layers; this assumption now can be experimentally validated.

In models of myocardial infarction, the mechanical prestretch around the infarct can be measured accurately, and any correlation between that mechanical abnormality and the propensity for focal ectopy and stable re-entry can be mapped. The ability of MRI to produce high-contrast, high-resolution, 3D images of the morphology of the infarct, in addition to the spatially registered strain maps, makes it the preferred method for studying the behavior of the infarcted heart.[56]

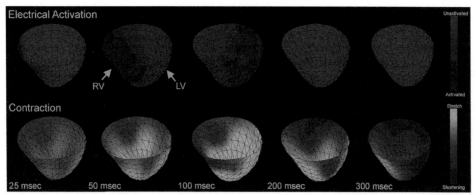

■ Figure 40-3 An example of coregistered mechanical contraction data and electrical activation data obtained from myocardial tagging and a 128-electrode sock array in a canine heart with left bundle branch block. The surface on which the gray levels are rendered represents the epicardial surface of the left (LV) and right (RV) ventricles. The dark gray area in the electrical activation data (top) shows the locus of points on the surface that have been activated after RV pacing. The bright gray region in the mechanical map of circumferential strain (bottom) shows a prestretch of the LV free wall at 100 msec, followed by contraction (dark gray). (See color insert.)

Summary

Although myocardial strain gives an incomplete picture of the forces developed during contraction of the heart, currently it is the most significant parameter that can be measured noninvasively over the entire heart when investigating local phenomena. Ideally, further research will yield methods for extracting fundamental parameters, such as the time of onset of local contraction and relaxation, and these parameters will be used in individual patients to estimate the risk for lethal events, guide interventions, and monitor recovery after therapy.

References

1. Reeder SB, McVeigh ER: The effect of high speed gradients on fast gradient echo imaging. Magn Reson Med 32:612–621, 1994.
2. Madore B, Glover GH, Pelc NJ: Unaliasing by Fourier-encoding the overlaps using the temporal dimension (UNFOLD) applied to cardiac imaging and fMRI. Magn Reson Med 42:813–828, 1999.
3. Pruessmann KP, Weiger M, Scheidegger MB, Boesiger P: SENSE: Sensitivity encoding for fast MRI. Magn Reson Med 42:952–962, 1999.
4. Kellman P, McVeigh ER: Adaptive sensitivity encoding incorporating temporal filtering (TSENSE). Magn Reson Med 45:846–852, 2001.
5. Larson AC, White RD, Laub G, et al: Self-gated cardiac cine MRI. Magn Reson Med 51:93–102, 2004.
6. McVeigh ER: MRI of myocardial function: Motion tracking techniques. Magn Reson Imaging 14:137–150, 1996.
7. Ozturk C, Derbyshire JA, McVeigh ER: Estimating motion from MRI data. Proc IEEE 91:1627–1648, 2003.
8. Morse OC, Singer JR: Blood velocity measurement in intact subjects. Science 170:440–441, 1970.
9. Zerhouni EA, Parish DM, Rogers WJ, et al: Human heart: Tagging with MR imaging—a method for noninvasive assessment of myocardial motion. Radiology 169:59–63, 1988.
10. Axel L, Dougherty L: MR imaging of motion with spatial modulation of magnetization. Radiology 171:841–845, 1989.
11. Axel L, Dougherty L: Heart wall motion: Improved method of spatial modulation of magnetization for MR imaging. Radiology 172:349–360, 1989.
12. Hennig J: Generalized MR interferography. Magn Reson Med 16:390–402, 1990.
13. Bolster BD Jr, McVeigh ER, Zerhouni EA: Myocardial tagging in polar coordinates with use of striped tags. Radiology 177:769–772, 1990.
14. Mosher TJ, Smith MB: A DANTE tagging sequence for the evaluation of translational sample motion. Magn Reson Med 15:334–339, 1990.
15. Pipe JG, Boes JL, Chenevert TL: Method for measuring three-dimensional motion with tagged MR imaging. Radiology 181:591–595, 1991.
16. Fischer SE, McKinnon GC, Maier SE, Boesiger P: Improved myocardial tagging contrast. Magn Reson Med 30:191–200, 1993.
17. McVeigh ER, Bolster BD Jr: Improved sampling of myocardial motion with variable separation tagging. Magn Reson Med 39:657–661, 1998.
18. Kuijer JP, Marcus JT, Gotte MJ, et al: Simultaneous MRI tagging and through-plane velocity quantification: A three-dimensional myocardial motion tracking algorithm. J Magn Reson Imaging 9:409–419, 1999.
19. Ryf S, Spiegel MA, Gerber M, Boesiger P: Myocardial tagging with 3D-CSPAMM. J Magn Reson Imaging 16:320–325, 2002.
20. Spiegel MA, Luechinger R, Schwitter J, Boesiger P: RingTag: Ring-shaped tagging for myocardial centerline assessment. Invest Radiol 38:669–678, 2003.
21. NessAiver M, Prince JL: Magnitude image CSPAMM reconstruction (MICSR). Magn Reson Med 50:331–342, 2003.

22. Aletras AH, Freidlin RZ, Navon G, Arai AE: AIR-SPAMM: Alternative inversion recovery spatial modulation of magnetization for myocardial tagging. J Magn Reson 166:236–245, 2004.

23. Reeder SB, Atalar E, Faranesh AZ, McVeigh ER: Multi-echo segmented k-space imaging: An optimized hybrid sequence for ultrafast cardiac imaging. Magn Reson Med 41:375–385, 1999.

24. Epstein FH, Wolff SD, Arai AE: Segmented k-space fast cardiac imaging using an echo-train readout. Magn Reson Med 41:609–613, 1999.

25. Herzka DA, Kellman P, Aletras AH, et al: Multishot EPI-SSFP in the heart. Magn Reson Med 47:655–664, 2002.

26. Herzka DA, Guttman MA, McVeigh ER: Myocardial tagging with SSFP. Magn Reson Med 49:329–340, 2003.

27. Peters DC, Epstein FH, McVeigh ER: Myocardial wall tagging with undersampled projection reconstruction. Magn Reson Med 45:562–567, 2001.

28. Peters DC, Ennis DB, McVeigh ER: High-resolution MRI of cardiac function with projection reconstruction and steady-state free precession. Magn Reson Med 48:82–88, 2002.

29. Fischer SE: Assessment of Human Heart Wall Motion by Magnetic Resonance Imaging (DISS. ETH No. 10926) [PhD thesis]. Zurich, Swiss Federal Institute of Technology, 1994.

30. Ennis DB, Thompson RB, Derbyshire JA, et al: Respiratory and cardiac gated 3D imaging for improved spatial and temporal resolution. Proc Intl Soc Magn Reson Med 10:1681, 2002.

31. Doyle M, Walsh EG, Blackwell GG, Pohost GM: Block regional interpolation scheme for k-space (brisk): A rapid cardiac imaging technique. Magn Reson Med 33:163–170, 1995.

32. Guttman MA, Prince JL, McVeigh ER: Tag and contour detection in tagged MR images of the left ventricle. IEEE Trans Med Imag 13:74–88, 1994.

33. Atalar E, McVeigh ER: Optimum tag thickness for the measurement of position with MRI. IEEE Trans Med Imag 13:152–160, 1994.

34. Amini AA, Chen Y, Elayyadi M, Radeva P: Tag surface reconstruction and tracking of myocardial beads from SPAMM-MRI with parametric B-spline surfaces. IEEE Trans Med Imaging 20:94–103, 2001.

35. Denney TS Jr: Estimation and detection of myocardial tags in MR image without user-defined myocardial contours. IEEE Trans Med Imaging 18:330–344, 1999.

36. Chen Y, Amini AA: A MAP framework for tag line detection in SPAMM data using Markov random fields on the B-spline solid. IEEE Trans Med Imaging 21:1110–1122, 2002.

37. Young AA: Model tags: Direct three-dimensional tracking of heart wall motion from tagged magnetic resonance images. Med Image Anal 3:361–372, 1999.

38. Young AA, Axel L: Three-dimensional motion and deformation of the heart wall: Estimation with spatial modulation of magnetization—a model-based approach. Radiology 185:241–247, 1992.

39. O'Dell WG, Moore CC, Hunter WC, et al: Displacement field fitting for calculating 3D myocardial deformations from tagged MR images. Radiology 195:829–835, 1995.

40. Denney TS, McVeigh ER: Model-free reconstruction of three-dimensional myocardial strains from planar tagged MR images. J Magn Reson Imag 7:799–810, 1997.

41. Declerck J, Denney TS, Ozturk C, et al: Left ventricular motion reconstruction from planar tagged MR images: A comparison. Phys Med Biol 45:1611–1632, 2000.

42. Huang J, Abendschein D, Davila-Roman VG, Amini AA: Spatio-temporal tracking of myocardial deformations with a 4-D B-spline model from tagged MRI. IEEE Trans Med Imaging 18:957–972, 1999.

43. Ozturk C, McVeigh ER: Four-dimensional B-spline based motion analysis of tagged MR images: Introduction and in vivo validation. Phys Med Biol 45:1683–1702, 2000.

44. Osman NF, Kerwin WS, McVeigh ER, Prince JL: Cardiac motion tracking using CINE harmonic phase (HARP) magnetic resonance imaging. Magn Reson Med 42:1048–1060, 1999.

45. Sampath S, Derbyshire JA, Atalar E, et al: Real-time imaging of two-dimensional cardiac strain using a harmonic phase magnetic resonance imaging (HARP-MRI) pulse sequence. Magn Reson Med 50:154–163, 2003.

46. Osman NF, Sampath S, Atalar E, Prince JL: Imaging longitudinal cardiac strain on short-axis images using strain-encoded MRI. Magn Reson Med 46:324–334, 2001.

47. Aletras AH, Ding S, Balaban RS, Wen H: DENSE: Displacement encoding with stimulated echoes in cardiac functional MRI. J Magn Reson 137:247–252, 1999.

48. Aletras AH, Wen H: Mixed echo train acquisition displacement encoding with stimulated echoes: An optimized DENSE method for in vivo functional imaging of the human heart. Magn Reson Med 46:523–534, 2001.

49. Kim D, Gilson WD, Kramer CM, Epstein FH: Myocardial tissue tracking with two-dimensional cine displacement-encoded MR imaging: Development and initial evaluation. Radiology 230:862–871, 2004.

50. McVeigh ER, Prinzen FW, Wyman BT, et al: Imaging asynchronous mechanical activation of the paced heart with tagged MRI. Magn Reson Med 39:507–513, 1998.

51. Wyman BT, Hunter WC, Prinzen FW, McVeigh ER: Mapping propagation of mechanical activation in the paced heart with MRI tagging. Am J Physiol 276(3 pt 2):H881–H891, 1999.

52. Wyman BT, Hunter WC, Prinzen FW, et al: Effects of single and bi-ventricular pacing on the temporal and spatial dynamics of ventricular contraction. Am J Physiol Heart Circ Physiol 282:H372–H379, 2002.

53. Faris OP, Evans FJ, Ennis DB, et al: Novel technique for cardiac electromechanical mapping with magnetic resonance imaging tagging and an epicardial electrode sock. Ann Biomed Eng 31:430–440, 2003.

54. Hsu EW, Henriquez CS: Myocardial fiber orientation mapping using reduced encoding diffusion tensor imaging. J Cardiovasc Magn Reson 3:339–347, 2001.

55. Surawicz B: U-wave: Facts, hypotheses, misconceptions, and misnomers. J Cardiovasc Electrophysiol 9:1117–1126, 1998.

56. Kim RJ, Wu E, Rafael A, et al: The use of contrast-enhanced magnetic resonance imaging to identify reversible myocardial dysfunction. N Engl J Med 343:1445–1453, 2000.

CHAPTER 41

Distributions of Myocyte Stretch, Stress, and Work in Models of Normal and Infarcted Ventricles

• • • •

Espen W. Remme, Martyn P. Nash, and Peter J. Hunter

A finite element model of the geometry and fibrous-sheet structure of the left ventricle (LV) and right ventricle (RV) of the pig heart has been developed.[1] Mechanical changes during the heart cycle are computed by solving the equations of motion under specified ventricular boundary conditions and using experimentally defined constitutive laws for the active and passive material properties of myocardial tissue. This work is an improvement to a previous study that used relatively simple boundary conditions.[2] The various phases of the cardiac cycle have been simulated using more physiologic boundary conditions. This chapter presents calculated regional cardiac coordinate stretch ratios, fiber stretch ratios, and stresses over the normal cardiac cycle, together with the fiber stress–strain work loops. This chapter also illustrates how these measures differ in the diseased heart, for which an infarcted region was incorporated into the ventricular model. Our data predict pronounced regional differences in the mechanical environment to which cells in different areas of the cardiac wall will be exposed, potentially contributing, via mechano-electric feedback (MEF), to mechanically induced heterogeneity in cardiac electrophysiologic behavior.

VENTRICULAR TISSUE STRUCTURE AND GEOMETRY

Cardiac tissue consists of discrete layers of muscle cells (approximately four to six cells thick), whose three-dimensional arrangement is associated with a complex hierarchy of extracellular connective tissue.[3] For modeling purposes, we assume the tissue to be a continuum

with orthotropic material properties[4]—that is, based on microstructural observations at any point within the myocardium, it is possible to define three material axes. One axis (the "fiber" axis) coincides with the muscle fiber direction; a second axis (the "sheet" axis) is in the plane of the muscle layer perpendicular to the fiber direction; and the third axis (the "normal" axis) is orthogonal to the other two, and thus perpendicular to the muscle layer (Fig. 41–1).

Detailed measurements of the LV and RV endocardial and epicardial surface geometries, together with the transmural variations in fiber and sheet axis orientations, have been used to formulate mathematical descriptions (on the basis of finite element methods) of the anatomic shape and microstructural architecture of the ventricles using smoothly continuous (tricubic-Hermite) interpolations of nodal parameters.[3,5–7] An article by Stevens and colleagues[1] contains a full

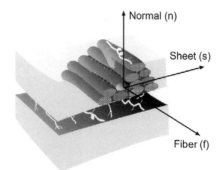

■ **Figure 41–1** Microstructural material axes used to describe myocardial tissue architecture. *(From LeGrice IJ, Smaill BH, Chai LZ, et al: Laminar structure of the heart: Ventricular myocyte arrangement and connective tissue architecture in the dog. Am J Physiol 269:H571–H582, 1995, with permission.)*

description of the mathematical model of the porcine ventricles used in this study. Figure 41–2 illustrates the ventricular geometry and the typical transmural rotation of the fiber axis direction.

The following sections describe some of the mathematical details of the model. (The reader who is more interested in the general aspects of this topic may skip the detailed explanation that follows and proceed at "Simulating the Ventricular Cycle.")

VENTRICULAR MECHANICS

During the heart cycle, myocytes undergo large, elastic deformations and typically change their lengths by up to 20%. Therefore, any analysis of cardiac mechanics must be based on finite deformation elasticity theory. The well-established stress equilibrium equations that govern the kinematics of soft, deformable materials are based on physical conservation laws (mass and momentum).[8,9] For ventricular mechanics, it is convenient to formulate terms in the governing equations with respect to an orthogonal system of curvilinear material coordinates aligned with the myocardial microstructural axes in the undeformed configuration.[4] The following section summarizes deformation,

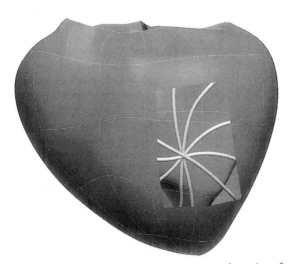

■ **Figure 41–2** Porcine ventricular geometry and rotation of the transmural myocyte orientation from roughly –60 degrees at the epicardial surface to +90 degrees at the endocardial surface (with respect to the circumferential direction; positive angles counterclockwise). (See color insert.)

stress, equilibrium equations, and boundary loads appropriate for analysis of regional deformation and stress of the porcine ventricles.

Material Coordinates, Deformation, and Stress

All soft biological tissues are anisotropic, displaying different material properties in different directions. Biaxial tension[5,10] and shear[11,12] experiments on sections of ventricular tissue have shown that the myocyte layers illustrated in Figure 41–1 have important implications for the mechanical behavior of cardiac tissue (Fig. 41–3). To encapsulate the anisotropic material behavior of cardiac muscle, we defined Lagrangian descriptions of tissue strain (Cauchy–Green strain tensor, $E_{\alpha\beta}$) and mechanical stress (second Piola–Kirchhoff stress tensor, $T^{\alpha\beta}$) with respect to the microstructural material coordinates (denoted v_α, where $\alpha \in$ (f, s, n); f, fiber; s, sheet; n, normal) using:

$$E_{\alpha\beta} = \frac{1}{2}\left(a_{\alpha\beta}^{(v)} - A_{\alpha\beta}^{(v)}\right) \tag{1}$$

$$T^{\alpha\beta} = \frac{1}{2}\left(\frac{\partial W}{\partial E_{\alpha\beta}} + \frac{\partial W}{\partial E_{\beta\alpha}}\right) - pa_{(v)}^{\alpha\beta} + T_a\frac{\partial V_\alpha}{\partial v_f}\frac{\partial V_\beta}{\partial v_f} \tag{2}$$

where $a_{\alpha\beta}^{(v)}$, $A_{\alpha\beta}^{(v)}$, and $a_{(v)}^{\alpha\beta}$ are metric tensors defined with respect to the microstructural material coordinates (see Reference 13 for further details); p is the intramural hydrostatic stress field; $\partial V_\alpha/\partial v_f$ are components of the inverse of the deformation gradient tensor $F_\alpha^\beta = \partial v_\beta/\partial V_\alpha$ defined with respect to the microstructural material coordinates (V_α = undeformed microstructural coordinate; v_β = deformed microstructural coordinate); and W and T_a are scalar functions defined to characterize the passive and active mechanical behavior of myocardial tissue, respectively (see next section). It is assumed that the active tension, T_a, is a Cauchy stress that is generated only along the deformed fiber axis (v_f), but the coordinate transformation (the last term in Eq. 2) distributes T_a across all components of the second Piola–Kirchhoff stress tensor.

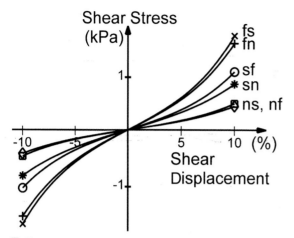

Figure 41–3 Experimental shear stress–strain data recorded from small blocks of porcine ventricular muscle (f, fiber; s, sheet; n, normal). *fs* denotes shearing in the fiber-sheet plane (i.e., a displacement in the sheet direction perpendicular to the fiber axis). The five other shear modes are labeled similarly. *(Regenerated from the raw data in Dokos S, Smaill BH, Young A, LeGrice I: Shear properties of passive ventricular myocardium Am J Physiol 283:H2650–H2659, 2002.)*

The extension or stretch ratios are computed from the Cauchy–Green strain components using the following equation:

$$\lambda_{\alpha\alpha} = \sqrt{2E_{\alpha\alpha} + 1} \quad \text{(no summation on } \alpha) \quad (3)$$

Stress Equilibrium and Incompressibility

In the absence of body forces and rigid body accelerations, the stress equilibrium equations that govern tissue mechanics can be formulated in terms of a set of nonoverlapping element integrals expressed in terms of finite element material coordinates (see Reference 4 for a more detailed discussion of this topic). The global system of nonlinear residual equations receives contributions associated with each of the spatial reference coordinates for each of the geometric parameters of the finite element model. Additional kinematic constraints are introduced to simulate the incompressible nature of the tissue. Fixed displacement constraints (e.g., rigid valve rings) eliminate the associated residuals from the global system, and pressure boundary constraints

(ventricular cavity pressures) can be applied to element surfaces by adding extra right-sided load terms.

All element integrals are evaluated numerically using Gaussian quadrature, for which the components of the second Piola–Kirchhoff stress tensor, $T^{\alpha\beta}$, are evaluated at the quadrature points using constitutive equations defined in the next section. The nonlinear residual equations are minimized with respect to the (unknown) deformed geometric parameters using full Newton iterations, which uses UMFPACK (LU factorization; University of Florida, Gainesville, FL)[14] to solve the resulting systems of linear equations. The finite element mesh of the porcine ventricles consists of a total of 5784 geometric degrees of freedom and 142 hydrostatic pressure degrees of freedom.

MYOCARDIAL MATERIAL PROPERTIES

There are three terms in the stress–strain relation (see Eq. 2). The passive deviatory components of stress are defined using derivatives of a scalar strain energy density function (SEDF), W. We used a pole-zero formulation of the SEDF as described in the following. The volumetric component involves setting up a scalar field to define the hydrostatic pressure field, p, with parameters that are obtained as a result of the solution process. It is assumed that the active contractile component of stress is only generated along the axis of the myocyte. The active tension is modeled using the steady-state Hunter-McCulloch-ter Keurs (HMT) model[15] described in the following. Mechanical properties of the tissue are contained within these descriptions of the SEDF and HMT models (see the following section).

Passive Mechanical Properties of Cardiac Tissue

To describe the passive deviatory properties of myocardium, the form of the SEDF has been defined using data from biaxial tension[5,10] and shear[11,12] mechanical tests on small sections of ventricular muscle (e.g., see Fig. 41–3). The general constitutive theory suggests that the six independent components of the stress tensor all depend on the six independent components of the strain tensor. However, the experimental results show a high degree of independence between a component of stress and the lateral strain components. For example, fiber stress was found to be nearly independent of the degree of lateral stretch along the sheet and normal axes.[10]

For each normal and shear mode of deformation, experimental stress–strain data typically exhibit non-linear properties (see Fig. 41–3) that are well represented using pole-zero type functions of the form:

$$W = k \frac{E^2}{(a - E)^b} \quad (4)$$

where E is a component of the Cauchy–Green strain tensor; and a, b, and k are the material parameters fitted to the experimental stress–strain data. The parameter a represents the elastic strain limit along a given material axis; b governs the curvature of the nonlinear stress–strain curve; and k is a scaling parameter (i.e., the relative contribution of a particular term to the total strain energy). Summing strain energy contributions for each of the six independent modes of deformation results in:

$$W = k_{ff} \frac{E_{ff}^2}{(a_{ff} - E_{ff})^{b_{ff}}} + k_{ss} \frac{E_{ss}^2}{(a_{ss} - E_{ss})^{b_{ss}}} +$$

$$k_{nn} \frac{E_{nn}^2}{(a_{nn} - E_{nn})^{b_{nn}}} + k_{fs} \frac{E_{fs}^2}{(a_{fs} - E_{fs})^{b_{fs}}} + \quad (5)$$

$$k_{fn} \frac{E_{fn}^2}{(a_{fn} - E_{fn})^{b_{fn}}} + k_{sn} \frac{E_{sn}^2}{(a_{sn} - E_{sn})^{b_{sn}}}$$

where $E_{\alpha\beta}$ are the components of the Cauchy–Green strain tensor (see Eq. 1), and the material parameters are identified by the indices associated with the deformation modes. Table 41–1 lists the parameter values used for this study. The derivatives of W with respect to the strain components are used to compute the passive deviatoric stress components in Equation 2.

Active Contractile Stress of Myocytes

Cardiac myocytes generate contractile forces when electrically stimulated. We used the steady-state HMT model[15] to simulate the active stress (T_a in Eq. 2) developed during contraction, as summarized in the following equation:

$$T_a = T_{ref} \left[1 + \beta_0 (\lambda_{ff} - 1) \right] z_{SS}$$

$$z_{SS} = \frac{[Ca]^n}{[Ca]^n + [Ca_{50}]^n}$$

$$n = n_{ref} \left[1 + \beta_1 (\lambda_{ff} - 1) \right] \quad (6)$$

$$Ca_{50} = 10^{(6 - pCa_{50})}$$

$$pCa_{50} = pCa_{50ref} \left[1 + \beta_2 (\lambda_{ff} - 1) \right]$$

The parameters used for the steady-state HMT model are summarized in Table 41–2. In the current simplified implementation of the HMT model used in this study, the β_1 and β_2 parameters are set to zero, making the Ca-dependent sigmoidal term (z_{SS}) factor independent of fiber stretch.

TABLE 41–1   Passive Material Parameters for the Pole-Zero Constitutive Law

Type	Axial Properties		Shear Properties	
Coefficients	k_{ff}	2.0 kPa	k_{fs}	1.0 kPa
	k_{ss}	2.0 kPa	k_{fn}	1.0 kPa
	k_{nn}	2.0 kPa	k_{sn}	1.0 kPa
Poles	a_{ff}	0.475	a_{fs}	0.8
	a_{ss}	0.619	a_{fn}	0.8
	a_{nn}	0.943	a_{sn}	0.8
Curvatures	b_{ff}	1.5	b_{fs}	1.2
	b_{ss}	1.5	b_{fn}	1.2
	b_{nn}	0.442	b_{sn}	1.2

See Equation 5.

TABLE 41–2   Active Material Parameters for the Hunter-McCulloch-ter Keurs Mechanics Model

T_{ref}	n_{ref}	pCa_{50ref}	β_0	β_1	β_2
100 kPa	3	6.3010	1.45	0	0

The value of pCa_{50ref} was found so that $Ca_{50} = 0.5$ (see Eq. 6).

SIMULATING THE VENTRICULAR CYCLE

Simulation of the cardiac cycle was started from the beginning of diastasis just after the rapid filling phase. During the rapid filling phase, the stored elastic energy in the wall from the fiber contraction during systole is released as an elastic recoil, and it is assumed that the myocardium is in its most unloaded state at the start of diastasis. In this unloaded reference configuration, residual strains[16] were included using the method of Rodriguez and colleagues.[17] The residual fiber strain was set to vary linearly with a 5% stretch at the epicardium and a 5% contraction at the LV endocardium[18] for the nodes between the basal and apical elements. During the simulation, all of the base nodes were fixed to avoid rigid body motion.

Because of numeric convergence problems caused by the tapered shape of the collapsed elements around the apex, these elements were treated differently than the rest of the mesh: the hydrostatic pressure term in Equation 2 was reduced, effectively relaxing the incompressibility constraint for this small ring of elements. The activation parameter was set to smaller values for the Gauss points in these elements, reducing the actively generated fiber tension in them. Compared with the value in the rest of the mesh, the Ca parameter value was set to 0%, 20%, and 60% for the three longitudinal rings of Gauss points from the apex and toward the base in these elements. At the same time, the scaling material parameter ($k_{\alpha\beta}$) for the various terms in Equation 5 was increased by up to a 10 times stiffer value in the apical elements to reduce their deformation. The developed stress and strain in the apical elements thus would be inaccurate; however, according to Saint-Venant's Principle,[19] the inaccurate stress and strain predictions are restricted to the apical region of the model. All results given in the following sections are for the equatorial elements of the model, well away from the apical region.

Passive Inflation

A pressure was applied to the endocardial surfaces of the ventricles to simulate the inflation by atrial contraction. From a zero pressure in the reference configuration at the beginning of diastasis, the LV and RV pressures were increased incrementally to 0.9 and 0.18 kPa, respectively, at end diastole (ED), resulting in an increase of the cavity volumes of 45% and 19%, respectively. During the passive inflation, the active tension was zero (Ca = 0 in Eq. 6).

Figure 41–4 shows the applied LV pressure during the various phases of the cardiac cycle, with the resulting volume and pressure–volume loop (the inflation phase is labeled A in the figure). The applied LV pressure shown in the figure is obtained from a Wiggers diagram (slightly modified from Reference 20). The time scale of the cycle is normalized to 1 sec. Because cycle time was not directly modeled (we have adapted a quasi-static approach), times for each deformation state due to specified endocardial pressures were determined from the pressure versus time graph in Figure 41–4.

Isovolumic Contraction

During systole, the Ca parameter was increased from zero to simulate the developed active fiber tension that caused the contractile deformation of the model. To simulate isovolumic contraction (IVC; when all of the ventricular valves are closed), the cavity volumes were held constant for each increment of Ca by iteratively adjusting the ventricular cavity pressures. The IVC phase is labeled B in Figure 41–4.

Ejection

The ejection phase was initiated when the LV pressure exceeded 10 kPa, representing the opening of the aortic valve. During ejection, the LV pressure was incremented to 15 kPa. The increments of the RV pressure were set to 20% of the LV increments. A specified LV volume was assigned for each LV pressure value during ejection based on the P-V loop in Figure 41–4. To obtain this volume the Ca parameter was iteratively adjusted for each pressure increment. (The phase of maximum ejection is labeled C in Fig. 41–4.)

The reduced ejection phase was simulated by keeping Ca fixed at the level of peak pressure and decreas-

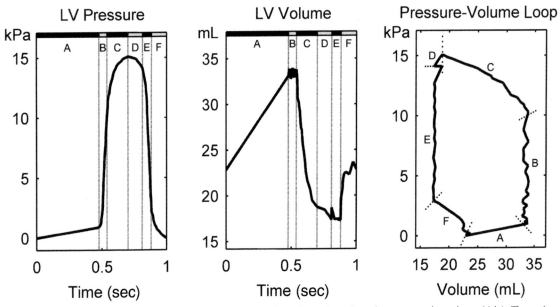

■ **Figure 41–4** Left ventricular (LV) endocardial pressure *(left)*, volume *(center)*, and pressure–volume loop *(right)*. The various cardiac phases are separated by *dotted lines*: A, passive inflation; B, isovolumic contraction; C, maximum ejection; D, reduced ejection; E, isovolumic relaxation; F, rapid filling.

ing the LV pressure in decrements to 14 kPa. The RV pressure was reduced by 0.2 kPa. The resulting LV and RV ejection fractions at the end of ejection were 48% and 52%, respectively. (The reduced ejection phase is labeled D in Fig. 41–4.)

Isovolumic Relaxation

The isovolumic relaxation (IVR) phase was simulated in a similar manner to the IVC phase, except that the Ca parameter was reduced. At each decrement, the cavity volumes were held constant at their volumes at the end of ejection by iteratively adjusting the cavity pressures. (The IVR phase is labeled E in Fig. 41–4.)

Rapid Filling

When the LV pressure decreased to less than 3 kPa (representing the pressure in the left atrium and the opening of the mitral valve), the Ca parameter and LV and RV pressures were synchronously reduced in decrements to reach zero simultaneously, concluding

the cardiac cycle. (The rapid filling phase is labeled F in Fig. 41–4.)

Simulating the Cardiac Cycle with an Infarcted Region

To examine the effects of myocardial infarction on ventricular deformation, one element at the anterior equatorial LV free wall was selected to represent an infarcted region associated with occlusion of a side branch of the left anterior descending coronary artery. The selected region had an approximate diameter of 25 mm, covered the entire transmural direction from epicardium to endocardium, and corresponded to 4.2% of the total myocardial LV and RV wall volume. The infarcted tissue was assigned significantly stiffer mechanical properties and did not generate active fiber tension. This was implemented in the model by multiplying the pole-zero coefficients $k_{\alpha\beta}$ for the various terms in Equation 5 by a factor of four and by setting the Ca parameter to zero throughout the whole cycle. The noninfarcted tissue retained the normal passive and active material properties. The cardiac cycle was simulated in a manner similar to the previous description.

ANALYSIS OF CARDIAC STRAINS, SARCOMERE LENGTH, AND FIBER STRESS

Transmural cardiac coordinate stretch ratios (calculated using Eq. 3) were analyzed at five locations around the equator of the ventricles. Figure 41–5 illustrates the circumferential, longitudinal, and radial stretch ratios at sub-endocardial, midwall, and sub-epicardial material points. Each row in Figure 41–5 is associated with a different circumferential location, as indicated by the diagram in the corresponding row of Figure 41–6. Sarcomere stretch ratios, fiber stresses, and fiber stress-stretch (work) loops also are illustrated in Figure 41–6. Comparing the wall and fiber strains in relation to the local wall geometry and fiber angles shown in the first column of Figure 41–6 may provide some understanding of the heterogeneity in regional mechanics that occurs during the cardiac cycle.

During the first filling phase, fiber stretch increases at all locations in the wall. During IVC, some regions experience further fiber stretch, whereas others contract, particularly sub-epicardial fibers. During ejection, the fibers shorten at all locations, but the sub-epicardial fibers shorten the most. During IVR and the rapid filling phase, the fibers lengthen at most locations. (See "Conclusions, Critique, and Current Directions" for further comment on regional disparity of fiber stretch.) The fiber stress changes do not always reflect fiber stretch, because lateral strains are different in different wall locations.

Effects of Myocardial Infarction on Stress and Stretch

The results at the five circumferential locations shown in Figures 41–5 and 41–6 remained relatively unchanged for the infarcted model, apart from small changes in the stretch and stress magnitudes of the two closest locations (see rows 2 and 3 in Figs. 41–5 and 41–6). The location of the infarcted region is shown in Figures 41–7 and 41–8. Within the infarct, there were some marked dif-

ferences. Figure 41–7 shows the fiber stretch, stress, and stress–stretch loop, together with the cardiac wall/coordinate stretch ratios before infarction. Figure 41–8 shows the same results after infarction. Myocardial infarction reversed the fiber stretch from predominantly compression (normal cycle) to elongation (infarcted) during systole, also referred to as paradoxical segment lengthening in the clinical setting. The fiber stress magnitude also increased significantly, and the fiber stress–stretch work loops tended toward pure passive stress–strain relations. The circumferential and longitudinal strains changed from predominantly compression

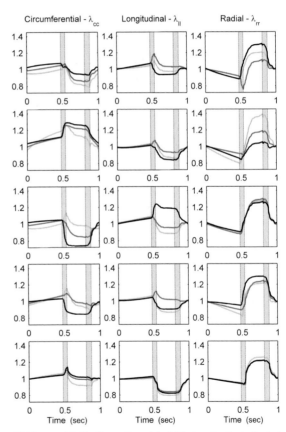

■ **Figure 41–5** Circumferential *(left)*, longitudinal *(center)*, and radial *(right)* stretch ratios, during the cardiac cycle at five circumferential locations around the equator of the ventricles, as indicated by the diagram in the corresponding row of Figure 41–6. *Light gray, dark gray,* and *black lines* represent subendocardial, midwall, and subepicardial locations, respectively. *Vertical bands* indicate the isovolumic contraction and relaxation phases of the cardiac cycle. (See color insert.)

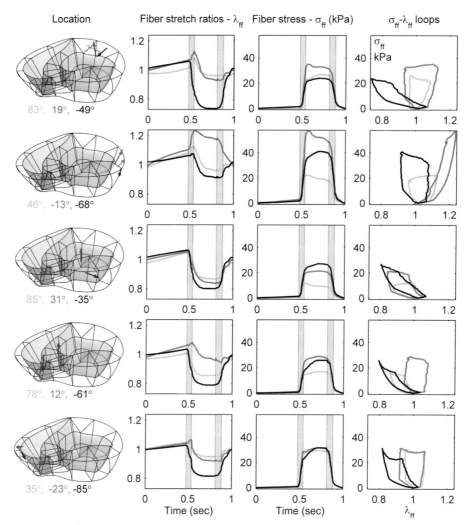

■ **Figure 41–6** Transmural sarcomere stretch ratio and stress during the cardiac cycle at five locations around the equator of the ventricles, illustrated on the *left* with fiber directions indicated by *arrows* and angles relative to the circumferential axis. *Light gray, dark gray,* and *black lines* represent subendocardial, midwall, and subepicardial locations, respectively. The *second column* shows the fiber stretch ratio through the heart cycle. The *third column* shows the developed fiber stress. The *right column* illustrates the resulting fiber stress–stretch loops. *Vertical bands* indicate the isovolumic contraction and relaxation phases of the cardiac cycle. (See color insert.)

to elongation during systole, whereas the large wall thickening was markedly reduced in the infarcted case.

CONCLUSIONS, CRITIQUE, AND CURRENT DIRECTIONS

The model of ventricular mechanics presented in this chapter includes accurate descriptions of ventricular

anatomy (although currently without papillary muscles; see the following) and an accurate description of the fibrous-sheet structure of myocardium. It does not currently contain the spatial distribution of the density of proteins such as collagen, although the framework has been established to incorporate this when the data become available. Measurements of collagen density currently are being undertaken and will be included in future versions of the model. Also, cellular electro-

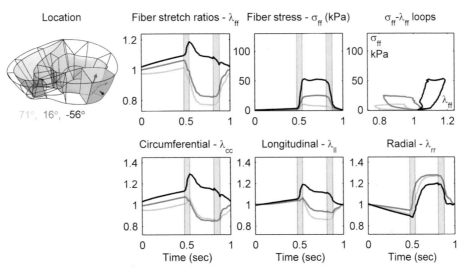

■ **Figure 41–7** Stretch and stress results in a left ventricular free wall anterior region *before* it is subject to infarction. The region is highlighted on the *left,* with fiber directions indicated by *arrows* and angles relative to the circumferential axis. The *top row* shows fiber stretch ratio and stress through the heart cycle and the resulting fiber stress-stretch loops. The *second row* shows corresponding stretch ratios in cardiac wall coordinates. *Light gray, dark gray,* and *black lines* represent subendocardial, midwall, and subepicardial locations, respectively. *Vertical bands* indicate the isovolumic contraction and relaxation phases of the cardiac cycle. (See color insert.)

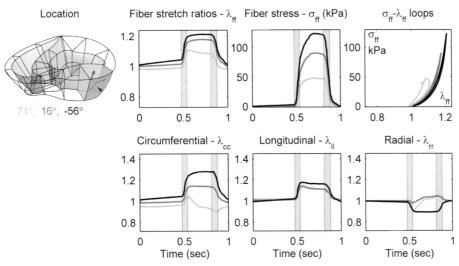

■ **Figure 41–8** Stretch and stress results from a left ventricular free wall anterior region subject to infarction. The region is highlighted on the *left,* with fiber directions indicated by *arrows* and angles relative to the circumferential axis. The *top row* shows fiber stretch ratio and stress through the heart cycle and the resulting fiber stress-stretch loops. The *second row* shows corresponding stretch ratios in cardiac wall coordinates. *Light gray, dark gray,* and *black lines* represent subendocardial, midwall, and subepicardial locations, respectively. *Vertical bands* indicate the isovolumic contraction and relaxation phases of the cardiac cycle. (See color insert.)

mechanical properties are assumed homogeneous, whereas there are significant transmural parameter gradients.[21,22]

The model of active force generation used in this chapter is a simplification of a more comprehensive model of myocyte mechanics.[15] Another limitation of the model is the assumption of instantaneous activation. In reality, activation of the ventricular myocardium takes about 50 msec to complete from the time of initial Purkinje fiber stimulation. We are currently modeling the activation sequence using ionic current models,[23] but these are not yet fully coupled to the whole-heart mechanics model. Similarly, the assumption of a spatially uniform pressure in the LV and RV is a simplification, because, in reality, pressure gradients develop during ejection. The current model is being coupled to a computational model of ventricular fluid dynamics to address this issue.

An accurate description of the papillary muscles and chordae tendineae is likely to be the main limitation, because the current model partially includes the base of the papillary model as a thickening of the LV free wall but does not model the connection to the mitral valve leaflets. The LV free wall in this region is therefore artificially thick compared with the adjacent regions, and this is reflected in the comparatively lower circumferential strains and stresses. If the papillary muscle attachment to the mitral valve were included in the model, it is likely that the longitudinal force balance would be affected during IVC, because the LV pressure acting on the mitral valve would produce a longitudinal force that is transferred to the apical end of the LV free wall through the chordae and papillary muscle.

The results presented in this chapter on the regional distribution of sarcomere length variation through the cardiac cycle are likely to be affected by these continuing improvements to the model, but they are unlikely to alter the overall patterns, because the major mechanical influences (anatomy, fibrous sheet structure, conservation laws for mass and momentum, and pressure–volume boundary conditions) have been accounted for. The effect that these sarcomere length changes may have on stretch-activated channels is discussed elsewhere in this textbook. For example, White (see Chapter 9) examines the influence of stretch-activated channels on MEF throughout the cardiac cycle, and Markhasin and Solovyova (see Chapter 22) examine the physiologic role of mechano-electric heterogeneity throughout the myocardium. Simulations such as those presented in this chapter will serve to integrate insight on cardiac mechano-electric interactions from pipette (single-cell level) to patient (whole-heart and clinical studies; see Chapter 40 for a discussion of noninvasive assessment of cardiac regional stresses and strains).

Acknowledgment

The authors thank Dr. Carey Stevens of the Auckland Bioengineering Institute for providing the original finite element mesh of the pig heart used in these simulations.

References

1. Stevens C, Remme E, LeGrice IJ, Hunter PJ: Ventricular mechanics in diastole: Material parameter sensitivity. J Biomech 36:737–748, 2003.
2. Stevens C, Hunter PJ: Sarcomere length changes in a model of the pig heart. Prog Biophys Mol Biol 82:229–241, 2003.
3. LeGrice IJ, Smaill BH, Chai LZ, et al: Laminar structure of the heart: Ventricular myocyte arrangement and connective tissue architecture in the dog. Am J Physiol 269:H571–H582, 1995.
4. Nash PM, Hunter PJ: Computational mechanics of the heart: From tissue structure to ventricular function. J Elasticity 61:113–141, 2000.
5. Nielsen PM, LeGrice IJ, Smaill BH, Hunter PJ: Mathematical model of geometry and fibrous structure of the heart. Am J Physiol 260:H1365–H1378, 1991.
6. LeGrice IJ, Hunter PJ, Smaill BH: Laminar structure of the heart: A mathematical model. Am J Physiol 272:H2466–H2476, 1997.
7. Hunter PJ, Smaill BH, Nielsen PM, LeGrice IJ: A mathematical model of cardiac anatomy. In: Panfilov AV, Holden AV (eds): Computational Biology of the Heart. West Sussex, UK, John Wiley & Sons, 1997, pp 171–215.
8. Malvern LE: Introduction to the Mechanics of a Continuous Medium. Englewood Cliffs, NJ, Prentice-Hall, 1969.
9. Eringen AC: Mechanics of Continua. New York, Krieger, 1980.
10. Smaill BH, Hunter PJ: Structure and function of the diastolic heart: Material properties of passive myocardium. In: Glass L, Hunter PJ, McCulloch AD (eds): Theory of Heart: Biomechanics, Biophysics, and Nonlinear Dynamics of Cardiac Function. New York, Springer-Verlag, 1991, pp 1–29.
11. Dokos S, Young A, Smaill BH, LeGrice IJ: A triaxial-measurement shear-test device for soft biological tissues. J Biomech Eng 122:471–478, 2000.
12. Dokos S, Smaill BH, Young A, LeGrice IJ: Shear properties of passive ventricular myocardium. Am J Physiol 283:H2650–H2659, 2002.

13. Hunter PJ, Nash MP, Sands GB: Computational electro-mechanics of the heart. In: Panfilov AV, Holden AV (eds): Computational Biology of the Heart. West Sussex, UK, John Wiley & Sons, 1997, pp 345–407.

14. Davis TA: UMFPACK Version 4.0 User Guide. Gainesville, FL, University of Florida, 2002. University of Florida CISE online: Available at http://www.cise.ufl.edu/research/sparse/umfpack.

15. Hunter PJ, McCulloch A, ter Keurs HEDJ: Modelling the mechanical properties of cardiac muscle. Prog Biophys Mol Biol 69:289–331, 1998.

16. Omens JH, Fung YC: Residual strain in the rat left ventricle. Circ Res 66:37–45, 1990.

17. Rodriguez EK, Hoger A, McCulloch AD: Stress-dependent finite growth in soft elastic tissue. J Biomech 27:455–467, 1994.

18. Costa KD, May-Newman K, Farr D, et al: Three-dimensional residual strain in midanterior canine left ventricle. Am J Physiol 273:H1968–H1976, 1997.

19. Malvern LE: Introduction to the Mechanics of a Continuous Medium. Englewood Cliffs, NJ, Prentice-Hall, 1969, p 508.

20. Katz AM: Physiology of the Heart, 2nd ed. New York, Raven Press, 1992, p 362.

21. Antzelevitch C: Transmural dispersion of repolarization and the T wave. Cardiovasc Res 50:426–431, 2001.

22. Taggart P, Sutton PMI, Opthof T, et al: Transmural repolarisation in the left ventricle in humans during normoxia and ischaemia. Cardiovasc Res 50:454–462, 2001.

23. Hunter PJ, Pullan AJ, Smaill BH: Modeling total heart function. Annu Rev Biomed Eng 5:147–177, 2003.

CHAPTER 42

Stretch Channel Blockers: A New Class of Antiarrhythmic Drugs?

• • • •

Frank Bode and Michael R. Franz

Evidence is growing for the existence of stretch-activated channels (SAC) in cardiac and noncardiac cells. These channels play a role in the cell response to mechanical stimuli—that is, in cell volume regulation, cell proliferation, baroreceptor activation, or generation of action potentials in cochlear cells. Given this list of examples, SAC are part of a greater family of "mechanosensitive channels" (see Chapter 1). In the heart, SAC have been suggested to mediate action potential changes and arrhythmic responses that can be observed during myocardial stretch. Pharmacologic blockers of SAC have been applied in experimental models to further define the contribution of such channels to cardiac electrophysiology. This chapter focuses on the role of SAC in atrial myocardium and on pharmacologic tools to block their function, especially in the context of stretch-facilitated atrial fibrillation (AF).

STRETCH-ACTIVATED CHANNEL BLOCKING SUBSTANCES

Currently, a heterogeneous group of substances has been found to inhibit stretch-activated membrane currents, including the diuretic amiloride, aminoglycoside antibiotics such as streptomycin, and the lanthanide gadolinium (Gd^{3+}). Gd^{3+}, a potent blocker of cationic SAC, shortens channel open time and increases closed time in a dose-dependent manner.[1] In isolated ventricles subjected to short stretch pulses, Gd^{3+} inhibits the generation of stretch-induced depolarizations and extrasystoles.[2] Afterdepolarizations that occur during increased atrial pressure are suppressed by Gd^{3+}.[3] These effects cannot be attributed to cross-reactivity of Gd^{3+}

with L-type calcium channels,[4] because specific calcium channel blockade does not interfere with arrhythmic responses.[2,3] The nonspecific SAC blocker, streptomycin, suppressed stretch-induced calcium influx into ventricular cells, but conventional calcium antagonists had no effect.[5] An increased intracellular calcium concentration is a key factor for the generation of afterdepolarizations.[5] In the isolated working rat heart, streptomycin reduces the occurrence of extrasystoles and complex ventricular arrhythmias during afterload and ventricular pressure increases.[6] Stretch-induced ventricular ectopy and action potential shortening are antagonized by streptomycin in isolated rabbit hearts.[7] Other substances such as amiloride have SAC-blocking activity in single-cell preparations with an affinity for SAC in the 100 µM range.[8] Application of these SAC blockers has been restricted to experimental settings, because in vivo use is hampered by side effects such as calcium channel block with gadolinium[4,9] or inapplicability of SAC-blocking dosages with streptomycin because of serious adverse effects such as loss of hearing.[6]

It has been reported that a peptide isolated from the venom of the Chilean tarantula *Grammostola spatulata* (Fig. 42–1) blocks SAC. It is a 4 kD peptide formed by 34 amino acids and is named Grammostola Mechanotoxin #4 (GsMTx-4). The peptide exhibits a specific block of cationic SAC in isolated cardiomyocytes and other cell types, whereas voltage-gated channels such as L-type calcium channels and K^+ channels are not affected.[10,11] GsMTx-4 has partial homology to other neuroactive peptides of the cysteine-knot family, which have been found to block various sodium, calcium, and potassium channels. GsMTx-4 had no detectable effect on the normal action potential

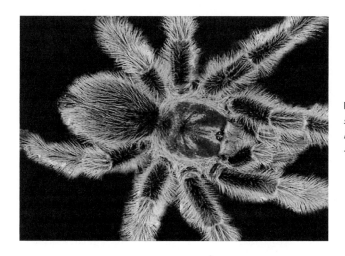

■ **Figure 42–1** The Chilean tarantula *Grammostola spatulata*. (See color insert.) *(From Bode F, Sachs F, Franz MR: Tarantula peptide inhibits atrial fibrillation. Nature 409:35–36, 2001, with permission.)*

in rabbit atrial cells (see Chapter 1) or rat astrocytes, and therefore could be of therapeutic interest.[11]

STRETCH-PROMOTING ATRIAL FIBRILLATION

AF is the most common sustained arrhythmia, yet the mechanisms that lead to AF are incompletely understood. The occurrence of AF often is associated with hemodynamic or mechanical disorders of the heart—that is, mitral valve disease, hypertension, or cardiac failure.[12] Likewise, atrial dilation is a common clinical finding and may play an important role for the susceptibility to AF.[13] The existence of mechano-electric feedback—that is, electrophysiologic changes in response to mechanical perturbations or changes in hemodynamic loading—has been established in human atrial myocardium. Atrial stretch caused by ventricular contraction modulates the atrial flutter cycle length in humans.[14] In the experimental setting, acute atrial dilation has been shown to facilitate the induction and maintenance of AF.[15]

We therefore hypothesized that SAC block by inhibitors such as Gd^{3+} and GsMTx-4 might antagonize proarrhythmic effects of myocardial stretch in the intact heart, and we tested those effects in a model of stretch-facilitated AF.[16,17]

Isolated Heart Preparation

To apply graded stretch to the atria, the heart was prepared according to a model described previously.[15] The caval and pulmonary veins were ligated. A Y-shaped manometer was inserted into the superior caval vein and a pulmonary vein to measure biatrial pressure. The interatrial septum was perforated to assure pressure equilibration between the left and the right atrium. Perfusion fluid left the heart exclusively through a cannula in the pulmonary artery. Atrial pressure and degree of atrial dilation were controlled by adjustment of the height of the pulmonary outflow cannula. To avoid atrial pressure changes caused by ventricular contractions, ventricular fibrillation was induced by burst pacing through a bipolar hook electrode attached to the left ventricle. The atrioventricular node was crushed to prevent retrograde atrial activation.

Electrophysiologic Measurements

Endocardial electrograms were recorded from the right and left midatrial free wall by bipolar 4F catheters introduced through the orifice of the inferior caval vein and a pulmonary vein. To test the inducibility of AF, burst pacing was performed through bipolar epicardial hook electrodes attached to both atrial appendages. Stimuli of 1-msec pulse duration and threefold diastolic pacing threshold were applied for 15 sec at 50 Hz.

Experimental Protocol

Intra-atrial pressure was increased progressively from 0 cm H_2O in steps of ~2.5 cm H_2O. Hearts were allowed to adapt to each new pressure level for 2 min before a burst pacing sequence was delivered. AF was defined as inducible when a fast irregular rhythm was maintained longer than 2 sec after cessation of burst pacing. Sustained AF was defined as a fast irregular rhythm that lasted for more than 60 sec after cessation of burst pacing and could only be terminated by decreasing pressure. The pressure level was increased until sustained AF was induced or a pressure level of 30 cm H_2O was reached.

Data Analysis

The probability of AF induction at different atrial pressures was analyzed by logistic regression analysis applying the function: $y = 1/(1 + exp(-(x-a)/b))$, where a and b are fitting parameters determined by an iterative procedure with a convergence criterion of a change of less than 0.01% for the two parameters. A dose–response relation was calculated for atrial pressures associated with 50% AF inducibility (P_{50}). P_{50} values for different drug concentrations were compared by t-test. AF durations and effective refractory periods (ERP) at different degrees of atrial dilation were statistically evaluated with the paired t-test. P values less than 0.05 defined statistical significance.

Effect of Acute Stretch on Atrial Fibrillation Inducibility

In the undilated atrium at a pressure of 0 cm H_2O, burst pacing did not induce AF. After an increase in atrial pressure, AF could be induced in each preparation (Fig. 42–2). The initial AF response seen during a stepwise pressure increase was predominantly non-sustained, whereas sustained AF emerged at greater pressure levels. AF inducibility in response to increas-

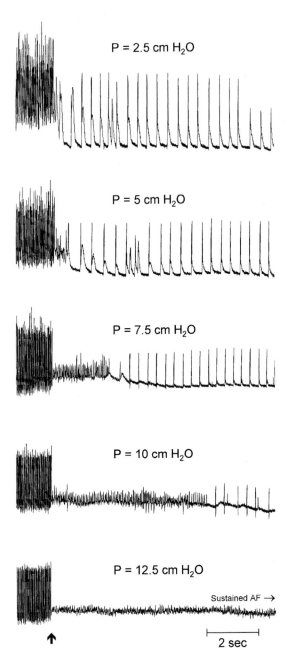

■ **Figure 42–2** Effect of atrial pressure (P) on atrial fibrillation (AF) inducibility and duration. Bipolar atrial electrograms after cessation of burst pacing during a stepwise increase in P. Although no AF response to burst pacing was observed at P = 2.5 cm H_2O, the atrium maintained AF progressively longer after adaptation to greater P. At P = 12.5 cm H_2O, AF became sustained. *(From Bode F, Sachs F, Franz MR: Tarantula peptide inhibits atrial fibrillation. Nature 409:35–36, 2001, with permission.)*

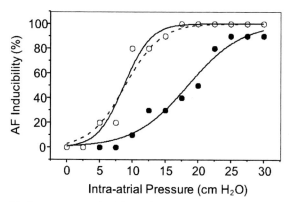

■ **Figure 42–3** Inducibility of AF (> 2 sec) plotted as a function of atrial pressure at baseline *(open circles)* and during application of 170 nM GsMTx-4 *(filled circles)*; n = 10. *(From Bode F, Sachs F, Franz MR: Tarantula peptide inhibits atrial fibrillation. Nature 409:35–36, 2001, with permission.)*

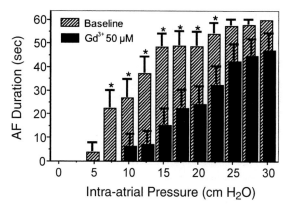

■ **Figure 42–4** Duration of induced AF in 16 hearts as a function of intra-atrial pressure (mean ± SEM). Administration of 50 μM Gd^{3+} decreased average AF duration compared with baseline. *$^*P < 0.05$. (From Bode F, Katchman A, Woosley RL, Franz MR: Gadolinium decreases stretch-induced vulnerability to atrial fibrillation. Circulation 101:2200–2205, 2000, with permission.)*

ing pressure followed a sigmoidal curve (Fig. 42–3). On average, intra-atrial pressure needed to be increased to 8.8 ± 0.2 cm H_2O (P_{50}) to produce AF after cessation of burst pacing. A further increase of intra-atrial pressure to 11.6 ± 0.6 cm H_2O ($P < 0.01$) was required to induce sustained AF (> 60 sec). Sustained AF terminated promptly on pressure release. Figure 42–4 demonstrates how the average duration of AF episodes lengthened as intra-atrial pressure was increased. Spontaneous AF occurred in five hearts when intra-atrial pressure increased to 13.8 ± 3.3 cm H_2O. Premature depolarizations often preceded runs of AF.

Effect of Gd^{3+} on Atrial Fibrillation Inducibility

Gd^{3+} at 50 μM suppressed AF inducibility in all hearts studied (Fig. 42–4). Subsequently, the dose dependence of Gd^{3+} effects on AF inducibility was examined by adding Gd^{3+} to the perfusate in serial concentrations of 12.5, 25, and 50 μM, allowing 15 min for equilibration. The AF response to burst stimulation with increasing atrial pressure was assessed at each concentration and after a 20-min washout period.

The intra-atrial pressure associated with P_{50} showed a linear correlation ($r = 0.99$; $P < 0.005$) with Gd^{3+} concentration over the 0 to 50 μM dose range. P_{50} increased by 0.15 cm H_2O/μM Gd^{3+}. P_{50} increased significantly during each step of increasing Gd^{3+} doses ($P < 0.01$). Each experiment lasted about 3 hours. Yet, time-related changes in the preparation could not have accounted for the observed reduction in AF vulnerability, because the effect of Gd^{3+} was largely reversible after 20 min of washout ($P < 0.01$ compared with 25 and 50 μM Gd^{3+}).

The effect of 50 μM Gd^{3+} was investigated in a total of 16 experiments. In each preparation, the lowest atrial pressure that had enabled AF induction in control hearts was no longer sufficient to maintain AF during Gd^{3+}. Instead, intra-atrial pressure needed to be increased to significantly greater levels to obtain AF. P_{50} for AF induction was shifted to 19.0 ± 0.5 cm H_2O ($P < 0.001$). On average, atrial pressure needed to be increased to 21.9 ± 0.4 cm H_2O to obtain sustained AF after Gd^{3+} ($P < 0.001$ vs. baseline). Gd^{3+} (50 μM) markedly decreased the average duration of induced AF at pressures between 7.5 and 22.5 cm H_2O ($P < 0.05$; see Fig. 42–4). Spontaneous AF was no longer observed during the stepwise increase in atrial pressure after Gd^{3+} was added.

Effect of Verapamil on Vulnerability to Atrial Fibrillation

Gd^{3+} has been reported to also block calcium, potassium, and sodium channels.[9,18] This chapter only addresses L-type calcium channels as possibly being responsible for AF vulnerability during stretch by administering verapamil in five studies.

Measurements were obtained before and 15 min after administration of 1 μM verapamil. After a 20-min washout period, 50 μM Gd^{3+} was applied to compare the effects of both substances. In isolated hearts, 1 μM verapamil achieved a marked block of Ca^{2+} channels,[2,19] by an amount expected to exceed the Ca^{2+}-channel blocking effects reported for Gd^{3+} with doses up to 80 μM.[3,20] Pacing thresholds were not affected by verapamil (0.21 ± 0.04 mA vs. 0.20 ± 0.03 mA at baseline). Verapamil did not inhibit AF induction during acute dilation. P_{50} was 6.3 ± 0.1 cm H_2O at baseline and 4.9 ± 0.2 cm H_2O after application of verapamil (P value not significant). In the same preparations, 50 μM Gd^{3+} increased P_{50} to 12.9 ± 0.5 cm H_2O ($P < 0.001$).

Effect of GsMTx-4 on Vulnerability to Atrial Fibrillation

After application of GsMTx-4 (170 nM) in 10 hearts, induction of AF required a significantly greater atrial pressure of 18.5 ± 0.5 cm H_2O ($P < 0.001$; see Fig. 42–3). This represented an increase of 9.7 ± 0.6 cm H_2O compared with baseline ($P < 0.001$). Sustained AF was obtained at 24.8 ± 0.6 cm H_2O after GsMTx-4, which was 13.2 ± 0.6 cm H_2O greater than baseline pressure ($P < 0.001$). The average duration of AF decreased significantly at intra-atrial pressures between 10 and 27.5 cm H_2O ($P < 0.05$), comparable with the effect of Gd^{3+} (50 μM) shown in Figure 42–4.[17] GsMTx-4 effects were reversible on washout.

Atrial Refractoriness

The effect of SAC blockade on atrial refractoriness was evaluated in 15 hearts. The free right atrial midwall was paced in close proximity to the recording electrode at twice diastolic threshold strength.

After a 10-beat train at 250-msec basic cycle length, a premature stimulus was introduced during electrical diastole. The coupling interval was shortened in 1-msec decrements until it failed to induce a propagated response, defining the ERP. Measurements were performed at increasing atrial pressure levels during baseline and after a 15-min period of perfusion with 50 μM Gd^{3+} (n = 8) and 170 nM GsMTx-4 (n = 7), respectively. Again, atria were given 2 min to adapt to each pressure level before ERP determination. The right atrial ERP progressively shortened with an increase in atrial pressure (Fig. 42–5). On average, ERP shifted from 78 ± 3 msec at 0.5 cm H_2O to 52 ± 3 msec at 20 cm H_2O ($P < 0.05$). After application of 50 μM Gd^{3+}, this ERP-pressure relation was maintained. ERP decreased from 73 ± 3 msec at 0.5 cm H_2O to 54 ± 2 msec at 20 cm H_2O. At each pressure step, ERP was unchanged from baseline.

Likewise, ERP was not significantly altered compared with baseline after application of GsMTx-4. However, there was a slight tendency toward longer ERP at atrial pressures greater than 2.5 cm H_2O (see Fig. 42–5).

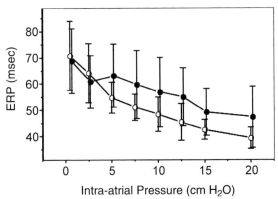

■ Figure 42–5 Right atrial effective refractory period (ERP) measured in seven hearts as a function of atrial pressure (mean ± SD). ERP progressively decreased with an increase in atrial pressure during control *(open circles)* and, similarly, after 170 nM GsMTx-4 *(filled circles, no significant difference to control)*. (From Bode F, Sachs F, Franz MR: Tarantula peptide inhibits atrial fibrillation. *Nature* 409:35–36, 2001, with permission.)

STRETCH-ACTIVATED CALCIUM BLOCKERS AS ANTIARRHYTHMIC AGENTS

Mechano-electric feedback has been well established in ventricular myocardium. It has been recognized in isolated heart preparations, in situ hearts, and humans. Ventricular stretch leads to a shortening of action potential duration and ERP. Acute ventricular dilation may induce premature depolarizations and trigger activity. SAC have been suggested to mediate these electrophysiologic phenomena. Currently, only a few studies have focused on the effect of SAC blockade in multicellular preparations. Gd^{3+} suppressed stretch-induced depolarizations in isolated canine ventricles when brief stretch was applied during electrical diastole.[2]

The role of SAC during sustained stretch has been studied in the working rat heart. Occurrence of ventricular premature beats because of increased left ventricular pressure was reduced by streptomycin.[6] In isolated rabbit hearts, streptomycin prevented stretch-induced shortening of ventricular action potentials.[7] Afterdepolarizations produced by constant stretch in atrial tissue were suppressed by Gd^{3+}.[3] SAC blockade by Gd^{3+} also was reported to reduce $[Ca^{2+}]_i$ during stretch[21] and to inhibit the release of atrial natriuretic peptide,[20] a substance that might contribute to action potential shortening during atrial stretch.[22]

In our studies, the most potent blockers of SAC, Gd^{3+} and GsMTx-4, reduced the vulnerability to AF during acute atrial dilation. They impeded electrical burst initiation of AF, hampered maintenance of burst-induced AF, and suppressed the generation of spontaneous AF during stretch. This is the first direct evidence that block of SAC counteracts the proarrhythmic effect of acute myocardial dilation on the inducibility and maintenance of a sustained arrhythmia. It is also the first report to prove that the GsMTx-4 peptide modulates electrical tissue properties when used in a whole-heart model.

The electrical vulnerability to stretch has been attributed to concurrent reductions in action potential duration and ERP, resulting in decreased wavelength of atrial excitation. A high correlation between ERP shortening and AF inducibility in a recent study by Ravelli and Allessie[15] supports this hypothesis. Our

data confirm these previous results by demonstrating a decrease in ERP and increased AF manifestation with progressive atrial stretch. Yet, we found the local atrial ERP response largely unaltered after application of Gd^{3+} and GsMTx-4, whereas the vulnerability to AF was significantly reduced. Apparently, shortening of ERP alone is insufficient to explain the increased susceptibility to AF during stretch. Acute atrial dilation increases the spatial dispersion of atrial refractoriness.[23] The inhomogeneous structure and wall thickness of the atria can create regional differences in wall stress during increased intra-atrial pressure. The nonuniform distribution of local atrial ERP caused by heterogeneous wall stress could provide a basis for the initiation and maintenance of atrial re-entry during stretch.[23] SAC block by Gd^{3+} or GsMTx-4 might interfere with local electrical properties dependent on the magnitude of regional wall stress and might reduce ERP dispersion.

The wavelength of the atrial impulse also is determined by myocardial conduction properties. The effect of acute myocardial stretch on intra-atrial conduction time recently has been evaluated in the rabbit atrium. Uniform conduction was observed in the unstretched atrium.[24] With an increase in atrial pressure, conduction velocity decreased in areas of delayed conduction, and local conduction block occurred. Alterations in conduction time depending on atrial load could influence the susceptibility to atrial re-entry. If SAC were to be involved in stretch-dependent changes in atrial conduction time, SAC block could be expected to mitigate them. However, this needs to be further elucidated.

The increased atrial irritability during stretch manifested in spontaneous onset of AF. An increase in atrial pressure elicited nonsustained runs of AF, initiated by premature depolarizations. This is in accordance with previous observations in dog hearts that developed spontaneous atrial arrhythmias on atrial balloon dilation.[25] A possible explanation for premature depolarizations is the occurrence of afterdepolarizations. Sustained atrial stretch induced afterdepolarizations that were abolished by SAC blockade.[3] Afterdepolarizations have been reported to account for the onset of polymorphic atrial tachycardia degenerating into AF.[26,27]

Conclusions

These studies show that SAC blockade modulates the electrical properties of the intact rabbit atrium during acute dilation, with minimal effects on normal excitability. Despite the differences in chemical structure, both GsMTx-4 and Gd^{3+} suppressed fibrillation in a similar manner without altering the stretch dependence of the ERP. A decrease in the stretch-induced vulnerability to AF was consistent with the concept that facilitation of AF is mediated by SAC. Blocking SAC may therefore represent a novel anti-arrhythmic approach to specifically diminish the proarrhythmic effect of acute atrial stretch toward AF. Whereas Gd^{3+} lacks specificity and cannot be used under physiologic conditions, GsMTx-4 should prove useful for studying mechanical transduction from the level of molecules to organisms, and it may be the first member of a new class of antiarrhythmic agents.

References

1. Yang XC, Sachs F: Block of stretch-activated ion channels in Xenopus oocytes by gadolinium and calcium ions. Science 243:1068–1071, 1989.
2. Hansen DE, Borganelli M, Stacy GP Jr, Taylor LK: Dose-dependent inhibition of stretch-induced arrhythmias by gadolinium in isolated canine ventricles. Evidence for a unique mode of antiarrhythmic action. Circ Res 69:820–831, 1991.
3. Tavi P, Laine M, Weckstrom M: Effect of gadolinium on stretch-induced changes in contraction and intracellularly recorded action- and afterpotentials of rat isolated atrium. Br J Pharmacol 118:407–413, 1996.
4. Lacampagne A, Gannier F, Argibay J, et al: The stretch-activated ion channel blocker gadolinium also blocks L-type calcium channels in isolated ventricular myocytes of the guinea-pig. Biochim Biophys Acta 1191:205–208, 1994.
5. Gannier F, White E, Lacampagne A, et al: Streptomycin reverses a large stretch induced increases in $[Ca^{2+}]_i$ in isolated guinea pig ventricular myocytes. Cardiovasc Res 28:1193–1198, 1994.
6. Salmon AH, Mays JL, Dalton GR, et al: Effect of streptomycin on wall-stress-induced arrhythmias in the working rat heart. Cardiovasc Res 34:493–503, 1997.
7. Eckardt L, Kirchhof P, Monnig G, et al: Modification of stretch-induced shortening of repolarization by streptomycin in the isolated rabbit heart. J Cardiovasc Pharmacol 36:711–721, 2000.
8. Lane JW, McBride DW Jr, Hamill OP: Amiloride block of the mechanosensitive cation channel in Xenopus oocytes. J Physiol (Lond) 441:347–366, 1991.
9. Caldwell RA, Clemo HF, Baumgarten CM: Using gadolinium to identify stretch-activated channels: Technical considerations. Am J Physiol 275:C619–C621, 1998.
10. Hu H, Sachs F: Mechanically activated currents in chick heart cells. J Membr Biol 154:205–216, 1996.
11. Suchyna TM, Johnson JH, Hamer K, et al: Identification of a peptide toxin from Grammostola spatulata spider venom that blocks cation-selective stretch-activated channels. J Gen Physiol 115:583–598, 2000.
12. Kannel WB, Abbott RD, Savage DD, McNamara PM: Coronary heart disease and atrial fibrillation: The Framingham Study. Am Heart J 106:389–396, 1983.
13. Henry WL, Morganroth J, Pearlman AS, et al: Relation between echocardiographically determined left atrial size and atrial fibrillation. Circulation 53:273–279, 1976.
14. Ravelli F, Disertori M, Cozzi F, et al: Ventricular beats induce variations in cycle length of rapid (type II) atrial flutter in humans: Evidence of leading circle reentry. Circulation 89:2107–2116, 1994.
15. Ravelli F, Allessie M: Effects of atrial dilatation on refractory period and vulnerability to atrial fibrillation in the isolated Langendorff-perfused rabbit heart. Circulation 96:1686–1695, 1997.
16. Bode F, Katchman A, Woosley RL, Franz MR: Gadolinium decreases stretch-induced vulnerability to atrial fibrillation. Circulation 101:2200–2205, 2000.
17. Bode F, Sachs F, Franz MR: Tarantula peptide inhibits atrial fibrillation. Nature 409:35–36, 2001.
18. Li GR, Baumgarten CM: Modulation of cardiac Na^+ current by gadolinium, a blocker of stretch-induced arrhythmias. Am J Physiol Heart Circ Physiol 280:H272–H279, 2001.
19. Hearse DJ, Yamamoto F, Shattock MJ: Calcium antagonists and hypothermia: The temperature dependency of the negative inotropic and anti-ischemic properties of verapamil in the isolated rat heart. Circulation 70:I54–I64, 1984.
20. Laine M, Arjamaa O, Vuolteenaho O, et al: Block of stretch-activated atrial natriuretic peptide secretion by gadolinium in isolated rat atrium. J Physiol (Lond) 480:553–561, 1994.
21. Sigurdson W, Ruknudin A, Sachs F: Calcium imaging of mechanically induced fluxes in tissue-cultured chick heart: Role of stretch-activated ion channels. Am J Physiol 262:H1110–H1115, 1992.
22. Kecskemeti V, Pacher P, Pankucsi C, Nanasi P: Comparative study of cardiac electrophysiological effects of atrial natriuretic peptide. Mol Cell Biochem 160-161:53–59, 1996.
23. Satoh T, Zipes DP: Unequal atrial stretch in dogs increases dispersion of refractoriness conducive to developing atrial fibrillation. J Cardiovasc Electrophysiol 7:833–842, 1996.
24. Eijsbouts SC, Majidi M, van Zandvoort M, Allessie MA: Effects of acute atrial dilation on heterogeneity in conduction in the isolated rabbit heart. J Cardiovasc Electrophysiol 14:269–278, 2003.
25. Solti F, Vecsey T, Kekesi V, Juhasz-Nagy A: The effect of atrial dilatation on the genesis of atrial arrhythmias. Cardiovasc Res 23:882–886, 1989.
26. Satoh T, Zipes DP: Cesium-induced atrial tachycardia degenerating into atrial fibrillation in dogs: Atrial torsades de pointes? J Cardiovasc Electrophysiol 9:970–975, 1998.
27. Kirchhof P, Eckardt L, Monnig G, et al: A patient with "atrial torsades de pointes." J Cardiovasc Electrophysiol 11:806–811, 2000.

Mechano-Electric Feedback: New Directions, New Tools

• • • •

Michael R. Franz, Frederick Sachs, and Peter Kohl

A large and seemingly never ending number of ion channels and ion exchangers is being identified and characterized throughout the heart, including Na^+, Ca^{2+}, Cl^-, and K^+ channels, the latter being identified in an ever-increasing multiplicity. Despite this arsenal of ion transporters that govern the cardiac action potential, there is a stunning paucity of information about the role of one type of ion channel: mechanosensitive channels (MSC).

This textbook summarizes the current state of knowledge on MSC. The channels are ubiquitous, occurring in all species and cell types, and appear to be one of the primary sensors involved in mechano-electric feedback (MEF).

The physiologic role of MSC in most tissues remains unclear. It is easy to understand the requirement for osmoregulation in blood cells, or even more so in microbes that have a need to respond to swelling or shrinkage depending on drastic changes in environmental milieu. MSC may be a direct means by which volume changes (and thus membrane tension) can be "sensed" and, by altered channel gating, lead to the requisite transport of osmolytes.

An important subgroup of MSC responds directly to changes in cell length or tension, rather than volume, and is termed *stretch-activated channels* (SAC). Smooth muscle probably benefits directly from such SAC. Extension of vascular or intestinal walls causes smooth muscle contraction, and SAC are probably involved. This is not to suggest that other metabolic (nitric oxide) or neurohumoral pathways (acetylcholine, norepinephrine) and Ca^{2+} homeostasis do not have a role.

The existence of SAC in *cardiac* cells has been well documented. The effect of stretch on myocytes has been measured by patch-clamp and action potential recordings using transmembrane or (extracellular) monophasic action potential probes. In experimental studies, stretch leads to diastolic membrane depolarization, early action potential shortening, late action potential lengthening, and appearance of "early afterdepolarization"-like potentials during terminal repolarization. Thus, stretch can elicit premature beats and more sustained arrhythmias, either as a result of direct, stretch-induced membrane depolarization or of increased heterogeneity of action potential durations, with both potentially contributing to re-entrant excitation.

It must be acknowledged, however, that the magnitude of global stretch applied in experimental settings is rarely experienced in the in situ beating human heart. The volume and pressure loading used in most studies far exceeds clinical conditions, even during severe afterload (aortic stenosis, hypertension) and severe preload (mitral regurgitation, congestive heart failure). The use of large stimuli in the laboratory is an experimental convenience to make the effects larger and faster, thereby guiding subsequent physiologic studies.

Although large strains are not common for the whole heart, in situ regional strains can be comparable. A myocardial infarct, a scar, or reduced local contractility introduces mechanical heterogeneity (and, subsequently, electrical heterogeneity). Stiff scar tissue, or more compliant ischemic areas, can cause large strains in the border zone between normal and ischemic myocardial segments. In the case of a consolidated scar, the stressed zone would be outside the nonviable myocardium, whereas in acute ischemia, the stressed zone may be within the border of the weakened, but still electrically active, muscle. Currently, only anecdotal evidence has been collected that would confirm this hypothesis. This is a key area for future research.

It is known that SAC normally inactivate with time, and the inactivation is dependent on cytoskeletal integrity. Disruption of the cytoskeleton can cause increased activity of MSC as inactivation is lost. Thus, large strains may not be the only manner in which SAC activity can influence arrhythmias.

Atrial fibrillation, shown to be facilitated by atrial distension, occurs experimentally only during non-physiologically high loading. Evidence for stretch-induced or stretch-facilitated ventricular arrhythmias under *clinical* conditions is still not strong, although this is to be expected if the key progenitor is local stress of susceptible tissue. Arrhythmogenesis by MEF is likely to go undetected in many patients, because no tools exist to identify and measure these effects.

The body surface electrocardiogram, for example, is notoriously inept at detecting slow, local depolarizations. Magnetocardiography may be a more useful approach, yet it is not widely available. Monophasic action potentials can resolve slow potential changes, but their invasive nature has hampered widespread clinical use in patients with acute infarcts. These patients require rapid therapeutic interventions, which makes additional catheter placement for research purposes difficult and ethically questionable. A new set of tools—highly specific and nontoxic SAC blockers (or, potentially, activators), such as GsMTx-4—may help in clarifying the association of cellular mechanisms with the clinical world.

Equally interesting, and an area for future investigations, is to identify the physiologic role of SAC. Cardiac SAC certainly have not been "invented" solely for the "purpose" of causing trouble. There are several potential physiologic roles for SAC in the heart.

First, there is the paracrine function of the heart to release natriuretic peptides into the bloodstream when the heart is experiencing an abnormally high volume load.

Second, there is the Frank–Starling effect, which increases contractility when preload increases. The Frank–Starling effect appears to involve greater Ca^{2+} sensitivity of extended myofilaments, greater Ca^{2+} influx through MSC (either directly or through the sodium-calcium exchanger), and altered Ca^{2+} handling by the sarcoplasmic reticulum.

Third, another role of SAC is probably to adjust the mechanical properties of the cytoskeleton. SAC activation depends on the status of the cytoskeleton, and SAC activation affects local ion concentrations, notably Ca^{2+}.

Fourth, SAC may serve as ligand-gated channels, responding to amphipathic second messengers, and direct mechanical sensitivity is merely a side effect.

Fifth, electrical cross talk among myocardial fibers is well established. It enables adaptation of action potential duration to better align ventricular repolarization with the sequence of ventricular activation. In this context, MEF may act to match the contractile performance of cells to their neighbors and to the overall hemodynamic demand (How else would the billions of cardiac cells know how to balance their Ca^{2+} load?). The matching of local mechanical performance to cardiac demand is essential in equilibrating right and left ventricular outputs, which are individually affected by changes in inflow and outflow.

Sixth, mechanically induced responses are undoubtedly involved in the development and structuring of cardiac tissue. Beating of the cardiac tube sets in during ontogenesis at the point when it starts to fill with fluid. It has been shown that a quiescent tube can be stimulated to beat simply by inflation. Mechanically induced "remodeling" may follow physiologically relevant programs for cell alignment and for setting the balance of myocytes and nonmyocytes. Fibroblasts are mechanosensitive, contain SAC, and are electrically coupled to myocytes.

MEF is an important facet of cardiac physiology. Although the underlying mechanisms are under intense scrutiny in the basic sciences, clinical evidence for the importance of MEF in arrhythmogenesis and sudden cardiac death is only emerging. We hope that this textbook will foster research into the rich and interdisciplinary field of MEF.

INDEX

Page numbers followed by 'f' indicate figures. Page numbers followed by 't' indicate tables.

Atrial fibrillation (*Continued*)
  dilated cardiomyopathy with
    acute atrial stretch, 234-235, 235f
    chronic atrial stretch, 235-236, 236f
    mechanisms underlying, 236-237
    overview of, 229
    remodeling from, 233-234
  electrical remodeling in, 145-146, 220, 230-231,
    230f, 231f
  mechanisms underlying, 229-230
  mitral regurgitation with, 222-223
  mitral stenosis, 222
  in mitral valve regurgitation, 222-223
  sinus node dysfunction with, 225-226
  stretch, 124-125
  stretch channel blockers, 394-397, 394f-396f
  stretch-related triggers for, 226-227
  structural remodeling in, 145-146, 232-233
Atrial fibrosis, 226
Atrial flutterm 235
Atrial natriuretic peptide (ANP), 6, 18, 166, 214, 242,
  350t, 367f, 397. *See also* B-type natriuretic peptide
  (BNP) and C-type natriuretic peptide (CNP)
  in congestive heart failure, 242-244, 242t, 243f
  stretch, 18
  structure of, 243f
Atrial refractoriness, 147t, 154, 157, 158f, 161, 226, 232,
  235, 396
Atrial refractory period, 146
  in atrial fibrillation, 230
Atrial remodeling
  age, 226
  atrial fibrillation, 225-226
  atrial stretch in
    acute, 220-221
    chronic, 221-227. *See also* Atrial stretch
  contractile, 231-232
    in atrial fibrillation, 145-146, 231-232
  electrical
    acute stretch in, 220-221
    in atrial fibrillation, 145-146, 230-231, 230f, 231,
     231f
    chronic stretch in, 221-227, 223f, 225f
  feedback loop for, 230f
  structural, in atrial fibrillation, 232-233
Atrial septal defect, 224-225
Atrial stretch154, 220, 221
  aging, 225-226
  in asynchronous pacing, 221-222
  atrial septal defect, 224-225, 225f
  chronic, 227

Atrial stretch (*Continued*)
  in congestive heart failure, 223-224
  in mitral regurgitation, 222-223, 223f
  in mitral stenosis, 222
  sinus node dysfunction, 225-226
  structure remodeling, 225-226
  triggers for, 226-227
Atrial stunning, 232
Atrioventricular block, 157, 236, 261
  complete, 261-262, 262f
Atrioventricular pacing delay, 358
Atropine, 281
Atrium. *See also* Atrial *entries*
  action potential duration in, 83, 192
  sinoatrial node pacemaker studies of, 76
Automaticity, abnormal, 286-287, 290
Axial fibrillation, 392
Axial flow pump, 343
Axial stretch, 78

B

BAD-triggered apoptosis, 168
Bainbridge reflex, 72, 177
Balloon pump, intra-aortic, 318-319
BAPTA-AM, 24
β-adrenergic receptor, 337
β-adrenergic stimulation, 347
β-blocker, 256, 282, 288, 326, 340, 351
  for heart failure, 288
  for reducing sudden death in heart failure, 254
  remodeling, 251-252
  in renin-angiotensin system, 250
β-catenin, 100-101
β₁ integrin, 23, 103
Bilayer, 33
  lipid, 42
Biological duplex, 201, 202f
Biventricular left ventricular pacing, 359
Block
  complete atrioventricular, 261-262, 262f
  left bundle branch, 261-262, 262f, 355-356, 355f, 356f
  right bundle branch, 356-357
Blood letting, 212
BQ123, 58
B-type natriuretic peptide. *See also* Natriuretic peptide
  in congestive heart failure
    in acutely ill patient, 245-246, 245f
    in ambulatory patient, 246-247
    in emergency care setting, 243-244
    as marker, 242t
    sudden death, 244-245